Diffusion MRI Outside the Brain

Antonio Luna • Ramón Ribes • Jorge A. Soto

Diffusion MRI Outside the Brain

A Case-Based Review and Clinical Applications

Springer

Authors
Antonio Luna, M.D.
Clinica Las Nieves
Sercosa
Carmelo Torres 2
23007 Jaén
Spain
aluna70@sercosa.com

Jorge A. Soto, M.D.
Radiology Department
Boston University School of Medicine
E. Newton St. 88
02118 Boston, MA
USA
jorge.soto@bmc.org

Ramón Ribes, M.D., Ph.D.
Department of Radiology
Case Western Reserve University
Euclid Ave. 111000
44106 Cleveland, OH
USA
ribesb@gmail.com

ISBN 978-3-642-21051-8 e-ISBN 978-3-642-21052-5
DOI 10.1007/978-3-642-21052-5
Springer Heidelberg Dordrecht London New York

Library of Congress Control Number: 2011933937

Printed on acid-free paper

Springer is part of Springer Science+Business Media (www.springer.com)

To both Marias, my wife and child, for their patience

Antonio Luna

To Rosario, my oldest daughter, for the priceless moments we share every day

Ramón Ribes

I dedicate this book to my wife, Ana, and my children, Andrea and Alejandro

Jorge A. Soto

Foreword

It is my pleasure to write the foreword for this book on Diffusion-Weighted Imaging (DWI) Outside the Brain, which we believe it is the first on this subject. This book is co-authored by three young and bright radiologists from two different continents but united by their quest for innovation in clinical Body-MRI. Drs. Luna, Ribes and Soto are practicing radiologists in different settings ranging from a large academic medical center in the USA such as in the case of Dr. Soto, to a large private practice multicenter group in Spain (Dr. Luna) and a hybrid of both in Dr. Ribes.

It is remarkable how the authors have been able to recruit a very comprehensive and talented team of collaborators from multiple locations in Europe, South America and the USA. The topics addressed cover the waterfront of Diffusion-Weighted Imaging (DWI). DWI is an emerging technique currently available in the majority of clinical MRI units and starting to generate a lot of interest because of its unique properties. Although DWI images are less pleasing to the eye than conventional T1-MRI and T2-MRI weighted images, DWI outside the brain holds the promise of quantification and in-depth functional information.

The contributors of this volume range from physicists and clinical scientists to practicing radiologists with obvious research tendencies including several M.D., Ph.D.s. This book contains a number of introductory chapters ranging from the physics basis for DWI to artifacts, quantification and pitfalls. A second component deals with DWI applied to different areas of the body from head to toe. Key chapters on pancreatic, hepatic, renal and adrenal; prostate, bladder and retroperitoneum; female pelvis, breast, GI tract, rectum, lung and heart; head and neck, musculoskeletal and whole body provide practical, clinical day-to-day applications for this technique. The reader will enjoy having in a single volume, a comprehensive compilation of the knowledge of DWI and its applications to all areas of the body. The volume is well illustrated and contains lessons learned from day-to-day practice.

Pablo R. Ros, M.D., M.P.H., Ph.D.
Theodore J. Castele University
Professors and Chairman
Department of Radiology
Case Western Reserve University
University Hospitals Case Medical Center

Preface

In 1827, the botanist Robert Brown described the presumably random drifting of particles suspended in a fluid. Nowadays, it is known as Brownian motion, which is a probabilistic process. In biological tissues, the extracellular water follows a Brownian motion, which is directly related to the tissue composition. Technological advances in magnetic resonance imaging (MRI) have made possible the detection of this microscopic motion by means of diffusion-weighted imaging (DWI). First used to detect brain ischemia, in the last decade, DWI has established as a robust imaging oncological biomarker with applications from head to toe. Its use outside the brain has been specially challenging due to the higher sensitivity of this technique to motion and susceptibility artifacts. However, the maturity of MRI technology has allowed its widespread use. Moreover, DWI forms part of today's clinical MR protocol in areas such as body, musculoskeletal, breast, or head and neck. This technique adds functional information about tissue composition to the conventional morphological sequences, with the advantage of need neither for intravenous contrast injection nor ionizing radiation.

Besides, DWI is fast and reproducible, showing a superb sensitivity to detect areas of high cellular content due to the restriction of extracellular water motion at this level. DWI is also a flexible technique that allows visual or quantitative assessment. Furthermore, the information of DWI may be added to vascular or metabolic information obtained by means of MR perfusion or MR spectroscopy. Therefore, in the era of functional imaging, DWI is one of the pillar which has converted MRI in a leading technique in this field.

Conversely, DWI has not still exploded its full potential. Available studies are still limited. At first, DWI was used as a detector of pathology, but now new oncological applications, as prediction of tumor response or early postreatment monitorization, have to be completely explored. Besides, new groundbreaking applications of DWI are developing as whole-body DWI or DWI neurography. Other areas of work and cooperation are the need of standardization of protocols and to discover the most appropriate model of diffusion signal decay and parameter of quantification according to the explored system and clinical use.

The idea to write this book was to summarize the author's experience dealing in a daily clinical environment with DWI. We intend to transmit the pros and cons of this technique in a case-based format in order to be easy and fast reading. We have enjoyed and learned a lot during this process, and we hope the readers may share some of our experiences working with DWI outside the brain.

Antonio Luna

Contents

List of Abbreviations

ADC	Apparent Diffusion Coefficient
ASTRO	American Society for Therapeutic Radiology and Oncology
AUC	Area under the curve
BAC	bronchioloalaveolar carcinoma
BF	Biochemical failure
BLADE	same sequence as propeller
BPH	Benign prostatic hyperplasia
BT	Brachyterapy
CC/Ci	Choline + creatine/Citrate
CEA	CarcinoEmbryonic Antigen
CHESS	Chemical Shift Selective pulses
CNR	contrast to noise ratio
COPD	chronic obstructive pulmonary disease
CRC	colorectal cancer
CT	computed tomography
D	true diffusion
D*	*perfusion contribution to signal decay*
DCE	Dynamic contrast enhanced
DCIS	Ductal carcinoma in situ
DDD	Degenerative disk disease
DIP	distal interphalangeal
DRE	digital rectal examination
DTI	Diffusion Tensor Imaging
DWI	Diffusion-Weighted Imaging
DWIBS	Diffusion Weighted whole body Imaging with body Background signal Suppression
EPI	Echo planar imaging
ETL	Echo Train Length
%fPSA	free prostatic specific antigen ratio
F	perfusión fraction
FA	Fibroadenoma
FA	Fractional Anisotropy
FASE	fast asymmetric SE
FDA	Food & Drug Administration
FDG	8-Fluor-deoxyglucose
FSE	Fast Spin-Echo
FIGO	International Federation of Gynecology and Obstetrics
FISP	Fast Imaging with Steady-state Precession

FOV	field of view
GE	Gradient-Echo
GIST	gastrointestinal stromal tumor
GRAPPA	Generalized Autocalibrating Partially Parallel Acquisition
GRASE	gradient spin-echo
HASTE	Half-Fourier Acquired Single-shot Turbo spin Echo
HCC	hepatocellular carcinoma
HIFU	high-intensity focused ultrasound
IVD	intervertebral disk
IVIM	Intra Voxel Incoherent Movement
LLC	lymphatic chronic leukemia
LSMFT	Liposclerosing myxofibrous tumor of bone
MALT	mucosa-associated lymphoid tissue
MCP	metacarpophalangeal
MIP	maximum intensity projection
MM	multiple mieloma
MNST	malignant nerve sheath tumor
MPR	multiplanar reconstructions
MRI	Magnetic Resonance Imaging
MRSI	MR spectroscopy imaging
NAC	neoadjuvant chemotherapy
NEX	*number of acquisitions*
NF-1	neurofibromatosis type 1
NPV	Negative predictive value
NSCLC	non-small-cell lung cancer
PC	prostate cancer
PCa	Prostate Cancer
PEG	polyethylene glycol
PET	Positron Emission Tomography
PIDC	perfusion-insensitive diffusion coefficient
PIP	proximal interphalangeal
PPV	Positive predictive value
PROPELLER	Periodically Rotated Overlapping ParallEL Lines with Enhanced Reconstruction
PSA	Prostatic specific antigen
PSIF	reverse fast imaging with steady-state precession
PSIR	Phase-Sensitive Inversion Recovery
PT	Phyllodes tumors
PPV	Predictive positive value
RA	Rheumatoid arthritis
RARE	Rapid Acquisition with Relaxation Enhancement
RCC	Renal Cell Carcinoma
RECIST	Response Evaluation Criteria in the Solid Tumor
RC	Rectal carcinoma
RF	radiofrequency
ROI	Region of interest
RP	radical prostatectomy
RT	Radiotherapy
SAR	specific absorption rate

SBP	solitary bone plasmocytoma
SCC	squamous cell carcinoma
SCLC	small cell lung cancer
SE	Spin-Echo
SENSE	Sensitivity Encoding
SNR	Signal-to-Noise Ratio
SP	solitary plasmocytoma
SPAIR	Spectral Attenuated Inversion Recovery
SPECT	single-photon-emission computed tomography
SPIR	Spectral Presaturation Inversion Recovery
SPLICE	split acquisition of fast spin-echo signals
SSEPI	Single Shot Echo Planar Imaging
SPIO	Small Particles of Iron Oxide
SSFP	Steady-State Free Precession
SSTSE	Single shot turbo spin echo
STIR	Short T1 inversion recovery
SUSHI	subtraction of unidirectionally encoded images for suppression of heavily isotropic objects
SV	seminal vesicles
SVI	seminal vesicle invasion
TACE	transcatheter arterial chemoembolization
TB	tuberculosis
TE	echo time
THRIVE	T1 High Resolution Isotropic Volume Excitation
true FISP	true fast imaging with steady-state precession
TR	repetition time
TSE	Turbo spin echo
TUR	Transurethral resection
UK	United kingdom
USPIO	Ultrasmall Particles of Iron Oxide
VIBE	Volumetric Interpolated Breath-hold Examination
WB-DWI	whole body DWI

Diffusion-Weighted Imaging: Acquisition and Biophysical Basis

1

Javier Sánchez-González and
Javier Lafuente-Martínez

1.1 Diffusion-Weighted Imaging: Physical Basis and Types of Acquisition

Molecules over 0°K (−273°C) experiment a random motion called Brownian movement. Water molecules are in constant motion, and the rate of movement or diffusion depends on the kinetic energy of the molecules which is temperature dependent. In biological tissues, diffusion is not truly random because of tissue structure. Cell membranes or vascular structures, for example, restrict the amount of diffusion.

In 1965 Stejskal and Tanner introduced an MRI sequence sensitive to this Brownian water motion in in vivo applications. This sequence (Fig. 1.1) is based on two lobe gradients that introduce signal diphase in the moving spins. After the RF excitation (Fig. 1.2.1), the first gradient lobe is applied (Fig. 1.2.2) producing a diphase in all the spins proportional to the gradient lobe area ($G\delta$). After this gradient lobe, the spins evolve freely. Those static spins remain in the same position while the moving spins change their relative position (Fig. 1.2.3). At the same time, a 180° pulse is applied changing the phase of all the spins 180°. Finally, a second gradient lobe of the same intensity and polarity of the first gradient, is applied (Fig. 1.2.4). In the case of static spins, after the second gradient lobe, all of them are in the same situation at the 90° pulse, neglecting any T2 effect. On the other hand, the moving spins do not recover the phase after the second gradient lobe because they have changed their position. Moreover, these gradients introduce a higher diphase among the spins. As a result, the acquired signal from the average moving spins is lower than the one from the static spins.

From Stejskal-Tanner sequence, the signal loss due to spins diphase can be controlled by a diffusion factor b that depends on acquisition parameters following Eq. 1.1:

$$b = \gamma^2 G^2 \delta^2 (\Delta - \tfrac{\delta}{3}), \qquad (1.1)$$

where γ is the gyromagnetic constant (42.57 MHz/T, for proton); G represents the gradient intensity; δ represents application time of the gradient lobes; and Δ represents the separation between applied gradient lobes. According to Eq. 1.1, the b factor is mainly affected by the gradient lobe area ($G\delta$). For example, an increase in a factor of 2 of the gradient area represents an increase in a factor of 4 in the b value. Therefore, in a higher gradient lobe area, the spins are more dephased and the signal decay due to their movement is also higher. On the other hand, the b factor is less affected by the evolution time between gradients (Δ). This relation represents the effect of the random change of position of the moving spins during the two gradients. This position variation causes the lack of rephasing of the spins after the second gradient producing a signal loss in the final acquired image.

J. Sánchez-González (✉)
Clinical Scientist, Philips Healthcare Iberia,
Madrid, Spain
e-mail: javier.sanchez.gonzalez@philips.com

J. Lafuente-Martínez
Chairman of Radiology Department,
Gregorio Marañon Hospital,
Madrid, Spain

A. Luna et al., *Diffusion MRI Outside the Brain*,
DOI 10.1007/978-3-642-21052-5_1, © Springer-Verlag Berlin Heidelberg 2012

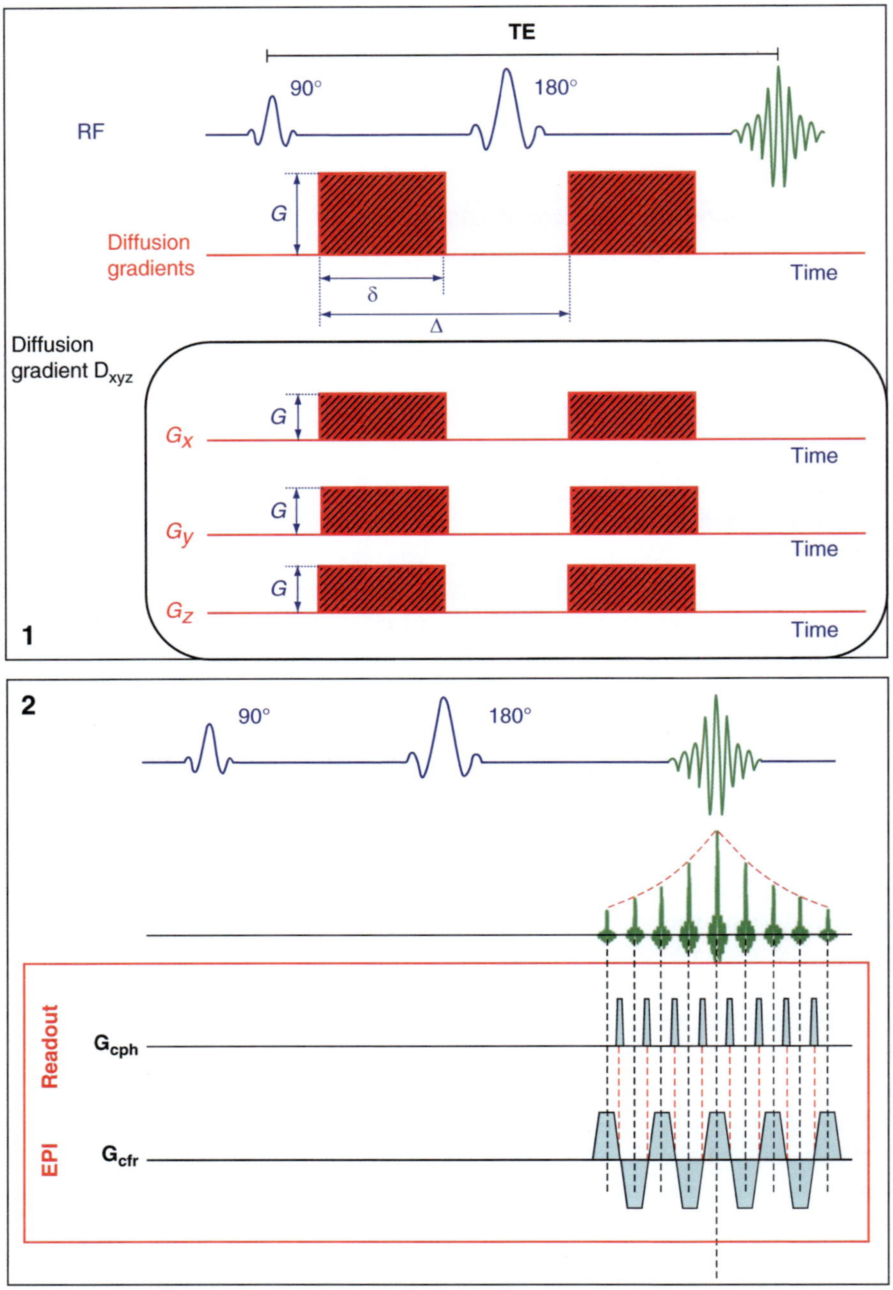

Fig. 1.1 Schematic representations of the DWI pulse sequence of Stejskal and Tanner and single-shot echo planar readout. In the upper part of Fig. **1.1.1**, there is a schematic representation of the pulse sequence introduced by Stejskal and Tanner in 1965. This sequence, which is based on two lobe gradients that introduce signal diphase in the moving spins is sensitive to Brownian water motion for in vivo applications. In the lower part of Fig. **1.1.1**, it can be appreciated that it is possible to obtain DWI in any spatial direction, just changing the combination of the gradient intensity of the X, Y, and Z gradients of the MR scanner. In Fig. **1.1.2**, there is a schematic representation of SS EPI readout that is the most common readout strategy for DWI. The pulse sequence read a whole image in a few milliseconds combining bipolar gradients in the frequency encoding direction with blip gradients in the phase encoding directions. EPI readout has advantages in terms of SNR and acquisition time, although it also shows some problems that are particularly relevant for body applications

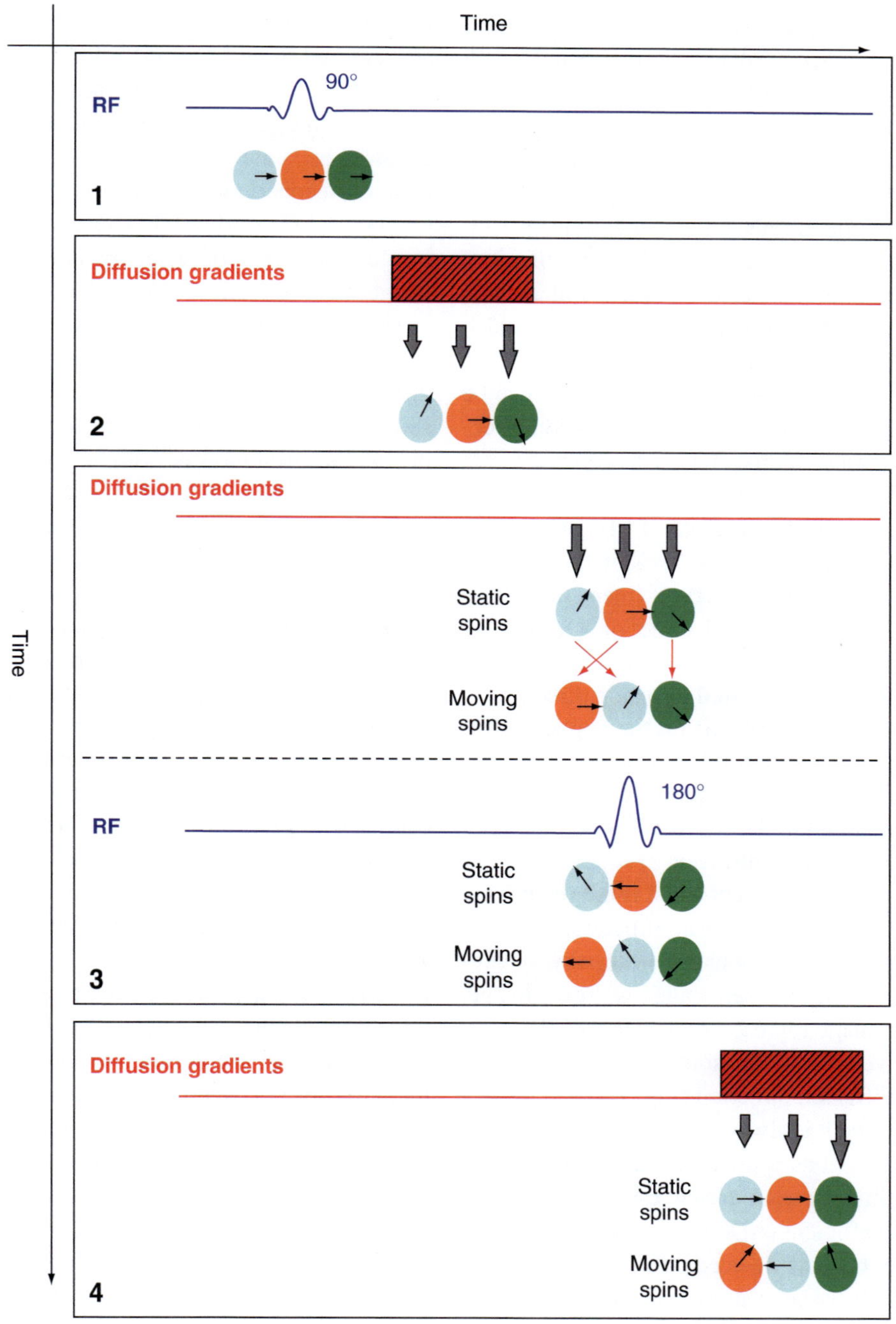

Fig. 1.2 Schematic representation of the phase evolution of the static and dynamic spins during the Stejskal-Tanner sequence. After the RF excitation, represented by the 90° pulse (**1.2.1**), the first gradient lobe is applied (**1.2.2**) producing a diphase in all the spins proportional to the gradient lobe area ($G\delta$). After this gradient lobe, the spins evolve freely. Static spins are in the same position while the moving spins change their relative position (*red arrows* in **1.2.3**). At the same time, a 180° pulse is applied flipping the phase of all the spins 180°. Finally, a second gradient lobe of the same intensity and polarity of the first gradient, is applied (**1.2.4**). Static spins after the second gradient lobe remain in the same situation neglecting any T2 effect. Conversely, the moving spins do not recover the phase after the second gradient lobe because they have changed their position between both gradient lobes. Moreover, these gradients introduce a higher diphase between the spins. As a result, the acquired signal from the average moving spins is lower than the one from of the static spins

From Eq. 1.1, it is easy to understand that the best approach to get higher b values is to increase the area of the gradient lobes. On the other hand, and taking into account the whole sequence, it is desirable to reduce as much as possible the echo time (TE) to reduce the signal loss due to T2 decay (Fig. 1.3). The most suitable option to reduce the whole sequence TE is to compact as much as possible the diffusion-weighted preparation part of the sequence increasing the gradient strength in order to reach the desired b value using the shortest sequence time.

Depending on the tissue structure, diffusion can be changed taking into consideration the diffusion direction. A clear example of this effect is the cerebral white matter where the water can move more easily along the axons than perpendicular to them. To be able to get DWI in different directions, the area of the gradient lobes can be composed by different intensities of the gradient lobes in each spatial direction (XYZ). By changing the area of the X, Y, and Z gradient, it is possible to get DWI for any desired diffusion direction.

Diffusion weighting depends on the applied diffusion direction (Fig. 1.4). For this reason, there are two types of possible diffusion studies according to the desired information. On the one hand, when the relevant information from the diffusion examination is just the amount of water movement and it is not required to obtain information about the tissue structure, just three orthogonal diffusion directions are necessary, obtaining a combined image of them called isotropic image. This isotropic image represents the effect of the average water movement in an isotropic tissue independently of the diffusion direction (Fig. 1.4.3). This is a tissue property and it is always equal, independently of the diffusion directions applied during the acquisition. This isotropic image can be used to estimate the apparent diffusion coefficient (ADC) (see in Chap. 3).

On the other hand, if we need information about the organization of a tissue, a more complex approach is required. In this case, it is important to estimate if the water can diffuse more easily in one direction than in the others, providing information of the tissue organization. For example, in the kidney, water can move more easily along the renal pyramid from nephrons to minor calyces than it could move in the cortex. In order to estimate this privileged diffusion direction, it is required to get the Diffusion Tensor Imaging (DTI). Although, a deep explanation of the DTI theory is beyond of the scope of this chapter, it is important to remark that at least six different diffusion directions are required to build the diffusion tensor (Fig. 1.4.1). In order to have a good estimation of this privileged direction, the diffusion-weighted images have to be acquired separately in the achievable most independent diffusion directions, covering a whole sphere. Of course, DTI studies allow us to obtain an isotropic image as the result of the combination of the diffusion images in all directions (Fig. 1.4.3).

Once the acquisition has been weighted in diffusion, it is necessary to acquire the image (Fig. 1.1.2). The diffusion-weighted images are normally based in single-shot Echo Planar Imaging (EPI) acquisitions to reduce the total acquisition time with an appropriate signal to noise ratio (SNR), although other readout techniques have also been proposed. In this sense, this chapter is going to be mainly focused on EPI readout although different readout strategies will be also commented later. Although, EPI readout has many advantages in terms of SNR and acquisition time, there are many problems that are particularly relevant for body applications.

The most important problem derived from EPI acquisition is the phase error accumulation during the single-shot readout mainly produced by two different causes. The first cause of phase error is produced by magnetic field inhomogeneities or local susceptibility, generating geometrical distortion in the acquired image (see a more detailed explanation in Chap. 2). This phase error accumulation can produce image distortion of the acquired image limiting the application of this technique in body studies. The best way to reduce this geometrical distortion is to reduce the phase accumulation error between different phase encoding steps. A good strategy to reduce the number of phase encoding steps is to combine a single-shot acquisition with parallel imaging techniques, such as Sensitivity Encoding (SENSE) and Generalized Autocalibrating Partially Parallel Acquisition (GRAPPA). Although there are substantially different technical details in the implementation of the parallel acquisition techniques, all of them are based on similar principles (Fig. 1.5). The general idea of these techniques is that it is possible to reduce the number of phase encoding steps during the acquisition phase using the sensitivity coil information to recover them during the reconstruction process.

The second cause of phase error during the single-shot EPI readout is produced by the chemical shift artifact, which shifts the fat signal several pixels from the

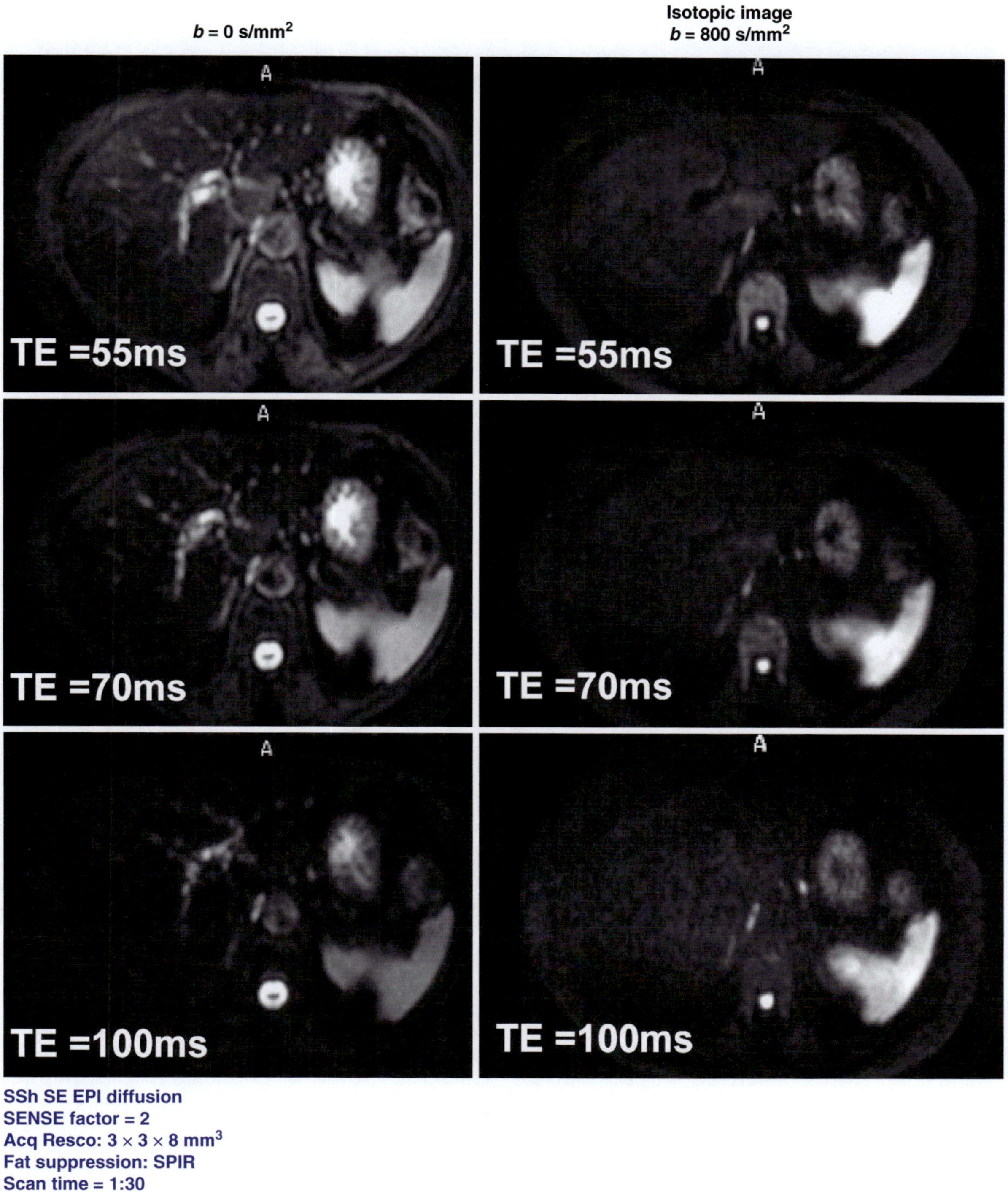

Fig. 1.3 Signal loss in DWI due to T2 effects. DWI is very prone to have low SNR due to signal loss derived from the diffusion-weighted part of the sequence. In this sense, any signal lost due to other image parameters like T2 effect must be avoided. This figure shows the results of the acquisition of three DWI sequences in the same volunteer maintaining the same scan parameters (TR=4,000 ms, voxel size=3.0 × 3.0 × 8.0 mm^3, fat suppression=SPIR) and only changing the applied TE (55, 70 and 100 ms), applying two different b values (0 and 800 s/mm^2). The acquisition was acquired under free breath conditions acquiring four averages in a total scan time of 90 s. All the scan images are displayed with the same window and level settings.In the acquisitions with higher TE, it is difficult to visualize the liver, even in the b=0 s/mm^2, due to signal decay of T2 effect. In the acquisition with TE of 100 ms and b value of 800 s/mm^2, there is a very important noise contamination which makes it very challenging to identify the underlying anatomy. On the other hand, when the TE is decreased, the signal from liver or other organs progressively improves, as it may be appreciated in the acquisition using a b = 800 s/mm^2 and a TE of 55 ms

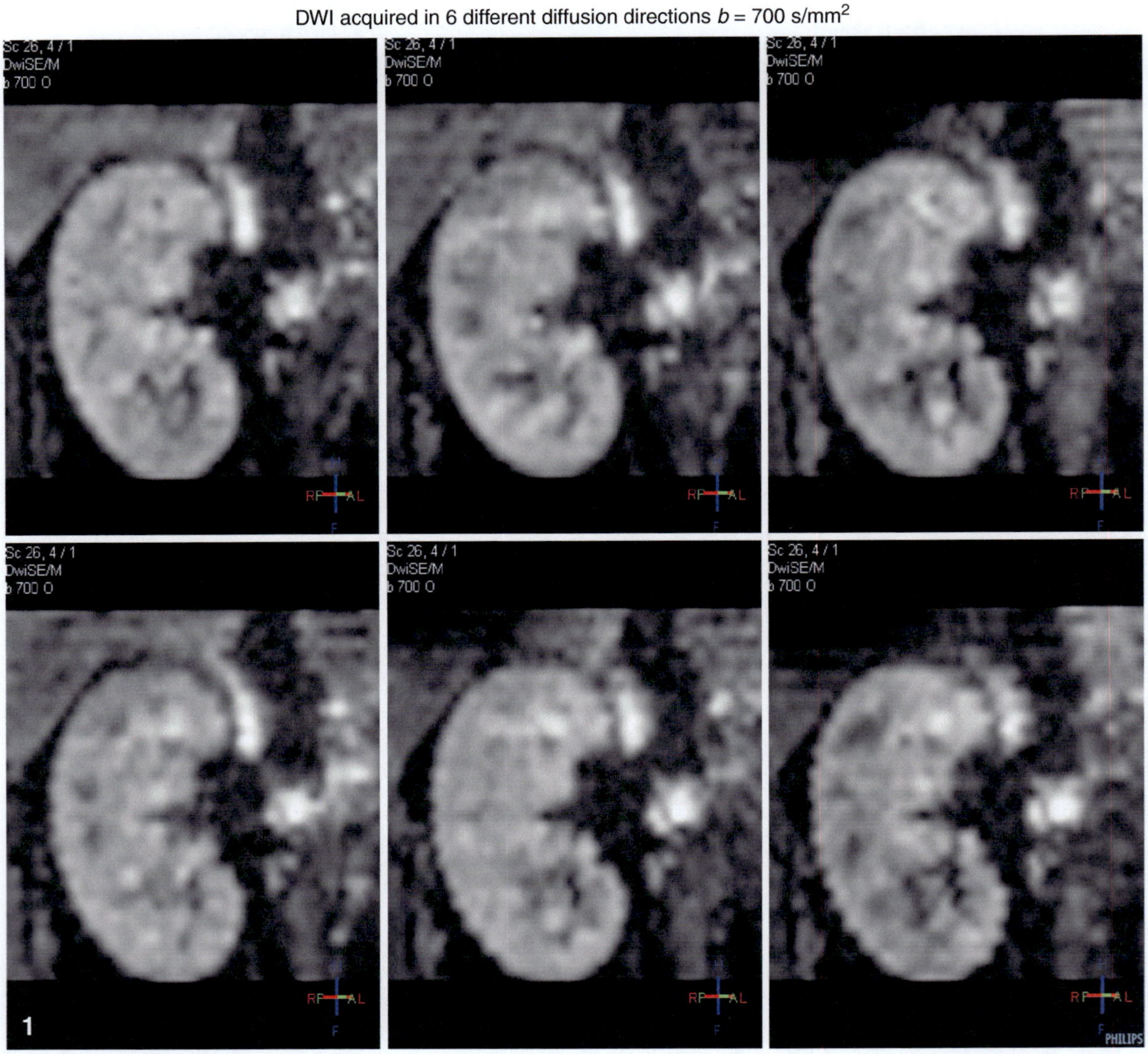

Fig. 1.4 **Effects of direction of the diffusion gradients in isotropic and anisotropic tissues**. The freedom of water molecules to freely move in any direction depends on the tissue organization in that direction. For this reason, water diffusion reflects the vectorial physical properties of the tissue. Therefore, the signal intensity of each pixel changes according to the direction of the applied diffusion gradients. In Fig. **1.4.1**, a diffusion experiment was acquired in six independent diffusion directions to build the DTI of a right kidney. These images are coronal reconstructions of an axial acquisition of the kidneys. The images were acquired under respiratory triggering with a *b* value of 700 s/mm^2 and a voxel resolution of $3.0 \times 3.0 \times 3.5$ mm^3. It can be appreciated that in those regions of the kidney, such as the cortex, that are not directionally organized in a cellular level and demonstrate quasi isotropic diffusion, there is not too much change in signal intensity between the different diffusion directions. Conversely, in those regions which are directionally organized, like the minor calyces, where the water flows more easily along the calyces than perpendicular to them, there are evident signal changes depending on the diffusion direction. Figure **1.4.2** represents the acquisition using a b value of 0 s/mm^2. Figure **1.4.3** shows the isotropic image of the six acquired diffusion directions with a *b* value of 700 mm^2/s

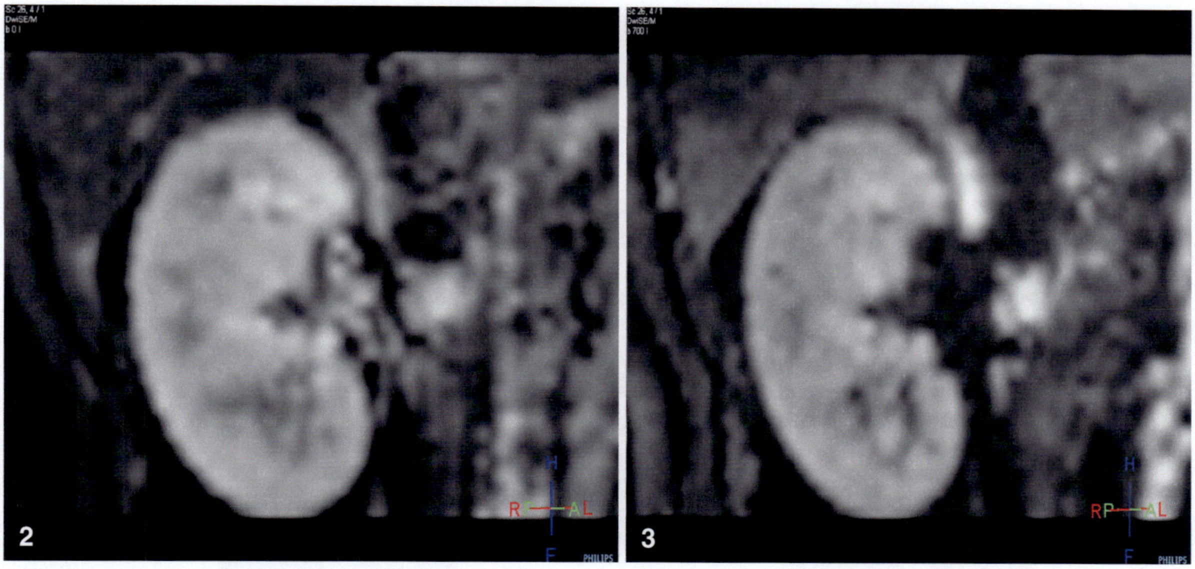

Fig. 1.4 (continued)

water signal in the phase encoding direction (Fig. 1.6). Moreover, fat signal has a low diffusion coefficient producing a severe variation in the estimation of the ADC in those pixels affected by the chemical shift artifact (see also in Chap. 3). In order to eliminate this artifact, it is mandatory to include in the acquisition fat suppression techniques. Although an intense overview of fat suppression techniques are beyond the scope of this chapter, different strategies are described briefly.

1.2 Fat Suppression Techniques

In order to get higher SNR at shorter acquisition times, spectral selected fat suppression techniques are performed such as Spectral Presaturation by Inversion Recovery (SPIR) (Fig. 1.7) or Spectral Attenuated Inversion Recovery (SPAIR) (Fig. 1.8). These techniques used inversion pulses tuned in the fat frequency to saturate the fat signal before the acquisition. The main difference between SPIR and SPAIR is the applied inversion pulse. While SPIR used normal Gaussian pulses, SPAIR uses adiabatic pulses to get a more homogeneous excitation for the whole field of view (FOV).[1] Although the excitation of adiabatic pulses is more homogenous, they have two main drawbacks. The first one is that these pulses require longer RF excitation increasing the Specific Absorption Rate (SAR) of the sequence. This effect has to be compensated by increasing the sequence TR and the total scan time. Moreover, these adiabatic pulses normally have a fix excitation angle of 90° or 180°, being necessary to spend more time until the fat signal becomes saturated. Both aspects make the acquisition time of sequences with SPAIR longer than those acquired with SPIR. For this reason, it is preferable to use SPAIR in those cases more prone to have B1 inhomogeneities such as 3T systems.

Both spectral saturation techniques are very sensible to magnetic field variations making it necessary to apply localized magnetic field shimming in the studied region. In some body applications, it is difficult to get a correct shimming, for example, when air regions must be included in the shimming region. In order to overcome this difficulty, a new shimming strategy, called image-based shimming, has been proposed. This new strategy is based on the acquisition of a reference image where the intensity of each pixel represents

[1] The efficiency of the adiabatic excitation pulses does not depend on the RF power but depend on the magnetization trajectory during the excitation.

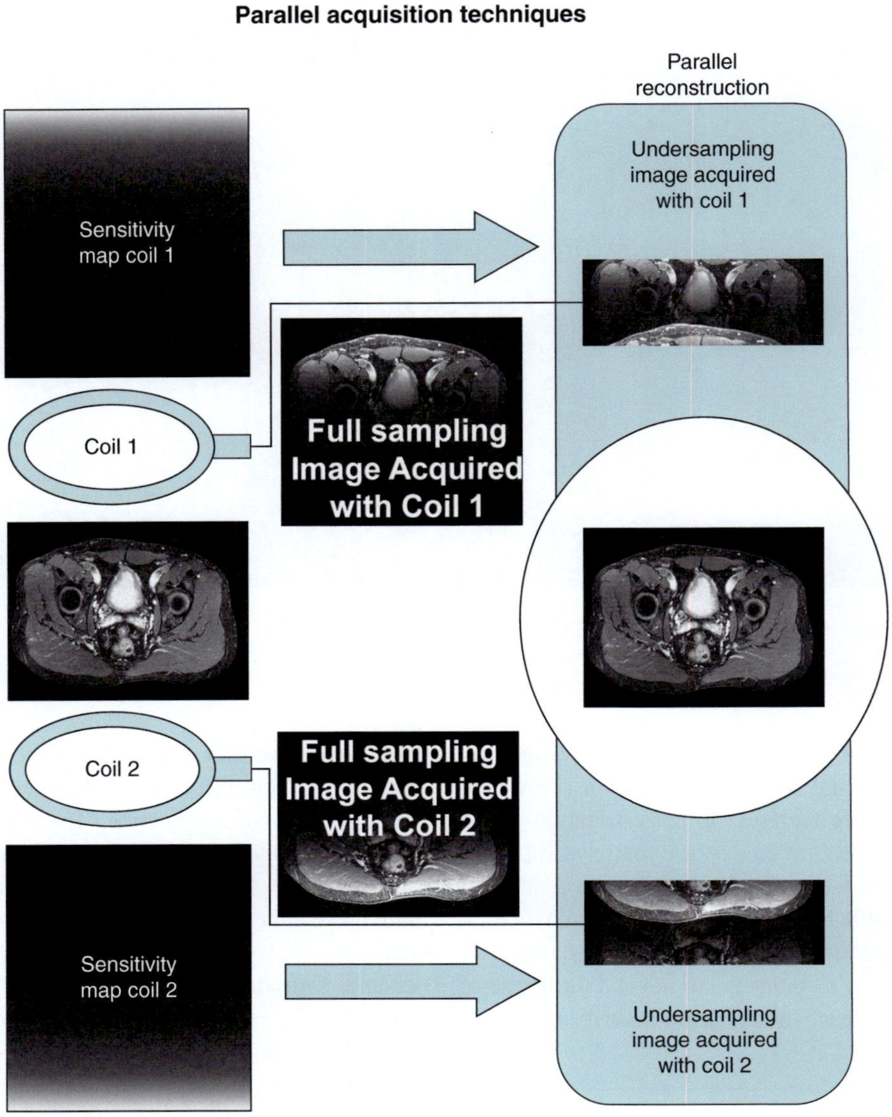

Fig. 1.5 Basis of parallel imaging. In this figure, two different coils are used to acquire the signal from the same anatomy (male pelvis). Each coil has a different sensitivity map, obtaining a higher signal close to the coil and receiving lower signal from the anatomy located further from the coil (sensitivity map of coils 1 and 2, respectively). On the one hand, if the image is acquired without any undersampling in the phase encoding direction, each coil will acquire an image where the signal intensity of each pixel will be the combination of the studied anatomy and the sensitivity map of each coil (*full sampling image acquired with coils 1 and 2*). On the other hand, if an undersampling version of the image is acquired skipping some phase encoding steps, each coil will obtain a foldover version of the Full Sampling Image Acquired with each coil (*undersampling image acquired with coils 1 and 2*). The parallel reconstruction algorithms combine the information of the sensitivity of the coils with the undersampling image of each coil in order to compose the full original image (*full image marked with a circle*)

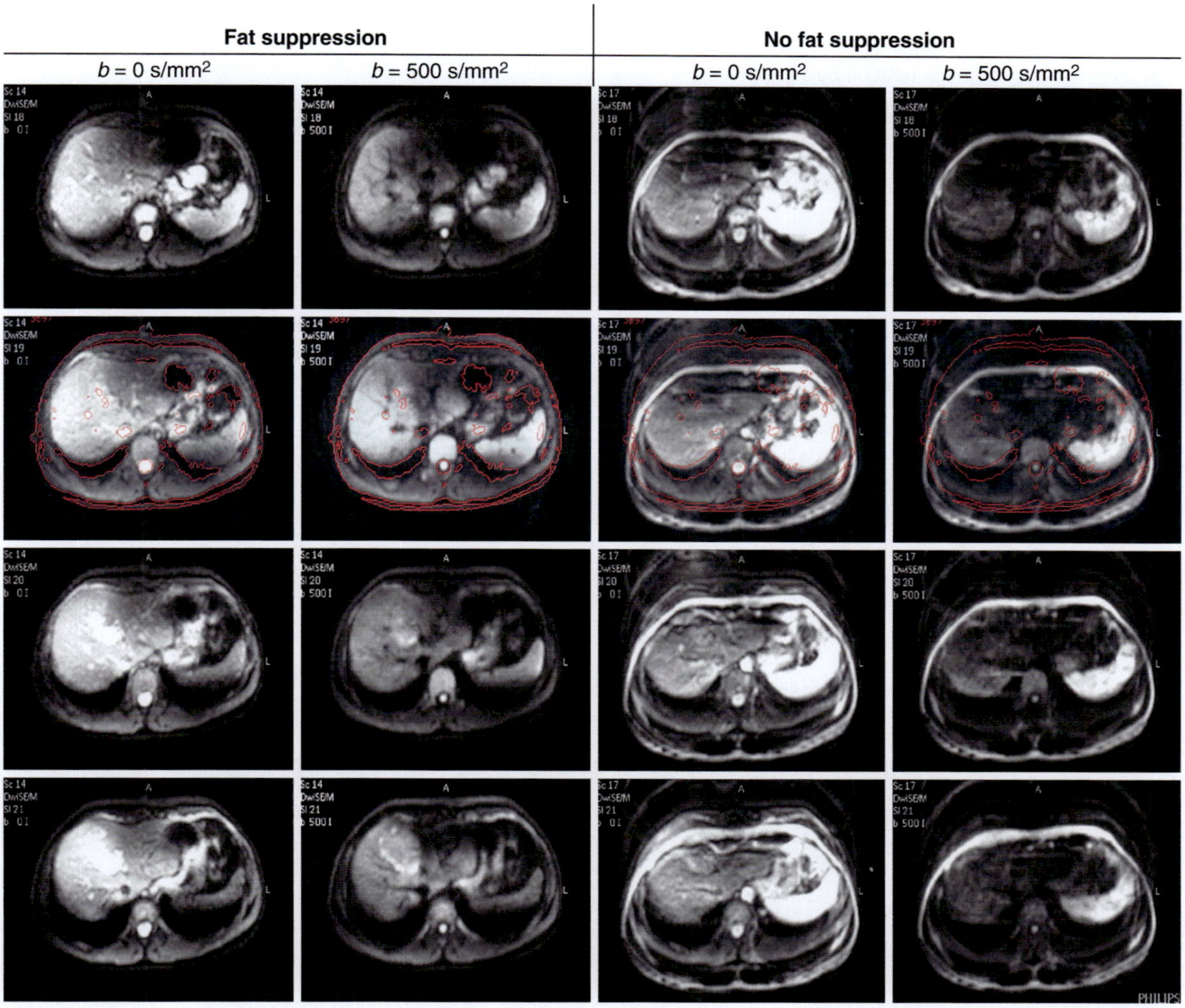

Fig. 1.6 **Effect of fat-shift artifact on**. DWI Two series of a liver DWI with and without fat suppression, using *b* values of 0 and 500 s/mm², are shown. There is a strong signal intensity in the middle of all the images obtained without fat suppression produced by chemical shift of the fat signal combined with the low diffusion coefficient of the fat signal. Besides, due to chemical shift artifact, there is an evident displacement of the fat with regard to the anatomical structures in the DWI without fat suppression compared to the one obtained with SPIR. Regions of interest (ROIs) were drawn to highlight this effect in all the acquisitions at one level

the magnetic field variation in that specific location. This information is used to adjust the shimming gradients during the sequence preparation phase to compensate the magnetic field variation.

If these sophisticated shimming strategies are not available in the scanner, it is preferable to use a conventional STIR acquisition. The disadvantage of STIR sequence is that the images acquired with this technique have a poorer SNR than those acquired with spectral selective fat suppression techniques, making necessary a higher number of averages to get an equivalent signal to noise ratio. Besides, this type of acquisition combining STIR suppression with DWI has provided a new image contrast, very popular in whole-body application, called Diffusion-Weighted Whole-body Imaging with Background body Signal suppression (DWIBS)

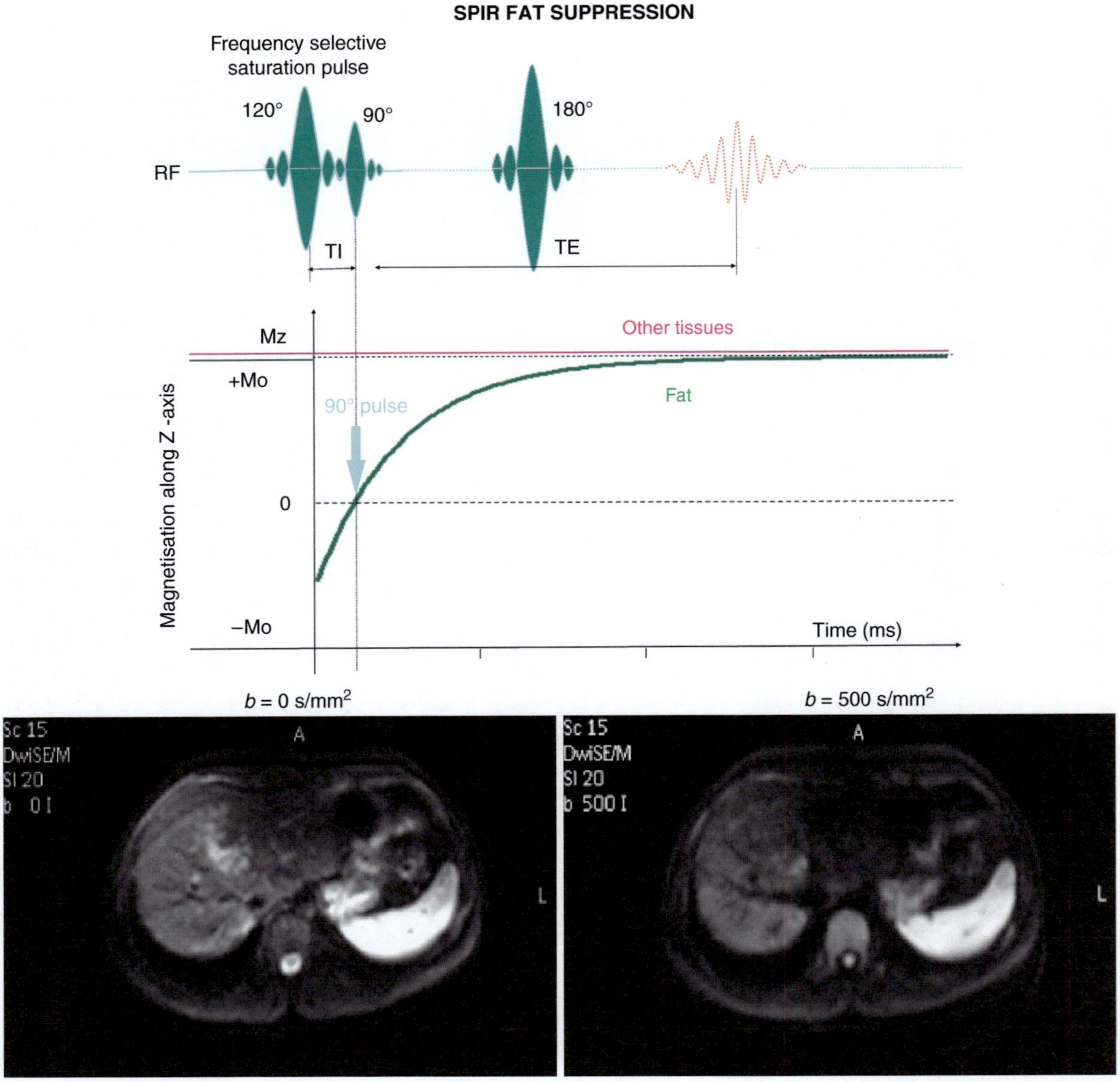

Fig. 1.7 **SPIR fat suppression**. In order to get a DWI acquisition with higher SNR in a shorter acquisition time, it is normally recommended to use spectral selected fat suppression techniques: e.g., spectral presaturation by inversion recovery (SPIR). This technique applies a 120° pulse tuned to fat frequency before the spin-echo acquisition to saturate just the fat signal leaving the rest of the water signal unaffected. This fat suppression signal has two principal advantages. First, the saturation pulse is normally a Gaussian pulse reducing the applied SAR over the patient. Second, the possibility to use a 120° pulse implies that it is necessary to wait a short period of time until the zero crossing of the fat signal, making the sequence faster than any other fat suppression technique. However, this fat suppression technique suffers from B1 inhomogeneities, like dielectric shielding or quadrupolar effect, obtaining a nonhomogeneous fat suppression over the whole anatomy, specially in very high magnetic fields. In this figure, three consecutive images of a DWI sequence with *b* values of 0 and 500 s/mm² at a 3T magnet. SPIR was used as fat suppression technique. The images correspond to a liver hemangioma. It can be appreciated that there is an inhomogeneous fat suppression, obtaining a better fat suppression from posterior-right to anterior-left direction than from anterior-right to posterior-left direction due to B1 inhomogeneity derived from quadrupolar effect. Notice how the inhomogeneous fat suppression is more evident with higher *b* values

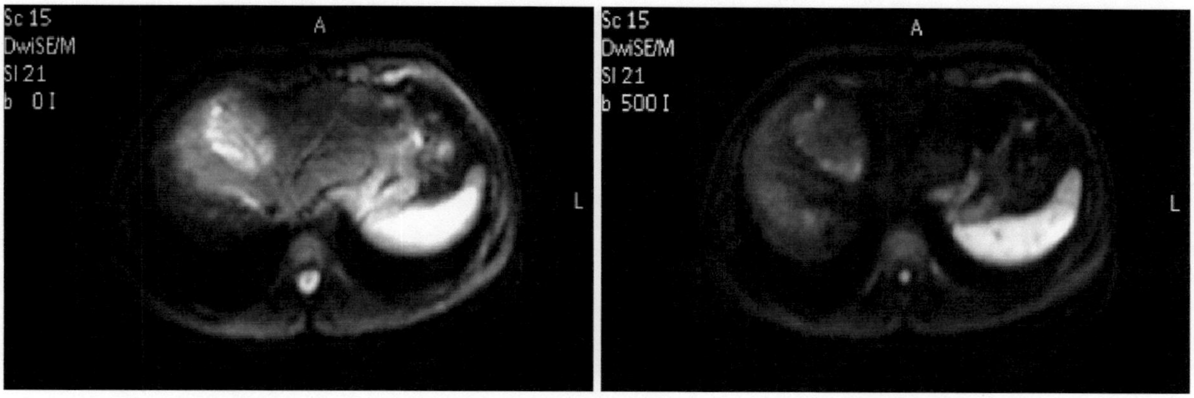

Fig. 1.7 (continued)

(Fig. 1.9). Furthermore, specific and breaking clinical applications have been explored using DWIBS, such as the visualization of neural roots in nervous plexi, also known as diffusion-weighted MR neurography (Fig. 1.10).

1.2.1 Advanced Fat Suppression Techniques

In combination with all these techniques, it is possible to add a new fat suppression strategy called gradient reversal. This technique is feasible in a sequence based on a spin-echo pulse. The base of this technique relies on the chemical shift artifact in the slice selection direction changing the polarity of the slice selection gradients between the 90° and 180° pulses. This change in the gradient polarity avoids the fat signal to be refocused after the whole excitation sequence, producing the fat signal suppression.

1.3 Motion Control

From the previous sections, it is clear that DWI studies the microscopic movement of the water applying movement sensitized gradients to a SE sequence. In this sense, any physiological motions such as cardiac pulsation or respiratory movement can affect the diffusion signal, producing an unexpected signal decay (see a more detailed explanation in Chap. 2). The easiest way to avoid this effect is to use respiratory and/or cardiac triggering for the DWI acquisition in abdominal applications. Breath-hold acquisitions may also be used, although they have a limited SNR and spatial resolution. In some scanners, it is also possible to acquire DWI images in combination with navigator echoes. This navigator can use the position information provided by the navigator echo signal to slightly move the slice excitation, acquiring images with higher consistency among different diffusion directions. It must be noticed that any kind of motion compensation is time consuming.

1.4 Non-Single-Shot EPI Acquisition

In order to avoid the artifacts associated with single-shot EPI acquisition, different strategies have been proposed. The most sensible one is to segment the echo-train length (ETL) of the EPI readout in different shots reducing the phase error accumulated during the readout. Although this approach has less geometrical artifacts, the acquisition time increases proportionally to the number of EPI shots.

A special application of the multi-shot EPI readout is the Periodically Rotated Overlapping el Parallel Lines with Enhanced Reconstruction acquisition (PROPELLER). This acquisition sequence organizes the segmented acquisition in a radial way around the center of the k-space. This approach has the advantage that the results are less sensible to motion artifacts reducing the necessity of synchronizing the acquisition with cardiac or respiration movements.

In order to reduce the phase errors during the EPI readout, it is also possible to use a gradient spin-echo

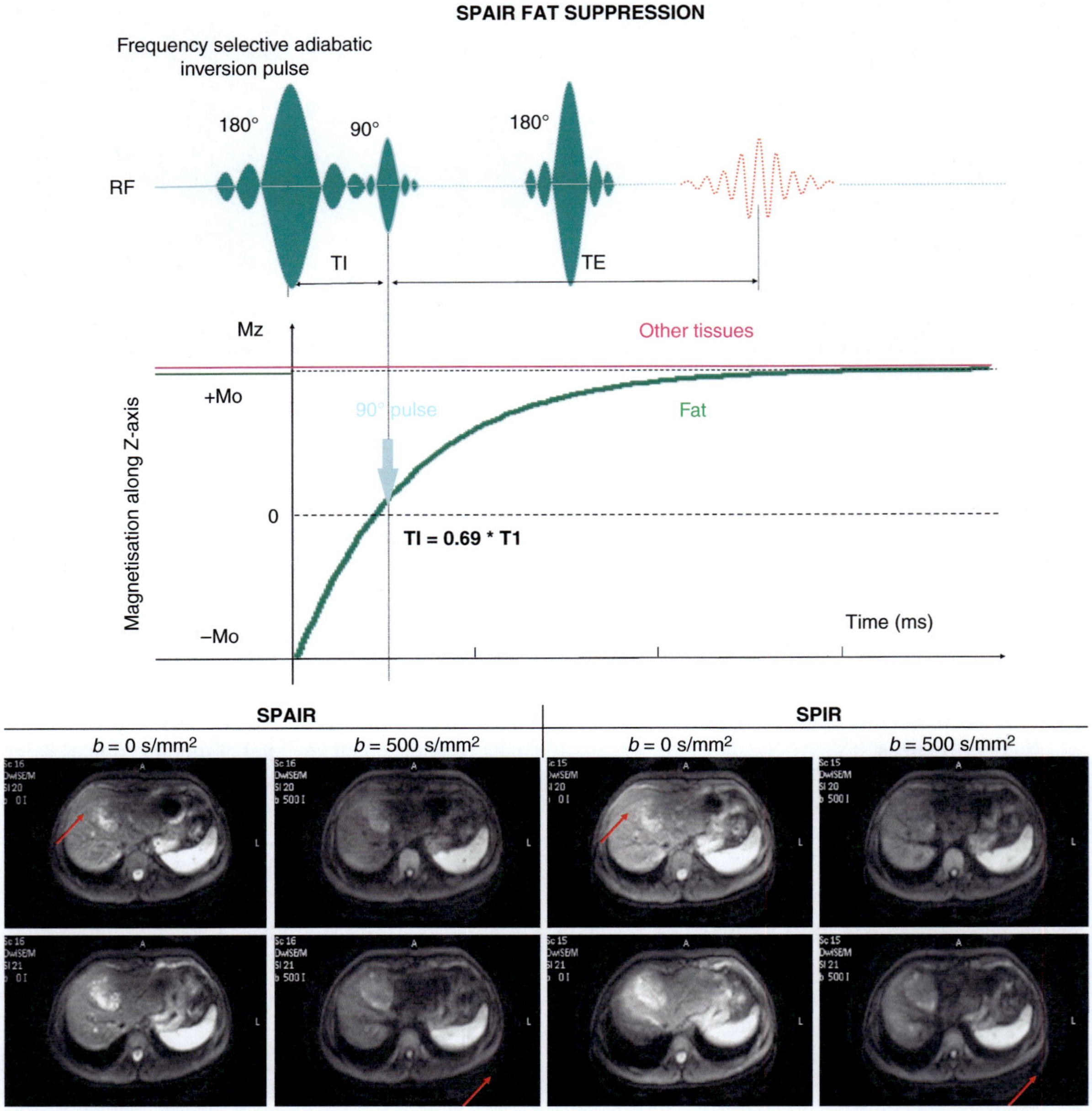

Fig. 1.8 **SPAIR fat suppression**. In order to avoid the fat saturation inhomogeneity of the SPIR sequence, Spectral Attenuated Inversion Recovery (SPAIR) was proposed. This spectral fat saturation technique replaces the 120° Gaussian pulse by a 180° adiabatic pulse to get a more homogeneous excitation for the whole FOV.[2] Although the excitation of adiabatic pulses is more homogenous, they have two main drawbacks. The first one is that this type of pulses require longer RF excitation increasing the SAR of the sequence. This effect has to be compensated increasing the sequence TR and the total scan time. The second reason is that these adiabatic pulses normally have a fixed excitation angle of 90° or 180°, being necessary to spend more time until the fat signal reach the zero crossing. Both aspects make the acquisition time with SPAIR fat suppression longer than those acquired with SPIR. However, it is preferable to use SPAIR as fat suppression technique in those cases more prone to have B1 inhomogeneities like 3T systems. In this figure, a comparison between SPIR and SPAIR DWI sequences of a liver hemangioma at a 3T magnet is shown. Notice the more homogeneous fat saturation with no B1 effect over the whole image using SPAIR than that obtained with SPIR. *Red arrows* show fat signal which is more evident on SPIR DWI acquisitions than on SPAIR acquisitions

[2] The efficiency of the adiabatic excitation pulses does not depend on the RF power but depend on magnetization trajectory during the excitation.

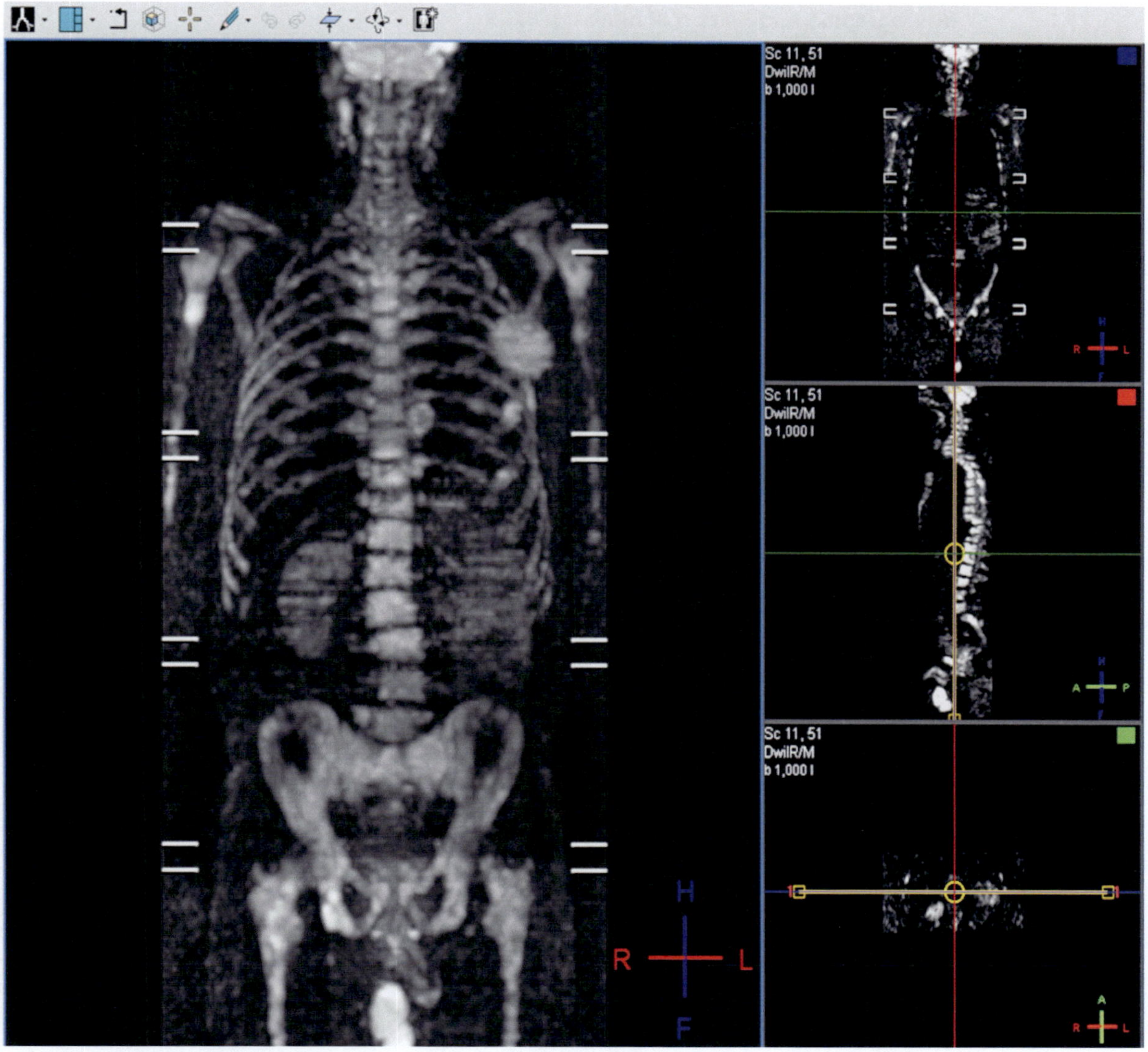

5 Different stacks acquired in 1.5T
SSh IR EPI diffusion
No SENSE factor
Acq Reso: $5 \times 5 \times 5$ mm^3
Fat suppression: STIR
b value = 1,000
Acquisition time per stack = 1:30 min

Fig. 1.9 DWIBS sequence. Diffusion imaging can also be used in whole body applications. In this case, a STIR acquisition tuned to reduce the fat signal contribution was applied in order to avoid magnetic field homogeneity problems. This combination of DWI with STIR acquisition is known as Diffusion-weighted whole-body imaging with background body signal suppression (DWIBS). Due to the high sensitivity of this type of image contrast to high cellular tissues, DWIBS is normally applied to look for metastases in whole-body exams. These sequences are normally acquired under free breath with many signal averages and with a high diffusion coefficient (*b* value between 600 and 1,000 s/mm^2). In whole-body applications, the sequence is obtained in different separated stacks, to cover the whole anatomy of interest, being necessary to move the patient table between them. The acquisition time is around 90–120 s per stack. In this figure, a coronal maximum intensity projection (MIP) of a whole-body exam performed at a 1.5T magnet of a patient with several soft tissue and bone metastases is shown. It was acquired in five different stacks. In the right part of the figure coronal, sagittal and axial MPR are shown

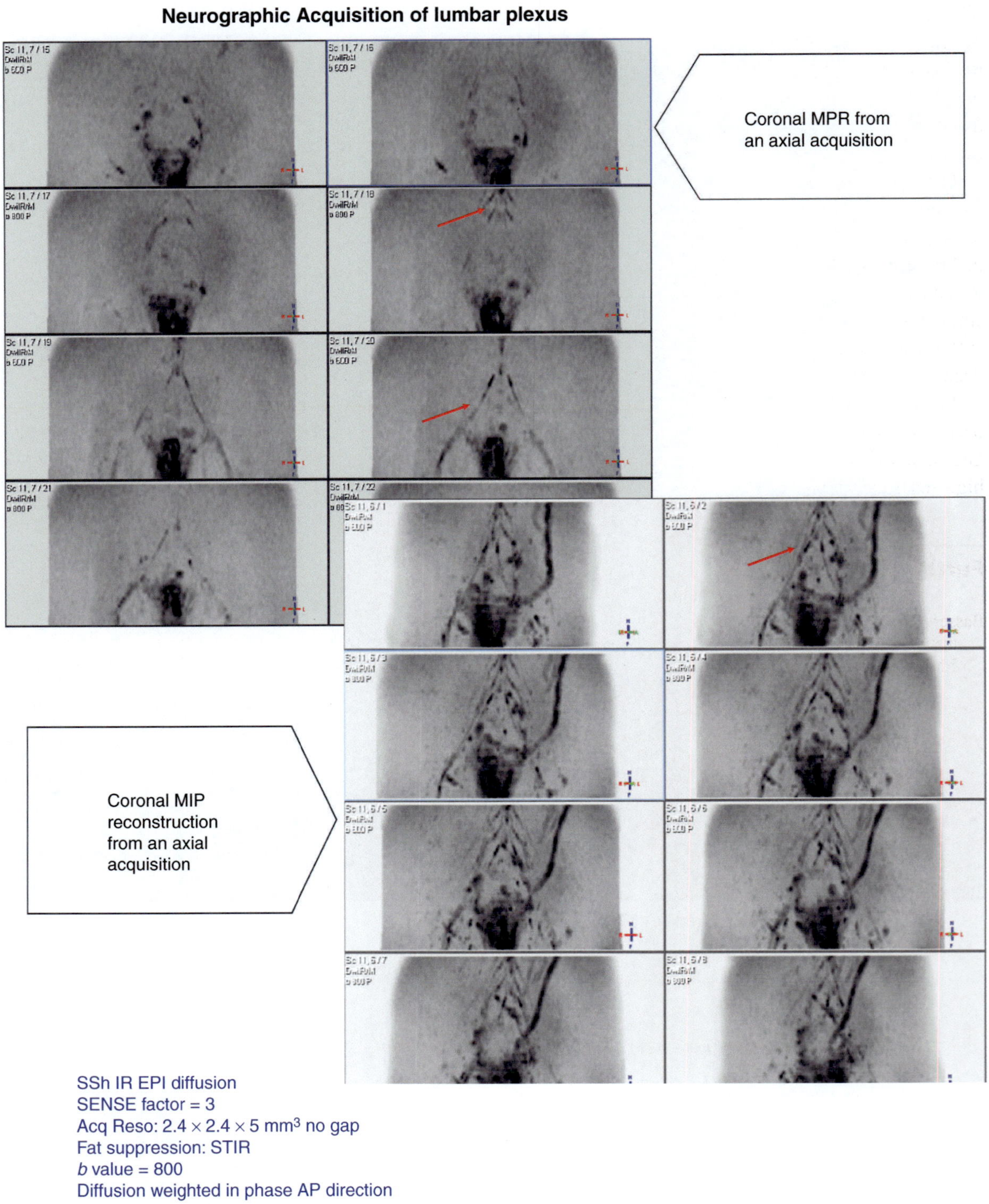

Fig. 1.10 **Neurography with DWIBS**. A special application of the DWIBS sequence is the obtainment of neurographic images in order to study neural roots and nerve plexi. It may be also used to obtain information from the peripheral nerves, using a high-resolution DWIBS sequence acquired with an adapted surface coil. In order to obtain a better contrast between the plexus and the rest of the surrounding tissues, a single diffusion direction is acquired in the anterior-posterior axis. In this figure, the lumbar plexus is studied with DWIBS acquired in a 3T magnet. In the upper-left aspect of the figure, different slices of a coronal MPR, obtained from an axial acquisition, are shown. In these images, the proximal nerve roots as well as its more distal portion (*red arrows*) are clearly depicted with low contamination from the surrounding soft tissue. In the lower-right aspect of the figure, a radial MIP reconstruction of the same acquisition is shown, which achieves a 3D reconstruction of the whole lumbar plexus

(GRASE) acquisition sequence that combines 180° pulses with different EPI readouts. This strategy makes feasible to use a single-shot acquisition approach controlling the image distortion. The problem of this approach is that it enlarges the TR of the sequence increasing the total acquisition time of the DWI sequence.

Other acquisition strategy to avoid image distortion is to use multishot or single-shot turbo spin-echo readouts. The main drawback of this strategy is the increase of TE losing SNR due to T2-relaxation effects. In order to reduce the signal loss by reducing the TE, half scan strategies can be applied. As a consequence, the images suffer from a blurring artifact produced by the T2 decay during the multi-echo acquisition.

Finally, in recent papers, the diffusion-weighted part includes a magnetization preparation of a Gradient Echo acquisition which is able to produce high-resolution DWI.

Further Reading

Basser PJ, Mattiello J, Le Bihan D (1994) Estimation of the effective self-diffusion tensor from the NMR spin echo. J Magn Reson 103:247–254

Bennett KM, Schmainda KM, Bennett RT et al (2003) Characterization of continuously distributed cortical water diffusion rates with a stretched-exponential model. Magn Reson Med 50:727–734

Dwyer AJ, Frank JA, Sank VJ et al (1988) Short-Ti inversion-recovery pulse sequence: analysis and initial experience in cancer imaging. Radiology 168:827–836

Griswold MA, Jakob PM, Heidemann RM et al (2002) Generalized autocalibrating partially parallel acquisitions (GRAPPA). Magn Reson Med 47:1202–1210

Haase A, Frahm J, Hanicke W et al (1988) 1H NMR chemical shift selective (CHESS) imaging. Phys Med Biol 30(4):341

Le Bihan D, Breton E, Lallemand D et al (1988) Separation of diffusion and perfusion in intravoxel incoherent motion MR imaging. Radiology 168:497–505

Mansfield P (1977) Multi-planar imaging formation using NMR spin-echo. J Phys C: Solid State Phys 10:55–58

Pruessmann KP, Weiger M, Scheidegger MB et al (1999) SENSE: sensitivity encoding for fast MRI. Magn Reson Med 42:952–962

Stejskal EO, Tanner JE (1965) Spin diffusion measurements: spin echoes in the presence of time-dependent field gradient. J Chem Phys 42(1):288–292

Takahara T, Imai Y, Yamashita T et al (2004) Diffusion weighted whole body imaging with background body signal suppression (DWIBS): technical improvement using free breathing, STIR and high resolution 3D display. Radiat Med 22:275–282

Takahara T, Hendrikse J, Kwee TC et al (2010) Diffusion-weighted MR neurography of the sacral plexus with unidirectional motion probing gradients. Eur Radiol 20(5):1221–1226

2 How to Identify and Avoid Artifacts on DWI

Javier Sánchez-González

DWI is currently considered a cancer biomarker and has a role in cancer detection and staging. DWI is also able to depict early posttreatment changes in oncological lesions treated with vascular disruptive drugs and useful for therapies that induce apoptosis. After these treatments, cellular death and vascular changes occur before changes in lesion size can be seen. Successful treatment is reflected by increases in ADC values. Rising ADC values with successful therapy have been noted in several anatomic sites, including breast cancers, primary and metastatic cancers to the liver, primary sarcomas of bone, and in brain malignancies.

These new applications make necessary to control the quality of DWI sequences which must be as accurate as possible for posterior quantitative analysis. In order to analyze the technical issues that can affect the quality of the diffusion images, it is necessary to decompose the typical diffusion acquisition scheme described in Chap. 1. This scheme is made up of two different parts. The first part of the sequence corresponds to the preparation phase of the magnetization, which is called the diffusion preparation part (Fig. 1.1.1). The second part is the readout scheme to acquire the images and will be referred as the acquisition part (Fig. 1.1.2). Although both parts are intimately related, the effect of them in the final image can be separated as well as their related artifacts.

J. Sánchez-González
Clinical Scientist, Philips Healthcare Iberia, Madrid, Spain
e-mail: javier.sanchez.gonzalez@philips.com

2.1 Optimization of Signal to Noise Ratio

Since DWI is prone to have low SNR, it is necessary to recover as much signal as possible. In order to increase the SNR, it is desirable to reduce the effective TE of the sequence to the minimum. The final TE of the diffusion sequence is affected by the total time of the diffusion preparation and the effective TE of the acquisition part.

As it was commented on in Chap. 1, in order to reduce the signal loss due to T2 effects, it is recommended to reduce the sequence time as much as possible (Fig. 1.3). In this sense, for a given *b* factor, it is recommended to use the maximum available gradient strength during the diffusion gradient lobes. In order to obtain the maximum available gradient strength, tetrahedral encoding or other simultaneous applications of gradient schemes (e.g., gradient overplus or three-scan trace) can be also used. These techniques do not use the diffusion-weighted gradients in pure X, Y, and Z direction. On the contrary, new diffusion directions are defined combining the maximum intensity of all the gradients at the same time. This approach allows to obtaining a maximum gradient strength that is the square root of three times higher than the gradient strength in a single X, Y, or Z pure direction. As a result, shorter effective TE can be reached improving the total SNR of the sequence (Fig. 2.1).

DWI normally has a low SNR especially for those anatomies that require high *b* values (e.g., prostate). To compensate this signal loss for high *b* values, it is desirable to increase the number of averages (Fig. 2.2). In order to reduce the scan time, "state-of-the-art" scanners

A. Luna et al., *Diffusion MRI Outside the Brain*,
DOI 10.1007/978-3-642-21052-5_2, © Springer-Verlag Berlin Heidelberg 2012

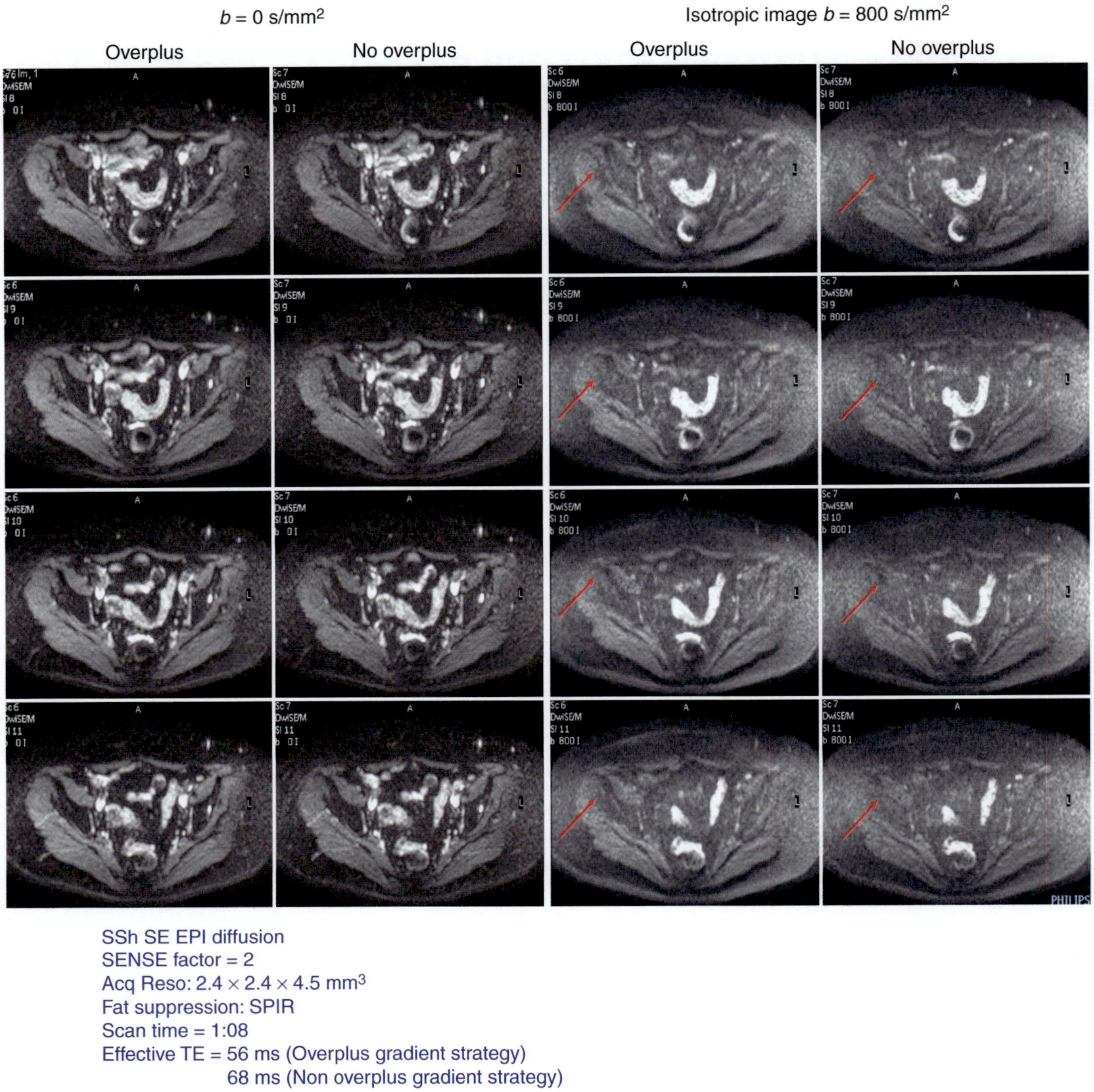

Fig. 2.1 SNR: gradient overplus use. In this figure, a pelvic diffusion-weighted SS SE EPI using SPIR sequence with *b* values of 0 and 800 s/mm^2 was acquired with and without gradient overplus strategy in the same volunteer. It can be appreciated that images acquired with overplus strategy have higher signal compared with those acquired with nonoverplus strategy due to the shorter TE. Notice increased depiction of the borders of the *right* acetabulum in the acquisition with high *b* value using gradient overplus compared to the one without gradient overplus (*red arrows*)

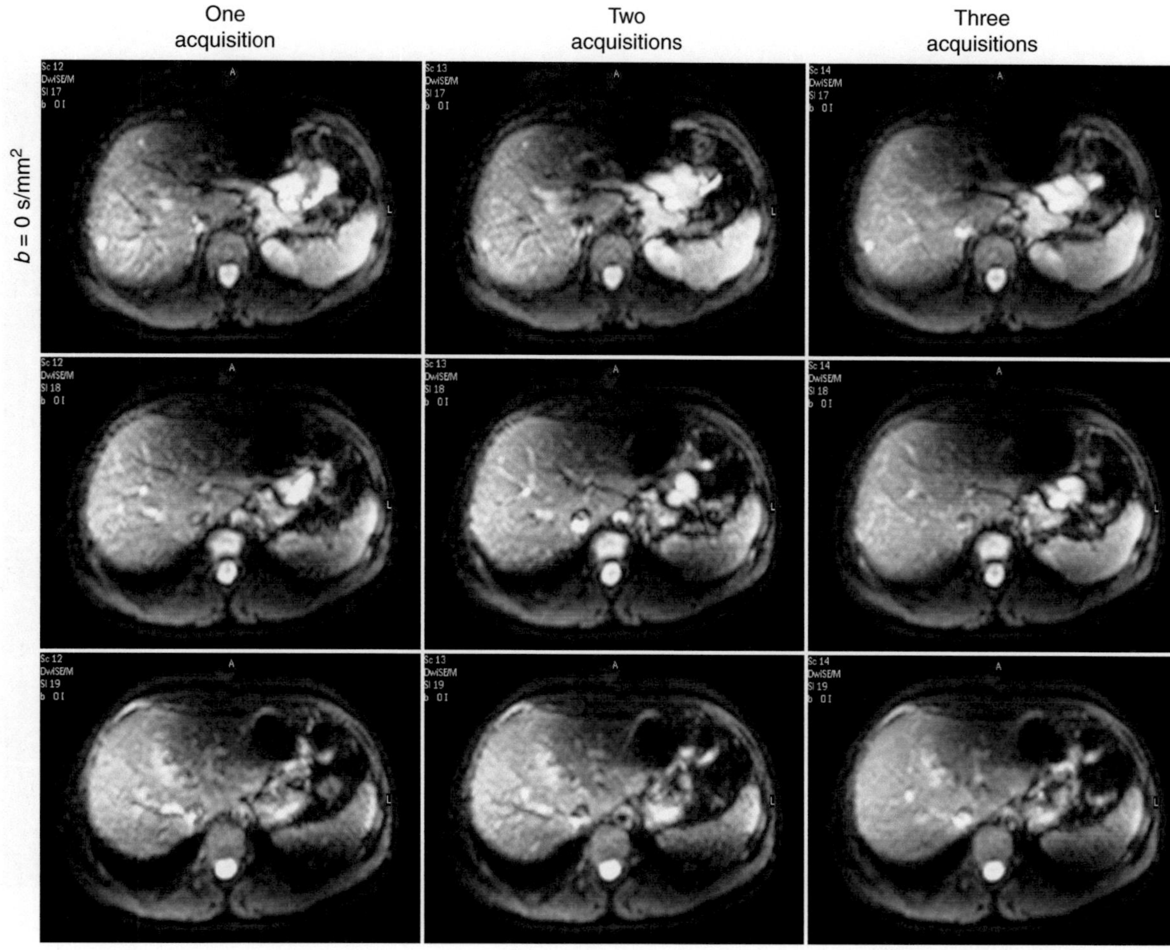

Fig. 2.2 SNR: effect of the number of signal average. In this figure, three liver DWI acquisitions in the same volunteer with different number of averages are shown. As it is expected, it can be noticed that SNR improves with the number of averages. An improved SNR will provide a better estimation of the ADC. In those cases where the gradients are not powerful enough or the tissue has a very high diffusion coefficient, the best way to increase the SNR is to increase the number of averages. The main problem of this strategy is that it is very time consuming. In order to reduce the scan time, modern scanners have the option to perform a variable number of averages according to the *b* value increasing the SNR just in those images with higher *b* values that are more prone to have low signal. This strategy makes feasible to maintain a good SNR in all the acquisitions with different *b* values in a reasonable scan time

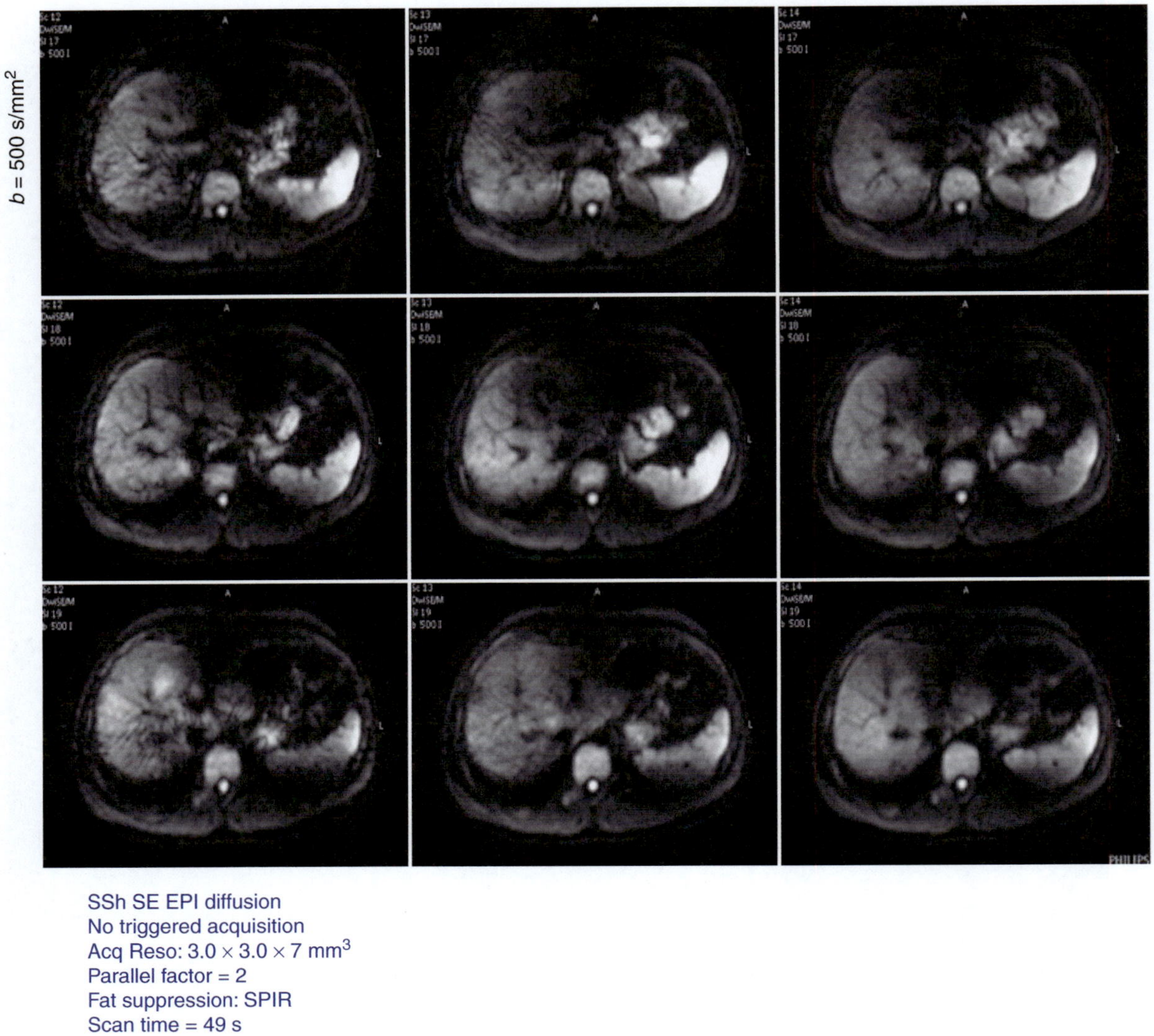

Fig. 2.2 (continued)

has the capability to perform variable number of averages according to the *b* value performed, increasing the SNR just in those images with high *b* values that are prone to have low signal. This approach makes it possible to have a reasonable SNR in all the acquisitions with different *b* values in a feasible scan time.

Fig. 2.3 **Bandwidth: noise artifacts**. A tool to improve the SNR is to adjust the acquisition bandwidth of the sequence. Schematic representations of the effect of the use of low and high bandwidth (1 and 2 respectively) on signal intensity are shown in the upper part of the figure. In both schemes, the *blue box* represents the total amount of the acquired image while the *black line* represents the noise level. In both cases, the total signal (area of the *blue box*) as well as the noise contamination is equal. Taking into account the definition of white noise, the same noise contamination is expected for all the bandwidth frequencies. In the low bandwidth acquisition (2.3.1), the *blue box* is spread in a narrow bandwidth obtaining a higher SNR compared with the high bandwidth acquisition (2.3.2). Besides, using high bandwidth, the signal is spread in more frequencies, including more noise in the acquired signal. Two series of a pelvic DWI with a *b* value of 500 s/mm^2 using different bandwidth frequencies in the same volunteer are shown in the lower part of this figure. The images acquired with low bandwidth show a higher SNR than those with high bandwidth (*red arrows*)

Another degree of freedom to improve the SNR is to change the received bandwidth during the acquisition (Fig. 2.3). This sequence parameter has to be treated carefully as lower bandwidth values increase the SNR of the sequence but produce higher image distortion as will be discussed in the distortion artifact section.

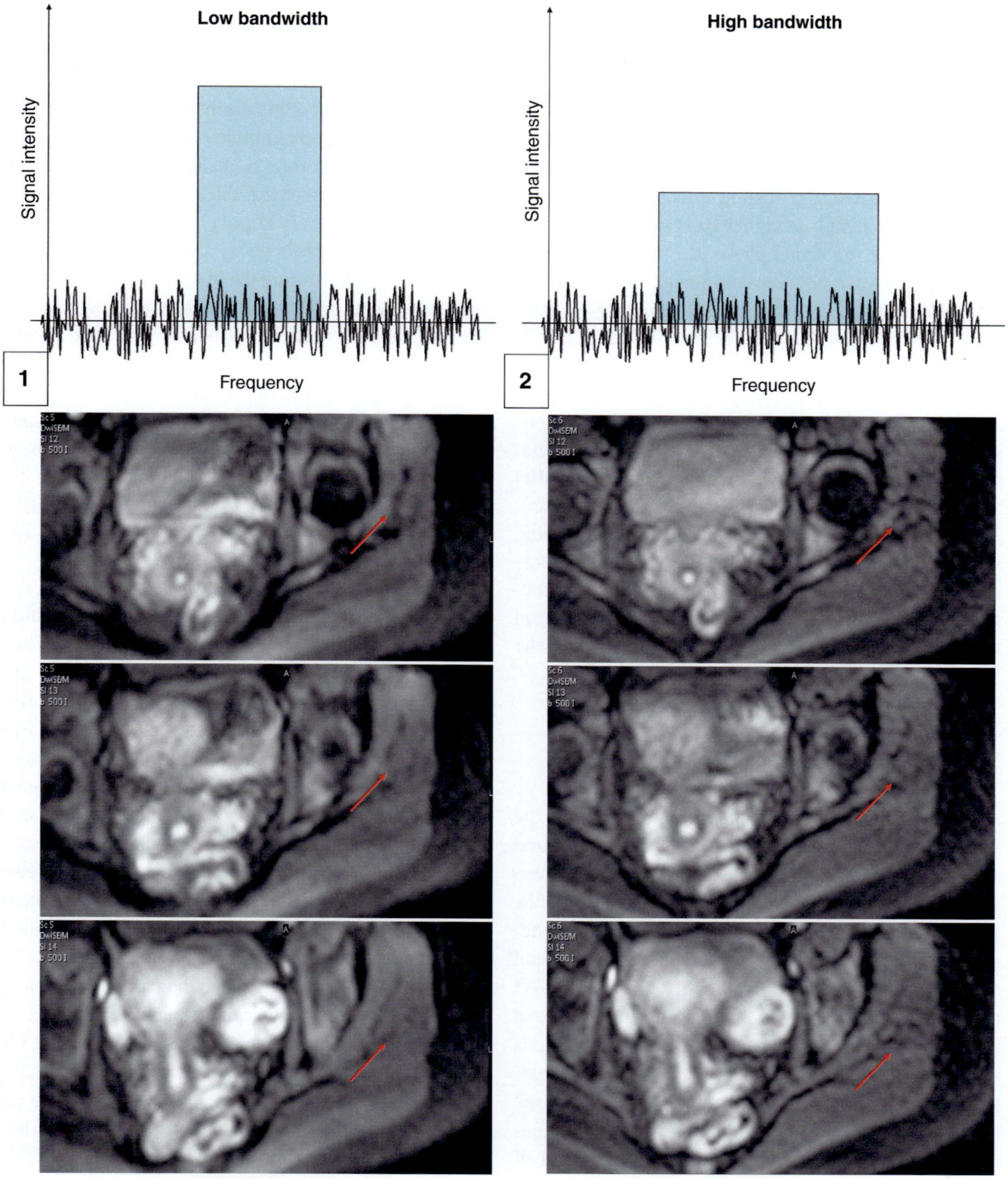

- SSh SE EPI diffusion
- Number of averages = 3
- *b* factor = 500 s/mm^2
- Acq Reso: 3.0 × 3.0 × 7 mm^3
- Parallel acquisition factor = 3
- Effective TE in both cases = 55 ms

2.2 Geometrical Distortion Artifacts

On DWI, some distortion is usually appreciated due to phase error accumulation during the EPI readout, although the MR scanner is perfectly adjusted. These geometric distortions can be reduced by increasing the readout bandwidth. Increasing the readout bandwidth has two effects. The first one is that the frequency difference between two consecutive phase encoding lines is higher, making that the phase error due to magnetic field inhomogeneities has less effect in the total readout. Moreover, the second effect is that a faster readout (equivalent to a higher bandwidth) leaves less time to change the signal phase due to magnetic field inhomogeneities producing less image distortion. For body applications, the difference between two phase encoding lines is typically between 1 and 2 kHz (Fig. 2.4). However, a higher readout bandwidth also increases the noise and Nyquist ghosting. Therefore, bandwidth or echo spacing settings should be optimized (Fig. 2.3). Another way to reduce the accumulation of phase error during the readout is to use parallel acquisition techniques (e.g., SENSE, GRAPPA, etc.). These techniques skip the readout of phase encoding steps that are compensated using the geometrical information of the coil sensitivity maps in the reconstruction process. As a consequence, this acquisition strategy reduces the effective echo spacing and the effect of image distortion (Fig. 2.5).

2.3 Motion Artifacts

Another problem involving the diffusion signal is the macroscopic movement produced by respiratory and cardiac motion which is critical in thoracic and abdominal acquisitions. In order to avoid these movements, different strategies have been proposed. These strategies have been carefully studied in the liver. Kandpal et al. demonstrated that respiratory triggered DWI acquisitions showed higher SNR in normal liver and higher CNR between normal liver and focal lesions than breath-hold sequences. Kwee and colleagues studied the effect of the heart motion on DWI of the liver, showing a strong degradation of those images acquired during the heart systole due to the effect of the heart movement (Fig. 2.6). Therefore, motion control mechanisms are necessary to reduce these artifacts (see Chap. 1 and Fig. 13.1).

2.4 Eddy Currents Artifacts

Eddy currents are generated by gradient switching producing changes in the static magnetic field. If the magnetic field variation produced by eddy currents disappears between the time of the applied field gradient and the image readout, a spatially dependent change in image phase with no discernible distortion will result. Diffusion encoding normally relies on the attenuation of the image magnitude rather than in the phase of the image. Therefore, a change in image phase of DWI does not change the diffusion measurement as long as the phase gradient per pixel is small. However, when the eddy currents decay slowly, a residual magnetic field remains during the image readout. This field behaves like an additional spatial encoding gradient field causing distortions or shifting of the image (Fig. 2.7).

From a technical point of view, eddy currents are compensated changing the gradient waveform in such a way that the final result is a very stable gradient on time. This technique is called pre-emphasis.

2.5 Fat Suppression Artifacts

Fat signal produces many difficulties in the acquisition of DWI in body applications, which are derived from the 3.4 parts per million shifting of the precession frequency of the fat signal from the water one. This frequency difference produces a water-fat shift in the EPI readout that can make the fat signal overlay in the studied region. Moreover, the contribution of the fat signal to the image is more pronounced for high *b* values, due to its very low diffusion coefficient. Under poor fat suppression conditions the combination of both effects produces ghosting artifacts, which can produce an inadequate estimation of the ADC, due to the combination of fat and tissue signal in the same voxel (Fig. 1.6).

Different strategies to reduce the fat contribution in the final diffusion image were reviewed in Chap. 1. When performing DWI over large FOVs on a 1.5-T system, STIR may be more useful than other methods in achieving uniform fat suppression due to its reduced sensitivity to magnetic field inhomogeneities. Unfortunately, diffusion studies based on STIR sequence show low SNR, making it necessary to increase the number of averages to recover signal. For targeted examinations to specific organs or anatomic

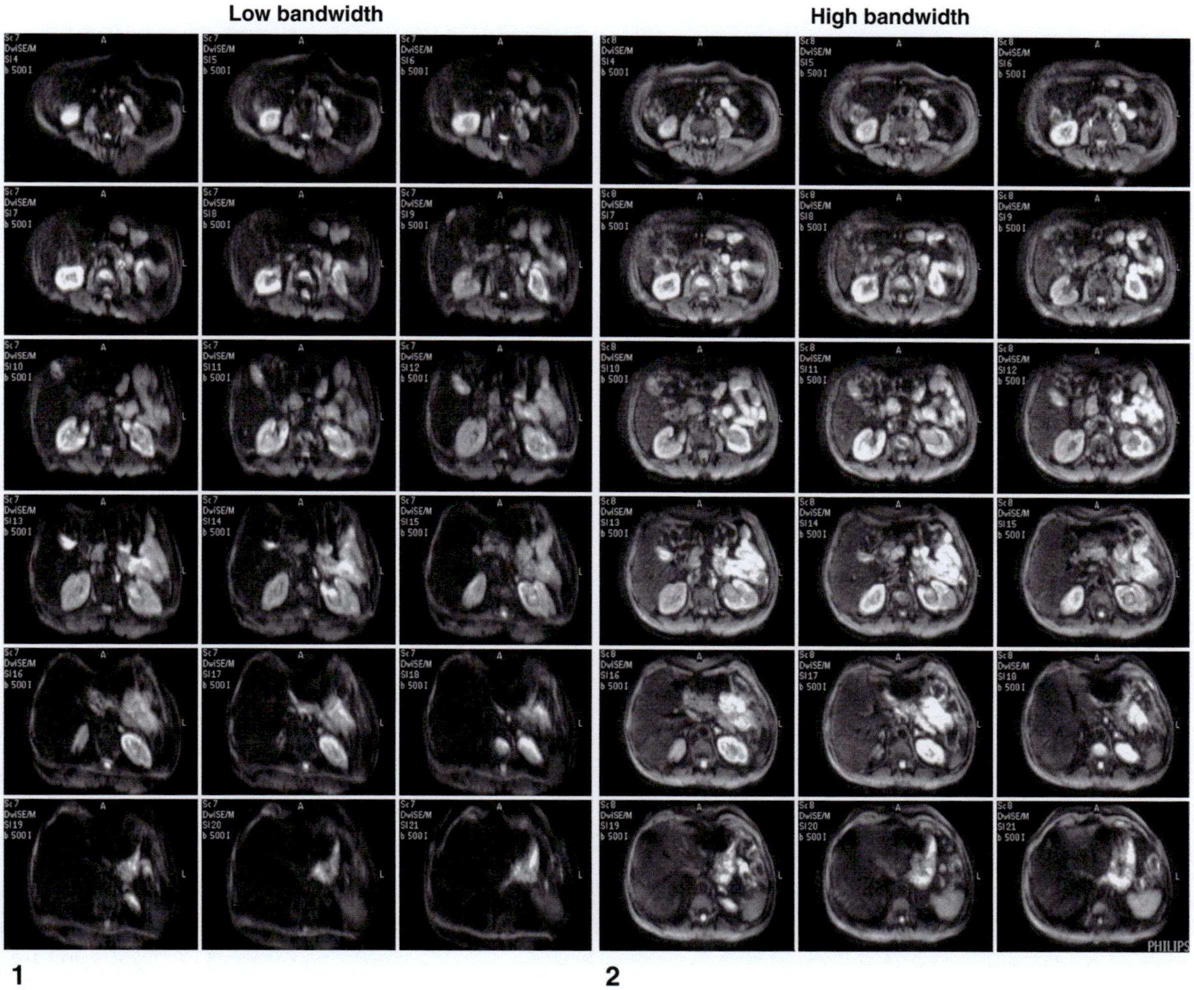

SSh SE EPI diffusion
Acq Reso: 3.0 × 3.0 × 7 mm^3
Fat suppression: SPIR
Scan time = 44 s
Number of averages = 3
b factor = 500 s/mm^2
Both acquisitions with gradient overplus strategy
Effective minimum TE in both cases = 71 ms (Low bandwidth)
49 ms (High bandwidth)

Fig. 2.4 Bandwidth: distortion artifacts. Two sets of DWI of the liver in the same volunteer are shown. Series number 1 was acquired with a low bandwidth (1,286 Hz per pixel) and series number 2 with a high bandwidth (3,632 Hz per pixel). The images of the series acquired with low bandwidth show strong distortions, mainly in the anterior aspect of the liver, which were minimized using high bandwidth. The increase of the bandwidth also reduced the effective TE, which helps to compensate the loss in SNR, due to a higher noise contamination proper of higher frequencies. Although reducing the acquisition bandwidth improves the SNR, it can also affect the geometrical distortion of the images due to the EPI readout. Some distortion can be expected on DWI due to phase error accumulation during the EPI readout. From the acquisition point of view, these geometric distortions can be reduced by increasing readout bandwidths. Increasing the readout bandwidth has two effects: the frequency difference between two consecutive phase encoding lines is higher, making the phase error due to magnetic field inhomogeneities less important in the total readout; and a faster readout (equivalent to a higher bandwidth) leaves a shorter time to change the signal phase due to magnetic field inhomogeneities producing less image distortion

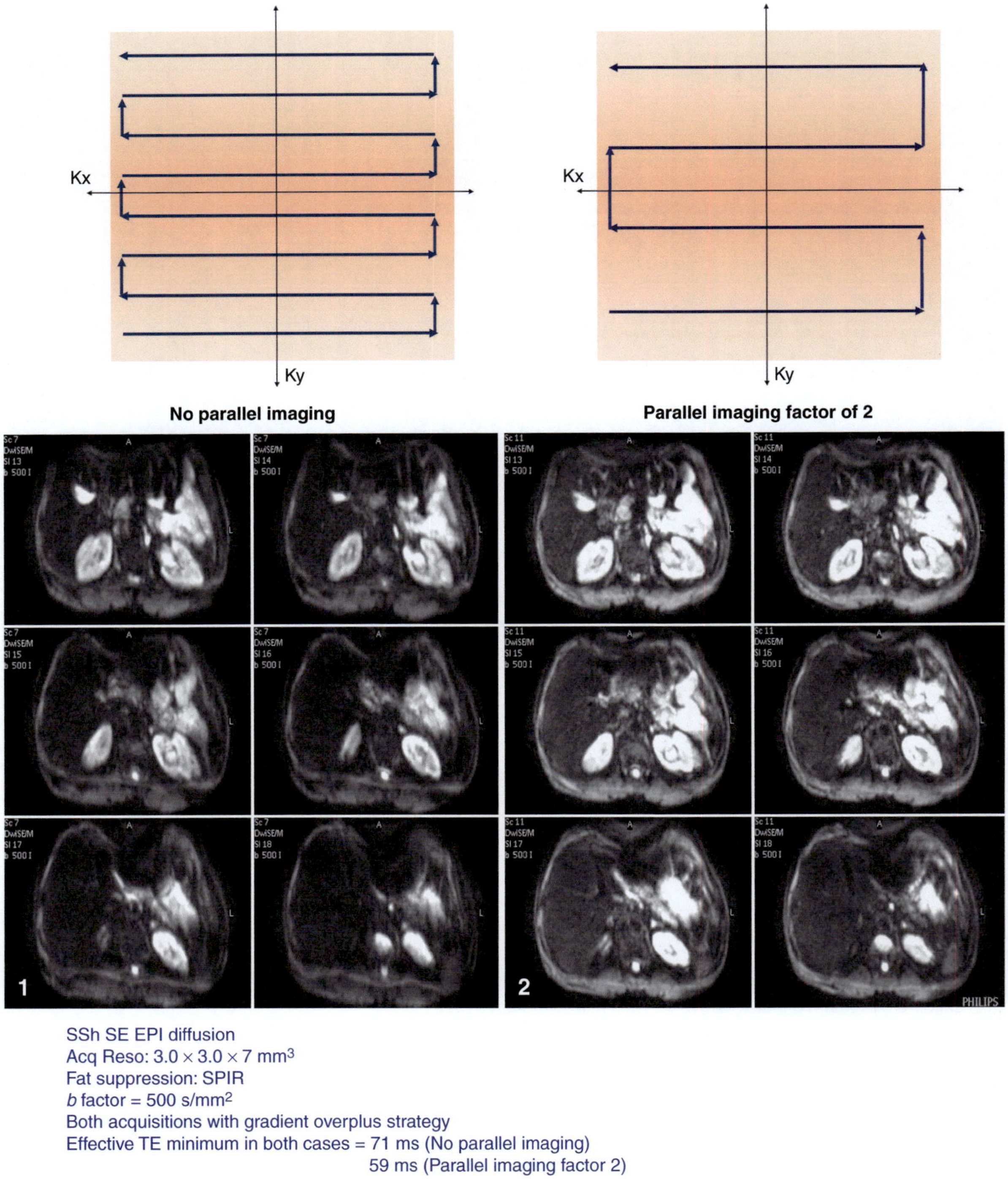

Fig. 2.5 **Use of parallel imaging for distortion artifacts**. Two series of a liver DWI in the same volunteer are shown. Series number 1 was acquired without parallel imaging and number 2 with a parallel factor of 2. This last sequence showed fewer artifacts in the anterior aspect of the liver, obtaining a more accurate geometrical representation of the studied anatomy, than the one without parallel imaging. As it was explained in Chap. 1, these image acquisition strategies skip some phase encoding lines replacing those non-acquired lines using the spatial information of the sensitivity maps of surface phased array coils (see schemes in the superior part of the figure). To skip some lines during the acquisition means to reduce the phase error accumulation and the associated image distortion

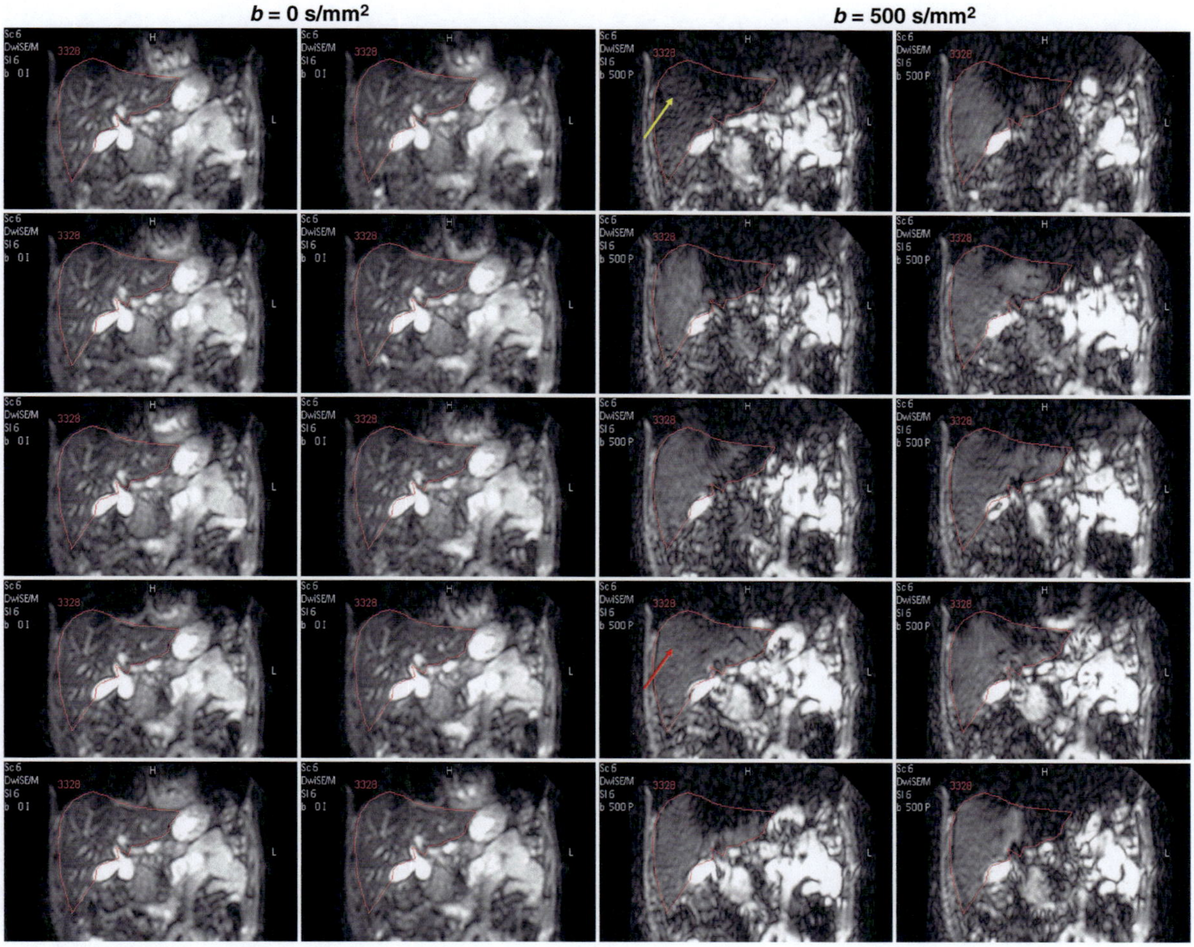

Fig. 2.6 Heart motion effects on DWI. In this figure, following the work of Kwee and colleagues, a dynamic DWI acquisition was performed in a volunteer under free breathing conditions. The acquisition included ten dynamics obtained in the coronal plane with two b values, that of 0 and 500 s/mm^2 (series 1 and 2, respectively). A single diffusion direction was acquired in foot-head direction for better evaluation of the influence of the heart movement. All the dynamics of a central slice of the acquisition using a b value of 0 s/mm^2 are shown in series number 1, and those acquired with $b = 500$ s/mm^2 in the series number 2. In all dynamics of series number 1, images are equivalent. However, in series number 2, there are several artifacts in different dynamics. *Yellow arrow* points an area where respiratory and heart movements completely destroy the signal from the liver. *Red arrow* shows the dynamic with a better signal of the liver as it was acquired during expiration and heart diastole. All the other images with $b = 500$ s/mm^2 show different areas of signal loss due to heart movement. ROIs surrounding the shape of the liver in all dynamics were drawn for easier visualization of the changes in signal

regions, the use of spectral spatial fat saturation techniques (e.g., SPIR or SPAIR) can be advantageous. SPIR produces nice results in a reasonable scan time, especially, on 1.5T magnets, due to the use of 120° pulses in the suppression reducing the required inversion time for zero cross of the fat signal. Conversely, on 3T systems, SPAIR technique has several advantages derived from the more homogenous excitation of the adiabatic pulses that reduce the effect of B1 inhomogeneities (dielectric or quadrupole artifacts).

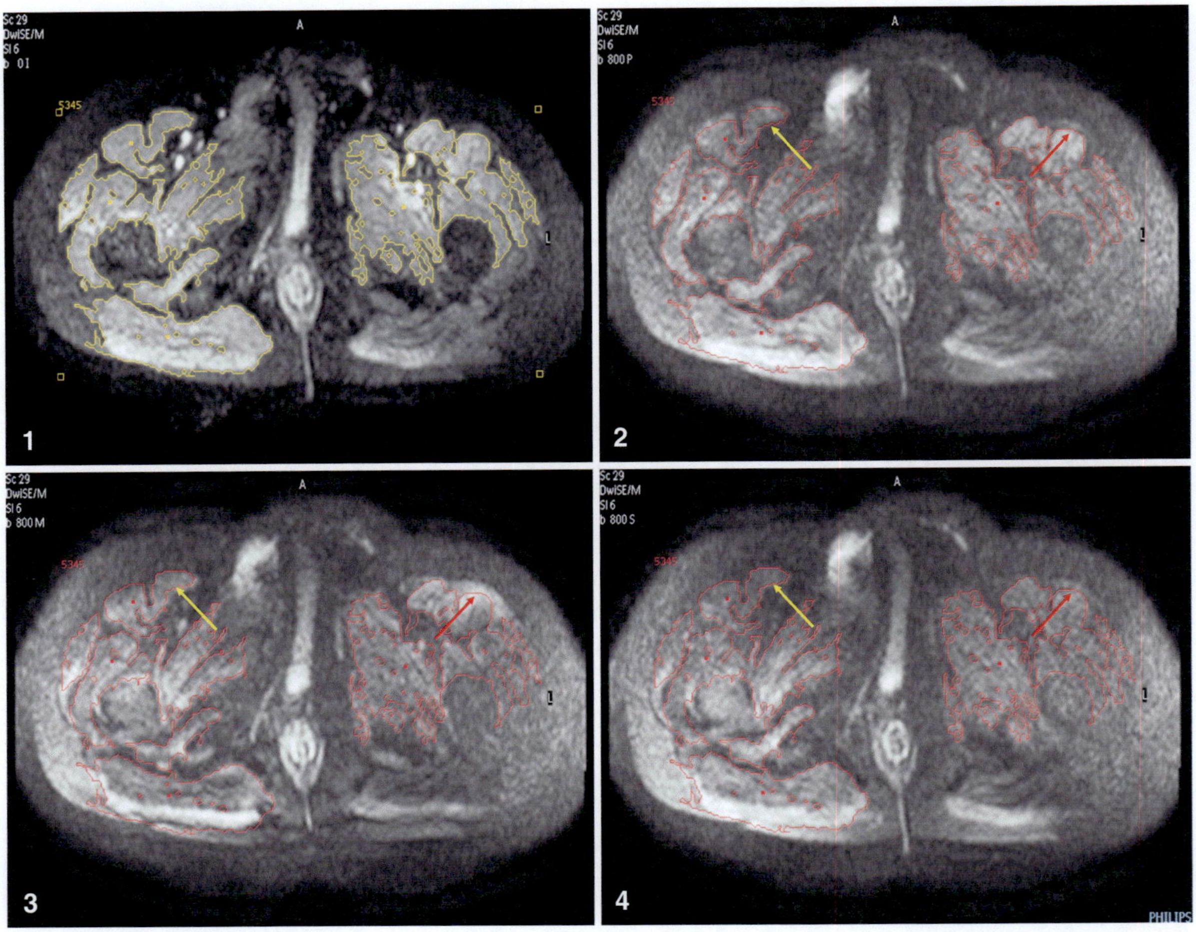

SSh SE EPI diffusion
Acq Reso: 2.0 × 2.0 × 7 mm^3
Fat suppression: SPIR
Scan time = 2:00 mn
Number of averages = 10
Maximum available gradient strength reaching an echo time = 49 ms
None gradient overplus strategy was applied to get X,Y and Z diffusion direction
$b = 0$ s/mm^2(1) and 800 s/mm^2 in phase, gradient and slice direction (2,3 and 4)

Fig. 2.7 Eddy currents artifacts. Different acquisitions of a pelvic DWI study with a *b* value of 800 s/mm² are shown, with the diffusion encoding in the phase, frequency, and slice direction (images 2, 3 and 4 respectively). Several ROIs were drawn in the $b=0$ s/mm² acquisition (image 1) and posteriorly overlaid in the other acquisitions with different diffusion directions in order to simplify the evaluation of image distortion. *Red* and *yellow arrows mark* those regions where the diffusion images do not perfectly fit with the *b* 0 image due to geometrical distortion produced by the eddy currents influence during the acquisition

Unfortunately, the adiabatic pulses require a high inversion time as these pulses need to excite a flip angle of 180°. Besides, the SAR of these pulses is also higher than that of the normal excitation pulses, requiring a longer TR in the sequence. Nowadays, the parallel excitation technology (Multi-Transmit) can also provide a homogeneous B1 excitation, allowing a uniform saturation using SPIR technique even in 3T systems.

Another challenge for spectral fat saturation is the magnetic field inhomogeneities especially in high magnetic fields. In order to compensate this difficulty, modern 3T systems are normally equipped with high order shimming (normally until second order) for better compensation of magnetic field variation along the high FOV used in body applications. Under poor magnetic field homogeneity conditions, it is possible to obtain two different effects. The first one is to have suboptimal fat signal suppression as it was shown in Fig. 1.6. The second effect is that some signal from the studied organ can become saturated losing information from those regions (Fig. 2.8).

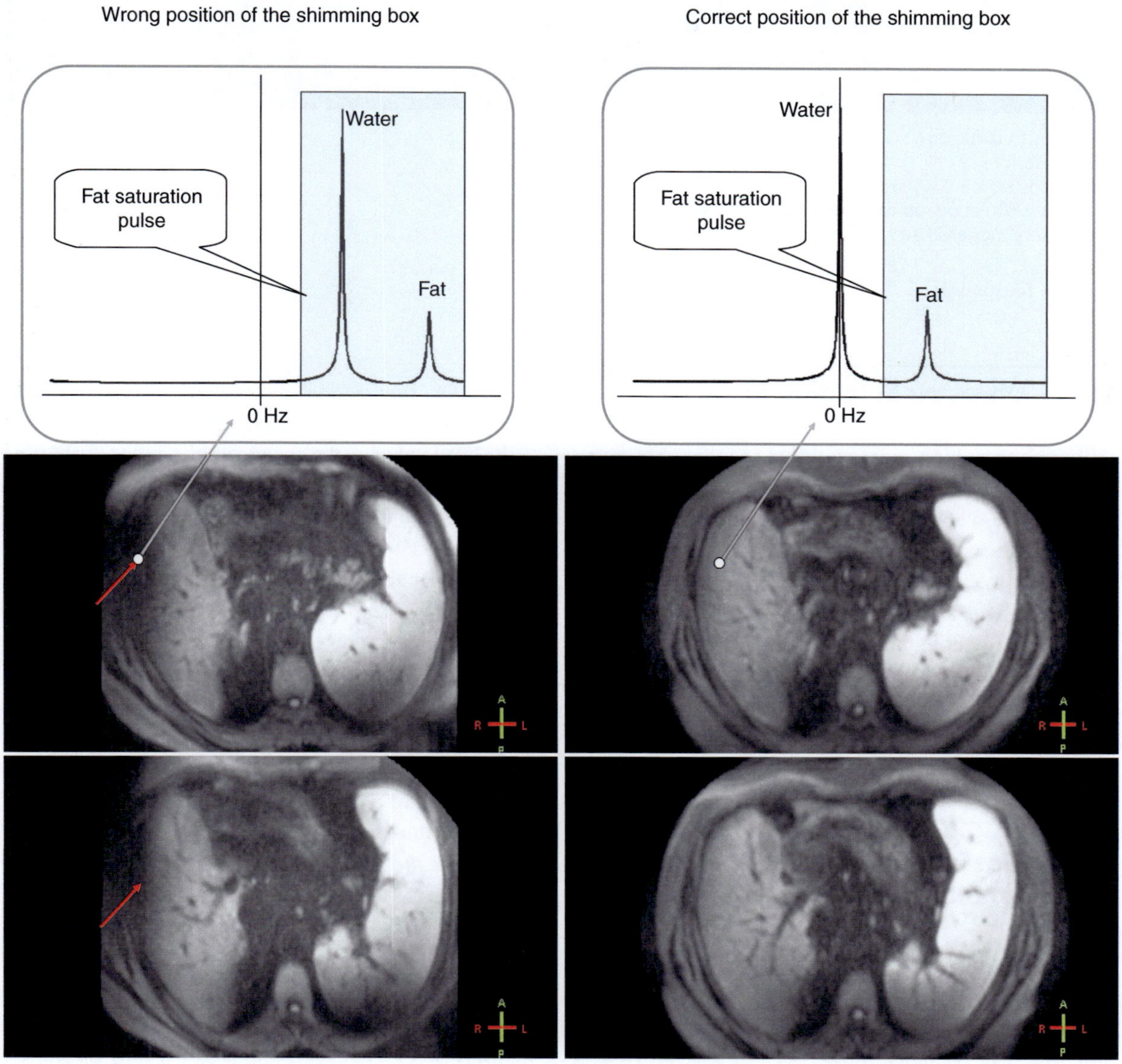

Fig. 2.8 Fat suppression artifacts: undesired tissue suppression. Fat suppression techniques can be divided into spectral and nonspectral selective techniques. In those techniques like SPIR or SPAIR, a good shimming is required in order to saturate properly just the spectral region of the fat signal. In this sense, a reduced region is selected to improve the magnetic field shimming of the region of interest. This region has to take into account the whole anatomy of interest or otherwise, the saturation pulse can destroy part of the signal from the region of interest. This figure shows a liver DWI acquisition where the shimming box was placed excluding some part of the right lobe of the liver (*left column*). As a result, the spectrum from a pixel in the right part of the liver is shifted due to magnetic field inhomogeneity and the saturation pulse completely destroys the signal from that region. On the *right column*, the same DWI sequence, but with the shimming box properly placed, shows how the saturation pulse only destroys the fat signal, achieving a homogeneous fat suppression. The spectrum of the same pixel in this case shows how tissue signal is completely preserved

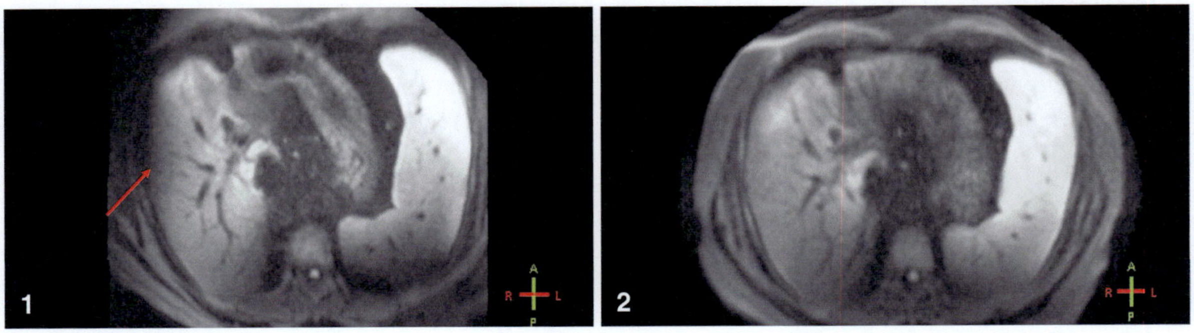

SSh SE EPI diffusion
SENSE factor = 2
Acq Reso: 3.0 × 3.0 × 7.0 mm^3
b values = 800 acquired with gradient overplus
Respiratory triggered and SPIR fat suppression

Fig. 2.8 (continued)

2.6 Dielectric Shielding Artifacts

Although very high magnetic field scanners have several advantages, they also present some technical challenges to be overcome. As it was explained in the fat suppression section, there is an inherent artifact associated to the 3T systems called dielectric artifact (Fig. 2.9). This artifact produces a nonuniform excitation of the whole anatomy due to the interaction between the radiofrequency wavelength of 3T systems and the shape of the patient. Therefore, depending on the patient shape, some regions may not be completely excited producing a focal signal loss (Fig. 2.10).

2.7 Tips in DWI Sequence Design for Body Applications

The image contrast at DWI relies on intrinsic differences in the water diffusion among tissues. Scanning parameters must be optimized in order to increase SNR and contrast to noise ratio (CNR). As previously described, DWI is prone to motion and magnetic susceptibility artifacts since the majority of DWI are based on EPI sequences. As a general rule, conventional DWI has a limited spatial resolution. Therefore, it is important to find the optimum equilibrium between scan time and spatial resolution. In order to increase the DWI sequence quality, several rules should be followed, which are a short resume of what has been detailed in chapters 1 and 2:

- *Use fat suppression techniques*: The use of fat suppression allows to increasing the dynamic range of the DWI reducing the chemical shift–induced ghosting artifacts. Although inversion-recovery approaches such as STIR are useful for imaging large areas, the use of chemical fat selective saturation is more appropriate for smaller areas of interest due to their better SNR.
- *Minimize T1 saturation*: TR should be long enough to avoid T1 saturation effects, which can result in falsely low ADC values.
- *Use short TE*: This can be done by increasing the gradient intensity in the gradient lobes, increasing the bandwidth and using parallel imaging the bandwidth (up to a maximum of 1,500 MHz) and using parallel imaging.
- *Increase the number of acquisitions (NEX),* because the noise is disruptive and the signal is additive, although it is time consuming.
- *Decrease FOV* to a minimum in the phase encoding direction.
- *Do not increase the resolution in plane* to levels where the noise increases significantly or image quality decreases severely because it will decrease the quality of ADC maps. Enlarging the FOV may have a similar result.
- *Trace approach/gradient overplus*: The use of three orthogonal motion-probing gradients to produce a single diffusion direction allows us to improve the gradient strength by square root of three. Therefore, this approach reduces the effective TE, increases the SNR and minimizes susceptibility, EPI, or motion artifacts.

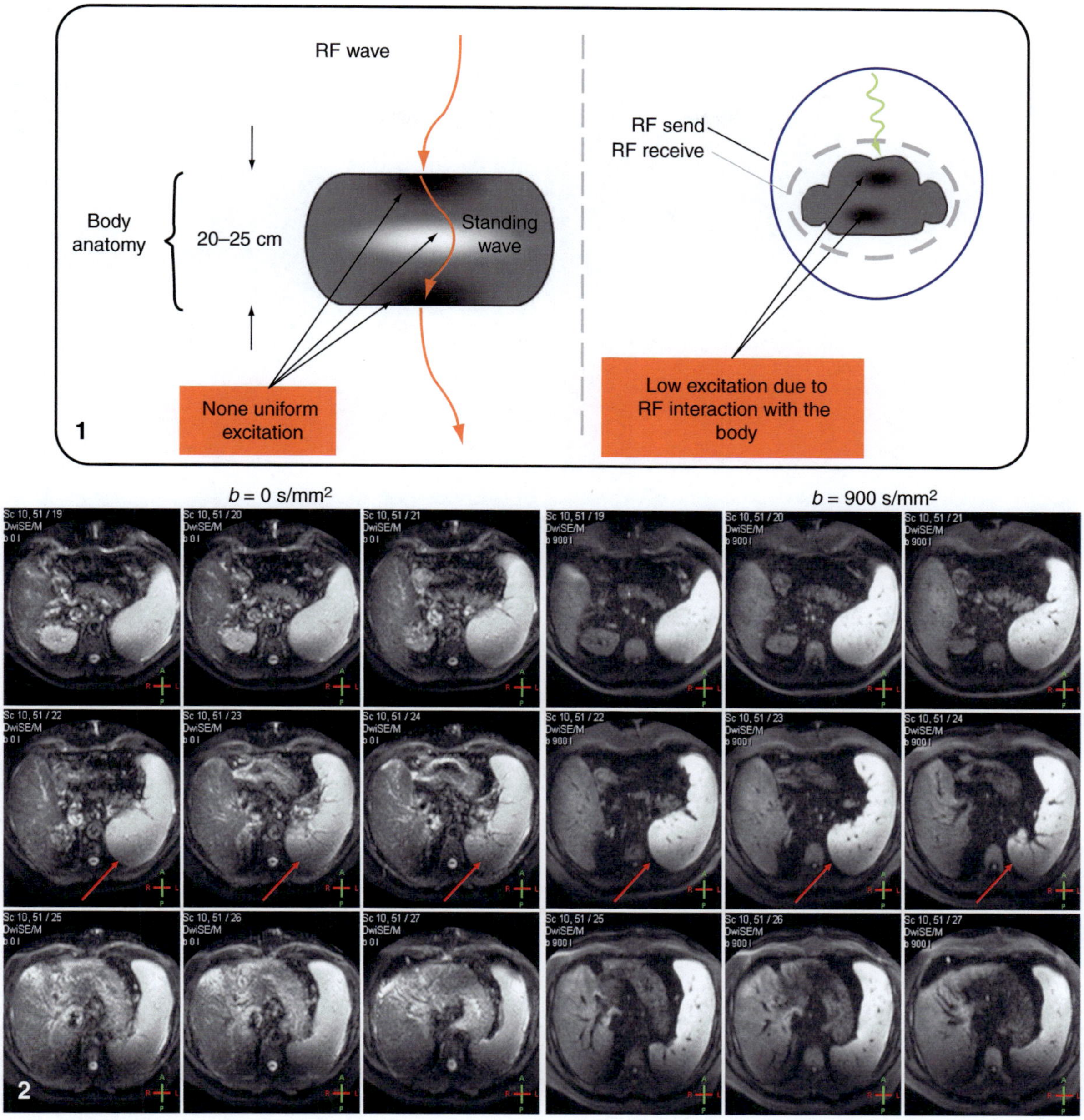

SSh SE EPI diffusion
SENSE factor = 2
Acq Reso: 3.0 × 3.0 × 7.0 mm^3
Effective TE = 59 ms
b values = 0.900 s/mm^2 acquired with gradient overplus
Respiratory triggered

Fig. 2.9 Dielectric artifacts. Dielectric artifacts are typical of 3T magnets. The schemes in the first part of the figure summarize their origin. These artifacts produce a nonuniform excitation of the whole anatomy due to the interaction between the RF excitation and the shape of the studied region producing a standing wave that can interact in a constructive and destructive manner. These interactions produce a nonuniform excitation of the sample (**2.9.1**). This effect is particularly relevant in 3T systems where the RF wavelength in the body is around 25 cm that fits with patient diameter. Therefore, depending on the patient shape, there are some regions that are not completely excited producing signal loss and other regions that are overexcited producing hot spots of signal. In the second part of this figure (**2.9.2**), a clinical example of a dielectric artifact in a liver DWI sequence is shown. Notice the signal loss in the spine region that reduces the signal in the spleen (*red arrows*) and in the posterior part of the liver, for both *b* values (0 and 900 s/mm^2). This signal loss produces a lower SNR

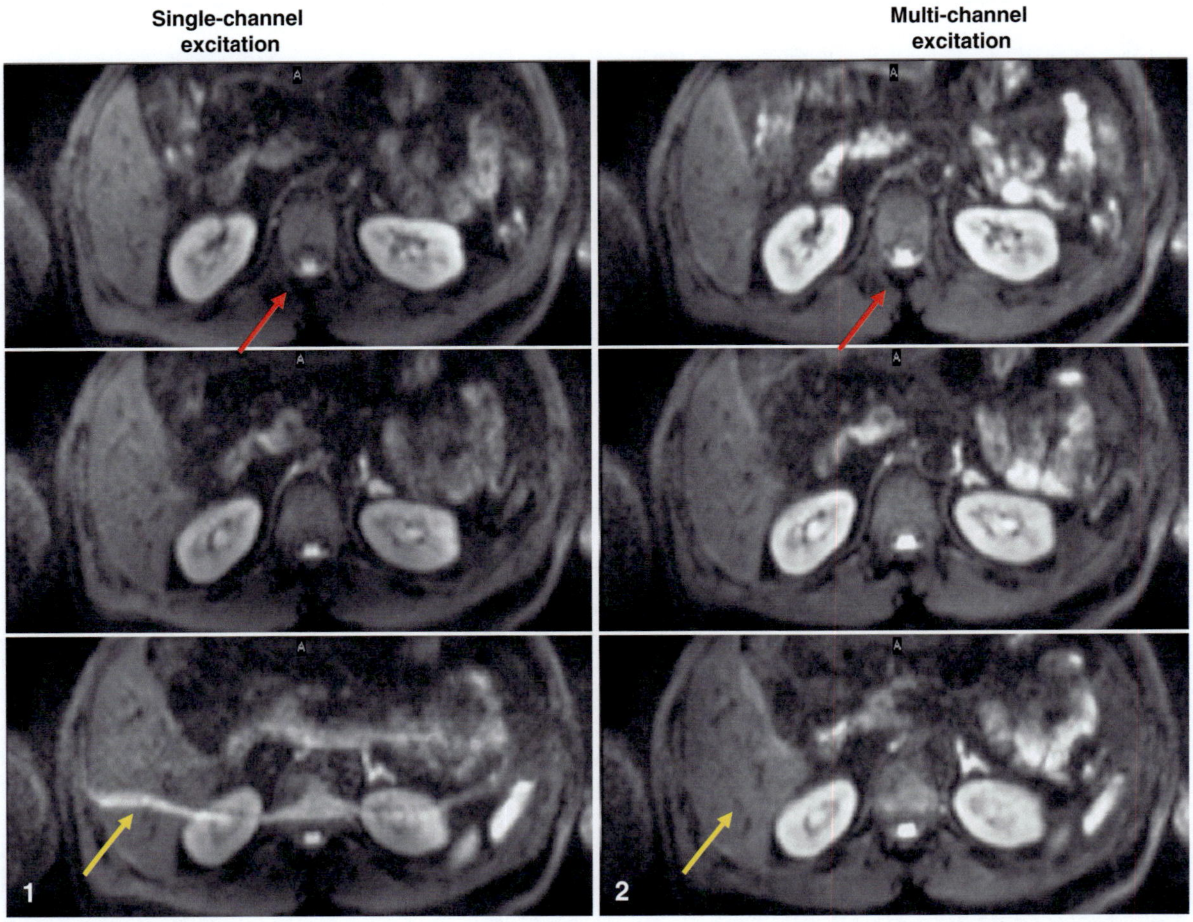

Fig. 2.10 Single channel versus multichannel excitation. In order to compensate the nonhomogeneous excitation of the entire FOV due to dielectric artifacts in high magnetic fields, it is necessary to look for new excitation strategies that allow a better RF distribution. The best way to ensure a more homogeneous excitation is to share the excitation between different RF excitation coils that can drive completely independent RF pulses (different amplitude, phase, frequency, and waveform) that allow an accurate excitation over the whole FOV, independently of the patient anatomy. Nowadays, there are 3T systems that allow excitation with completely independent RF excitation sources as well as patient adaptive strategies that ensure a homogeneous excitation over the whole FOV independently of the patient shape. This figure shows the results of two single breath-hold DWI acquisitions of the same patient using a single-channel (**2.10.1**) or multichannel acquisition strategies (**2.10.2**). Both images were acquired with the same acquisition parameters and displayed with the same window level and width for comparison. In these images, *red arrows* showed a dark signal region in the spine in the single-channel excitation acquisition (**2.10.1**) while a more homogeneous excitation is appreciated in the whole FOV for multichannel excitation (**2.10.2**). Finally, *yellow arrows* showed some fat artifacts in the single-channel excitation acquisition, that were not present in the multichannel acquisition, due to wrong excitation in the SPIR fat suppression

- *SNR may be increased* by using higher field strength (3T magnets), reducing TE, applying higher gradient power, using a short EPI train, and using phase-array coils with more number of elements.

Further Reading

Hamstra D, Rehemtulla A, Ross BD (2007) Diffusion magnetic resonance imaging: a biomarker for treatment response in oncology. J Clin Oncol 25:4104–4109

Hayashida Y, Yakushiji T, Awai K et al (2006) Monitoring therapeutic responses of primary bone tumors by diffusion-weighted image: initial results. Eur Radiol 16:2637–2643

Kamel IR, Reyes DK, Liapi E et al (2007) Functional MR imaging assessment of tumor response after 90Y microsphere treatment in patients with unresectable hepatocellular carcinoma. J Vasc Interv Radiol 18:49–56

Kandpal H, Sharma R, Madhusudhan KS et al (2009) Respiratory-triggered versus breath-hold diffusion-weighted MRI of liver lesions: comparison of image quality and apparent diffusion coefficient values. Am J Roentgenol 192:915–922

King AD, Ahuja AT, Yeung DKW et al (2007) Malignant cervical lymphadenopathy: diagnostic accuracy of diffusion-weighted MR imaging. Radiology 245:806–813

Kwee TC, Takahara T, Niwa T et al (2009) Influence of cardiac motion on diffusion-weighted magnetic resonance imaging of the liver. MAGMA 22:319–325

Mardor Y, Pfeffer R, Spiegelmann R et al (2003) Early detection of response to radiation therapy in patients with brain malignancies using conventional and high b-value diffusion-weighted magnetic resonance imaging. J Clin Oncol 21(6): 1094–1100

Merkle EM, Brian MD (2006) Abdominal MRI at 3.0T: the basics revisited. Am J Roentgenol 186:1524–1532

Padhani AR, Liu G, Koh DM et al (2009) Diffusion-weighted magnetic resonance imaging as a cancer biomarker: consensus and recommendations. Neoplasia 11(2):102–125

Patterson DM, Padhani AR, Collins DJ (2008) Technology insight: water diffusion MRI – a potential new biomarker of response to cancer therapy. Nat Clin Pract Oncol 5(4):220–233

Pickles MD, Gibbs P, Lowry M et al (2006) Diffusion changes precede size reduction in neoadjuvant treatment of breast cancer. Magn Reson Imaging 24:843–847

Shen SH, Chiou YY, Wang JH et al (2008) Diffusion-weighted single-shot echo-planar imaging with parallel technique in assessment of endometrial cancer. Am J Roentgenol 190(2): 481–488

Sumi M, Sakihama N, Sumi T et al (2003) Discrimination of metastatic cervical lymph nodes with diffusion-weighted MR imaging in patients with head and neck cancer. Am J Neuroradiol 24:627–1634

Takahara T, Imai Y, Yamashita T et al (2004) Diffusion weighted whole body imaging with background body signal suppression (DWIBS): technical improvement using free breathing, STIR and high resolution 3D display. Radiat Med 22(4): 275–282

Theilmann RJ, Borders R, Trouard TP et al (2004) Changes in water mobility measured by diffusion MRI predict response of metastatic breast cancer to chemotherapy. Neoplasia 6:831–837

Thoeny HC, De Keyzer F, Vandecaveye V et al (2005) Effect of vascular targeting agent in rat tumor model: dynamic contrast-enhanced versus diffusion-weighted MR imaging. Radiology 237:492–499

Uhl M, Saueressig U, van Buiren M et al (2006) Osteosarcoma: preliminary results of in vivo assessment of tumor necrosis after chemotherapy with diffusion- and perfusionweighted magnetic resonance imaging. Invest Radiol 41:618–623

Yankeelov TE, Lepage M, Chakravarthy A et al (2007) Integration of quantitative DCE-MRI and ADC mapping to monitor treatment response in human breast cancer: initial results. Magn Reson Imaging 25:1–13

3 Quantification and Postprocessing of DWI

Javier Sánchez-González and Antonio Luna

3.1 Biophysical Basis

MRI allows the "in vivo" study of the effective displacement of water molecules for a given time by means of diffusion-weighted sequences. Even more, measurements of water diffusion are possible with this technique, calculating the Apparent Diffusion Coefficient (ADC). Current MRI technology allows us to measure the diffusion in a fraction of time between 40 and 80 ms with a spatial resolution of millimeters.

There are several factors influencing the "in vivo" diffusion properties of a tissue such as temperature, cell size, tissue structure and organization, water exchange between intracellular and extracellular compartments, cell density, flow and perfusion, and macroscopic motion. Differences in temperature are not a critical factor on DWI. Bulk motion may be compensated by using motion correction techniques, as previously described in Chap. 1. The influence of perfusion and flow in diffusion quantifications can be reduced if the signal from *b* values smaller than 100 s/mm^2 is obviated in DWI measurements, according to the intravoxel incoherent motion model (IVIM), as it will be explained later in this chapter. The calculation of a minimum high *b* value is necessary to minimize the perfusion effect over diffusion in tissues with a rich vascularity, which varies from tissue to tissue. Therefore, to perform DWI measurements, it is necessary to calculate at least a low and a high *b* value which should be adjusted to the studied anatomy.

The rest of factors limiting free water diffusion in the extravascular space are related to the characteristics of cells and tissue structure. Therefore, a strong negative correlation between ADC values and cell density and size within a tissue has been demonstrated in several organs and diseases, which has made DWI a robust cancer biomarker. However, this correlation is clearer in tumors such as gliomas, round-cell tumors, or lymphomas than in adenocarcinomas due to the fact that each tumor and tissue exhibit different multiexponential signal decay over a broad range of *b* values and the definitive biophysical basis of diffusion is not totally understood at this moment.

3.2 Estimation of Quantitative Data

3.2.1 ADC and eADC Estimation with Two and Multiple *b*-Values

DWI is an MRI strategy that allows the visualization of the microscopic movement of the water inside a voxel. Assuming that the diffusion image voxel can be interpreted as an average of all kinds of different water behaviors, the amount of water movement can be represented according to a single parameter known as ADC (Fig. 3.1). This parameter represents the exponential decay of the diffusion signal while increasing the *b* values as an average single water component, as previously explained in the physical basis section of Chap. 1. The estimation of ADC values compensates the T2

J. Sánchez-González (✉)
Clinical Scientist, Philips Healthcare Ibéria, Madrid, Spain
e-mail: javier.sanchez.gonzalez@philips.com

A. Luna
Chief of MRI, Health Time Group, Jaén, Spain
e-mail: aluna70@sercosa.com

A. Luna et al., *Diffusion MRI Outside the Brain*,
DOI 10.1007/978-3-642-21052-5_3,

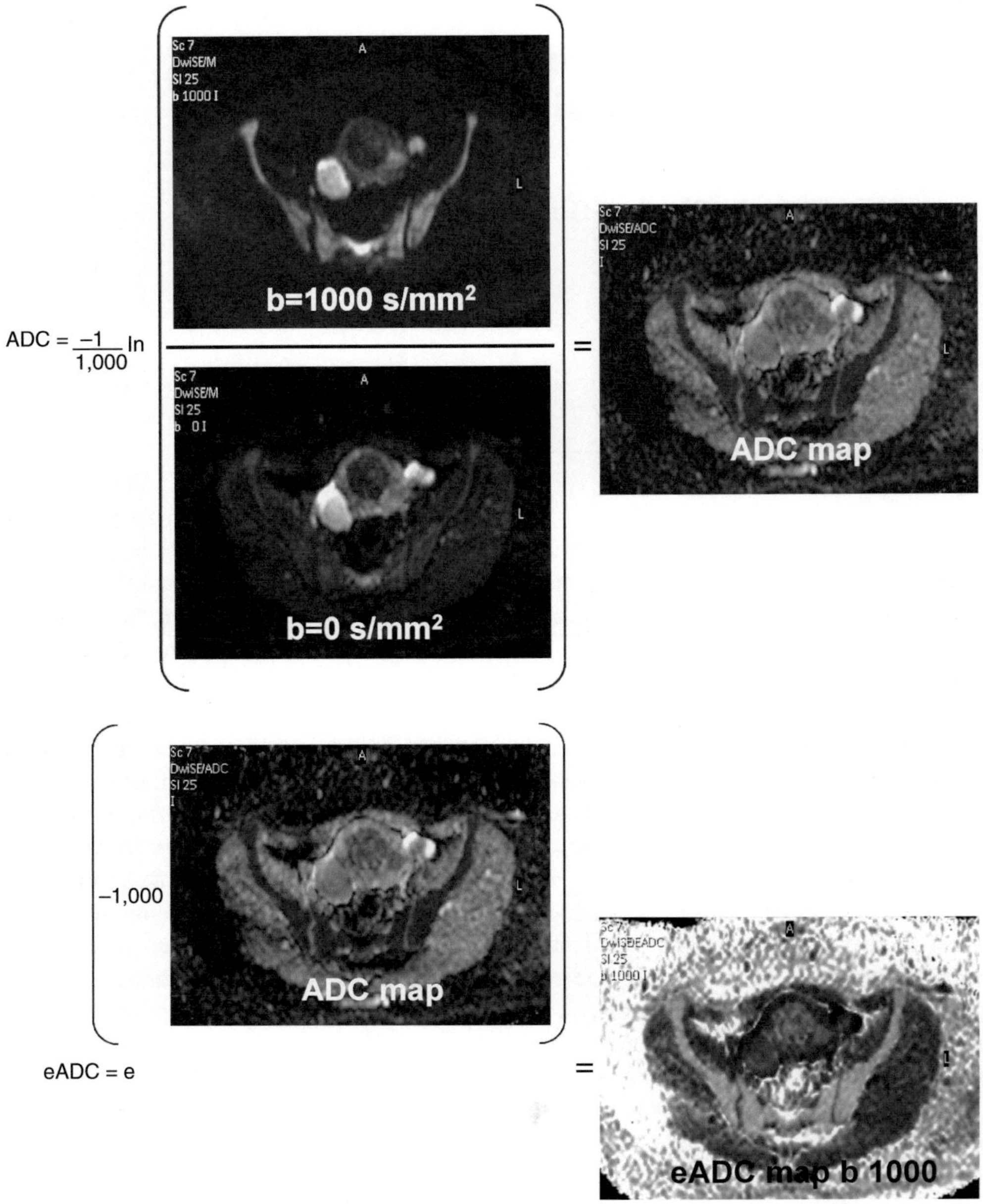

Fig. 3.1 ADC and e-ADC calculation. ADC represents the exponential decay of a single component of DWI according to the theory described in Chap. 1. Assuming that the rest of sequence parameters remain equal between the images with different *b* values, this parameter can be estimated using only two *b* values as:

$$\mathrm{ADC} = -\frac{1}{b_2 - b_1}\ln\left(\frac{S_2}{S_1}\right),$$

where $b_2 > b_1$ in the special case where b_1 is equal to zero, this equation becomes in the most known expression:

$$\mathrm{ADC} = -\frac{1}{b_2}\ln\left(\frac{S_2}{S_0}\right),$$

where S_i represents the signal intensity of the acquired images and includes the T_1 and T_2 effects of the signal. Once the ADC map is estimated, this information can be used to calculate the exponential ADC (eADC). This quantity is calculated as $\mathrm{eADC} = \exp(-b \times \mathrm{ADC})$, where the values has to be established for a given *b* value, for example, for a *b* value of 1,000 s/mm^2, the eADC value will be estimated as: $\mathrm{eADC}_{1000} = \exp(-1000 \times \mathrm{ADC})$

effect in the evaluation of the water restriction. In lesions with very long T2 values, the T2 effects of the signal may produce high signal even in acquisitions with high *b* values, although there is no real diffusion restriction (Fig. 4.8). This effect is known as T2 shine-through, one of the most important pitfalls on DWI. This effect is avoided using ADC quantifications. Besides, due to the very short T2-effect of some tissues (e.g., hemorrhagic lesions), there may be regions that completely lose the signal on DWI images independently of the diffusion properties of the tissue and of the acquired *b* value. This effect is called dark-through effect (Fig. 4.8).

In order to get a good estimation of the ADC, it is necessary to acquire at least two *b* values, which should provide enough signal difference to reduce the noise effect in the ADC estimation (Fig. 3.2). Besides, if the highest *b* value is too high, the acquired images may show very low SNR, making the obtained ADC maps of very poor quality due to noise contamination. Taking these two concepts into account, it is necessary to define the final image protocol with an adequate balance between the maximum acquired *b* value and an appropriate SNR in an appropriate scan time. Padhani et al estimated the most appropriate maximum *b* value for studying different organs outside the brain on 1.5 T magnets which are summarized in Table 3.1.

A better estimation of the ADC value is obtained when more than two *b* values are acquired. In this manner, the intensity values of the whole range of *b* values are fitted to a monoexponential decay model where the decay constant represents the estimated ADC value (Fig. 3.3).

When more than two *b* values are acquired, it is also possible to get more information from the diffusion signal. Theoretically, the amount of visible movement of the water molecules in the acquired image can be controlled by the *b* factor. For high *b* values, those molecules with high movement do not significantly contribute to the final image signal and only those water molecules with restricted movement can provide signal. Furthermore, water molecules with high displacement contribute to the signal of the final image of DWI when acquiring low *b* values. In this sense, the *b* value may be considered as a control parameter to decide the water molecules' range of movement contributing to the final image.

3.2.2 Multiexponential Modeling of Diffusion

In a simplified version of the water behavior inside a voxel of a diffusion image, we could consider four different compartments: free water, intravascular water, and water located in the extracellular and intracellular spaces. This approach delineates four compartments with four different diffusion properties of the water movement. The water within the vessel is flowing due to heart beating, the liquid water has no barriers for the movement and finally the extracellular and intracellular waters have more restrictions to the movement due to presence of membranes and cells. Although a direct relation between these compartments and the diffusion signal is not straightforward, there are some reports that established some relationship between these compartments and the diffusion signal at different *b* values. Considering this approach and measuring the diffusion signal with many *b* values, it is possible to get different microscopic behaviors of the tissue that can be interpreted according to the *b* values used during the acquisition. If we have to study the fast movement of the water, low *b* values have to be measured. Conversely, if we have to analyze the slow diffusion component, we will need to acquire high *b* values according to the region of interest.

3.2.2.1 Intravoxel Incoherent Motion

It is possible to measure the water movement in the blood stream (perfusion). For this, many DWI acquisitions with *b* values lower than 100 s/mm^2 and some DWI series with *b*-values between 100 s/mm^2 and the maximum *b*-value are required. The rest of the imaging parameters should remain constant for all DWI acquisitions. This theory, called Intravoxel Incoherent Motion (IVIM), was proposed by LeBihan to evaluate the microcirculation of brain tumors, but its application has been extended to the evaluation of liver cirrhosis and also to other organs such as muscle, brain, lung, and pancreas. The idea behind this theory is that the blood that flows in the arteries provides a visible diffusion signal for very low *b* values and has no contribution for higher *b* values. A further explanation of this model can be obtained in Fig. 3.4.

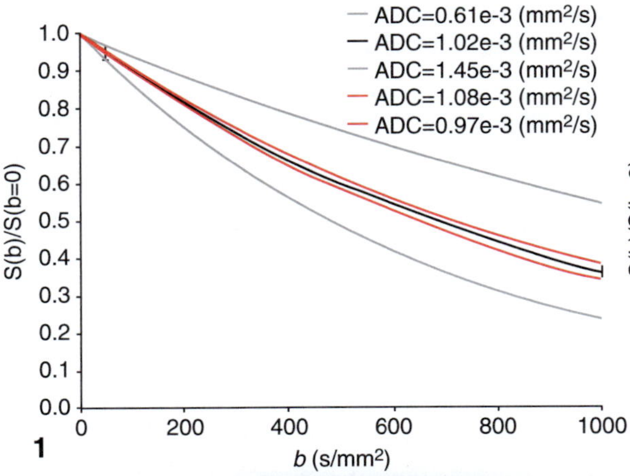
ADC=0.61e-3 (mm²/s)
ADC=1.02e-3 (mm²/s)
ADC=1.45e-3 (mm²/s)
ADC=1.08e-3 (mm²/s)
ADC=0.97e-3 (mm²/s)
S(b)/S(b=0)
b (s/mm²)
1.0
0.9
0.8
0.7
0.6
0.5
0.4
0.3
0.2
0.1
0.0
0
200
400
600
800
1000

1

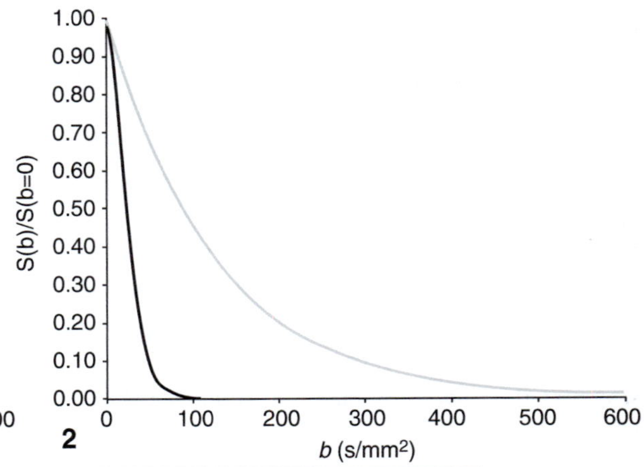
S(b)/S(b=0)
b (s/mm²)
1.00
0.90
0.80
0.70
0.60
0.50
0.40
0.30
0.20
0.10
0.00
0
100
200
300
400
500
600

2

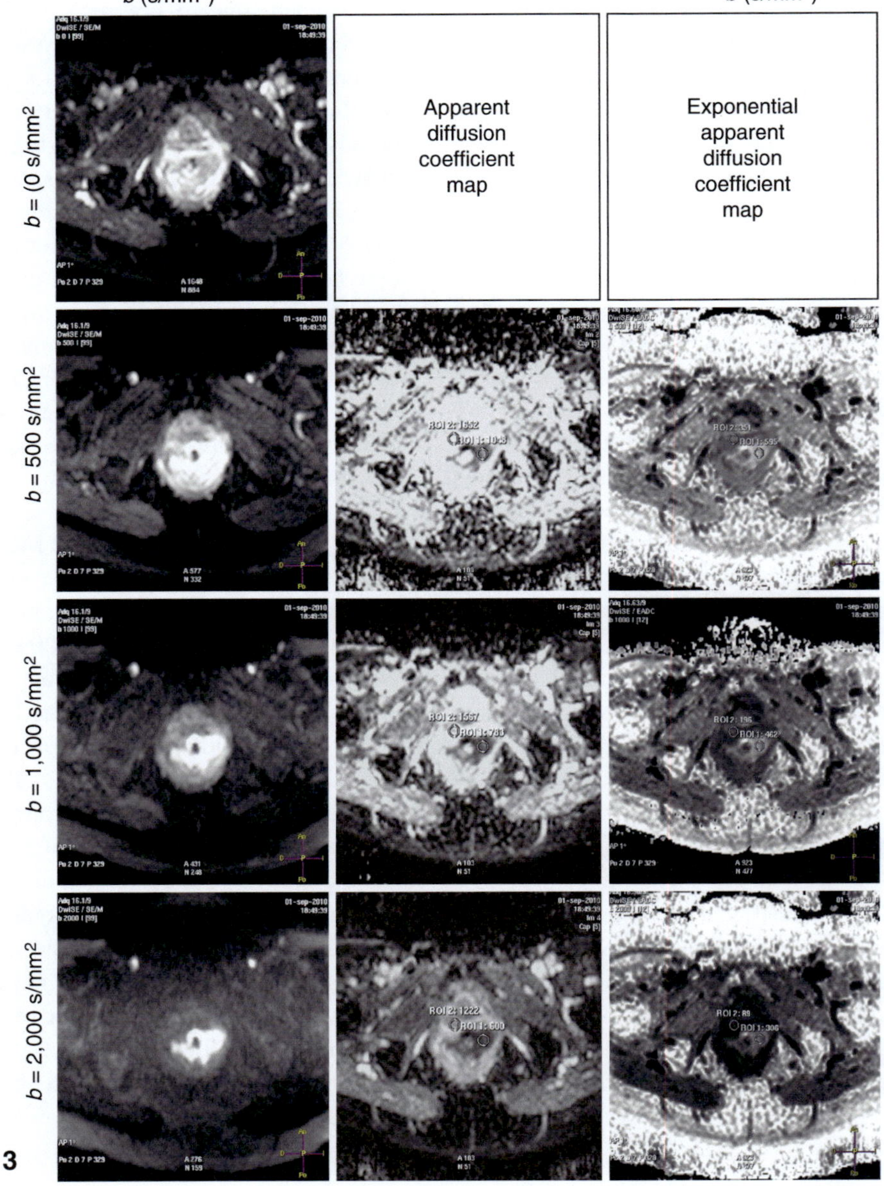
b = (0 s/mm²
b = 500 s/mm²
b = 1,000 s/mm²
b = 2,000 s/mm²
Apparent diffusion coefficient map
Exponential apparent diffusion coefficient map

3

Fig. 3.2 Selection of b values on ADC Maps. In order to obtain a reliable ADC estimation from the DWI study with two different *b* values, it is necessary to choose the correct *b* values. In the case where the difference between both *b* values is very low, the difference in the signal intensity (SI) has small variations being very sensible to noise effects. In the top left of this figure (**3.2.1**), a graph of the expected exponential signal decay with the variation of the *b* values is shown. In order to simplify the explanation, the signal has been normalized to the signal intensity of $b=0$ s/mm². The black line represents the real value of the tissue. The gray lines represent the limits of the variation due to the noise in the ADC estimation for a *b* value of 50 s/mm², if it is applied a variation of 0.02 in the SI of *b* 50/ SI of *b* 0 ratio. The *red lines* represent the result in the ADC for the same variation for *a b* value of 1,000 s/mm². In this graph, it can be appreciated how the highest error in the ADC calculation is produced when lower b-values are used for ADC estimation due to noise contamination. If the selected *b* values are too high for the studied organ, the result can also be wrong. In Fig. **3.2.2**, the signal for a pixel of a tissue with very high ADC value is studied. As in the other graph, the signal is normalized to the signal intensity of $b=0$ s/mm². If a very high *b* value is used to estimate the ADC value for this pixel (*gray line* in the graph), it is not possible to distinguish it from those signals with a higher ADC value, because the signal disappears for lower *b* values. However, if the signal is measured using a lower *b* value, a better estimation of higher *b* values will be obtained. Finally, in the lower part of this figure (**3.2.3**), a DWI series of a rectal cancer acquired with different high *b* values are shown. Notice how the limits of the lesion are better depicted with higher *b* values. The results of the estimation of the ADC and e-ADC maps with $b=0$ s/mm² and different maximum *b* values are also presented in both normal rectal wall and rectal cancer, according to the ROIs drawn. It can be appreciated a change in the ADC values of both tissues normal and tumoral rectal wall, depending on the maximum *b* value used for ADC calculation, as shown in Table 3.2

Table 3.1 Optimum highest *b* values in body DWI at 1.5 T, Modified from Padhani et al. (2009)

b values (s/mm²)	Anatomic regions
>1,000	Prostate, uterus, cervix, lymph nodes
750–1,000	Breast, chest, general abdomen (including colorectal, pancreas, kidneys, peritoneum), pelvis (ovaries, bladder), whole-body imaging with DWIBS
500–750	Liver (primary and metastatic disease)
20–60	Use as a black-blood technique for focal liver lesion detection

Table 3.2 ADC variation regarding to the *b* values used in the estimation

b 0 s/mm² and		*b* 500 s/mm²	*b* 1,000 s/mm²	*b* 2,000 s/mm²
ADC(mm²/s)	Healthy tissue	1.65×10^{-3}	1.57×10^{-3}	1.22×10^{-3}
	Cellular tissue	1.05×10^{-3}	0.78×0^{-3}	0.60×10^{-3}

3.2.3 Diffusion Tensor Imaging

The diffusion signal from a DWI experiment depends on the direction of the applied diffusion gradients (Fig. 1.4), as the diffusion information of a tissue is a vectorial property. For this reason, describing the molecular movement of the water in a tissue requires a tensor, *D*, which fully describes the molecular mobility along each direction and correlation between these directions:

$$\mathrm{ADC}=\begin{pmatrix}\mathrm{ADC_{XX}} & \mathrm{ADC_{XY}} & \mathrm{ADC_{XZ}}\\ \mathrm{ADC_{YX}} & \mathrm{ADC_{YY}} & \mathrm{ADC_{YZ}}\\ \mathrm{ADC_{ZX}} & \mathrm{ADC_{ZY}} & \mathrm{ADC_{ZZ}}\end{pmatrix}, \tag{3.1}$$

This tensor is symmetric ($\mathrm{ADC}_{ij}=\mathrm{ADC}_{ji}$, with $i, j=$X, Y, Z). It is important to note that by using diffusion encoding gradient pulses along only one direction, say X, the signal attenuation not only depends on the diffusion effects along this direction, but it may also include contribution from other directions, say Y and Z. In order to obtain independent information from each direction, it is necessary to obtain the matrix transformation from the MR coordinate system (Fig. 3.5.1) to a new coordinate system where all the elements of the tensor described in Eq. 3.1 will be equal to zero, except those in the diagonal ($i=j$) (Fig. 3.5.2). The estimation of this transformation is called diagonalization.

As it is difficult to display tensor data with images (multiple images would be necessary), the concept of diffusion ellipsoids has been proposed. An ellipsoid is a three-dimensional representation of the diffusion distance covered in space by molecules in a given diffusion time (*Td*). These ellipsoids, which can be

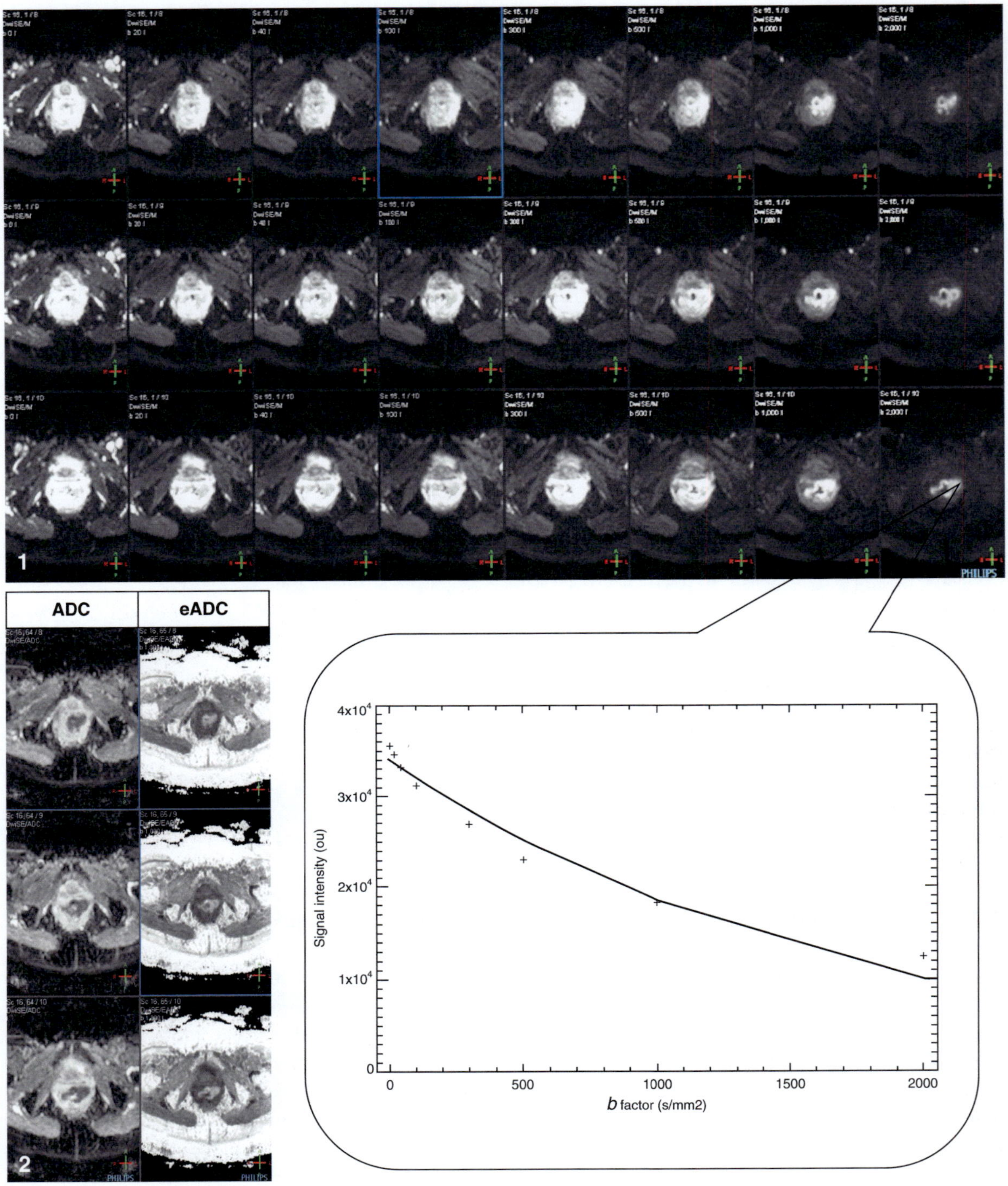

Fig. 3.3 **Use of several b values for DWI measurements.** In order to avoid bias in the ADC and e-ADC estimation due to the used *b* values, it is recommended to measure more than just two *b* values to calculate the ADC maps. Therefore, the ADC is obtained as a result of fitting the signal intensity for all the *b* values to a monoexponential model as it was described in Chap. 1. In this approach, the ADC is obtained as the decay constant of the exponential model after the fitting process, which has several advantages. The first one, the results are less sensible to the relative SNR of each image due to the estimation of all the *b* values used. The second one, if the *b* values are properly chosen, it is possible to properly estimate the ADC values from tissues with very fast signal decay to areas of slow water movement, being sensible for a higher range of ADC values. In the *top* of this figure (**3.3.1**), a DWI acquisition of a rectal cancer with eight different *b* values ranging from 0 to 2,000 s/mm^2 at three different levels is shown. In the lower part of the figure (**3.3.2**), the estimated ADC and eADC maps for a maximum *b* value of 1,000 s/mm^2 at those three levels are presented after calculation of the fitting of the signal intensity of the *b* values to an exponential decay. The graph of Fig. **3.3.2** shows the result of fitting the signal to a monoexponential decay model

displayed for each voxel of the image, are easily calculated from the diffusivities (λ_1, λ_2, and λ_3) in three main directions X′, Y′, and Z′, referred to the frame of the main diffusion direction of the tensor (Fig. 3.6.2). These eigen diffusivities represent the unidimensional diffusion coefficients in the main directions of diffusivities of the medium.

From the main diffusivity values (λ_1, λ_2, and λ_3), different value properties of the tissue can be calculated. The most establish one is the Fractional Anisotropy (FA) that can be calculated as (Fig. 3.5.3):

$$FA = \frac{\sqrt{3\left[\left(\lambda_1 - \langle\lambda\rangle\right)^2 + \left(\lambda_2 - \langle\lambda\rangle\right)^2 + \left(\lambda_3 - \langle\lambda\rangle\right)^2\right]}}{\sqrt{2\left(\lambda_1^2 + \lambda_2^2 + \lambda_3^2\right)}}, \quad \text{where } \langle\lambda\rangle = \frac{\lambda_1 + \lambda_2 + \lambda_3}{3} \tag{3.2}$$

The values of FA ranging from 0 (completely isotropic) to 1 (completely anisotropic).

Furthermore, if at least six independent diffusion directions are acquired, it is possible to obtain more detailed information from the tissue microstructure applying the Diffusion Tensor Theory (Fig. 3.5). From these experiments, it is possible to obtain the FA information and an estimation of water pathways where the water can move more easily, which is known as tractography (Fig. 3.6).

3.3 DWI Analysis and Postprocessing

3.3.1 Diffusion Registration

In order to overcome the shift due to the eddy current effects (Fig. 2.7) or to imperfect alienation due to motion effects, it is recommended to apply a registration of the images before the application of any quantification step (Fig. 3.7).

In an image-based registration scheme, one uses a cost function Q to measure how well the images are spatially aligned. First, a target image is chosen as a reference for all other images in the data set (source images). Because it is usually less distorted and has a higher SNR than the heavily DWI images, the image acquired with no diffusion sensitization (the *b* 0 image equivalent to a T2-weighted image) is usually used as the target image for registering DWI images. Next, using a spatial transformation model, one aligns all other images to the target image by optimizing a cost function. Image-based registration schemes differ from each other in terms of (1) the definition of Q, and (2) the types of transformations applied to the image in search of the maximum of Q.

Haselgrove and Moore proposed the first image-based registration method to correct eddy current–induced distortions. They used the undistorted T2-weighted image, as a target image for the registration of the DWI images. Q was based on the cross-correlations between the source image and the target image. Unfortunately, cross-correlation performs poorly as a measure of alignment when the contrast of the source and target images differs significantly. Cost functions based on mutual information are more robust than those based on correlation for registering images with significantly different contrasts.

From the transformation point of view, normally, an affine transformation is applied to compensate the image distortion. This transformation maintains the straight lines straight after the transformation.

3.3.2 DWI Analysis and Postprocessing

Axial orientation is usually preferable to obtain DWI images in body applications in order to acquire reduced FOV in the phase encoding direction and to apply parallel imaging techniques to reduce EPI artifacts. Unfortunately, some anatomical structures are better visualized in sagittal or coronal orientations. To overcome this limitation, it is possible to perform Multi-Planar Reconstruction (MPR) or Maximum Intensity Projection (MIP) of the DWI data to visualize the anatomical information in other orientations (Fig. 3.8). Furthermore, volume rendering is also feasible which helps to identify the 3D structure of a lesion and to calculate its volume. As the signal is nonquantitative, DWI may be shown as inverted grayscale (PET-like) images.

Depending on the applied *b* value in the DWI acquisition, only those regions with very restricted diffusion have enough signals to be visualized, losing most of the anatomical information. For better image evaluation, it

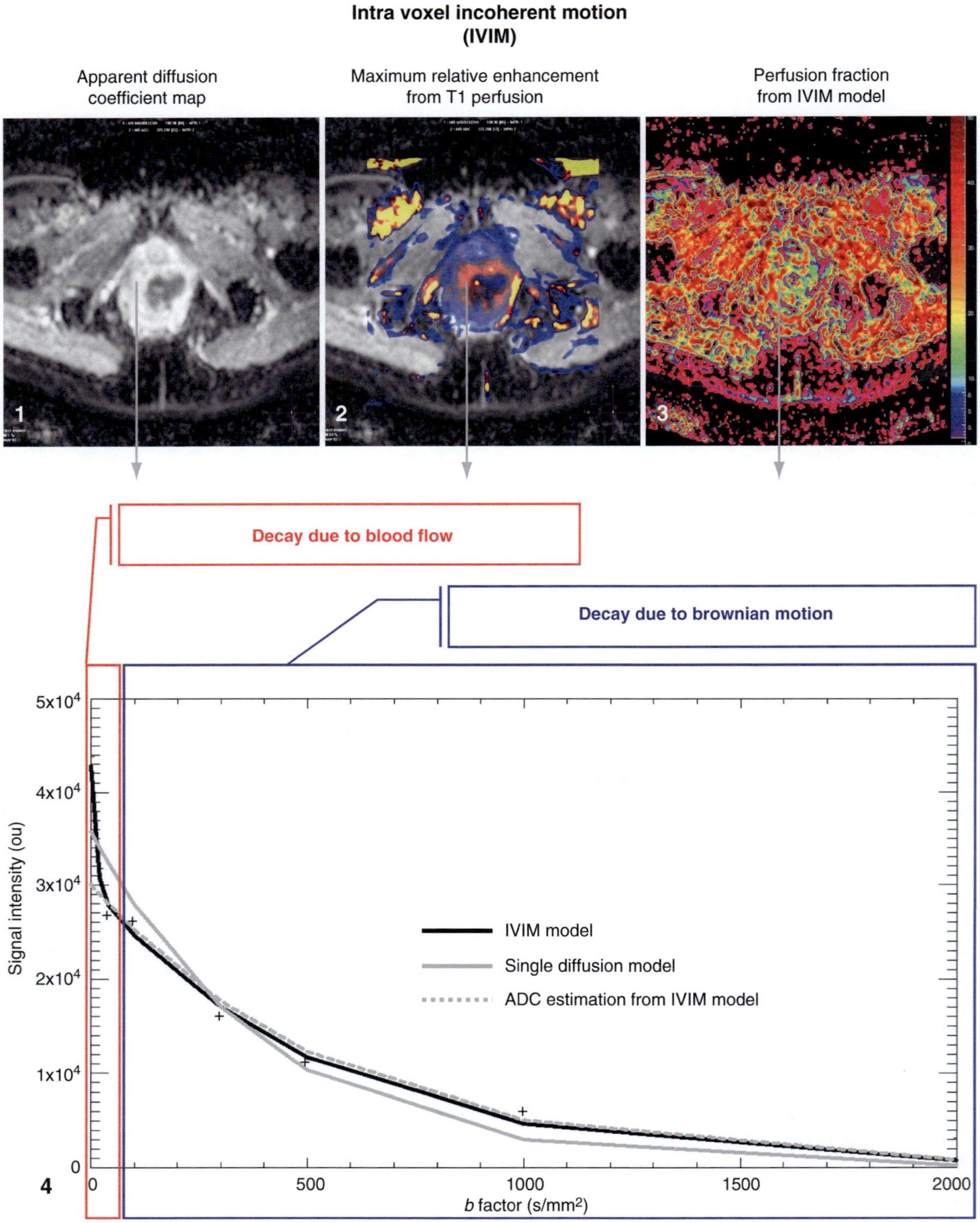
Intra voxel incoherent motion
(IVIM)
Apparent diffusion
coefficient map
Maximum relative enhancement
from T1 perfusion
Perfusion fraction
from IVIM model
1
2
3
Decay due to blood flow
Decay due to brownian motion
Signal intensity (ou)
5x10^4
4x10^4
3x10^4
2x10^4
1x10^4
0
IVIM model
Single diffusion model
ADC estimation from IVIM model
4
0
500
1000
1500
2000
b factor (s/mm2)

is desirable to overlay the DWI images over a more anatomical image for better spatial localization (Fig. 3.9). This process is known as fusion. Fusion software first performs a superimposition of DWI and anatomical data sets, which does not require to be acquired in the same orientation or with the same spatial resolution. After this, complex computer algorithms allow for alignment using anatomical landmarks of reference. Finally, the merging of the gray-scale anatomical images with pseudocolor *b* values images is performed, which may be further balanced and adjusted. Misregistration of the different data sets may need additional corrections.

In the era of multiparametric analysis, it is also possible to integrate the functional diffusion information not only with morphological series if not with other functional MRI techniques as MR perfusion or spectroscopy. Furthermore, new software allow to merge DWI with other techniques such as CT and PET. The fusion of different functional imaging techniques better reflects the functional heterogeneity of a lesion, which has been defined as a characteristic of more aggressive lesions with more resistance to chemoradiation.

3.3.3 ADC Analysis

As previously exposed in this chapter, the monoexponential ADC is only a rough approximation of the true diffusion coefficient, because diffusion exhibits multiexponential signal decay in biologic tissue. Other proposed models as the biexponential model and the stretched-exponential model are probably more accurate for some tissues, although their use is limited in clinical practice due to the necessity to acquire multiple *b* values and the absence of postprocessing software prepared for the clinical arena.

Most commonly, ADC is measured using ROIs in daily clinical practice (Fig. 3.10.1). There is a lack of standardization in ROI analysis, which is prone to errors since it is operator dependent. The number and size of ROIs varies from series to series. There is also no consensus based on if it is more appropriate to use the mean, median, or minimal ADC value. The mean ADC, representing the average magnitude of diffusion of water molecules in a volume of tissue, is the best validated metric of diffusion. Mean ADC allows comparison between series for lesional characterization and the evaluation of changes after treatment of the same lesion, although changes in shape or size have occurred. As a lesion may be heterogeneous, mean ADC may not appropriately reflect this property. For example, necrosis combined with solid areas can increase the mean ADC value. Therefore, two lesions may show the same mean ADC, but one may be completely solid and the other show combined necrotic and solid areas. The solid areas of the lesion with necrosis will be more hypercellular than the first completely solid lesion, as both show the same mean ADC.

Fig. 3.4 **IVIM model**. When more than two *b* values are acquired, it is also possible to get more information from the diffusion signal. From Intravoxel Incoherent Motion (IVIM) theory, it is possible to obtain perfusion information from diffusion signal. For this, many DWI acquisitions with *b* values lower than 100 s/mm^2 and some DWI series with *b*-values between 100 s/mm^2 and the maximum *b*-value are required. The rest of the imaging parameters should remain constant for all DWI acquisitions. The idea behind this theory is that the blood that flows in the arteries can be modeled as a diffusion signal providing signal for very low *b* values, while it has no contribution for higher *b* values.The graph in Fig. **3.4.4** represents the signal decay for the acquired *b* values within the pixel pointed in the ADC map of a rectal cancer at a 3T magnet (**3.4.1**, same case than Fig. 3.2). In this graph, two different regions may be clearly distinguished according to the IVIM model (*black line*). One located in the left part of the graph, represented with red lines, with a fast signal decay, where the diffusion signal is mainly affected by the blood (perfusion effect). The second one, located in the right part of the graph with blue lines, shows a slower signal decay due only to the Brownian movement of the water (real diffusion effect). Notice the difference, mainly with low *b* values, in the signal decay of the IVIM model (*black line*) compared to the monocompartmental model of the diffusion (*gray line*) or the ADC estimated from the IVIM model (discontinuous *gray line*). This behavior can be mathematically represented by the expression proposed by LeBihan:
$\frac{S_b}{S_0} = (1-f)\exp(-b \times D) + f\exp\left[-b \times (D + D^*)\right]$, where the S_b and S_0 represent the signal intensity for each *b* value including the T_1 and T_2 relaxation effects; *D* and *D** represent the signal decay due to the Brownian and blood movement, respectively; and *f* represents the fraction of signal decay due to the blood movement and it is called perfusion fraction. At the top, the comparison between the perfusion fraction map (**3.4.3**) obtained for the IVIM analysis of the DWI and the maximum relative enhancement parametric map (**3.4.2**) obtained from a *T*1 perfusion study (dynamic contrast enhanced THRIVE acquisition) of a rectal scan is shown. A good agreement in the tumoral perfusion in both maps may be appreciated

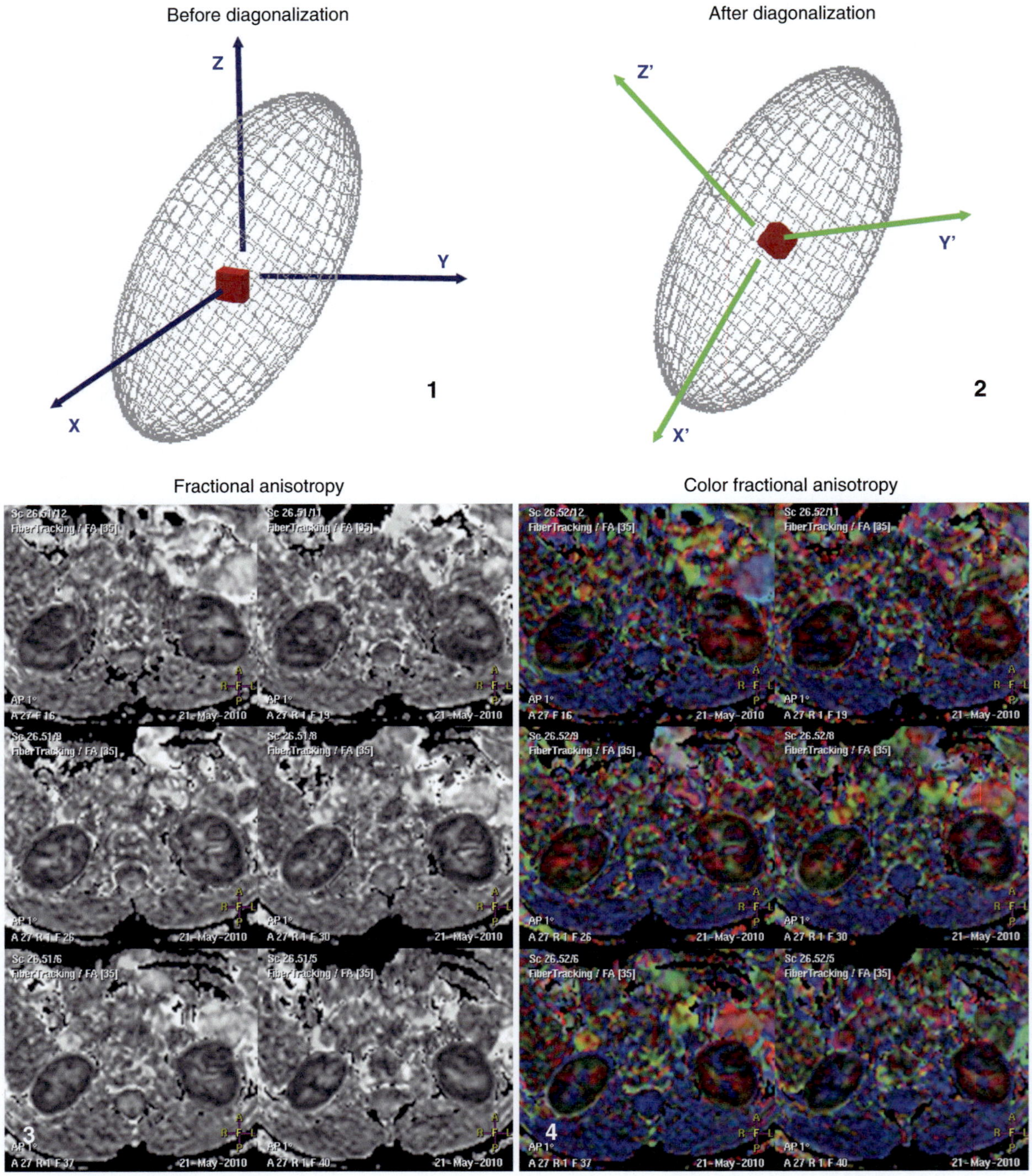

Fig. 3.5 Fractional anisotropy and colored fractional anisotropy. As it was previously described, the diffusion signal from a DWI experiment depends on the direction of the applied diffusion gradients. Normally, the diffusion information in one direction is affected by the diffusion information in the other directions. This effect can be represented in the diffusion space as an ellipsoid (**3.5.1**), that represent the relation of one diffusion direction with the other directions. If the correlation between different diffusion directions disappears, by means of a diagonalization of the diffusion tensor, a new reference system is obtained (**3.5.2**) where just three completely independent directions are shown (X′, Y′ and Z′) in the main direction of the axis of the diffusion ellipsoid. These independent directions represent the direction of the maximum diffusion. Figure **3.5.3** shows the FA map of an axial acquisition of the kidneys at six different consecutive levels obtained from a DWI acquisition with six different diffusion directions, previously shown in Fig. 1.4. A colored version of this FA map is shown in Fig. **3.5.4** where the color information represents the most important diffusion direction. *Blue* for FH (foot to head) direction. *Red* for RL (*right* to *left*) direction. *Green* for AP (anterior to posterior) direction

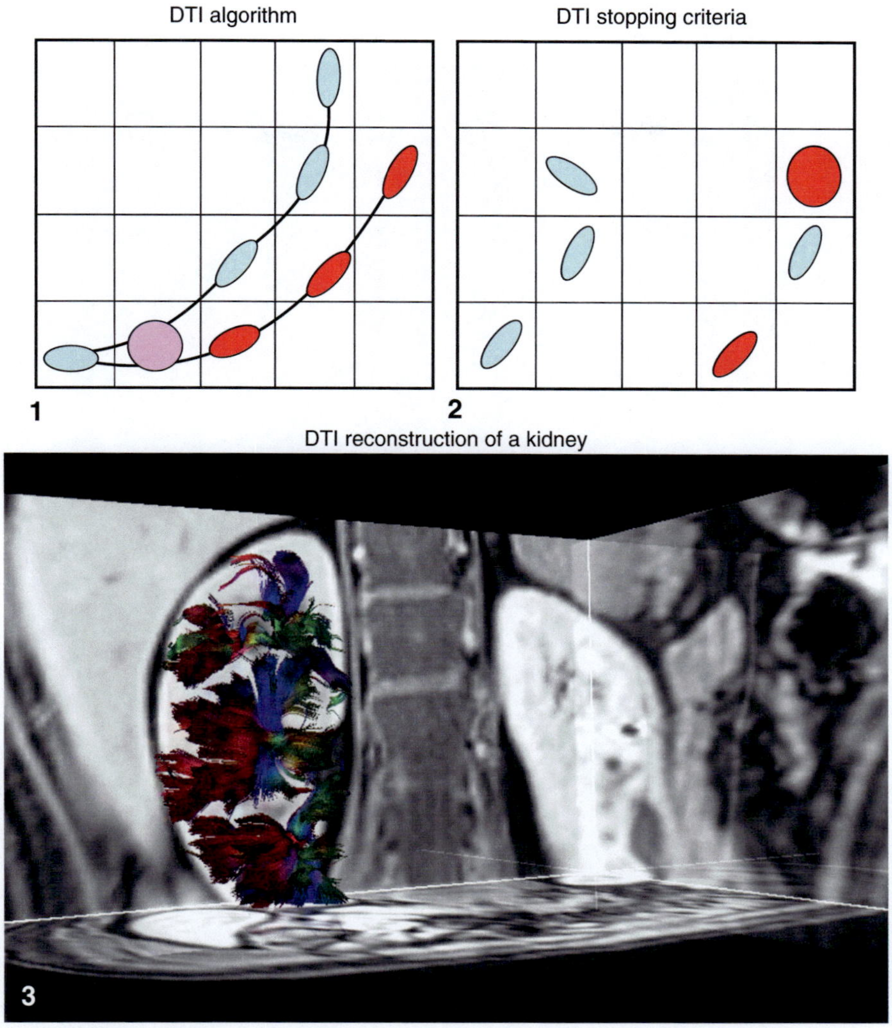

Fig. 3.6 Diffusion tensor imaging. Following the ellipsoid description, the main axis of the ellipsoid represents the main diffusion direction in the voxel (coinciding with the direction of the fibers). The eccentricity of the ellipsoid provides information about the degree of anisotropy. In the theorical case of a tissue with a completely isotropic diffusion, the ellipsoid will become a perfect sphere. If this ellipsoid is built for all the pixels in an image, then it is possible to link those pixels where the main diffusivity direction will be equivalent (**3.6.1**) in order to build the most suitable pathway of a ROI or to link the pixels between two different ROIs. This information between pixels can be linked following some rules (**3.6.2**). It is not possible to establish a pathway with an angular change higher than certain limits, being possible to link different consecutive pixels until a region, which is not sufficiently anisotropic, is reached. In Fig. **3.6.3**, a DTI reconstruction of a kidney is presented. The water pathway has been estimated following the theoretical path from the cortex to the medulla, being able to represent in images the pathways of the renal collecting system. The color of the pathways follows the same code described in the previous colored FA map (Fig. 3.5.4)

Therefore, another single metrics has been proposed to quantify diffusion, as the minimal ADC which informs of the areas with the highest cellularity within a volume of tissue. For example, in a recent series, minimum ADC demonstrated significant differences for evaluating the chemotherapeutic response of osteosarcoma, as the patients with a good response had a significantly higher minimum ADC ratio than those with a poor response. This difference was not achieved with the average ADC value of 3 ROI positioned in each tumor.

Another approach is to calculate the ADC in a pixel-by-pixel basis, which permits to analyze every single component of a lesion, although it is complex and time

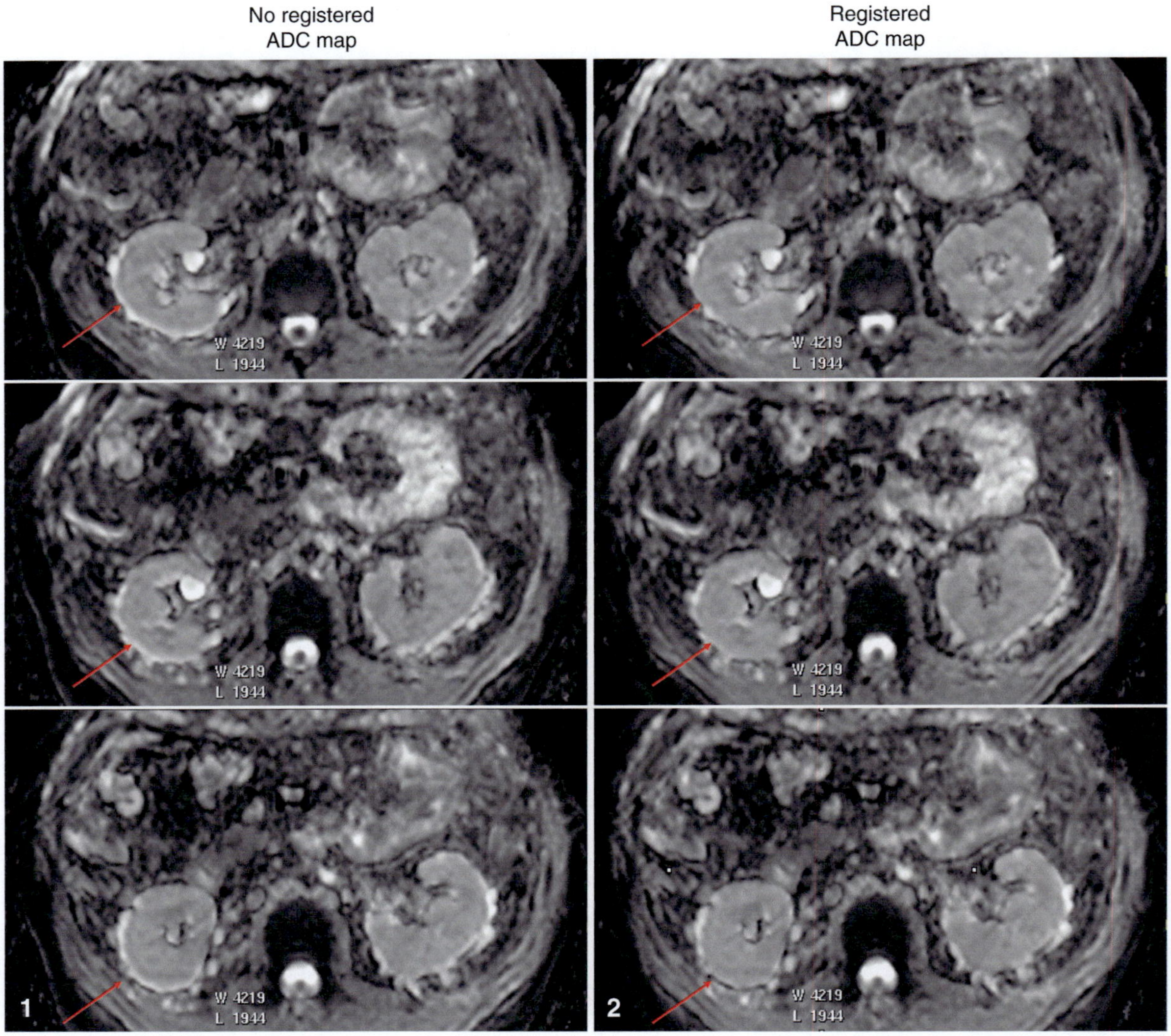

Fig. 3.7 **Diffusion registration**. This figure shows a comparison of the ADC maps at three different levels using the raw DWI images and the images after the registration process. *Red arrows* point bright lines around the kidneys in the ADC calculated with the original data, secondary to areas of misregistration, that almost completely disappear in the registered ADC map. Before any DWI quantification, it is desirable to avoid as much as possible misregistration between the diffusion images obtained with different *b* values. In order to compensate artifacts from movements or eddy currents, an affine registration is applied between the different diffusion acquisitions

consuming. Besides, the analysis of regions smaller than the voxel-size of the DWI sequence may lead to partial volume effects and unreliable quantifications.

Heterogeneous diffusion properties of a lesion benefit in their analysis of the use of histograms to represent the different ADC values within the ROI, which allows a more precise knowledge of the structural changes in ADC within a lesion (Fig. 3.10.2). In ADC histogram, the x-axis represents the ADC value and the y-axis the number of voxels for every ADC value. In this manner, ADC histogram may differentiate lesions with a similar mean ADC but different distribution of ADC values. ADC histogram also allow for easy intraindividual comparison over time, as they do not need correlation of all the voxels of a lesion. ADC histogram is limited by loss of the spatial distribution of the heterogeneity of a lesion, although it may be expressed through different parameters such as range, standard deviation, centile values, skewness, entropy, or kurtosis. In any case, if the standard deviation of the ROI is high (it has been

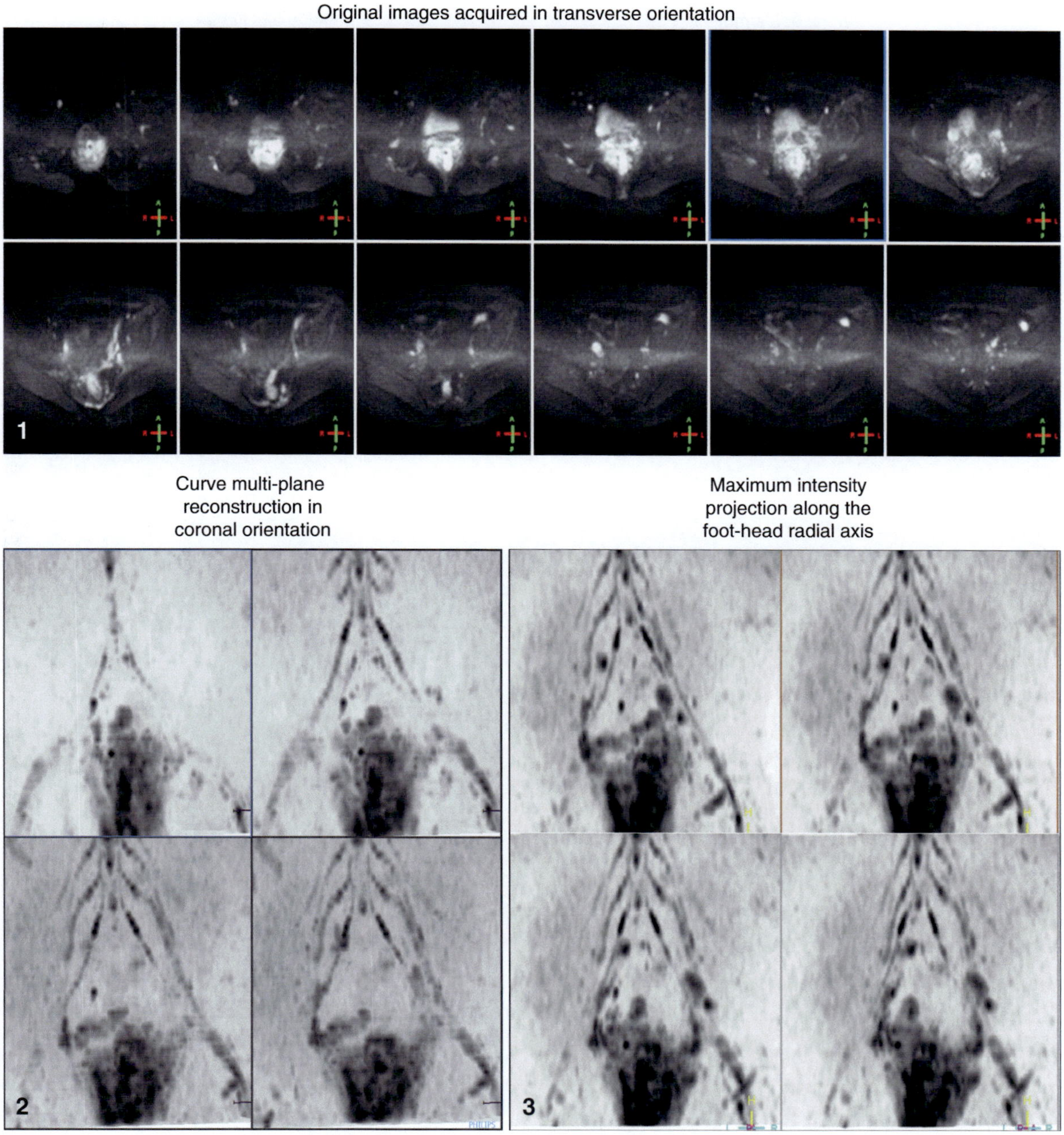

Fig. 3.8 **MPR and MIP reconstructions**. In order to reduce the image distortion, the DWI images are normally acquired in transverse direction to facilitate the possibility to applied parallel acquisition techniques, as shown in the DWI-neurography acquisition of the lumbar plexus with a *b* value of 800 s/mm^2 (**3.8.1**). Once the DWI volume is acquired, different postprocessing techniques can be applied for better visualization of the organ of interest in different orientations. If the images are acquired with sufficient resolution in all directions, MPR can be performed to obtain coronal and sagittal orientations (**3.8.2**). MPR can also be applied to ADC and e-ADC maps. These techniques are especially interesting in whole-body applications where a multi-stack acquisition in the transverse direction is normally used. After the acquisition, different MPR orientations can be obtained from the whole image data set. Besides, in order to get volumetric information, Maximum Intensity Projections (MIP) of the volume can also be performed in different orientations (**3.8.3**)

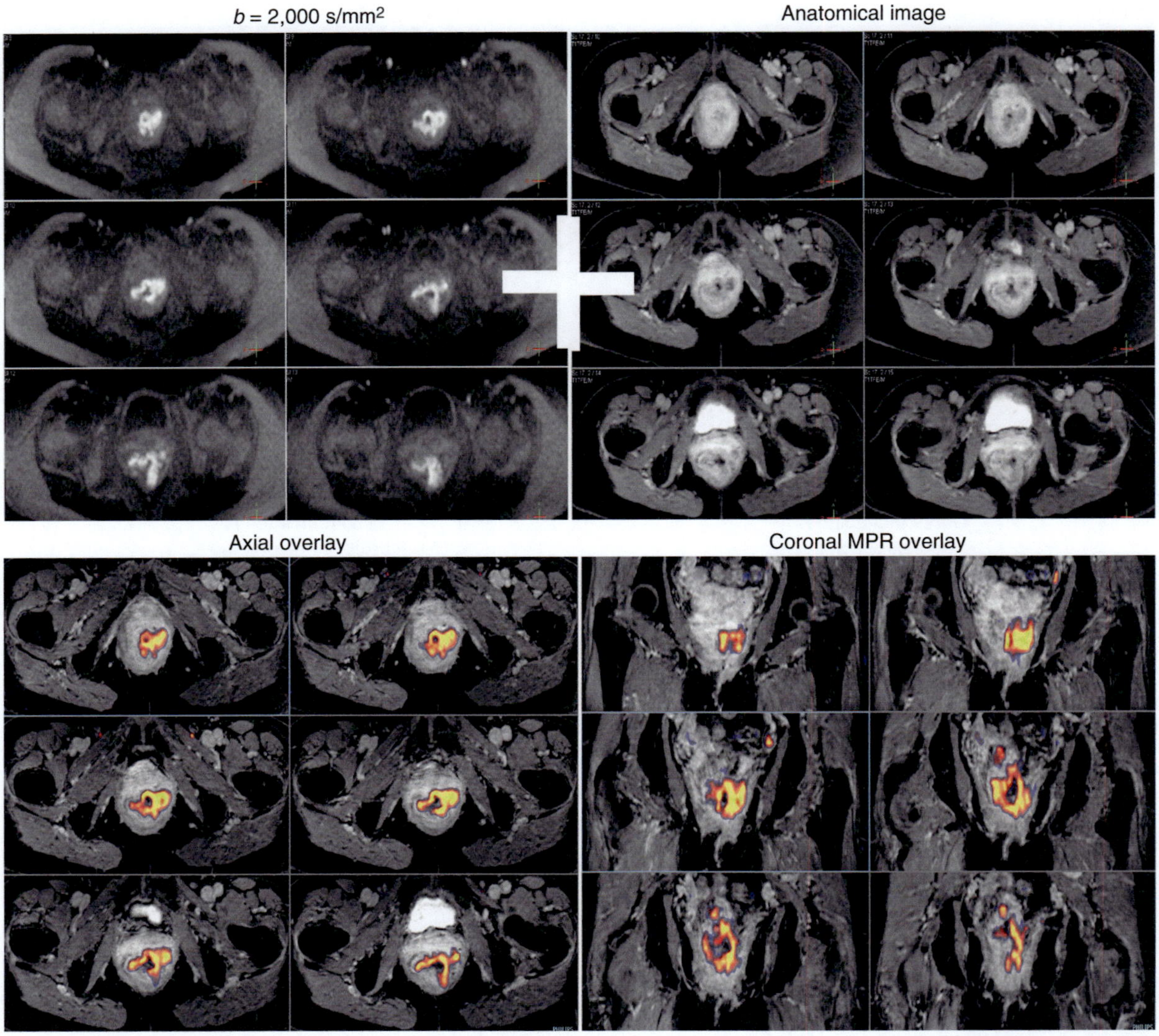

Fig. 3.9 Fusion of DWI and anatomical images. Most commonly, when very high b values are applied during the DWI acquisition, most of the anatomical information is lost, as only very high cellular tissues show sufficient SNR to be visualized while the information of the rest of the tissues disappears (background suppression). This is specially relevant in Inversion Recovery acquisition approaches that are more prone to have low SNR. In order to facilitate the anatomical localization of the structures, it is possible to fuse the DWI information with anatomical images. At the *top* of Fig. 3.9., the DWI acquisition with a b value of 2,000 s/mm^2 and an axial postcontrast THRIVE is fused to obtain the colored axial overlaid series, which nicely depicts the restriction of diffusion of a rectal tumor. The obtained series may be postprocessed as any other original acquisition, as shown in the coronal MPR

proposed 20% or higher of the calculated ADC), the ROI should be repositioned to avoid insufficient reliability of ADC measurements. Furthermore, complex software to track the changes of ADC values with therapy is a work-in progress, known as threshold or functional diffusion map or ADC parametric map. Registration of pre- and post-therapy morphological sequences and ADC maps is necessary using sophisticated software. Therefore, a color map is generated where statistically significant changes in voxels according to a threshold ADC change value are shown. Initial experience with this approach in brain, head, and neck and bone has been promising, although its clinical application is challenging due to its limited access, problems in registration in areas with physiological movement or EPI distortion (e.g., chest, abdomen and breast), and changes in size and shape of the lesion during treatment.

Areas of necrosis and with susceptibility artifacts should be avoided in ADC measurements. In cases where they are present, it is better to perform analysis with several ROIs avoiding these regions, than one ROI surrounding the whole lesion. Furthermore, it may be challenging to define the limits of a lesion and to position the ROI directly in an ADC map due to poor SNR. It is preferable to position the ROI directly on the original DWI acquired with high *b* value, and then, to copy and paste the ROI in the ADC map. Anatomical images can be also used to position the ROI, if they were acquired with the same orientation than the DWI series. In cases of bone marrow lesions, sometimes, the ADC map allows a better depiction of lesional borders than the original DWI image.

Another potential source of error in DWI measurement is misregistration of the images with different *b* values, or the presence of patient motion or image distortion, which cause variations of the ADCs. This can be partially solved using registration software that improves the alignment of DWI series with different *b* values.

To overcome the limitations of ADC, several semiquantitative measurements have been proposed, as the lesion-to-spinal cord ratio, that represents the ratio of lesion signal intensity to spinal cord signal intensity. These semiquantitative approaches do not suffer from misregistration and may complement or even replace ADC, although their clinical feasibility has still to be shown.

1. ROI DRAWING

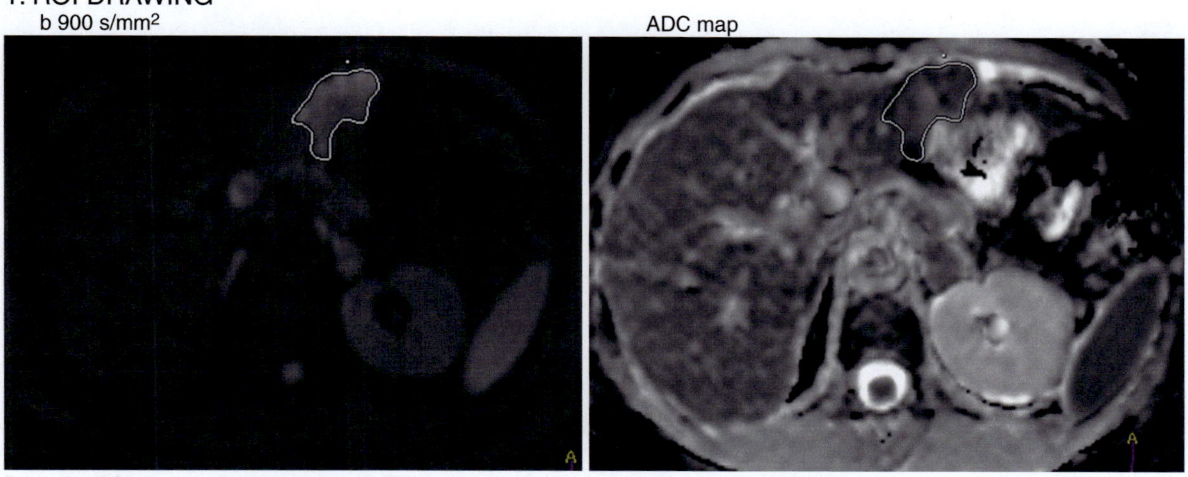

Draw the ROI surrounding the lesion on DWI with high b value and copy it to the ADC map

Fig. 3.10 **ADC analysis (3.10.1)**. The first part of this figure shows how it is better to draw the ROI surrounding the whole lesion on the DWI with high *b* value or even in an anatomical image acquired in the same location than directly in the ADC map, as they allow better depiction of the lesional limits. Then, the ROI can be copied and pasted to the ADC map. In this case, the lesion in segment 2 of the liver corresponds to a metastasis of a previous resected pancreatic adenocarcinoma. (**3.10.2**) The second part of the figure shows different strategies for ADC analysis. The first one is to locate several small ROIs in different areas, trying to assess the different components of the lesion. In the left image, the ROI is positioned in the central area of the lesion with a mean ADC value of 1.2×10^{-3} mm^2/s, minimal ADC of 1.1×10^{-3} mm^2/s and maximum ADC of 1.38×10^{-3} mm^2/s. In the *right* image, a second ROI of the same size is located peripherally in an area with higher restriction, indicating the heterogeneous composition of the lesion (mean ADC value of 0.57×10^{-3} mm^2/s, minimal ADC of 0.7×10^{-3} mm^2/s and maximum ADC of 0.96×10^{-3} mm^2/s). The second exposed strategy is to analyze the whole lesion with a ROI. This approach has the advantage to assess completely the studied lesion, although may not accurately reflect the heterogeneity of the lesion, and may include in the ADC measurements areas of susceptibility artifact or necrosis that may affect the ADC value in a significant manner, as shown in the left ADC map. In this case, the ADC values of the whole lesion are: mean ADC value of $0{,}9 \times 10^{-3}$ mm^2/s, minimal ADC of 0.4×10^{-3} mm^2/s and maximum ADC of 1.38×10^{-3} mm^2/s. There is controversy on which one of these ADC metrics is the most appropriate to characterize a lesion. The minimal ADC value reflects the area with more restriction, probably representing the area with the highest cellularity. Conversely, the maximal ADC corresponds to the area with the least restriction of free water. Mean ADC is affected by the heterogeneity of the lesion, as shown in this example. An approach that is interesting to avoid these limitations is the use of histogram analysis which allows to evaluating the ADC of the different components of the lesion, as shown on the *right* image

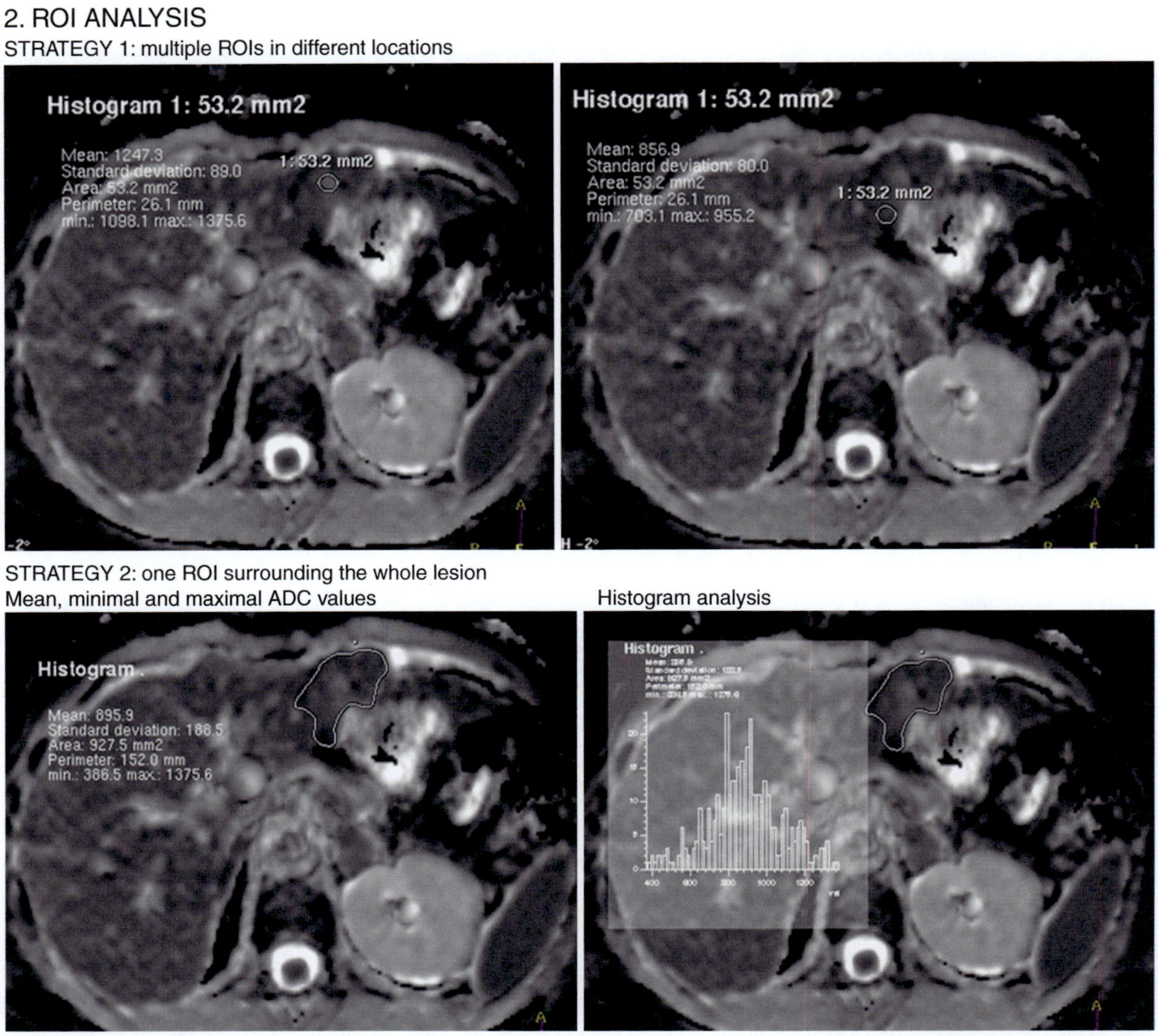

Fig. 3.10 (continued)

Further Reading

Basser PJ, Mattiello J, Le Bihan D (1994) Estimation of the effective self-diffusion tensor from the NMR spin echo. J Magn Reson 103:247–254

Basser PJ, Mattiello J, Le Bihan D (1994) MR diffusion tensor spectroscopy and imaging. Biophys J 66:259–267

Bastin ME (1999) Correction of eddy current-induced artifacts in diffusion tensor imaging using iterative cross-correlation. Magn Reson Imaging 17:1011–1024

Haselgrove JC, Moore JR (1996) Correction for distortion of echo-planar images used to calculate the apparent diffusion coefficient. Magn Reson Med 36:960–964

Herneth AM, Mayerhoefer M, Schernthaner R et al (2010) Diffusion weighted imaging: lymph nodes. Eur J Radiol 76:398–406

Le Bihan D, Breton E, Lallemand D et al (1986) MR imaging of intravoxel incoherent motions: application to diffusion and perfusion in neurologic disorders. Radiology 161(2): 401–407

Le Bihan D, Delannoy DJ, Levin RL (1988) Temperature mapping with MR imaging of molecular diffusion: application to hyperthermia. Radiology 171:853–857

Low RN (2009) Diffusion-weighted MR imaging for whole body metastatic disease and lymphadenopathy. Magn Reson Imaging Clin N Am 17(2):245–261

Oka K, Yakushiji T, Sato H et al (2010) The value of diffusion-weighted imaging for monitoring the chemotherapeutic response of osteosarcoma: a comparison between average apparent diffusion coefficient and minimum apparent diffusion coefficient. Skeletal Radiol 39(2): 141–146

Padhani AR, Koh DM (2011) Diffusion MR imaging for monitoring of treatment response. Magn Reson Imaging Clin N Am 19(1):181–209

Padhani AR, Liu G, Koh DM et al (2009) Diffusion-weighted magnetic resonance imaging as a cancer biomarker: consensus and recommendations. Neoplasia 11(2):102–125

Provenzale JM, Engelter ST, Petrella JR et al (1999) Use of MR exponential diffusion-weighted images to Erradícate T2 "shine-through" effect. AJR Am J Roentgenol 172: 537–539

Schafer J, Srinivasan A, Mukherji S (2011) Diffusion magnetic resonance imaging in the head and neck. Magn Reson Imaging Clin N Am 19(1):55–67

Whittaker CS, Coady A, Culver L et al (2009) Diffusion-weighted MR imaging of female pelvic tumors: a pictorial review. Radiographics 29(3):759–774

4 DWI at 3 T: Advantages, Disadvantages, Pitfalls, and Advanced Clinical Applications

Javier Sánchez-González and Antonio Luna

4.1 DWI at 3 T

DWI benefits from the higher SNR derived from the use of higher magnetic field in clinical scanners. A theoretical two-fold increase of SNR is expected from 1.5 to 3 T magnets, although T1 and T2 properties of the tissues are also modified by this two-fold signal increase. For example, a signal improvement of 50% has been reported in kidney studies when comparing 3 T and 1.5 T within the same acquisition time. The increase of signal of 3 T magnets may be used in order either to get higher resolution or to reduce scan time. Furthermore, this increase in SNR can allow us either to increase the highest *b* value up to 3,000 s/mm^2 with adequate SNR and image resolution (Figs. 3.3 and 4.9) or to acquire similar *b* values than at 1.5 T magnets, faster or with improved spatial resolution (Fig. 4.1). As it was explained in Chap. 3, caution is necessary when using ultrahigh *b* values, as noise contamination in higher *b* values, due to a poor SNR, has a significant influence in ADC estimations.

A magnetic field variation is a common problem for MRI. Although the MRI systems have a magnetic field variation under 1 ppm for a 50 cm diameter sphere, this value changes markedly when the patients are placed in the center of the main magnetic field, producing field variations due to different susceptibility properties of body tissues. As a consequence, the additional magnetic fields of the materials inside the magnet are superimposed to the originally homogeneous B_0, field, resulting in decreased overall field homogeneity. This magnetic field variation can be partially compensated by shimming of the magnetic field but the remaining field variation produces artifacts in the acquired images. Unfortunately, the effect of susceptibility variations is proportional to the main magnetic field strength B_0, producing a two-fold frequency variations when comparing 3 T to 1.5 T magnets. Therefore, all kind of susceptibility artifacts appear much more pronounced at 3 T MRI than at lower field strengths. These susceptibility variations have a very strong influence in an SS EPI readout, like in DWI, producing geometric distortions at interfaces between soft tissue and bone or air, which may be critical in anatomical areas such as skull base, neck, or chest (Fig. 4.2). As it was explained in Chap. 2, these distortions can be reduced by decreasing the echo spacing of the readout train (e.g., by increasing the receiver bandwidth) (Fig. 2.4) or by applying parallel imaging techniques to reduce the echo-train length (Fig. 2.5). It is important to maintain the TE as shorter as possible in DWI acquisitions at 3 T, to reduce susceptibility artifact and signal loss due to T2 decay on these long echo-train acquisitions. The higher gradient performance at higher magnetic fields and the chance to apply higher parallel acquisition factors, due to its higher SNR, can be also used to compensate the higher image distortion at 3 T systems. Susceptibility artifacts are exacerbated by the presence of metal, which completely destroy the DWI signal (Fig. 4.3.1). A similar effect, although not so extreme, may be found in diseases such as hemochromatosis, where the iron deposition increases locally in a significant manner in some tissues (Fig. 4.3.2).

J. Sánchez- González (✉)
Clinical Scientist, Philips Healthcare Iberia,
Madrid, Spain
e-mail: javier.sanchez.gonzalez@philips.com

A. Luna
Chief of MRI, Health Time Group,
Jaén, Spain
e-mail: aluna70@sercosa.com

A. Luna et al., *Diffusion MRI Outside the Brain*,
DOI 10.1007/978-3-642-21052-5_4, © Springer-Verlag Berlin Heidelberg 2012

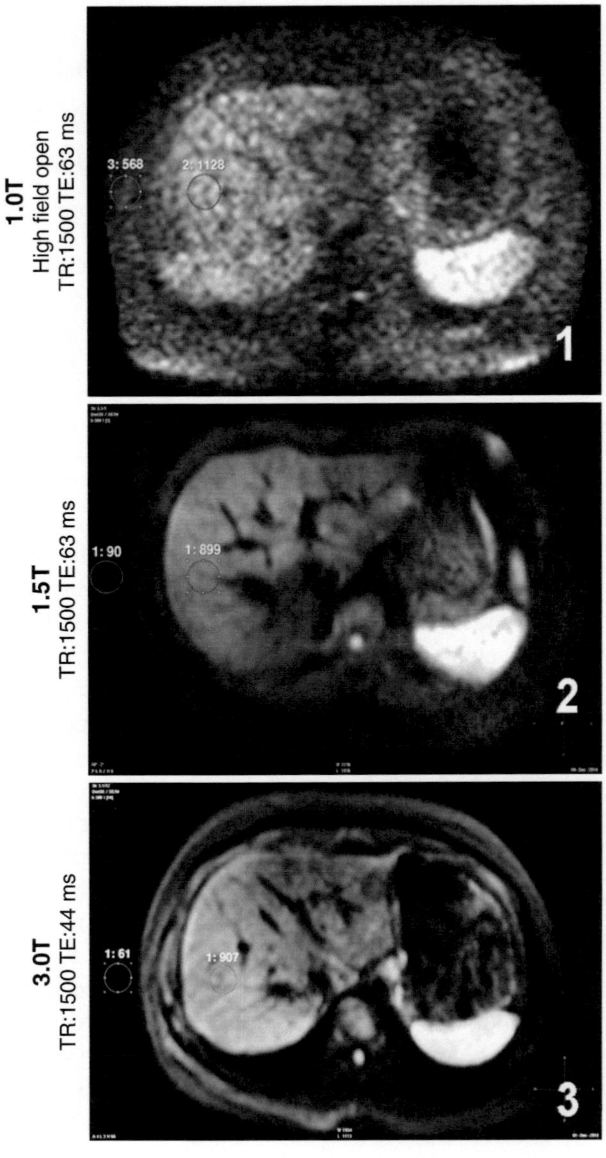

Fig. 4.1 **Signal to noise ratio of DWI at different magnetic fields**. The use of higher magnetic field produces an increase in SNR. DWI sequence of the liver on the same volunteer, with a *b* value of 500 s/mm^2 acquired under breath-hold condition. From top to bottom, the images were acquired in different magnetic fields. The top image was acquired in a 1.0 T High Field Open magnet, the image in the middle was performed in a 1.5 T cylindrical bore magnet and the bottom one in a 3.0 T cylindrical bore magnet. All these acquisitions were acquired with equivalent parameters limiting the TR to 1,500 s and the TE to the lowest available limited by the gradient strength. In order to estimate the SNR in all images, two ROIs where placed, one in the liver and the other in the image background. SNR was calculated as the fraction between mean values of each ROI (which are represented in the value adjacent to each ROI). The resulting values were 2.1 for 1.0 T, 13 for 1.5 T, and 18 for 3 T systems. These values demonstrate the benefit of increasing the magnetic field in terms of SNR for DWI. It should be taking into account that on breath-hold acquisitions, the use of shorter TR highly affects the SNR due to saturation effect, especially at higher magnetic fields, where the T1 value of tissues is longer

4.1.1 Advanced Clinical Applications at 3 T Magnets

In order to solve the lack of spatial resolution of DWI sequences, the use of higher field magnets as 3 T has been proposed for body applications. The acquisition problems inherent to DWI increase in 3 T magnets, due to higher magnetic field variation and susceptibility artifacts, which produce image distortion, and SAR limitations. All these factors make more difficult to obtain a homogeneous fat supression. These limitations can be overcome using appropriately the higher strength of the gradient systems of 3 T scanners in combination with parallel imaging and advanced fat suppression sequences. In our experience, all these tools make also feasible to acquire body DWI studies in 3 T systems. Furthermore, advanced clinical applications, such as DWIBS-based neurography or DTI, take full advantage of the increase in SNR, which also benefits from sophisticated models of analysis of the diffusion signal decay.

4.1.1.1 DWI Neurography

DWI neurography using DWIBS is a new approach for visualizing abnormalities of peripheral nerves, which demonstrates peripheral nerves with high conspicuity

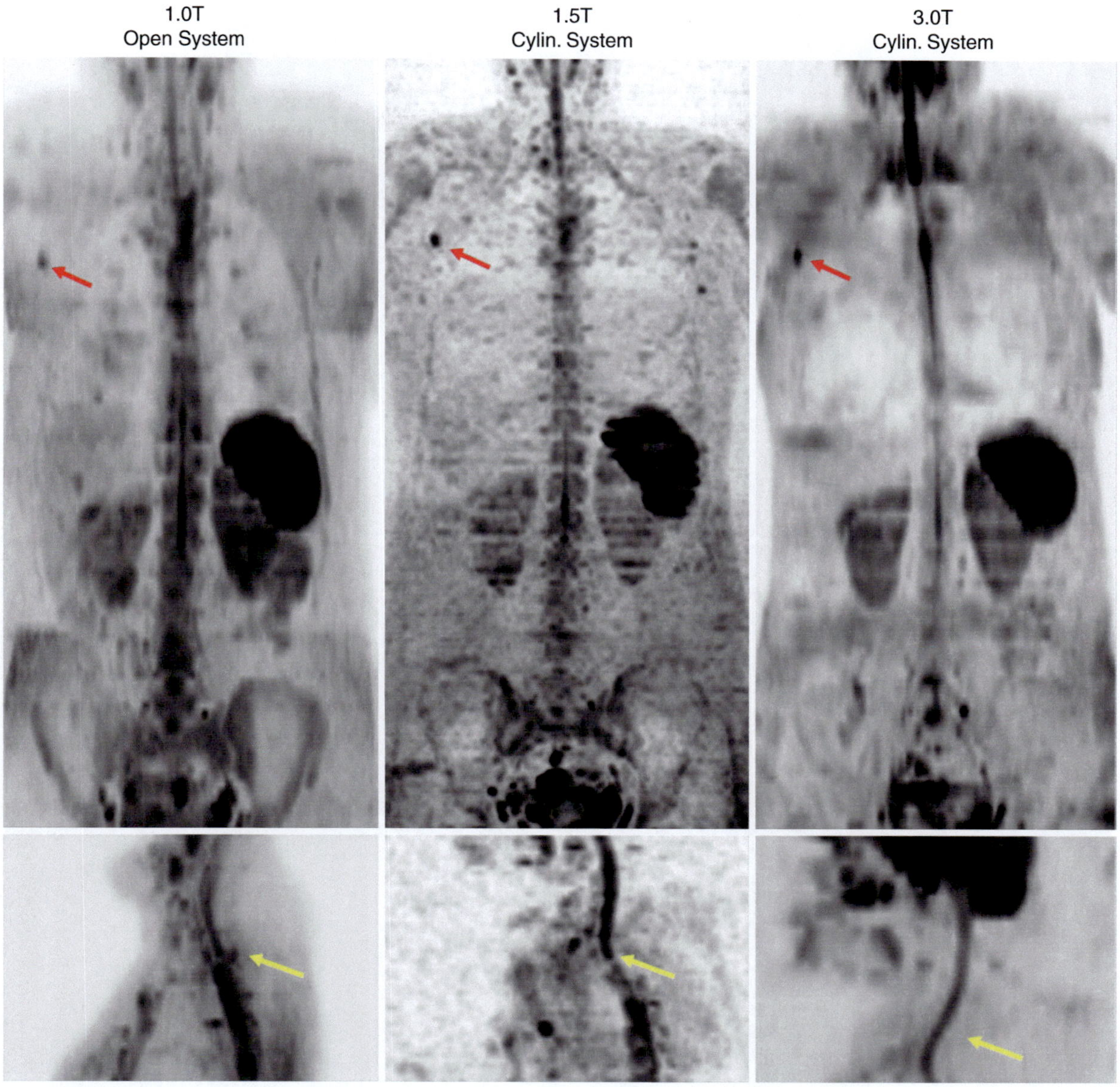

Fig. 4.2 **DWIBS acquisition at different field magnets.** DWIBS imaging has an increasing role for whole-body staging purposes in oncologic patients. Whole-body DWI has been traditionally performed at 1.5 T systems, which less clinical experience in other systems, like 3 T or even high-performance open magnets. DWIBS at 3 T potentially offers higher SNR, since it increases linearly when increasing the field strength. In contrast, susceptibility artifacts also increase exponentially when increasing the field strength, which will degrade DWI and DWIBS acquisitions. A recent feasibility study reported that DWIBS at 3 T provided a better lesion-to-bone tissue contrast, compared with DWIBS at 1.5 T. In the same report, STIR proved to offer the best fat suppression for DWI acquisitions in all body regions at 3 T. However, larger susceptibility-induced image distortions and signal intensity losses, stronger blurring artifacts, and more pronounced motion artifacts degraded the image quality at 3 T. Thus, further investigations concerning DWIBS at 3 T should be undertaken. On the contrary, DWIBS application at high-performance 1 T open system has the drawback of lower SNR (Fig. 4.1), but this limitation can be overcome increasing the acquisition time in order to obtain successful results.

Imaging Findings DWIBS acquisition of the same volunteer at three different magnetic fields. In the upper row of images, the left one represents a coronal MIP reconstruction with inverted gray scale of a DWIBS acquisition, using a b value of 1,000 s/mm^2, in a High Field 1 T Open system. The middle image shows the same type of acquisition in a 1.5 T cylindrical bore and the right one, the corresponding acquisition in a 3 T system. In order to compensate the lower SNR of 1 T open bore magnet, the double acquisition time per stack (total scan time per stack, 3 min) than at 1, 5 and 3 T magnets was employed in order to obtain a similar SNR. In all images, the presence of a low-intensity lesion can be seen (red arrows) representing a small axillary lymph node. In the bottom row, a sagittal MIP of the neck stack is shown in the three system. The foot-head coverage in the 3 T acquisition was smaller than in the 1 T and 1.5 T in order to control the geometrical distortions. Even though, higher distortion in the neck region can be observed in the 3 T images (yellow arrows), due to magnetic field inhomogeneities

1

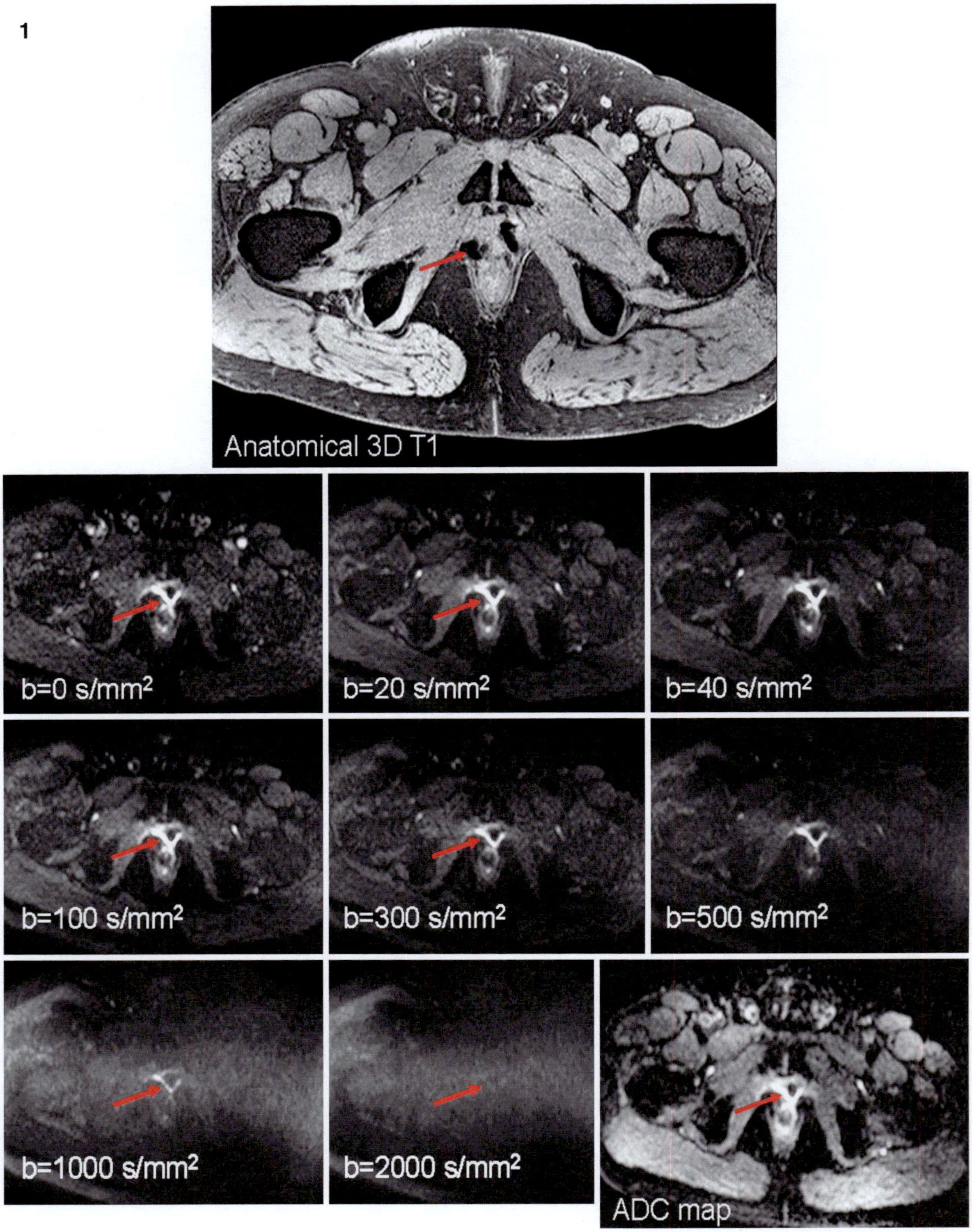
Anatomical 3D T1
b=0 s/mm2
b=20 s/mm2
b=40 s/mm2
b=100 s/mm2
b=300 s/mm2
b=500 s/mm2
b=1000 s/mm2
b=2000 s/mm2
ADC map

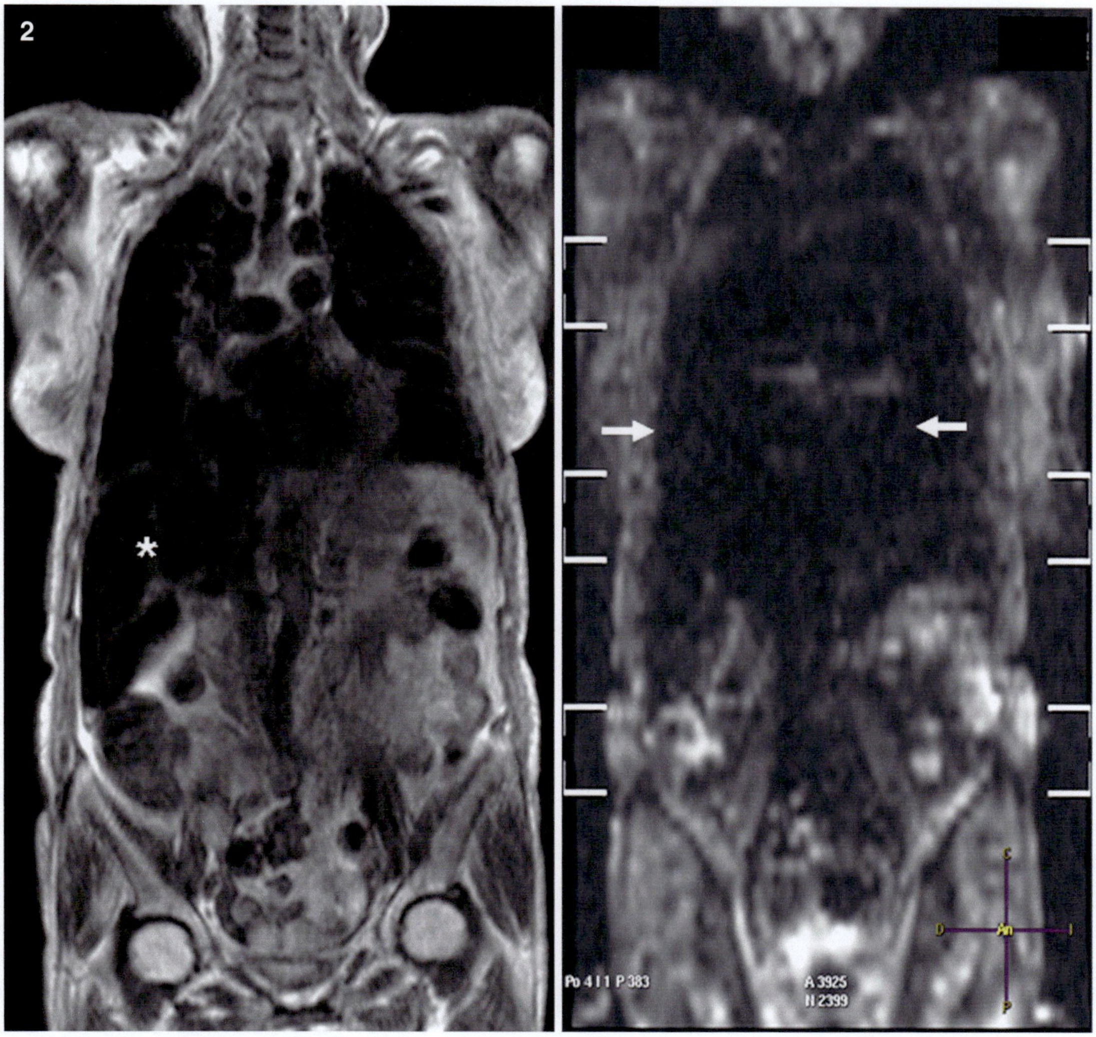

Fig. 4.3 (continued)

Fig. 4.3 Ferromagnetic and iron deposition artifacts. All metallic implants produce a magnetic field distortion due to susceptibility artifacts causing image distortions. In the anatomical fat-suppressed GE T1-weighted images, the magnetic field inhomogeneities produced by the surgical clips are shown as an area of abnormal signal intensity (**4.3.1**). This magnetic field variation produces a wrong location of the signal image in the DWI, producing abnormal bright and dark signals in the images (*red arrows* in **4.3.1**). This signal variation is more pronounced in DWI based in EPI readout due to phase error accumulation during the image acquisition. In the ADC estimation, these artifacts normally appear as areas of bright signal (*arrow*).

In pathological diseases with increased iron deposition in some tissues, such as hemochromatosis or transfusional iron overload, local variation in the magnetic field strength may occur. The increased levels of iron cause local signal loss in all sequences, which are more pronounced in sequences with higher magnetic susceptibility, as EPI ones, and also in T2-weighted sequences. This effect will also increase with higher magnetic fields. Therefore, DWI of the liver, or tissues with iron deposit, in patients with hemochromatosis will show signal loss and an increase in artifacts. This artifact has been exploited to increase liver lesion detection by means of superparamagnetic iron oxide particles. These particles, which are taken up by Kupffer cells, decrease the signal intensity of normal liver on DWI, increasing the relative signal intensity of lesions without Kupffer cells as metastases. Figure 4.3.2 shows the effect of severe iron deposit in the liver on DWI acquisitions, in a patient with hemochromatosis. In the upper left, a coronal whole-body HASTE sequence shows decreased signal intensity on the liver (*asterisk*), which is more pronounced, causing a severe susceptibility artifact, in a whole-body DWIBS acquisition with a b value of 800 s/mm^2 (*arrows*). In the left bottom row, severe local distortion of the magnetic field is demonstrated at T2* sequence consistent with severe iron deposit. In the right bottom image, a DWIBS acquisition using a b value of 800 s/mm^2 demonstrates severe signal loss and AP distortion (white circle)

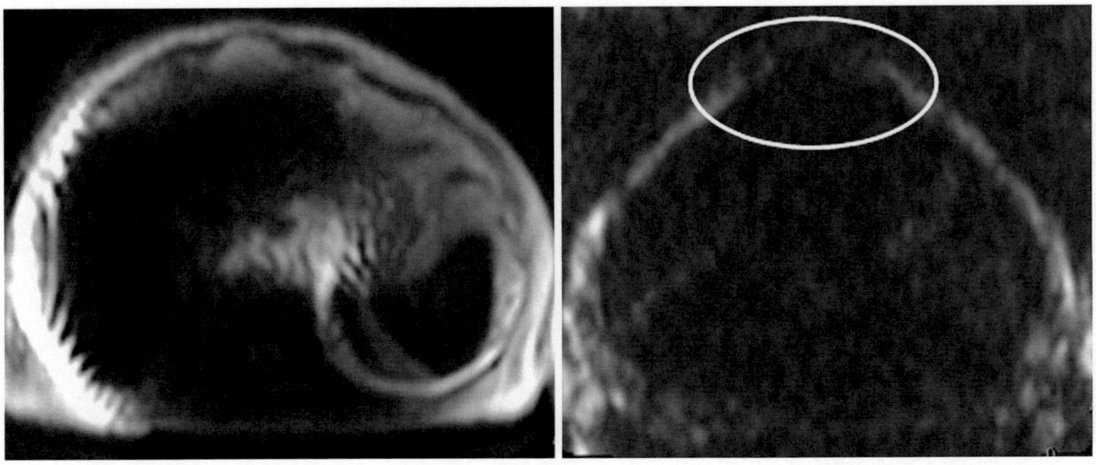

Fig. 4.3 (continued)

(Fig. 1.10). The technique is similar to that of DWIBS used in whole-body acquisitions for oncological staging. DWI neurography applies stronger gradients which maintain the signal from the highly cellular peripheral nerves while suppressing the signal from surrounding tissues. Acquisitions are performed in a volumetric data set with many thin sections which allowed 3D reconstructions, such as MPR and MIP, being especially useful in the coronal plane to depict a long trajectory of a peripheral nerve. This type of sequence usually uses a STIR pre-pulse due to robust fast suppression than spectral fat suppression and is usually acquired under free breathing. As peripheral nerves are anisotropic, diffusion is more restricted in a plane perpendicular to the nerves than in any other direction, being minimal parallel to their course. Therefore, the highest signal intensity of the peripheral nerves can be obtained by applying only one pair of motion probing gradients perpendicular to the course of nerves, as confirmed by Takahara and colleagues in their study of sacral plexus and sciatic nerve. In a recent report by Zandieh and colleagues, a b value of 500 s/mm^2 on a 1.5 T MRI system allowed to obtain optimal qualitative and quantitative indexes for DWI neurography of the brachial plexus compared to b values of 1,000 and 1,500 s/mm^2.

DWI neurography has been investigated in several regions, especially in the lumbosacral and brachial plexi. This technique allows the visualization of the spinal cord, ganglia, postganglionic nerve roots, and peripheral nerves due to their high cellular content with an organized structure. Other normal hypercellular structures, such as lymph nodes, bone marrow, veins showing slow flow, mucosa of small bowel, endometrium, adnexa, or tonsils, are also visualized in DWI neurography, and they may superimpose to neural structures. Therefore, they should be deleted during the postprocessing to facilitate the visualization of the peripheral nerves alone. In this task, the use of the soap-bubble MIP reconstruction better allows the visualization of the nerve plexus over its entire length and eliminates the overlap of anatomical structures, using a user-defined curved subvolume, as reported by Takahara and colleagues. Furthermore, sophisticated subtraction techniques such as subtraction of unidirectionally encoded images for suppression of heavily isotropic objects (SUSHI) have been proposed, demonstrating better depiction of the sciatic, common peroneal, and tibial nerves, but being less useful for brachial plexus imaging.

The use of 3 T allows the use of higher spatial resolution or faster acquisitions at the same resolution than 1.5 T magnets, despite higher susceptibility to artifacts and image distortion (Fig. 4.4). The use of 3 T magnet opens the door for acquisition of smaller and distal peripheral nerves.

In the limited available series, DWI neurography has shown potential for several clinical applications. Eguchi et al. described that in lumbar nerve roots compressed by herniated disks, mean ADC values were significantly higher in the compressed dorsal root ganglia and distal spinal nerves than in the uninvolved ones, related to the presence of edema and Wallerian degeneration within compressed nerve roots. In the

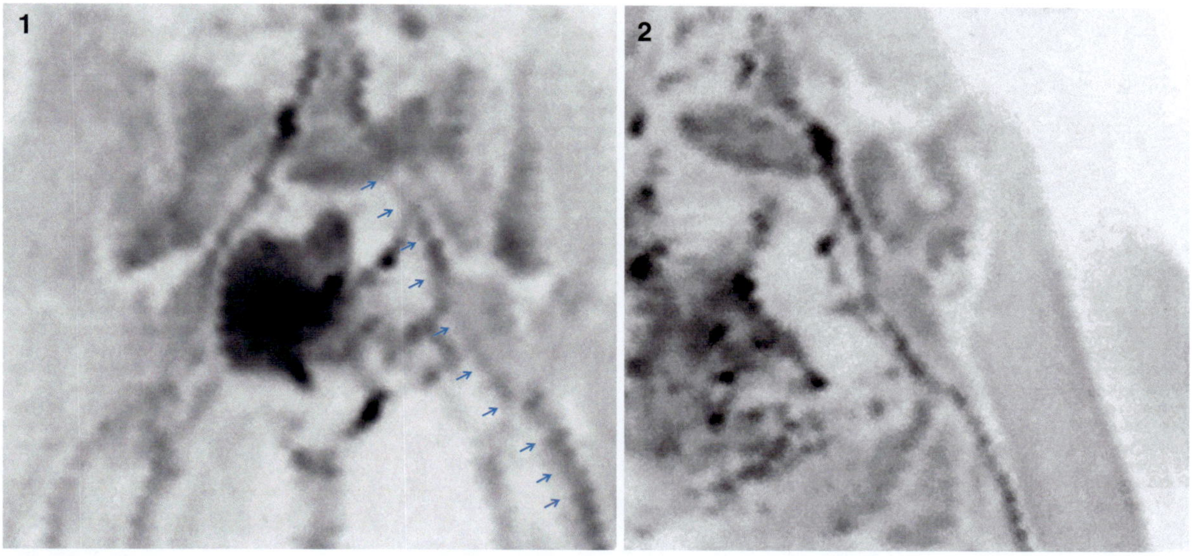

Fig. 4.4 DWI and DTI neurography: evaluation of pyramidal syndrome. A 47-year-old female with persistent deep pain in left buttock and hip regions was referred to our department for a MRI neurography of sciatic nerves. Clinically a piriform syndrome was suspected after a negative lumbar spine MRI. **Imaging Findings** Coronal mini-MIP of a DWI neurography using a DWIBS sequence with a *b* value of 800 s/mm^2 of both sciatic nerves with inverted gray scale demonstrated a thickened left sciatic nerve (*arrows* in Figure **4.4.1**). This finding is better visualized in the curve MPR of both sciatic nerves (**4.4.2** – left sciatic nerve; **4.4.3** – right sciatic nerve). The compression of the left piriformis muscle over the left sciatic nerve is depicted in a sagittal-oblique fusion image of a TSE T2-weighted image and a DWI neurographic acquisition (**4.4.4**). The thickening of the left sciatic nerve was also confirmed in a DTI sequence as shown in the coronal MPR of the FA map overlaid on a T1-weighted sequence (**4.4.5**) and in the coronal tractographic reconstruction overlaid on a TSE T2-weighted sequence shown in Fig. **4.4.6**. The FA value of left sciatic nerve was lower than that of the right one, demonstrating also an increase ADC value (**4.4.7**). Mean FA value of left sciatic nerve: 0.39 ± 0.11, mean FA value of right sciatic nerve 0.44 ± 0.11, mean ADC value of left sciatic nerve: $1.55 \pm 0.27 \times 10^{-3}$ mm^2/s, mean ADC value of right sciatic nerve: $1.33 \pm 0.33 \times 10^{-3}$ mm^2/s. In Fig. **4.4.7**, it should be noticed the uncommon course of the left sciatic nerve through the piriformis muscle in the greater sciatic foramen and the normal course of right sciatic nerve at the same level. Figure **4.4.8** shows an axial image of the FA map of both sciatic nerves overlaid on a TSE T1-weighted sequence confirming once again the difference in thickness of both structures (*arrows*). **Comments** Piriformis syndrome is a controversial entity which has been proposed as a cause of sciatica with an origin distal to the lumbosacral foramina. In occasions, the sciatic nerve or one of its divisions may lie above or through the piriformis muscle in the greater sciatic foramen, although the sciatic nerve is usually located in the infrapiriformis portion of this foramen. Alterations in the piriformis muscle, such as inflammation, spasm, contracture, hematoma, fibrosis, or hypertrophy, may cause compression of the sciatic nerve, causing a sciatic pain with or without associated weakness, paresthesias, or numbness. Treatment of this syndrome is initially conservative with surgical release of the sciatic nerve reserved for refractory cases. The diagnosis of piriformis syndrome is predominantly clinical as electromyography is not definitive due to the deep location of the sciatic nerve. MRI has been used in its diagnosis. MR neurography with STIR sequence has been demonstrated as a valuable tool, demonstrating thickening and high signal intensity in the involved sciatic nerve compared to the contralateral one. Besides, hypertrophy of the ipsilateral piriformis muscle may increase the diagnostic confidence, altogether with the above-described alterations in the sciatic nerve, although the size of the piriformis muscle should not be used as the unique criterion to establish a diagnosis of piriformis syndrome because different grades of asymmetry in piriformis muscle have been described in healthy volunteers. In the series by Filler et al., signs of sciatic nerve edema were present in 88% of patients with reproducible signs of piriformis syndrome. The combined presence of high signal intensity in the sciatic nerve and enlargement of the involved piriformis muscle raised up the diagnostic sensitivity and specificity in this series up to 64% and 93%, respectively. These results were posteriorly confirmed by Lewis and colleagues. DWI neurography and DTI have been used in the evaluation of peripheral nerve compression in cases of carpal tunnel syndrome and lumbar nerve compression by disc herniation. Despite the scarce available data, decreased FA values and increased ADC values have been demonstrated in the involved nerve distally to the compression site, probably related to segmental demyelination, Wallerian degeneration, and at a late stage of axonal damage. This case demonstrates the potential application of DWI neurography and DTI to diagnose piriformis syndrome

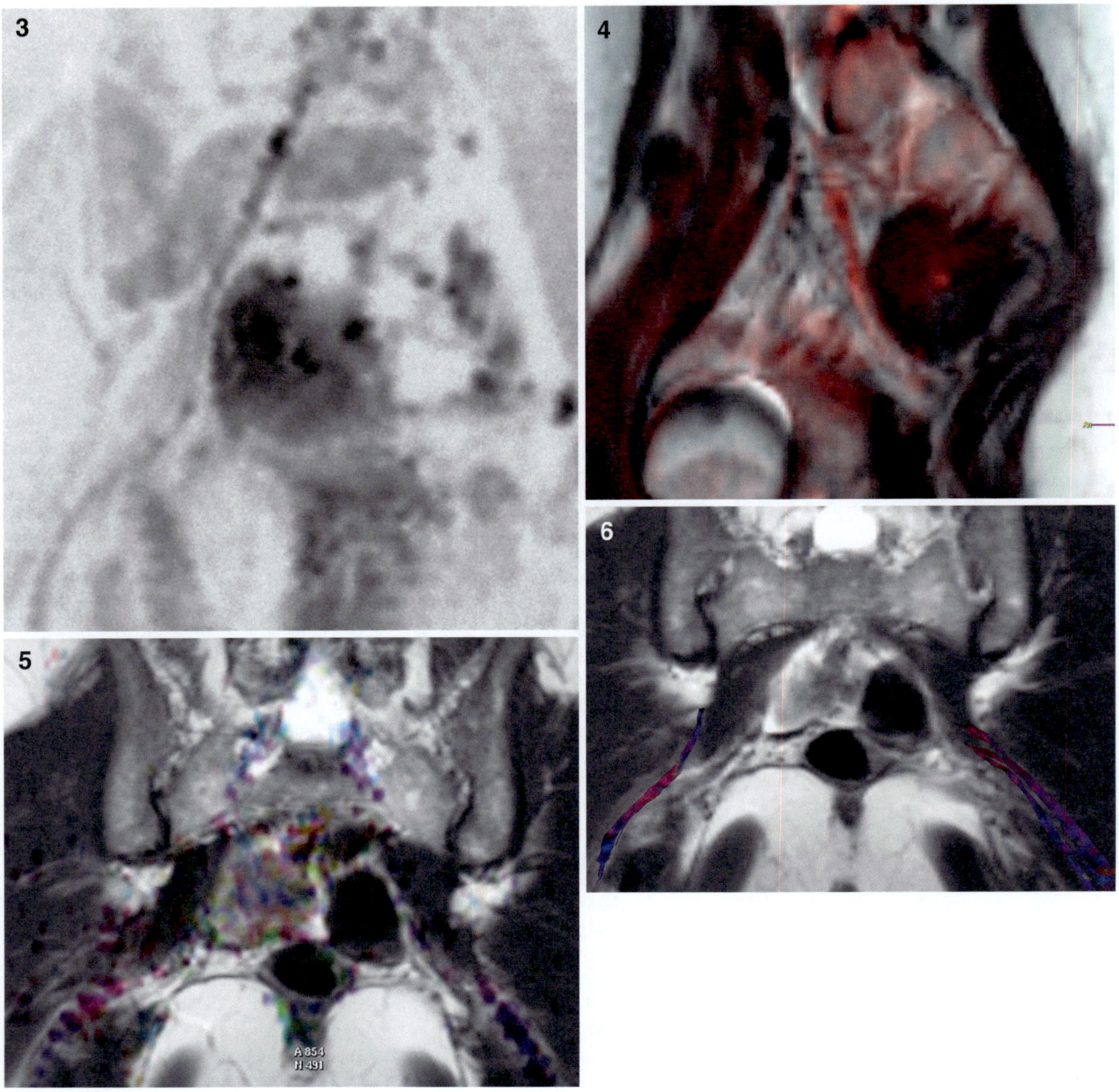

Fig. 4.4 (continued)

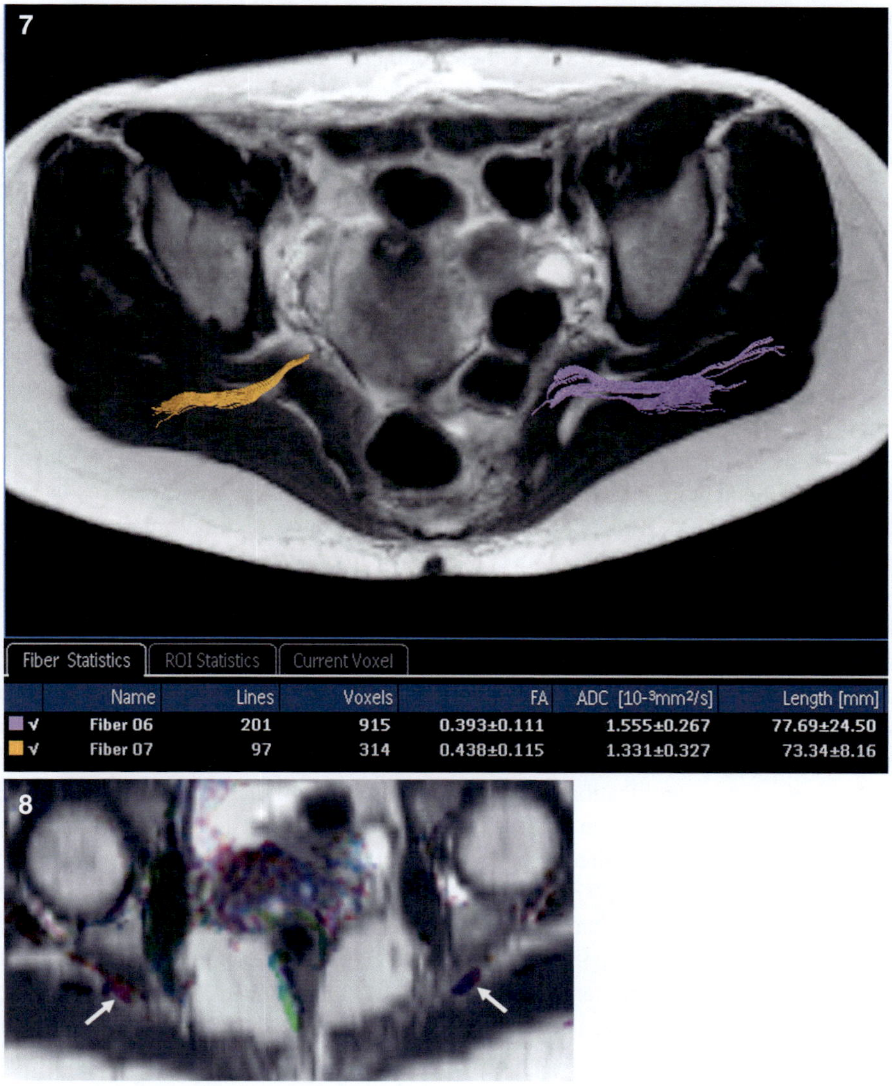

Fig. 4.4 (continued)

same series, DWI neurography allowed to depict nerve swelling at and bellow the compression site. Other main clinical application of DWI neurography is the assessment of the relationship between tumor and adjacent neural structures, being capable to exclude displacement, deformation, or interruption of nerve fibers. Abnormal decreased signal intensity in DWI neurographic acquisitions in postganglionic traumatic plexus injury, which may indicate axonal injury, has also been proposed as an area of research for this technique.

DWI neurography does not usually employ motion probing gradients in more than three orthogonal directions, which prevents tracking the anisotropy of the nerve. In order to study the anisotropy of the nerve fibers, it is necessary to obtain at least six different diffusion directions by means of DTI. This approach has been also proposed for the study of peripheral nerves, as diffusion is slightly higher along axons in the peripheral nerves. The application of DTI in the brain and spinal cord is well known being possible to perform fiber tracking following lines of fast diffusion related to the axonal architecture. Besides, measurements derived from the diffusion tensor allow us to obtain fractional anisotropy (FA) maps and quantifications. It still remains unclear which are the optimum parameters for clinical brain DTI, including number of directions, spatial resolution, and maximum *b* value. The physical basis of this approach was explained in Chap. 3.

DTI of peripheral nerves has been applied in vivo for brachial, lumbar, and sacral plexi, and median, ulnar, radial, sciatic, tibial, and peroneal nerves. The use of tractography reveals adequately the course of the nerve, and the use of FA quantifications allows a better functional assessment of the neural anisotropy and microstructure. Limited by short clinical data, potential applications of this technique are similar to those described for DWI neurography, such as acute nerve injuries, monitorization of posttraumatic neural lesions, evaluation of chronic nerve entrapments, and evaluation of the relationship between masses and peripheral nerves or plexus. In this sense, preliminary reports in animal models suggest that a decrease in FA values after an acute peripheral nerve injuries indicates the presence of Wallerian degeneration and that quantitative measurements, such as FA, axial diffusivity, and radial diffusivity, may be good indicators of peripheral nerves regeneration. Chronic damage to a nerve may produce several combinations of segmental demyelination, Wallerian degeneration, and axonal damage, along with intrafascicular edema and an increase of the fibrous tissue at the endoneurium and perineurium. Therefore, chronic entrapment syndromes may change neural diffusion, with decrease in mean FA values, as demonstrated in several in vivo research in animals and humans. This has been especially studied for carpal tunnel syndrome, although there is still lack of consensus about the normal FA values of the median and other peripheral nerves. Besides, FA values of the tibial nerves were significantly lower in patients with chronic inflammatory demyelinating polyradiculoneuropathy than in healthy volunteers. Assessment of the involvement or no involvement of peripheral nerves or neural plexus in a tumor, such as perineuromas or neurogenic ones, may be of interest in the planning of surgery or therapeutic management. Preliminary data has shown the potential of DTI in this task.

4.1.1.2 Extracranial Applications of DTI

With the advent of multichannel radiofrequency coils and parallel imaging, high-resolution DTI has been possible at 3 T magnets, solving their greater EPI susceptibility artifacts. Furthermore, improvements in gradient technology have allowed its application not only for peripheral nerve evaluation, but in organs such as prostate (Fig. 4.5), heart (Fig. 13.10), kidney (Figs. 3.5 and 3.6) and muscle (Fig. 4.6), with increased image quality than acquisitions at 1.5 T magnets. The use of 3 T allows to either shortenning the acquisition time with similar technical parameters or increasing the spatial resolution or number of obtained directions of diffusion in a similar scan time.

4.1.1.3 IVIM Approach

In a similar manner, the increase in SNR of 3 T magnet permits to acquire more *b* values in a similar scan time than 1.5 T magnets. The use of multiple *b* values is especially useful when the biexponential model of diffusion signal decay, also known as intravoxel incoherent motion (IVIM), is applied. This approach is under investigation in several organs such as lung, liver, pancreas, kidney, prostate, muscle, and brain, although with very few clinical series. Its physical basis was also explained in detail in Chap. 3. This model is able to separate the effect of tissue perfusion on the diffusion signal. To obtain the perfusion information, it is necessary to

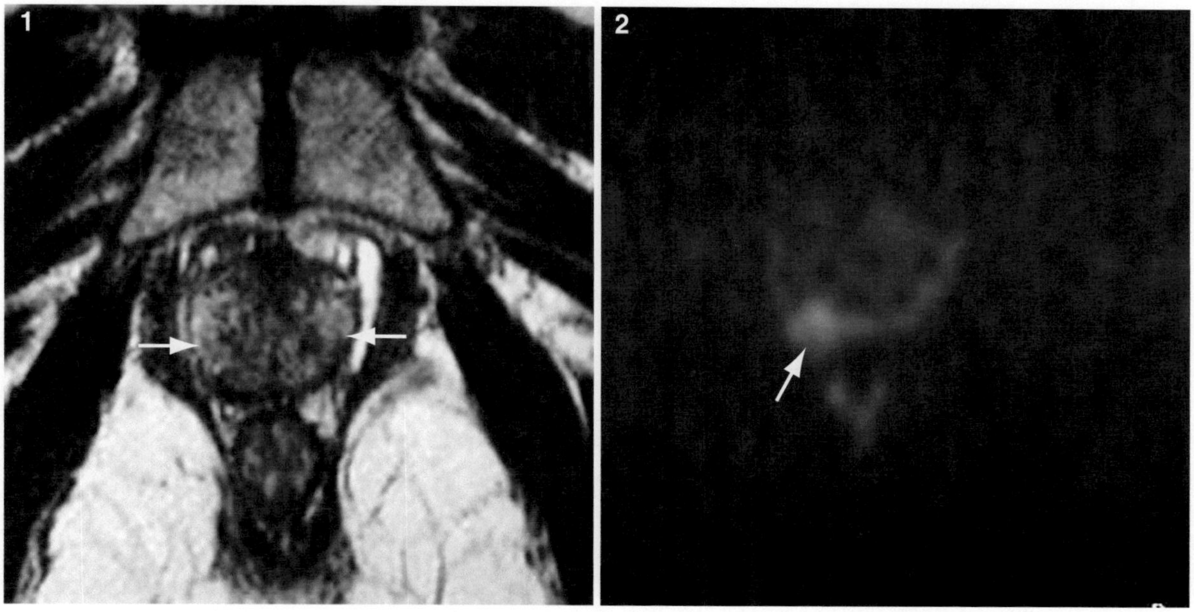

Fig. 4.5 **DTI of persistent prostate cancer**. A 57-year-old male with prostate cancer D stage in treatment with androgen suppression for 1 year was submitted to our department. MRI at a 3 T magnet was performed as part of the surveillance workup. **Imaging Findings (4.5.1)** Axial TSE T2-weighted image at the level of prostatic apex shows nonspecific ill-defined low-intensity area within the peripheral zone (*arrows*). (**4.5.2**) DWI with a b value of 2,000 s/mm^2 demonstrates a persistent tumor in right apical peripheral zone as a foci of high signal intensity (*arrow*). (**4.5.3**) ADC map demonstrates the true restriction of diffusion of the tumor (*arrow*), which presents a mean ADC value of 0.7×10^{-3} mm^2/s. (**4.5.4**) FA map at the same level showed a FA value for prostatic cancer of 0.54 (*arrow*) and 0.47 for normal peripheral zone.

Comments Improved SNR at 3 T may be of benefit for prostatic DWI, as its application may overcome the limitations on spatial resolution of DWI. It must be noticed that differences between cancer and normal and peripheral zones have also been confirmed at 3 T. A report by Kim and colleagues at 3 T found that an ADC cutoff value of 1.67×10^{-3} mm^2/s had 0.97 area under the curve (AUC) in the prediction of peripheral zone cancer and for the prediction of transitional zone cancer, an ADC cutoff value of 1.61×10^{-3} mm^2/s showed 0.92 AUC. The 3 T magnets also favor the use of ultrahigh b values, as shown in this case, that allow to clearly depict the tumor against a totally suppressed background, improving tumor delineation.

Different diffusion and anisotropy properties have been demonstrated for peripheral and central gland using DTI. The central gland shows different components, such as stroma, smooth muscle fibers, and organized ductal structures, which causes diffusion anisotropy. Besides, the less structured peripheral zone shows less anisotropy. DTI is able to detect these microstructural differences by means of the fractional anisotropy (FA) value, as the diffusion properties of the tissues are studied in at least six different gradient directions. With the available data, a significant difference between prostate cancer and normal peripheral zone can be assumed, although with contradictory results. For example, in the series by Gibbs et al., Rischauer et al., and Gürses et al., the FA values were significantly higher in prostate cancer than in normal peripheral zone. However, the contrary has been observed by Manenti et al. In most of these series, prostate cancer shows higher FA values than normal prostatic tissue, as in the case shown. Recently, a significant difference in the FA values of chronic prostatitis and cancer has also been reported. FA is more sensitive to noise than ADC, which limits its clinical applicability as a repeatable marker compared to ADC. Further research is needed to define the role of DTI in prostatic cancer diagnosis

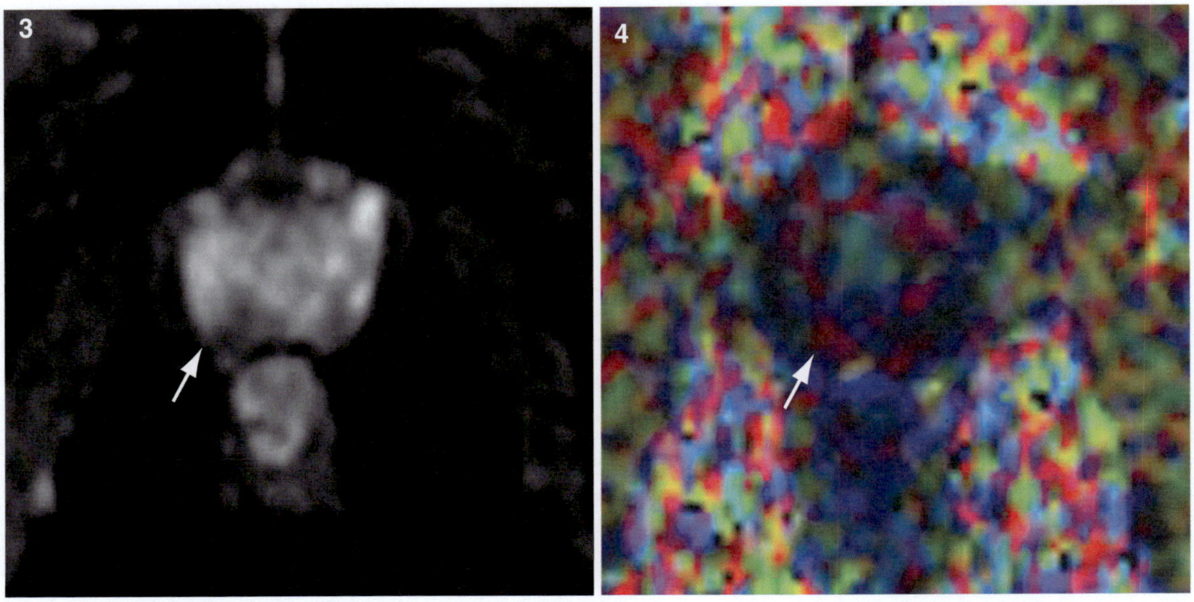

Fig. 4.5 (continued)

obtain several *b* values between 0 and 100 s/mm^2. Besides, the acquisition of several *b* values over 100 s/mm^2 permits to model the true diffusion signal decay. This approach is more accurate as more *b* values are obtained. Therefore, scanning time will increase making the examination prone to movement artifacts. In our own experience, the use of 3T magnets for this kind of approach is a clear advantage to reduce scan time increasing the number of *b* values obtained (Figs. 4.5, 4.7, 8.1, 13. 2 and 14.2).

Fig. 4.6 **Muscle DTI**. In Fig. 4.6, a tractography reconstruction of the vastus medialis of the quadriceps femoris muscle in a normal volunteer is presented. It can be appreciated that it is possible to study the microstructure of the muscle showing the fiber orientation inside the muscular belly.

Muscular DTI has been proposed for several clinical applications. First of all, DTI may have a role in the assessment of muscular microstructure. DTI is a more accurate technique than ultrasound to study muscular pennation, a concept related to the obliquity between the muscles fibers and the main axis of the muscle. The pennation of some muscles, as the quadriceps femoris is heterogeneous, and muscles with a heterogeneous structure will show a lesser grade of anisotropy and decreased FA values compared to perfectly oriented ones. Furthermore, Kan and colleagues reported a significant variation in the pennation of the quadriceps muscle in patients with lateral patellar dislocation compared to healthy volunteers, suggesting the potential role of DTI to create biomechanical models for this pathological condition and healthy subjects. Besides, the evaluation of muscle function might benefit from DTI and tractography. In this sense, Deux and colleagues reported ADC and FA changes in calf muscles during rest and contraction in volunteers. These changes occurred in opposite directions in opposite functional muscular groups during dorsal and plantar flexions. Therefore, the tibialis anterior muscle, which is active during dorsal flexion, increased the three eigen values and ADC, whereas all these parameters were decreased in the medial grastrocnemius muscle. According to DTI data, several authors have reported that the changes in water diffusion during muscular contraction occur in different directions to the main fiber one. Furthermore, tractography allows the visual assessment of muscle in different functional states (contraction or rest) and diseases. In the review by Khalil and colleagues, DTI and tractography were proposed as a new tool in the evaluation of muscle function and in the monitorization of muscle function impairment. Besides, changes in diffusivity have been related to pathological conditions, such as a decrease of FA and increase of ADC to acute muscle tear, increase in ADC after muscle denervation or even increase in FA values secondary to minimal muscle fatigue or damage

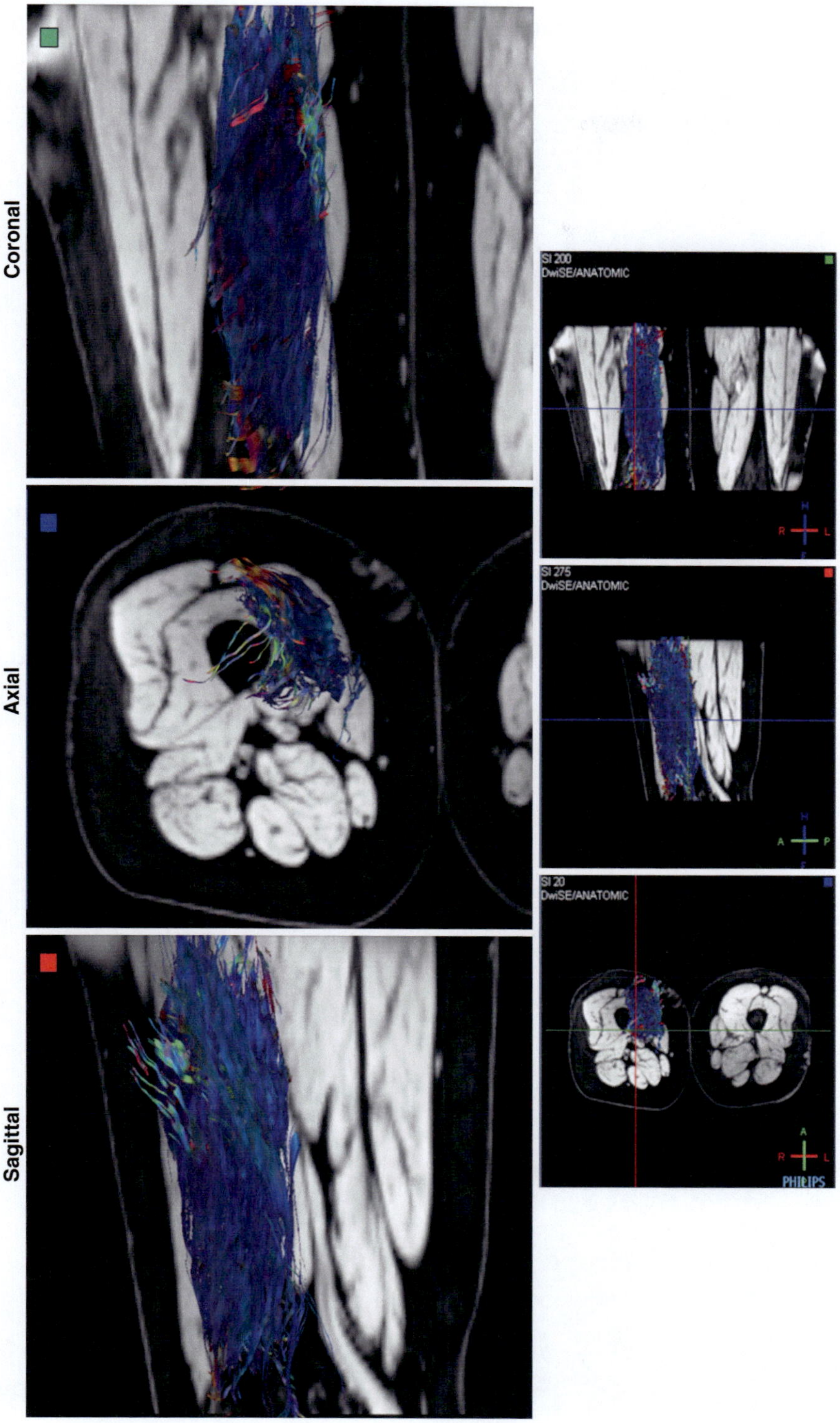
Coronal
Axial
Sagittal
SI 200
DwiSE/ANATOMIC
H
R
L
SI 275
DwiSE/ANATOMIC
H
A
P
SI 20
DwiSE/ANATOMIC
A
R
L
PHILIPS

1 **Monocompartimental model**

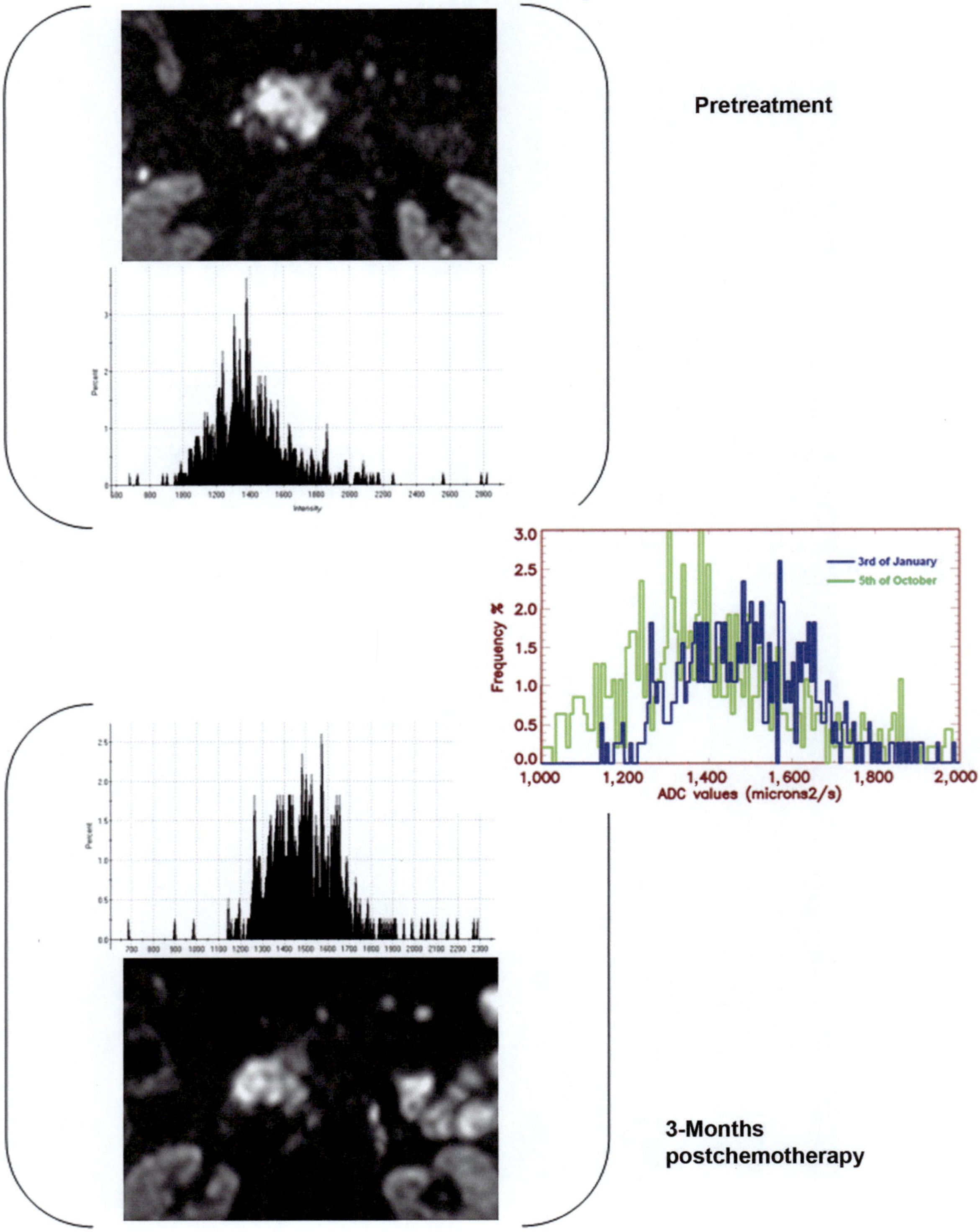

2 **Bicompartimental model**

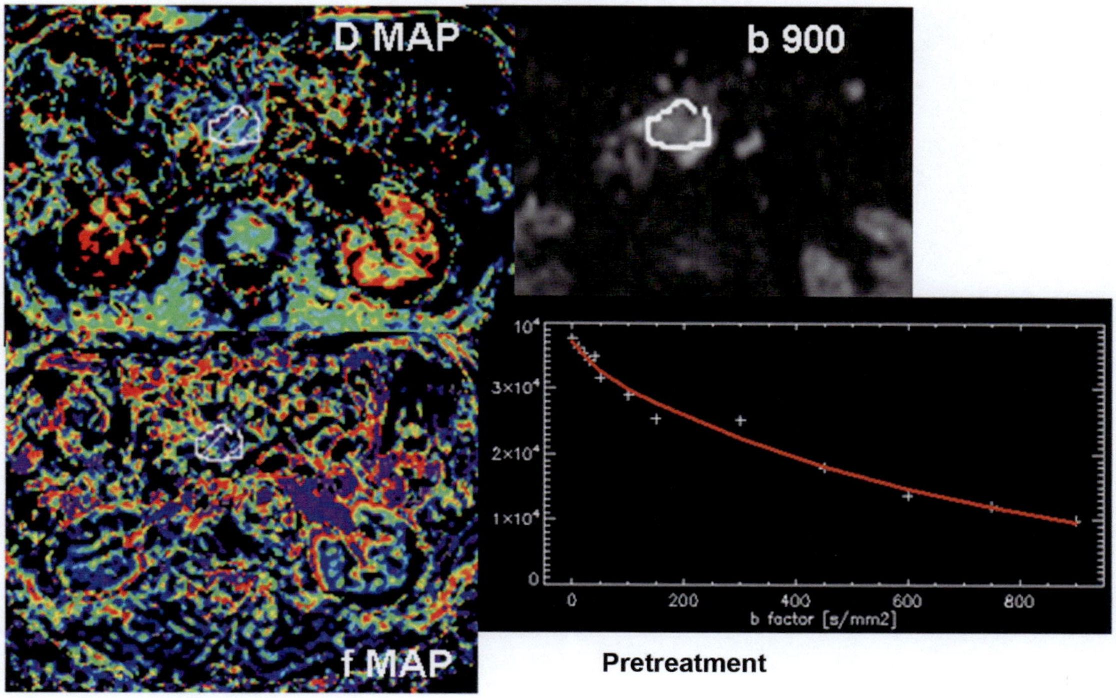

Fig. 4.7 (continued)

Fig. 4.7 IVIM model: monitorization of treatment response of pancreatic cancer. A 65-year-old male with unresectable pancreatic cancer in treatment with chemotherapy. MRI studies in a 3 T magnet were performed before and 3 months after the start of treatment for monitorization of response.

Imaging Findings Figure **4.7.1** shows the comparison between pre- and posttreatment DWI and ADC maps of pancreatic cancer at approximately the same level. DWI was analyzed with a monocompartmental approach. The mass demonstrated in both studies a similar volume, although the ADC values of the lesion increased between both studies indicating a partial response to treatment, as it may be visualized in the overlay of the ADC histogram of both studies, showing a displacement to the right of the ADC values in the follow-up MRI. Pretreatment mean ADC value: 1.36×10^{-3} mm^2/s. Posttreatment mean ADC value: 1.51×10^{-3} mm^2/s Figure **4.7.2** shows the comparison between pre- and posttreatment DWI of the pancreatic cancer at approximately the same level. DWI was analyzed with a bicompartmental approach. Parametric maps of true diffusion (**D**) and perfusion fraction (**f**) demonstrate a decrease in tumoral perfusion, but with stability of true diffusion values (pretreatment **D** value: 1.40 ± 0.1×10^{-3} mm^2/s; postreatment **D** value: 1.47 ± 0.2×10^{-3} mm^2/s; pretreatment f: 6.2 ± 7%; postreatment **f**: 3.3 ± 4.1%). In the signal decay graphics, it may be also noticed that the drop of the slope of the first fast decay of the diffusion signal in the follow-up MRI compared to the pretreatment one indicates less influence of the perfusion on the diffusion measurement. Therefore, the differences in ADC values may be mainly related to the decrease in tumoral perfusion.

Comments Very recently, the IVIM approach has demonstrated to be feasible in the pancreas. Klauss and colleagues evaluated its role in the differentiation between pancreatic cancer and mass-forming chronic pancreatitis. ADC values of mass-forming chronic pancreatitis were significantly higher than those of pancreatic cancer. However, no significant differences were found for the true diffusion values (**D**) but perfusion fraction (**f**) was significantly higher in pancreatitis compared with pancreatic carcinoma. Therefore, differences in ADC could be attributed mainly to differences in perfusion. DWI has demonstrated to be of benefit in monitoring therapy in other tumor entities but there is no published data for pancreatic cancer. This example shows the potential of DWI and the IVIM approach in the evaluation of response to treatment of pancreatic cancer. In this case, the differences in ADC values were related to the decreased perfusion of the tumor after chemotherapy as there was a decrease in the perfusion fraction between both studies but the true diffusion values remained almost unchanged

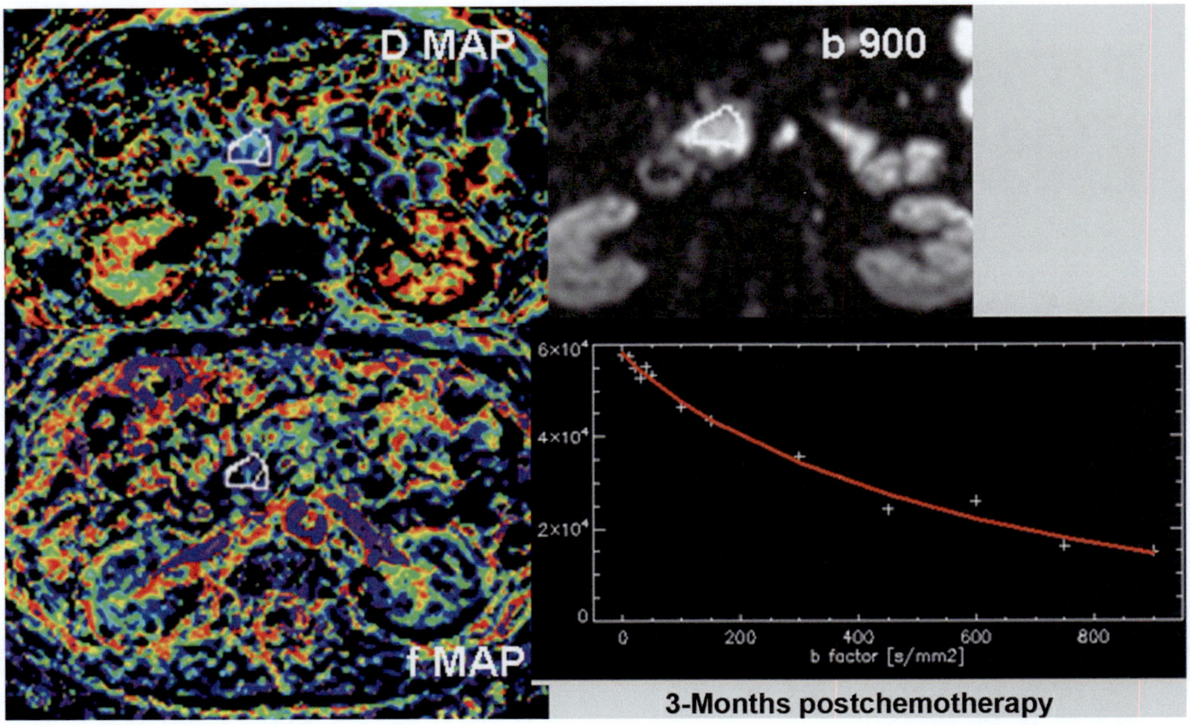

Fig. 4.7 (continued)

4.2 Pitfalls in DWI

In this section, the most common pitfalls of DWI are resumed, which may be found not only in 3 T magnets, if not in any kind of scanners, and in most of anatomic areas.

4.2.1 T2 Shine-Through

DWI signal is mainly related to restriction in the movement of interstitial free water and relaxation times on T2-weighted sequences of the tissue, as DWI is intrinsically a T2-weighted sequence. Therefore, lesions or tissues with long T2 values may be hyperintense on DWI even with high *b* values. ADC and exponential ADC maps allow to avoid this pitfall, as lesions without true diffusion restriction may not show hypointensity on ADC maps or hyperintensity on exponential ADC maps, as lesions with true restriction of free water movement would (Fig. 4.8). Furthermore, ADC measurements may give additional information to differentiate lesions with and without true restriction of water movement.

4.2.2 T2 Dark-Through

This term, also known as T2-blackout, is related to hypointensity of a lesion on DWI secondary to low signal on T2-weighted sequences. It is commonly seen in cases of hemorrhage due to local susceptibility effect, although in other conditions such as melanoma metastases, it can also occur. It should be noticed that ADC measurements should be avoided in areas with local susceptibility effects due to local field distortions. In the case of hemorrhagic lesions, there are always different grades of susceptibility effect according to the moment of evolution of blood, because of the paramagnetic properties of blood products, except in the hyperacute stage, as oxyhemoglobin is diamagnetic.

Shine through

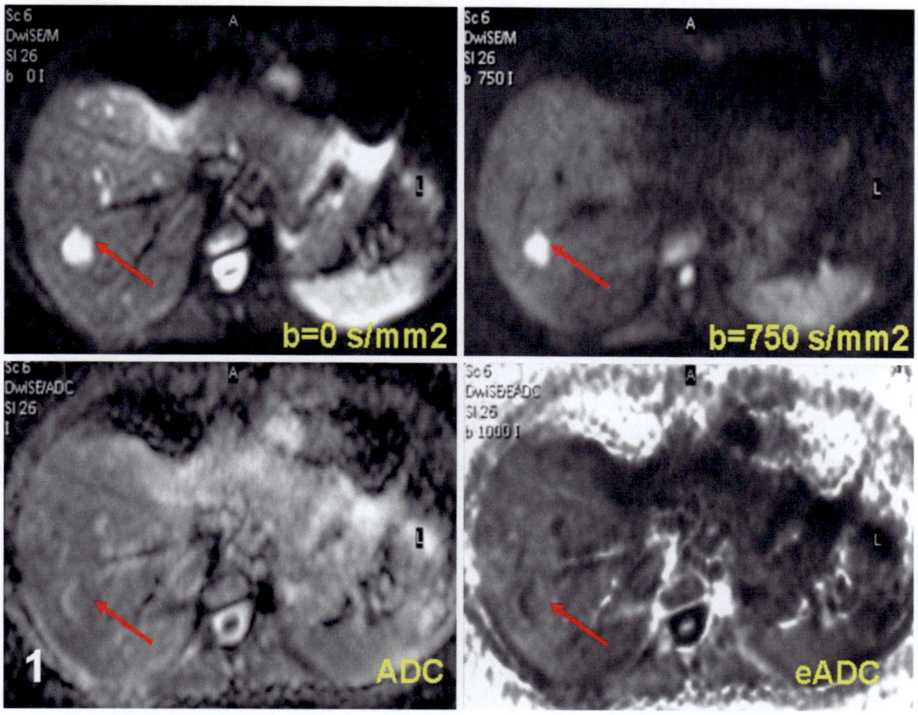

Fig. 4.8 **Shine-through and dark-through pitfalls**. A common source of error is derived from those tissues with very long TE producing a bright signal even in the images with high diffusion values falsely appearing as regions of restricted diffusion. However, when the ADC and eADC are obtained, this difference disappears showing the right diffusion properties of the tissue. At the top of this figure, an example of shine-through effect is shown. A liver hemangioma demonstrates high signal on the DWI obtained with *b* values of 0 and 750 s/mm^2 (*arrows*), consistent with diffusion restriction. However, in the corresponding ADC and eADC maps, the absence of true restricted diffusion compared with the surrounding tissue can be appreciated, as the hemangioma is mildly hyperintense on the ADC image and hyperintense on the e-ADC map (*arrows*). Therefore, routine quantification of ADC and e-ADC is recommended, as lesions with "true restriction" will show low signal on ADC maps and high signal on e-ADC maps, which will increase along with the degree of diffusion restriction.

There are regions in the acquired images that may show low signal due to the very low T2 values for some tissues (e.g., hemorrhagic tissues). These areas do not represent the fast diffusion properties of the tissue, this effect is known as dark-through. At the bottom of this figure, a dark-through example of a left ovarian endometrioma is shown. This lesion demonstrates low signal on DWI acquired with both b values of 0 and 1,000 s/mm^2 (red arrows). It can also be appreciated that the lesion does not present, as should be expected, high signal on the ADC map and low signal on the e-ADC map

Dark through

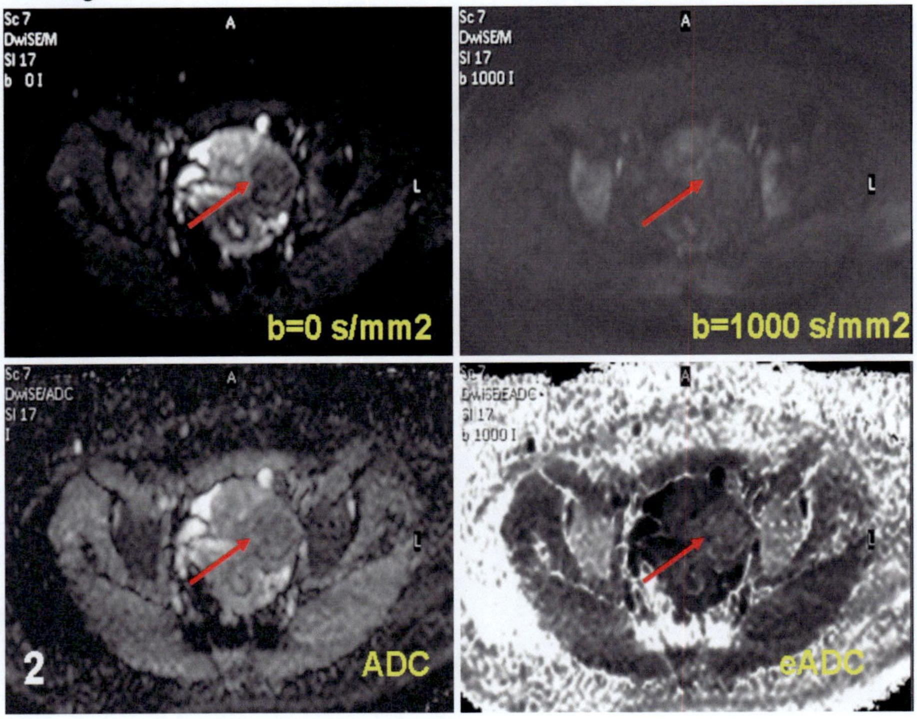

Fig. 4.8 (continued)

4.2.3 Restriction of Normal Structures

Normal hypercellular tissues may show hyperintensity on DWI even with high *b* values. Therefore, endometrium, adnexa, normal lymph node, small bowel mucosa, or spleen usually may simulate hypercellular lesions. Radiologists must be aware of this potential pitfall, which may be partially solved using ADC maps and anatomical sequences.

4.2.4 Iron Overload

A pathological increase in iron deposit within a tissue may result in local signal loss on DWI due to magnetic susceptibility effect. This alteration may diminish the capability to detect lesions of DWI. This is typical in patients with hemochromatosis, especially for those studied at 3 T magnets (Fig. 4.3.2). ADC measurements will not be accurate in this situation because of the susceptibility effects produced by local field inhomogeneity.

4.2.5 Nonmalignant Lesions with Apparent Restrictions on DWI

Feuerlein and colleagues explored 231 patients with an abdominal MRI including a DWI sequence with a higher *b* value of 1,000 s/mm^2 and ADC quantification. In this series, 21.8% of the lesions showing restricted diffusion (12 of 55 lesions) were benign, excluding the presence of lymph nodes in their analysis. The authors were aware of a number of benign lesions which may simulate malignancy on DWI. Inflammatory lesions, benign tumoral lesions with high cellularity, such as liver adenomas or focal nodular hyperplasia or ovarian teratomas, lesions with mucinous or hemorrhagic content may be a potential pitfall on DWI (Fig. 4.9). Most of the time, correlation of DWI findings with morphological MRI sequences, clinical history, and other imaging studies may avoid them.

The presence of macromolecules is the cause of this appearance in lesions with high protein content. The restriction of abscesses on DWI has been related to the presence of viscous fluid containing bacteria,

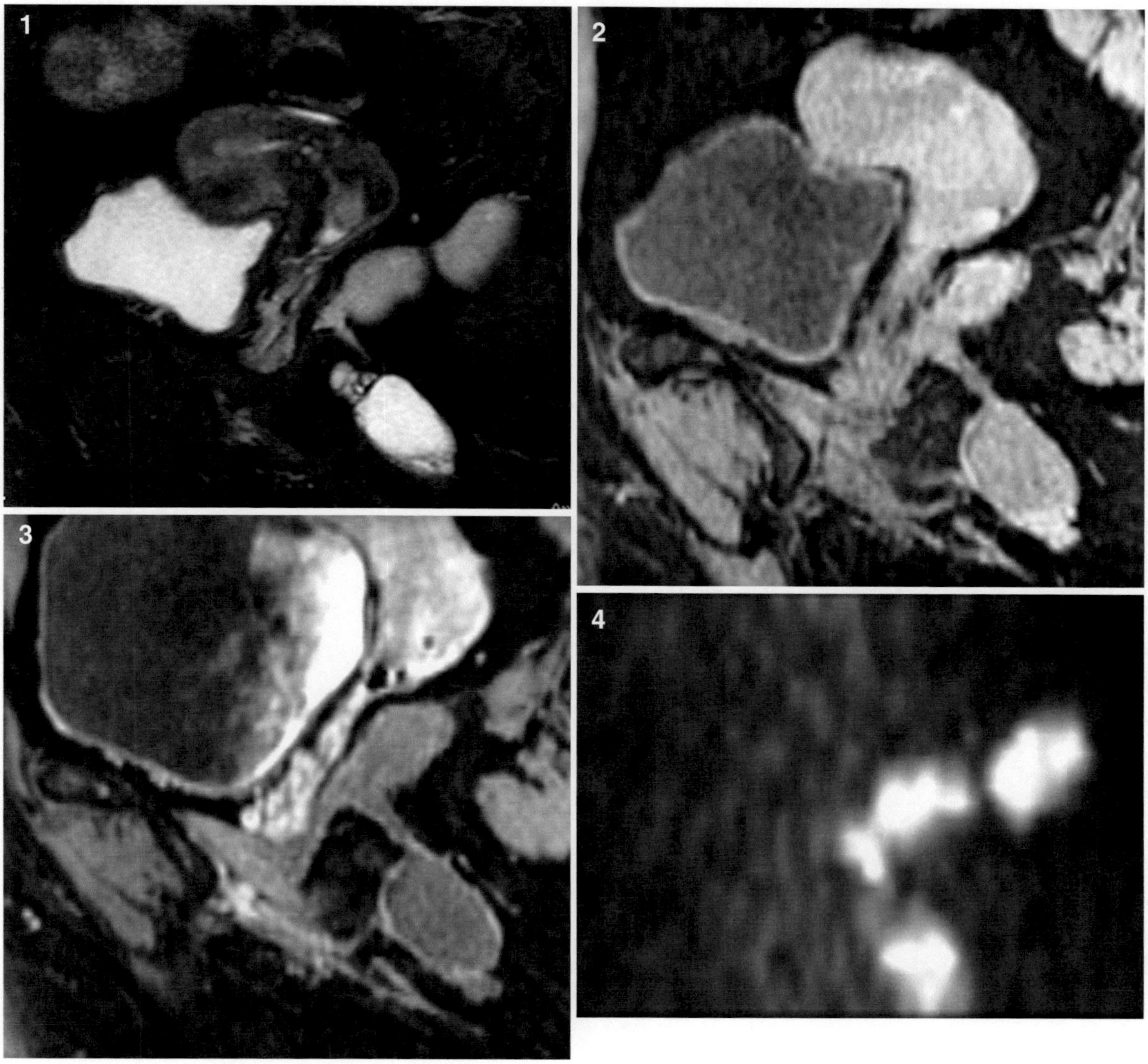

Fig. 4.9 False restriction of DWI pitfall: tailgut cyst with mucin content. A 61-year-old female with mass sensation and pain in anal region. A 3 T MRI was performed as part of the clinical workup.

Imaging Findings (4.9.1–4.9.3) Sagittal fat-suppressed TSE T2-weighted, pre- and postcontrast THRIVE sequences show a multiloculated cystic mass in the mesorectal space and right ischiorectal fossa, which present areas of hyperintensity on precontrast T1-weighted sequences related to mucinous content. (**4.9.4–4.9.6**) Sagittal MPR of DWI with a **b** value of 3,000 s/mm^2, fusion image of **4.9.1** and **4.9.4** and sagittal MIP of DWI with a **b** value of 3,000 mm^2/s nicely demonstrate the topography of the mass which shows high signal on ultrahigh **b** values suggesting diffusion restriction. (**4.9.7**) ADC map shows a mean ADC value of 0.81×10^{-3} mm^2/s suggesting a hypercellular lesion, although in this case, it was a pitfall due to the high proportion of mucin within the lesion.

Comments The tailgut cysts are a rare congenital tumor included in the group of the enteric cysts which originates from embryonic tissue located in the presacral space. They are more common in middle-aged women. These tumors usually are multicystic in appearance, demonstrating well-defined borders. It may show mucinous content, which demonstrates high signal intensity on T1-weighted and T2-weighted sequences. The presence of mucinous material is a key feature for its characterization. The presence of tiny calcifications is rare. Peripheral wall enhancement after gadolinium administration may be found. To our knowledge, the characteristics on DWI of tailgut cyst have not been reported. In this case, the tumor showed severe restriction, with low ADC values and high signal even in DWI with ultrahigh **b** values. This false restriction was due to the presence of mucinous content which is a known cause of false restriction related to the presence of macromolecules

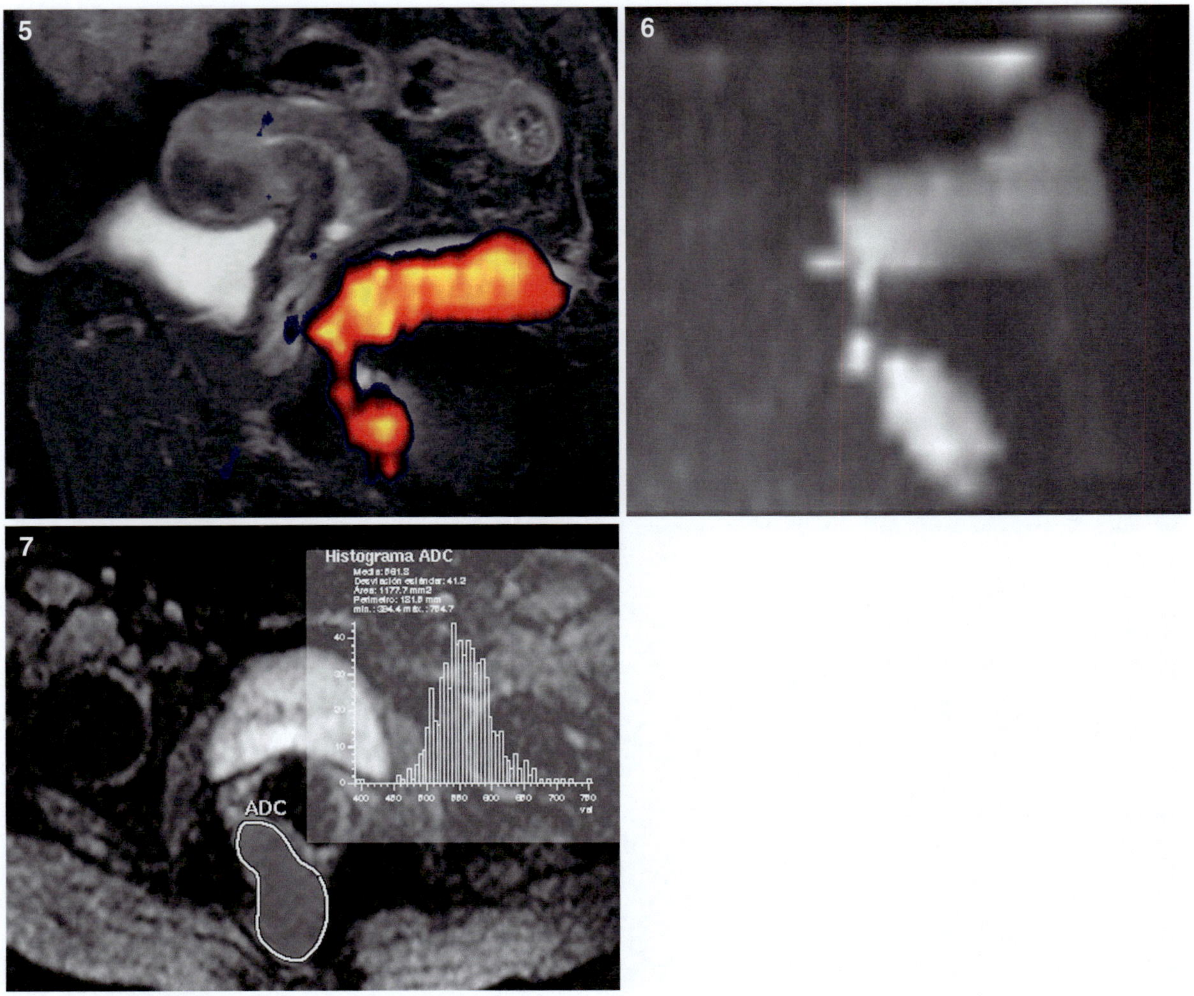

Fig. 4.9 (continued)

inflammatory cells, mucoid proteins, and cellular debris. This appearance has been used for their differentiation form cystic lesions in liver or brain, with the potential to avoid the use of intravenous contrast agents. Furthermore, the restriction on DWI usually occurs during the acute phase, because in their evolution, they increase their ADC value in the central area secondary to liquefaction. This has also been proposed as a sign of response to treatment and good evolution.

Sometimes the perfusion effect on DWI in lesions such as liver hemangiomas may produce the appearance of a lesion with restriction of DWI, with high intensity on DWI with high *b* values and even low intensity on ADC maps. As explained above, the use of an IVIM approach may reduce this effect and avoid this pitfall, although in clinical practice, it is enough with the correlation of DWI with morphological MRI sequences to easily characterize liver hemangiomas, although atypical sclerosing hemangiomas may also show restriction on DWI and may be harder to characterize on conventional MRI sequences.

4.2.6 Tumors with Low Cellular Density

DWI is a functional oncological technique, which is able to detect areas of restriction to water diffusion secondary to hypercellular areas. In hypocellular tumors, such as low-grade tumors, restriction to water diffusion may be minimal. Therefore, hypocellular tumors may not be depicted using DWI (Fig. 4.10).

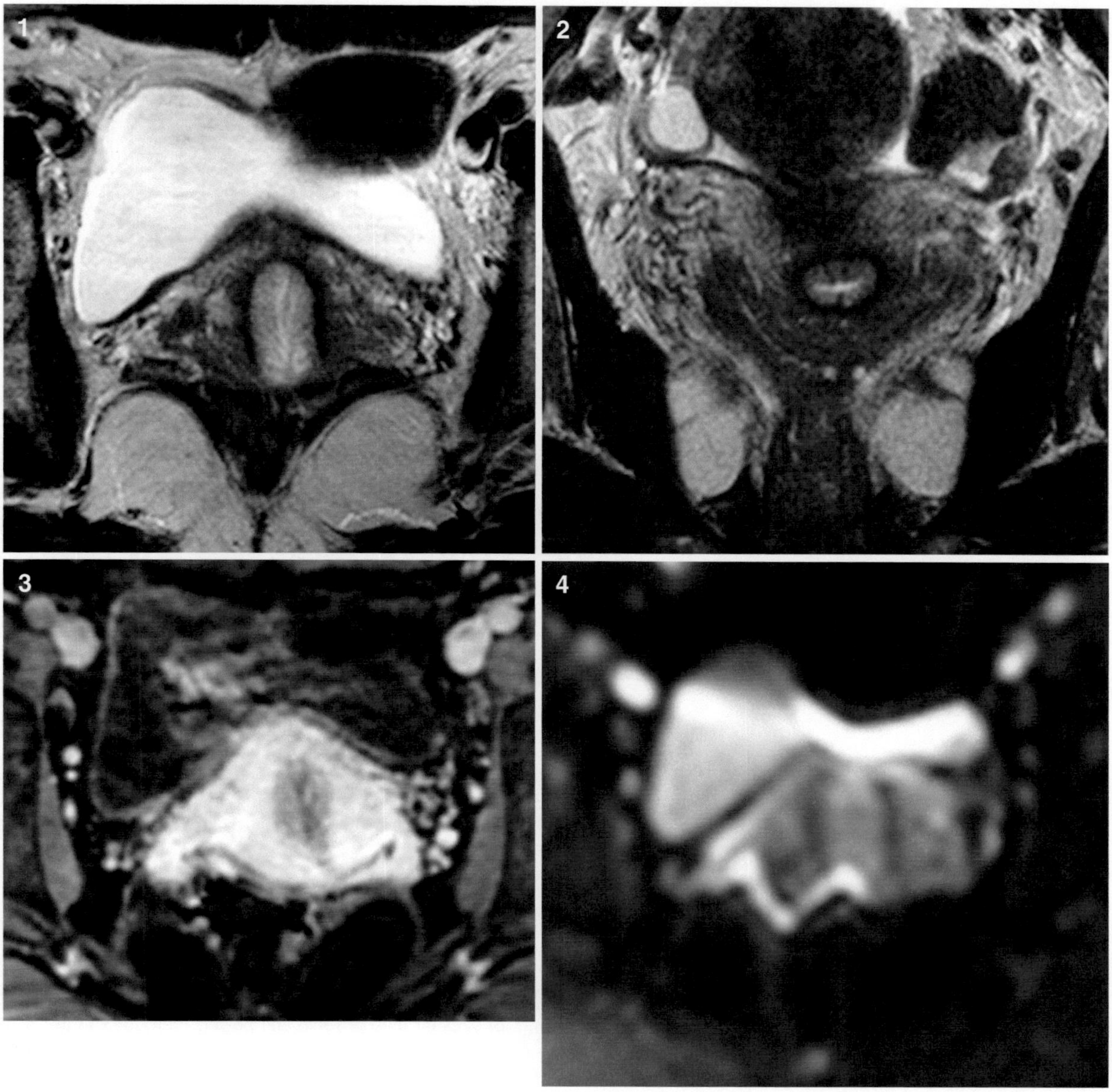

Fig. 4.10 Low-grade epidermoid cervical cancer. A 42-year-old female with positive Papanicolau smear for cervical intraepithelial neoplasia was submitted to our department for preoperative staging MRI in a 3 T magnet.

Imaging Findings (**4.10.1–4.10.3**) Axial and coronal TSE T2-weighted and axial postcontrast fat-suppressed THRIVE sequences do not depict any tumor or lesion in uterine cervix. Stroma is intact. (**4.10.4–4.10.6**) Axial DWI with **b** values of 0 and 1,000 s/mm^2 and corresponding ADC map confirm the absence of any detectable lesion. Hysterectomy was performed and a cervical intraepithelial neoplasia was confirmed.

Comments Studies have found that the mean ADC values can be used to differentiate between normal and cancerous tissue in the uterine cervix, with little overlap. Squamous cell carcinoma tends to have lower ADC values than adenocarcinoma and normal tissue has higher ADC values than both primary malignancies: cervical carcinoma $0.88–1.11 \times 10^{-3}$ mm^2/s vs. normal tissue $1.5–1.8 \times 10^{-3}$ mm^2/s, according to several series. ADC values can also provide information about the histology of the tumor. Tumors with higher cellular density and higher histologic grade show a tendency toward lower ADC values compared with those of tumors with lower histologic grade and lower cellular density, which have higher ADC values. Even in cases of stage 1 cervical cancer, DWI has demonstrated a significant difference in ADC values between well/moderately and poorly differentiated tumors. This suggests that DWI and ADC values of uterine cervical cancer may indirectly characterize the cellular density of the tumor. However, in cases of low-grade tumors demonstrating low cellularity, the restriction of free water diffusion may be minimal or even absent, making tumoral detection with DWI very challenging. Therefore, as in the case presented, the absence of areas of restriction on DWI does not always allow exclusion of malignancy, especially if an in situ or low-grade carcinoma occurs

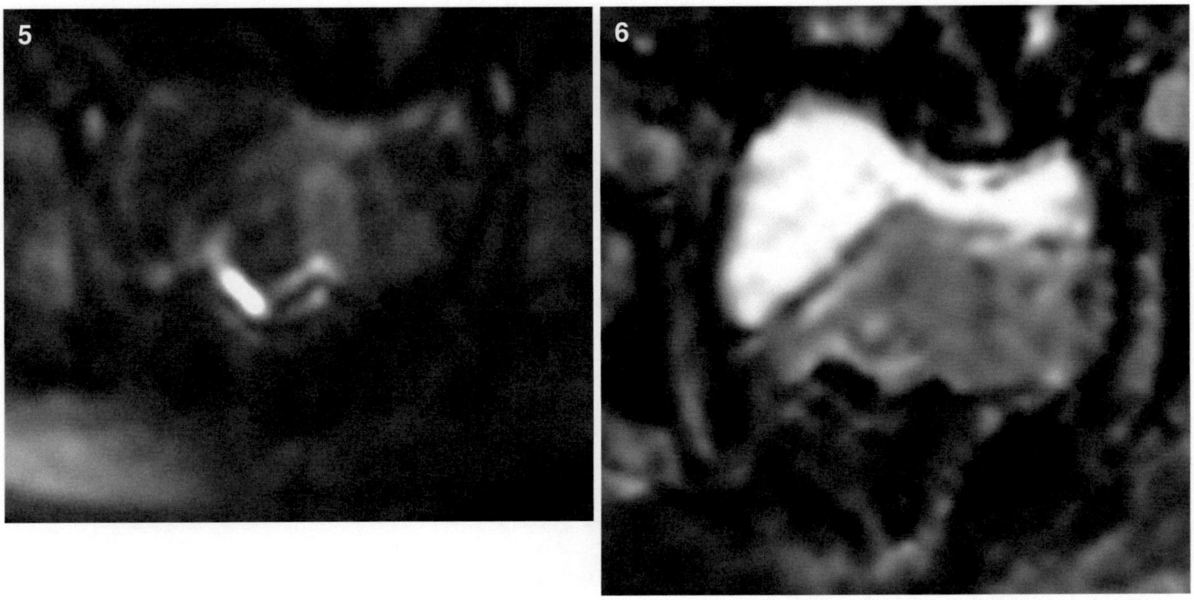

Fig. 4.10 (continued)

4.3 Conclusions

DWI at 3 T benefits of the increase of SNR in several manners, such as improvement in image quality and faster acquisitions. Although it is technically demanding, the advent of body DWI at 3 T scanners allows to using advanced applications compared to 1.5 T magnets, as DWI neurography, applications of DTI outside the brain, and the analysis of the bicompartmental model of diffusion signal decay. Radiologists should be aware of potential pitfalls in DWI at both 1.5 and 3 T magnets, in order to diminish both false-positive and false-negative results.

Further Reading

Balbi V, Budzik JF, Duhamel A et al (2011) Tractography of lumbar nerve roots: initial results. Eur Radiol 21(6):1153–1159

Bernstein MA, Huston J III, Ward HA (2006) Imaging artifacts at 3.0 T. J Magn Reson Imaging 24(4):735–746

Chandarana H, Lee VS, Hecht E et al (2011) Comparison of biexponential and monoexponential model of diffusion weighted imaging in evaluation of renal lesions: preliminary experience. Invest Radiol 46(5):285–291

Deux JF, Malzy P, Paragios N et al (2008) Assessment of calf muscle contraction by diffusion tensor imaging. Eur Radiol 18(10):2303–2310

Eguchi Y, Ohtori S, Yamashita M et al (2011) Diffusion weighted magnetic resonance imaging of symptomatic nerve root of patients with lumbar disk herniation. Neuroradiology 53(9):633–641

Feuerlein S, Pauls S, Juchems MS et al (2009) Pitfalls in abdominal diffusion-weighted imaging: how predictive is restricted water diffusion for malignancy. Am J Roentgenol 193(4): 1070–1076

Filler AG, Haynes J, Jordan SE et al (2005) Sciatica of nondisc origin and piriformis syndrome: diagnosis by magnetic resonance neurography and interventional magnetic resonance imaging with outcome study of resulting treatment. J Neurosurg Spine 2:99–115

Fitts RH, McDonald KS, Schluter JM (1991) The determinants of skeletal muscle force and power: their adaptability with changes in activity pattern. J Biomech 24(Suppl 1):111–122

Galban CJ, Maderwald S, Uffmann K et al (2005) A diffusion tensor imaging analysis of gender differences in water diffusivity within human skeletal muscle. NMR Biomed 18(8): 489–498

Gibbs P, Pickles MD, Turnbull LW (2006) Diffusion imaging of the prostate at 3.0 tesla. Invest Radiol 41(2):185–188

Grünberg K, Grenacher L, Klauß M (2011) Diffusion-weighted imaging of the pancreas. Radiologe 51(3):186–194

Gurses B, Tasdelen N, Yencilek F et al (2011) Diagnostic utility of DTI in prostate cancer. Eur J Radiol 79(2):172–176

Hiwatashi A, Kinoshita T, Moritani T et al (2003) Hypointensity on diffusion-weighted MRI of the brain related to T2 shortening and susceptibility effects. Am J Roentgenol 181(6): 1705–1709

Holl N, Echaniz-Laguna A, Bierry G et al (2008) Diffusion-weighted MRI of denervated muscle: a clinical and experimental study. Skeletal Radiol 37(12):1111–1117

Kakuda T, Fukuda H, Tanitame K et al (2011) Diffusion tensor imaging of peripheral nerve in patients with chronic inflammatory demyelinating polyradiculoneuropathy: a feasibility study. Neuroradiology. Feb 12 [Epub ahead of print]

Kan JH, Heemskerk AM, Ding Z et al (2009) DTI-based muscle fiber tracking of the quadriceps mechanism in lateral patellar dislocation. J Magn Reson Imaging 29(3):663–670

Khalil C, Budzik JF, Kermarrec E et al (2010) Tractography of peripheral nerves and skeletal muscles. Eur J Radiol 76(3): 391–397

Kim CK, Park BK, Han JJ et al (2007) Diffusion-weighted imaging of the prostate at 3 T for differentiation of malignant and benign tissue in transition and peripheral zones: preliminary results. J Comput Assist Tomogr 31: 449–454

Klauss M, Lemke A, Grünberg K et al (2011) Intravoxel incoherent motion MRI for the differentiation between mass forming chronic pancreatitis and pancreatic carcinoma. Invest Radiol 46(1):57–63

Kuhl CK, Textor J, Gieseke J et al (2005) Acute and subacute ischemic stroke at high-field-strength (3.0-T) diffusion-weighted MR imaging: intraindividual comparative study. Radiology 234:509–516

Kwee TC, Takahara T, Ochiai R et al (2008) Diffusion-weighted whole-body imaging with background body signal suppression (DWIBS): features and potential applications in oncology. Eur Radiol 18:1937–1952

Lewin JS, Duerk JL, Jain VR et al (1996) Needle localization in MR-guided biopsy and aspiration: effects of field strength, sequence design, and magnetic field orientation. Am J Roentgenol 166(6):1337–1345

Lewis AM, Layzer R, Engstrom JW et al (2006) Magnetic resonance neurography in extraspinal sciatica. Arch Neurol 63(10):1469–1472

Luna A, Sánchez-Gonzalez J, Caro P (2011) Diffusion-weighted imaging of the chest. Magn Reson Imaging Clin N Am 19(1):69–94

Manenti G, Carlani M, Mancino S et al (2007) Diffusion tensor magnetic resonance imaging of prostate cancer. Invest Radiol 42(6):412–419

McVeigh PZ, Syed AM, Milosevic M et al (2008) Diffusion-weighted MRI in cervical cancer. Eur Radiol 18: 1058–1064

Merkle EM, Dale BM (2006) Abdominal MRI at 3.0 T: the basics revisited. Am J Roentgenol 186(6):1524–1532

Morisaki S, Kawai Y, Umeda M et al (2011) In vivo assessment of peripheral nerve regeneration by diffusion tensor imaging. J Magn Reson Imaging 33(3):535–542

Murtz P, Krautmacher C, Traber F et al (2007) Diffusion-weighted whole-body MR imaging with background body signal suppression: a feasibility study at 3.0 Tesla. Eur Radiol 17:3031–3037

Notohamiprodjo M, Dietrich O, Horger W et al (2010) Diffusion tensor imaging (DTI) of the kidney at 3 tesla-feasibility, protocol evaluation and comparison to 1.5 tesla. Investig Radiol 45(5):245–254

Okamoto Y, Kunimatsu A, Miki S, Shindo M, Niitsu M, Minami M (2008) Fractional anisotropy values of calf muscles in normative state after exercise: preliminary results. Magn Reson Med Sci 7(3):157–162

Petchprapa CN, Rosenberg ZS, Sconfienza LM et al (2010) MR imaging of entrapment neuropathies of the lower extremity. Part 1. The pelvis and hip. Radiographics 30(4): 983–1000

Qayyum A (2009) Diffusion-weighted imaging in the abdomen and pelvis: concepts and applications. Radiographics 29(6): 1797–1810

Reischauer C, Wilm BJ, Froehlich JM et al (2010) High-resolution diffusion tensor imaging of prostate cancer using a reduced FOV technique. Eur J Radiol. Jul 15 [Epub ahead of print]

Schenck JF (1996) The role of magnetic susceptibility in magnetic resonance imaging: MRI magnetic compatibility of the first and second kinds. Med Phys 23(6):815–850

Takahara T, Hendrikse J, Yamashita T et al (2008) Diffusion-weighted MR neurography of the brachial plexus: feasibility study. Radiology 249(2):653–660

Takahara T, Hendrikse J, Kwee TC et al (2010) Diffusion-weighted MR neurography of the sacral plexus with unidirectional motion probing gradients. Eur Radiol 20(5):1221–1226

Takahara T, Kwee TC, Hendrikse J et al (2011) Subtraction of unidirectionally encoded images for suppression of heavily isotropic objects (SUSHI) for selective visualization of peripheral nerves. Neuroradiology 53(2):109–116

Tamai K, Koyama T, Saga T et al (2007) Diffusion-weighted MR imaging of uterine endometrial cancer. J Magn Reson Imaging 26(3):682–687

Vargas MI, Viallon M, Nguyen D et al (2010) New approaches in imaging of the brachial plexus. Eur J Radiol 74(2): 403–410

Wang J, Yu T, Bai R et al (2010) The value of the apparent diffusion coefficient in differentiating stage IA endometrial carcinoma from normal endometrium and benign diseases of the endometrium: initial study at 3-T magnetic resonance scanner. J Comput Assist Tomogr 34(3):332–337

Whittaker CS, Coady A, Culver L et al (2009) Diffusion-weighted MR imaging of female pelvic tumors: a pictorial review. Radiographics 29(3):759–774

Zandieh S, Berna R, Steinbach S et al (2011) The optimal B value in diffusion-weighted magnetic resonance neurography of the brachial plexus. Internet J Radiol 13(1)

Zaraiskaya T, Kumbhare D, Noseworthy MD (2006) Diffusion tensor imaging in evaluation of human skeletal muscle injury. J Magn Reson Imaging 24(2):402–408

DWI of the Liver

5

Antonio Luna and Luis Luna

5.1 Background

DWI has expanded its applications outside the brain in the last years because of technological improvements in gradient strengths and sequences. Nowadays, DWI forms part of state-of-the-art liver MRI protocols. There is great variability in DWI sequence designs according to different vendor or institution approaches. The number of *b* values and the post-processing to calculate ADC maps increase the lack of standardization. All these different strategies make it difficult to have clear cutoff values in ADC maps to characterize liver disease and make it necessary for every institution to have their own ADC map values of reference in order to exploit the quantification capabilities of DWI.

In this chapter, we analyze the main technical parameters of DWI of the liver in order to choose the most appropriate type of sequence according to the magnet and patient status. The characteristics on DWI of focal and diffuse liver disease are also summarized, outlining the currently established and potential clinical applications of this functional technique.

A. Luna (✉)
Chief MRI Section, Health Time Group,
Jaén, Spain
aluna70@sercosa.com

L. Luna
MRI Section, Clínica Las Nieves, SERCOSA,
Carmelo Torres 2,
Jaén, Spain
luisluna@sercosa.com

5.2 DWI: Basic Concepts

DWI reflects the diffusion of water in the body. The net motion of water molecules is directly related to the motion of water in the extra- and intracellular and intravascular space. DWI provides an indirect estimation of tissue cellularity and cell membrane integrity. Diffusion in a normal tissue is isotropic, as water molecules move in a random manner in any direction similarly to a bull entering the bull-fighting arena. When the water molecules are forced to move in one predetermined direction, as occurs in the nerve fibers similarly to a horse during a race, it is called anisotropic diffusion. DWI in the normal liver is isotropic. In hypercellular lesions the motion of water molecules is restricted compared to that of hypocellular lesions and normal liver. Therefore, impeded water diffusion may occur in lesions other than oncological ones. After treatment, solid tumors usually show a variable restriction of diffusion depending on the proportion of viable tumoral cells, necrosis and fibrosis. All these concepts were extensively described in previous chapters.

5.3 DWI: Basic Sequence Design

The image contrast on DWI relies on intrinsic differences in the water diffusion between tissues. Scanning parameters must be optimized to increase the SNR and CNR. DWI is a very sensitive sequence that is prone to motion and magnetic susceptibility artifacts, especially those of the echo-planar family. As a rule, conventional DWI has a limited spatial resolution, which is more evident in the liver. Several types of sequences have

A. Luna et al., *Diffusion MRI Outside the Brain*,
DOI 10.1007/978-3-642-21052-5_5, © Springer-Verlag Berlin Heidelberg 2012

been used for liver DWI, although the single-shot spin-echo echo-planar imaging (SS SE EPI) sequence is the most commonly performed. This sequence is relatively insensitive to macroscopic patient motion because of its very fast readout of the complete image data, within about 100 ms. DWI using a PROPELLER (periodically rotated overlapping parallel lines with enhanced reconstruction) multi-shot sequence (blade sequence) has also been used in several series. It improves image quality, reducing geometric distortions and artifacts. ADC values of abdominal organs increase their values with the PROPELLER sequence compared to DW-SE-EPI sequences. Therefore, it is important to find the optimum equilibrium between scan time and spatial resolution. In order to increase the DWI sequence quality, several rules should be kept in mind:

- *Fat suppression technique*: fat signal has a very low diffusion coefficient, which makes it very relevant for high *b* values. Besides, the difference in precession frequency between the water and the fat produces a water-fat shift of several voxels in the phase-encoding direction of the EPI readout (Figs. 1.6 and 2.8). Due to both factors, the fat signal usually overlaps on the studied anatomy, making applying fat suppression techniques mandatory. Its use allows us to reduce the chemical shift-induced ghosting. Inversion recovery (STIR) is a valid approach that has been most commonly used as a fat suppression technique in sequences such as DWIBS, especially for whole-body application. The main problem of sequences using STIR is the low signal-to-noise ratio (SNR) due to water signal reduction after the inversion pulse. For the liver the use chemical fat selective saturation (SPIR, SPAIR, CHESS, etc.) is more appropriate because of the superior SNR to those of acquisitions using STIR.
- *Selection of TR and TE*: TR should be long enough to avoid T1 saturation effects, which can result in falsely low ADC values. A TR over 2,500 ms is usually recommended. The shortest possible TE should be performed in order to improve the image quality and SNR (Fig. 1.3). This can be done by increasing the bandwidth (Figs. 2.3 and 2.4) and using parallel imaging (Fig. 2.5).
- *Spatial resolution*: this should be enough to allow detection of small focal liver lesions. It can be improved by increasing the number of acquisitions (NEX), although this is time consuming (Fig. 2.2). The field of view (FOV) should be reduced in the phase-encoding direction to a minimum. The resolution in plane should be kept at levels where the noise does not increase severely, as this will make ADC maps of reduced quality.
- *DWI encoding technique:* because water diffusion in tumors and livers is isotropic, the motion-probing gradient can be applied in a single direction. However, the trace approach has been proposed for some vendors to improve the SNR of DWI in the liver (Fig. 5.1). Increasing the number of obtained diffusion directions, there will be a net increase in the SNR because the noise is disruptive and the signal additive. The use of three orthogonal motion-probing gradients to yield both directional and trace DWI images allows improvement in the SNR by a square root of 3 in isotropic regions. The analysis of the original directional DWI images also allows us to minimize susceptibility, EPI and motion artifacts. Furthermore, tetrahedral encoding has been proposed to increase DWI quality in the liver, permitting the reduction of the TE. It should be taking into account that the diffusion encoding technique affects the ADC measurements.
- *Relationship to contrast media:* several series have documented that the performance of DWI before or after the injection of contrast media, such as gadoxetic acid or gadopentetate dimeglumine, does not alter liver ADC values. When possible, it is preferable to perform this before gadolinium chelate injection.

Fig. 5.1 Effects on diffusion encoding and respiratory synchronization in liver DWI. Four different approaches to liver DWI in a healthy volunteer are presented. All of them are a SS EPI DWI with a *b* value of 600 s/mm^2. At the top of the figure, a breath-hold TRACE approach is presented. Three orthogonal motion-probing gradients were applied to yield both directional (three top images) and trace DWI images (TRACE breath-hold DWI image). This approach allows the improvement in SNR in isotropic regions, as can be demonstrated in the direct comparison with the breath-hold DWI image using only one motion-probing gradient. In addition, a comparison between different mechanisms of respiratory synchronization is presented at the bottom of the figure. In the same volunteer a monopolar SS EPI DWI with a *b* value of 600 s/mm^2 was acquired with breath-holding (acquisition time: 27 s), respiratory triggering (acquisition time: 5 min and 16 s) and free breathing (acquisition time: 3 min and 24 s). These different acquisitions allow different ways of balancing acquisition time and SNR

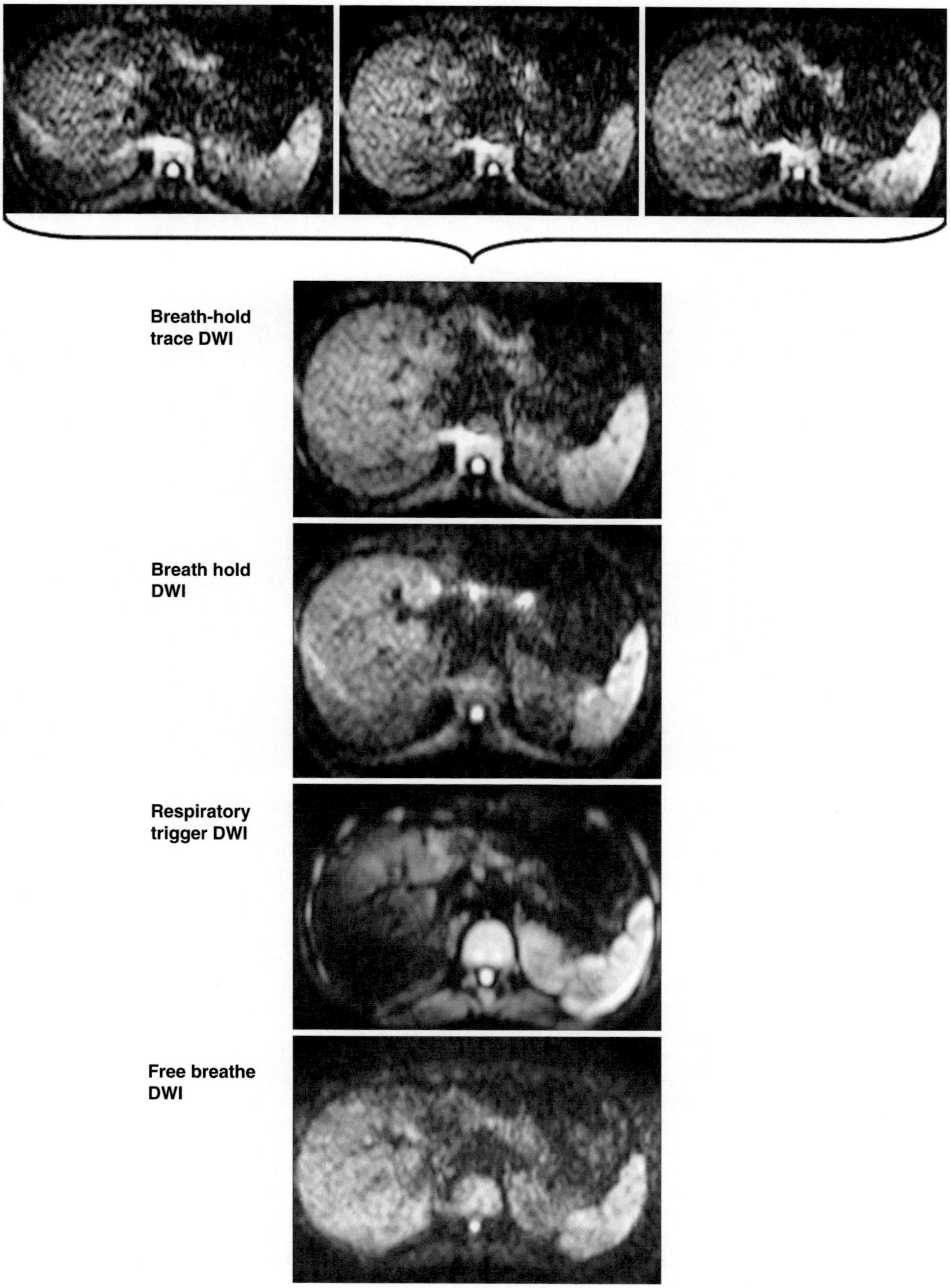
Breath-hold
trace DWI
Breath hold
DWI
Respiratory
trigger DWI
Free breathe
DWI

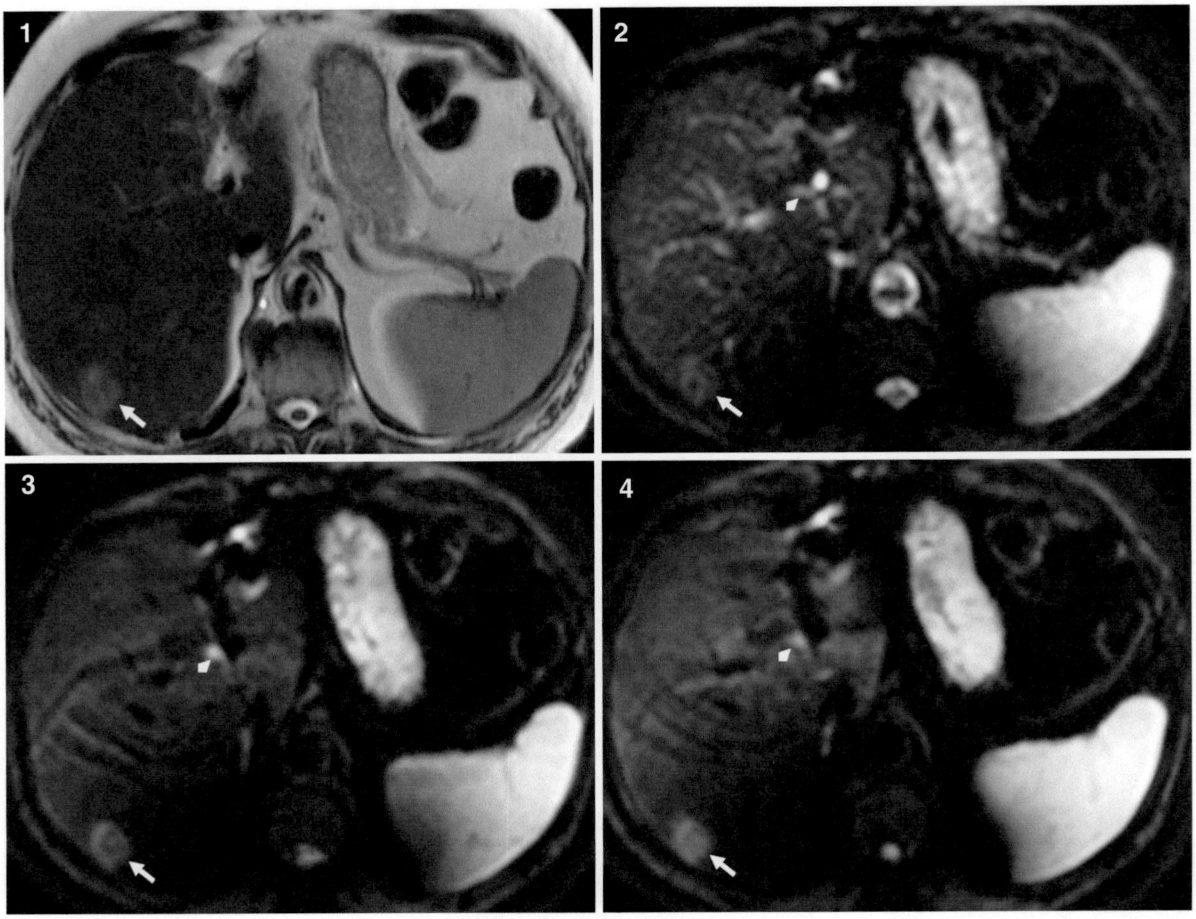

Fig. 5.2 Detection of focal liver lesions with black-blood DWI with a low *b* value. A 69-year-old male with previous history of colon carcinoma and resection of liver metastasis was submitted to our department for follow-up MRI of the liver with a 3-T magnet.

Imaging Findings Axial HASTE showed a liver metastasis in segment 7 (*arrow* in **5.2.1**), which is confirmed as lesion with restricted diffusion in the DWI images (*arrows*) with *b* values of 0, 10, 40, 600 and 900 s/mm^2 (**5.2.2–5.2.6**, respectively), which are part of our IVIM DWI sequence. Besides, in the DWI series a small hyperintense lesion adjacent to the hepatic hilum is identified in the black-blood DWI with low *b* value (10 and 40 s/mm^2, arrowhead in **5.2.3** and **5.2.4**). Notice how it is hardly depicted with a *b* value of 0 s/mm^2 (*arrowhead* in **5.2.2**) because of the presence of blood flow signal, which is completely suppressed with low *b* values. This lesion corresponded to a hepatic cyst as demonstrated in postcontrast series (not shown); this is why it disappears with high *b* values (*arrowhead* in **5.2.5** and **5.2.6**). Figures **5.2.7** and **5.2.8** show ADC maps calculated with all *b* values (**5.2.7**) and all *b* values over 100 s/mm^2 (**5.2.8**). Notice how the metastasis shows increased restriction of diffusion in Fig. **5.2.8**, as the perfusion effect over diffusion has been diminished by excluding *b* values under 100 s/mm^2. In both ADC maps, the cyst shows absence of impeded water motion diffusion.

Comments DWI increases detection of liver metastases compared to T2-weighted sequences, including fat-suppressed and STIR sequences. The most sensitive approach is the use of a low *b* value (between 10 and 50 s/mm^2), which depicts solid focal liver lesions with high signal intensity against a background with the signal of vessels completely suppressed. DWI is especially useful in the detection of lesions smaller than 1 cm and those adjacent to vascular structures. The use of a low *b* value outperforms DWI with a *b* value higher than 500 s/mm^2 for metastases detection. DWI in combination with conventional T2- and T1-weighted sequences has been demonstrated to be superior to SPIO MRI in the counting of hepatic metastases. DWI in combination with manganese, gadoxetic acid or SPIO-enhanced MRI in the study of hepatic metastases has improved the results of their counterparts alone. Furthermore, DWI outperforms multislice CT in the detection of liver metastases in patients with either colorectal or pancreatic cancers. However, Shimada et al. reported higher accuracy in the detection of small metastases with gadoxetic acid-enhanced MRI than with DWI, although they used a *b* value of 500 s/mm^2 and not a black-blood DWI sequence, which is an important limitation. According to these data, liver DWI can be considered a reasonable alternative to gadolinium chelates or hepatospecific contrast media in patients at risk for nephrogenic systemic fibrosis for focal lesion detection

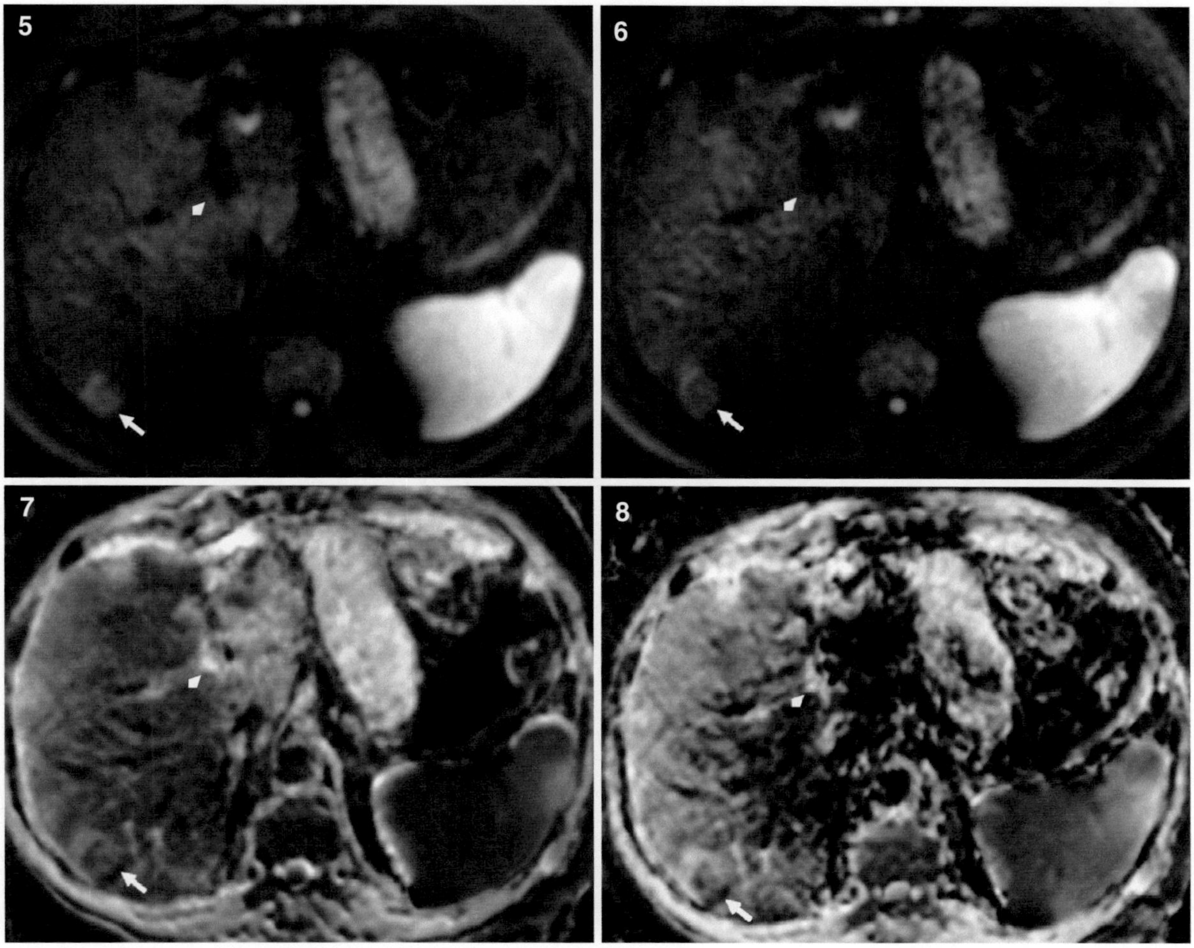

Fig. 5.2 (continued)

- *3-T magnets*: DWI benefits from the increase in signal of high field magnets because of the secondary increase in the SNR. For example, a signal improvement of 50% has been reported in kidney studies when comparing 3 T and 1.5 T within the same acquisition time. However, the magnetic susceptibility is also doubled and the magnetic field variation higher, making DWI at 3 T even more prone to artifacts and image distortion. Parallel imaging is crucial to reduce scan time and to diminish susceptibility effects. Besides, the use of a higher strength of 3-T scanner gradient systems in combination advanced fat suppression sequences allows 3-T magnets to perform DWI adequately in the liver.
- *Selection of b values*: DWI in the liver can be used for lesional detection and/or characterization purposes. The use of a low *b* value is very useful for detection of focal liver lesions, as there is a black-blood effect that renders blood vessels black and remaining focal liver lesions bright. This increases the depiction of smaller liver lesions (Fig. 5.2). The optimum low *b* value for lesion detection is still under debate, although it should be somewhere between 10 and 50 s/mm^2. For characterization, it is necessary to acquire at least one low and another high *b* value, which also permits ADC measurements. First published series used a maximum *b* value between 400 and 600 s/mm^2. In the last years, an increase in the maximun *b* value has been possible because of technological improvements. The increase in *b* values allows a better differentiation between benign and

malignant liver lesions, reduces the chance of T2 shine-through, although the T2 relaxation time of the liver is short, and improves lesion characterization (Fig. 3.2). The optimum high *b* value should range between 600 and 1,000 s/mm^2 in order to maintain a sufficient SNR. In our experience, an accurate ADC quantification is critical for lesion characterization. The more *b* values obtained, the more accurate the ADC will be (Fig. 3.3). However, each acquired *b* value increases the acquisition time. Therefore, the optimum set of *b* values for liver DWI still has to be defined. Our routine liver DWI sequence includes five *b* values: 0, 50, 100, 500 and 800 s/mm^2.

- *Synchronization*: another problem involving the diffusion signal is the macroscopic movement produced by the respiratory motion and heart beat, which are critical in liver acquisitions. In order to avoid these movements different strategies have been proposed for the liver, as for other areas (Figs. 5.1 and 13.1). Kwee et al. reported good agreement in the estimation of ADC values comparing breath-hold and free-breathing sequences, while respiratory-triggered acquisitions systematically showed an overestimation of the ADC values. In contrast, Kandpal et al. found good agreement in the ADC values acquired with respiratory triggered and breath-hold strategies for normal liver and focal lesions, although respiratory-triggered acquisitions showed higher SNR in normal liver and higher CNR between normal liver and focal lesions than breath-hold sequences. Finally, in another report, Kwee and colleagues also studied the effect of heart motion on DWI of the liver, showing a strong degradation of those images acquired during heart systole because of the effect of heart movement. Although in this paper the effect of cardiac movement in the ADC estimation was not studied, the authors suggest that the signal loss in DWI images should affect the ADC estimation.

Breath-hold single-shot acquisitions are the most common approach to DWI of the liver. If the patient is collaborative, the breath-hold sequences are preferred as misregistration is avoided, the examination time reduced and the sensitivity to bulk motion diminished. Geometric distortions and poor image quality are the shortcomings of breath-hold DWI sequences. Cardiac pulse triggering can reduce the cardiac pulsatile artifact over the left lobe, but increase scan time, the number of breath-holds needed and probably motion artifacts (Figs. 2.6 and 13.1). The acquisition of *b* values is limited with this approach, reducing the correct calculation of ADC maps. Breath-hold DWI with a low and a high *b* value can be performed in less than 30 s, which is optimal for screening.

Respiratory-triggered DWI allows us to scan a greater volume of tissue and avoid breath-holding, which may be of interest for severely ill, obese or non-collaborative patients. The use of multi-shot interleaved EPI with parallel imaging reduces distortions and allows increasing the spatial resolution. Motion-related phase error from shot to shot, which interferes with sensitivity encoding, is the major disadvantage of this technique. Cardiac gating and navigator echoes have been added to this technique in order to reduce motion artifacts. Acquisition time is related to the type of breathing, and on occasion it may be long.

Free-breathing multiple averaging DWI allows shorter acquisitions than respiratory trigger sequences, although this technique allows less spatial resolution, tissue contrast and positional information than respiratory-triggered DWI. The calculated ADC map will show an increased scattering of values in the free-breathing sequences compared to the respiratory-triggering ones. On the contrary, the spatial resolution is improved, and the number of acquired *b* values may be increased compared to the breath-hold approach. ADC maps obtained from non-breath-hold sequences are less optimal to evaluate small liver lesions because of volume averaging, although the use of coregistration software may solve this problem (Fig. 3.8). Multiplanar and MIP reconstructions are possible with free breathing acquisitions, allowing fusion imaging, which are not easily feasible with the breath-hold approach.

5.4 Quantification

The T2 shine-through effect is secondary to the high signal intensity that tissues with long T2 relaxation tissues can show in DWI because of its intrinsic T2 weighting. It is one of the most common pitfalls of false restriction on DWI.

ADC maps (apparent diffusion coefficient maps) are necessary to avoid the T2 shine-through effect that can falsely be confounded with restricted diffusion. The ADC map determines the average diffusion on a pixel-by-pixel basis. It is necessary to acquire two or more images with a different gradient duration and amplitude (*b* values). The contrast in the ADC map depends on the spatially distributed diffusion coefficient of the acquired tissues and does not contain T1 and T2* values. The use of ADC maps using only *b* values superior to 100 s/mm^2 has been proposed to obtain a more accurate estimate of the real water diffusion without the perfusion effect when the IVIM approach is not performed. ADC maps allow quantification of diffusion. If only low *b* values are acquired, the diffusion weighting of the sequence decreases and the ADC value of the liver increases. With low *b* values, the perfusion and T2 time modify the ADC measurements in an important manner. This is why several authors prefer to calculate the ADC maps excluding *b* values lower than 100. When increasing the *b* values, the image quality decreases, making ADC evaluation more difficult.

For accurate quantification of DWI, it is very important to keep several rules for ROI drawing in mind. These rules were reviewed in Chap. 3 (Fig. 3.10).

5.5 Other Techniques

- *DWIBS* (diffusion weighted imaging with background body signal suppression): this sequence uses only two *b* values (typically 0 and 600–1,000 s/mm^2), being designed only for qualitative analysis. STIR and high *b* values are necessary to increase background suppression. The main clinical application is whole-body imaging (Fig. 1.9). The presentation of the images is usually performed using a MIP reconstruction with inverted gray scale to look like PET. Most of normal tissues are suppressed, although normal organs, such as the spleen, prostate, testes, ovaries, endometrium and spinal cord, may remain visible. In cases where the objective is to rule out metastatic disease in several regions or the search for a primary tumor, DWIBS can be used as the primary tool. Its reduced spatial resolution may preclude the visualization of small liver lesions, although it has been shown to depict more liver metastases than PET in several series.
- *IVIM* (intravoxel incoherent motion MR imaging): this method was developed by Le Bihan and coworkers to quantitatively assess the microscopic translational motions that occur in each image voxel at MRI. Le Bihan also demonstrated that pure molecular diffusion and microcirculation (also known as blood perfusion) can be distinguished by means of IVIM using multiple *b* values lower and higher than 100 s/mm^2, in order to assess the biexponential signal decay of the signal intensity in the abdominal organs while increasing *b* values (Fig. 3.4). There is initial rapid signal attenuation with *b* values of about 100 s/mm^2 followed by a more gradual descent in signal attenuation with the increase in *b* values. The first fast decay is due to diffusion and perfusion effects (*b* values lower than 100 s/mm^2), and the real diffusion of water molecules demonstrates a slower decay. Until the advent of respiratory-triggering DWI sequences, IVIM had not been applied in the evaluation of the liver. Recently, Luciani et al. showed the presence of restricted diffusion in patients with cirrhosis related to decreased perfusion and alteration in pure water diffusion (Fig. 5.3). To adequately calculate this biexponential signal decay, at least three *b* values should be obtained, optimally acquiring multiple *b* values under and over 100 s/mm^2. Calculation and quantification of D* (perfusion contribution to signal decay), D (real diffusion of H_20 molecules) and f (perfusion contribution to the diffusion signal) are possible with this approach. D is a more reliable marker of tissue diffusion than ADC, even when calculated using only the *b* values inferior to 100 s/mm^2. The IVIM approach can also be used to evaluate the diffusion and perfusion of focal liver lesions.

5.6 Clinical Applications in Liver Disease

5.6.1 Focal Liver Lesion Detection

DWI is one of the most sensitive noninvasive imaging techniques to detect focal liver lesions. As previously mentioned, the use of a DWI acquisition using a low *b* value (between 10 and 50 s/mm^2) increases detection of focal liver lesions, as solid lesions keep their high signal intensity against a background with the signal of

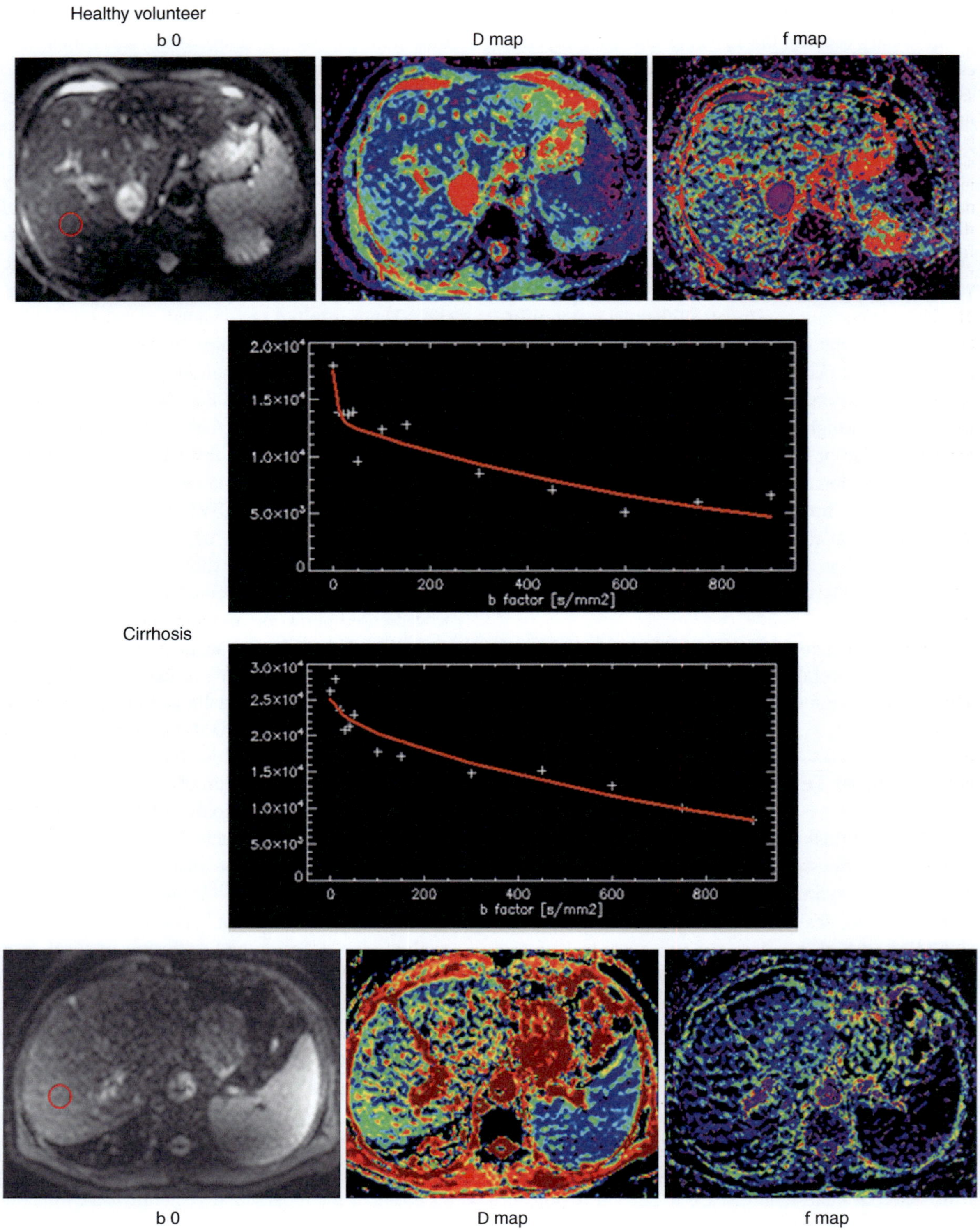
Healthy volunteer
b 0
D map
f map
2.0×10⁴
1.5×10⁴
1.0×10⁴
5.0×10³
0
0
200
400
600
800
b factor [s/mm2]
Cirrhosis
3.0×10⁴
2.5×10⁴
2.0×10⁴
1.5×10⁴
1.0×10⁴
5.0×10³
0
0
200
400
600
800
b factor [s/mm2]
b 0
D map
f map

Fig. 5.3 Evaluation of cirrhosis with an IVIM sequence. In this figure, a comparative study with a IVIM sequence of a healthy liver (*top part* of the figure) and a cirrhotic one (F4 stage) secondary to virus C hepatitis (*bottom part* of the figure) is presented. The IVIM sequence was performed in a 3-T magnet, including 12 *b* values (0, 10, 20, 30, 50, 60, 100, 150, 300, 450, 600, 750 and 900 s/mm^2). In the normal liver, the graph of the signal decay of DWI in the right lobe (area marked with the ROI in the *b* 0 s/mm^2 image) demonstrates an early fast decay of signal for *b* values under 100 s/mm^2, which is flattened in the cirrhotic liver. This difference is also reflected in the perfusion fraction parametric map (*f* maps) of both livers. *D* value of normal liver was 1.18×10^{-3} mm^2/s and in the cirrhotic one of 1.10×10^{-3} mm^2/s. Both of them were inferior to ADC values. The contribution of perfusion to diffusion signal decay was greater in the healthy liver compared to the cirrhotic one (25% vs. 9%). All these findings are in concordance with the report by Luciani and colleagues, who compared the results of applying an IVIM sequence on a 1.5-T magnet to the livers of 12 patients with documented cirrhosis and 25 healthy patients. ADC and *D** were significantly reduced in the cirrhotic liver group compared with those in the healthy liver group, but not *D* or *f* parameters. They concluded that restricted diffusion observed in patients with cirrhosis may be related to *D** variations, which reflect decreased perfusion, as well as alterations in pure molecular water diffusion in cirrhotic livers. In a more recent report by Patel and colleagues, *f*, *D**, *D* and ADC values were significantly lower in cirrhotic than in healthy livers. They compared 14 patients with cirrhosis to 16 non-cirrhotic patients using an IVIM DWI sequence and also a dynamic contrast-enhanced (DCEI) sequence. Several parameters derived from either a monocompartmental or a bicompartmental analysis of the dynamic contrast-enhanced series were increased in cirrhotic livers. The combination of ADC with distribution volume and time to peak provided 84.6% sensitivity and 100% specificity for the diagnosis of cirrhosis, although there was no correlation between IVIM- and DCE-MRI parameters. Therefore, the combination of parameters derived from diffusion and dynamic contrast-enhanced sequences may provide accurate diagnosis of cirrhosis

vessels completely suppressed. DWI in combination with conventional T2- and T1-weighted sequences has been demonstrated to be superior to SPIO MRI in the counting of hepatic metastases. DWI has also been shown to be superior to different T2-weighted sequences (Fig. 5.2), including fat-suppressed and STIR sequences, in the detection of focal liver lesions and metastases, being especially useful in the detection of lesions smaller than 1 cm and those adjacent to vascular structures. The increase of detection of hepatocellular carcinoma (HCC) with DWI compared to T2-weighted sequences is still under debate. Therefore, DWI has replaced STIR or fat-suppressed T2-weighted sequences in many institutions.

DWI in combination with manganese-enhanced MRI in the study of hepatic metastasis, with SPIO in the detection of HCC and metastases along with dynamic contrast imaging in the detection of small hepatocellular lesions has improved the results of their counterparts alone. Very recently, DWI has shown the potential to increase sensitivity for the detection of liver metastases in addition to gadoxetic acid-enhanced MRI, but not for detecting HCC. Shimada et al. reported higher accuracy in the detection of small metastases with gadoxetic acid-enhanced MRI than with DWI, although they used an acquisition with a *b* value of 500 s/mm^2, not a black-blood DWI sequence, which is an important limitation. Previous reports have highlighted the superiority of black-blood DWI in the detection of focal liver lesions compared to acquisitions with higher *b* values (Fig. 5.2). According to these data, DWI may be considered a reasonable alternative to gadolinium chelates or hepatospecific contrast media in patients at risk for nephrogenic systemic fibrosis.

Furthermore, DWI outperforms multislice CT in the detection of liver metastasis in patients with either colorectal or pancreatic cancers.

5.6.2 Characterization of Focal Liver Lesions

DWI is very useful in the distinction between benign and malignant focal liver lesions and in the differentiation between hemangiomas and metastases. Visual inspection of high *b* value (over 600 s/mm^2) images allows a fast assessment of the presence of solid lesions, as the cyst tends to disappear on DWI with high *b* values (Fig. 5.2). For further characterization of solid focal liver lesions, it is necessary to perform ADC measurements. Benign lesions tend to show higher ADC values and lower signal intensity with high *b* values than malignant ones. Etturk et al., using a DWI sequence with a maximum *b* value of 1,000 s/mm^2, showed a sensitivity of 91% and a specificity of 94% in the differentiation between hemangiomas and metastases with an ADC threshold of 1.45×10^{-3} mm²/s. In the same series, using a cutoff ADC value of 1.63×10^{-3} mm²/s, the distinction between benign and malignant focal lesions was possible with a sensitivity of 95% and specificity of 91%. These results are similar to those of previous series using different DWI sequences and *b* values, with the ADC cutoff range proposed to be between 1.4 and 1.6 63×10^{-3} mm²/s in the distinction between benign and malignant lesions, with reported sensitivity and specificity between 74% and 100%. However, an important overlap exists in the ADC value of benign and malignant lesions, especially of focal nodular hyperplasia (FNH) and adenomas with HCC and metastasis, as will be described in the next section. The presence of intratumoral necrosis, areas of cystic degeneration or mucinous content may falsely increase the ADC values of malignant lesions, with the potential of a false-negative result. Therefore, DWI cannot be used alone for the characterization of focal liver lesions, although improvements in accuracy can be expected if it is used in combination with information from morphological and perfusion sequences.

5.6.3 Benign Focal Liver Lesions

The most common benign hepatic lesions, cysts and hemangiomas, are easily identified with DWI. Cysts show the highest ADC values (mean ADC values in different series between 3 and 3.7×10^{-3} mm²/s) and disappear on DWI with *b* values superior to 400 s/mm² (Fig. 5.2). Hemangiomas show the second highest ADC values of all focal liver lesions at between 1.9 and 2.95×10^{-3} mm²/s (Fig. 4.8). A small overlap between ADC values of cysts and hemangiomas has been described. Commonly hemangiomas lose signal and disappear with high *b* values; in our experience, hemangiomas tend to show T2 shine-through, with ADC quantification being necessary in order to exclude other hypercellular lesions as metastases. Both typical and atypical hemangiomas do not show a significant restriction of water molecule motion.

FNH typically shows restricted diffusion, with their ADC values in several series being intermediate between benign and malignant lesions (between 1.4 and 1.75×10^{-3} mm²/s) (Fig. 5.4). An overlap of the ADC value of FNH with that of malignant hepatocellular has been reported. Adenomas typically demonstrate similar behavior to FNH on DWI.

Fig. 5.4 Focal nodular hyperplasia. A 45-year-old female with several focal liver lesions detected on a ultrasound exam was submitted to our MRI unit to eliminate the possibility of liver metastasis.
Imaging Findings A slightly hyperintense lesion was identified on the axial TSE T2-weighted sequence (**5.4.1**), demonstrating a highly hyperintense central scar, located in segment III (*arrow*). In the dynamic contrast-enhanced series (Figs. **5.3.2–5.3.5**, corresponding to precontrast, arterial, portal and equilibrium postcontrast phases, respectively), this lesion showed the typical behavior of an FNH, a homogeneous early enhancement during arterial phase, with a rapid washout, being nearly isointense to the liver in the equilibrium phase. The scar demonstrated a slowly progressive enhancement. On the delayed hepatocellular phase with gadolinium-BOPTA (**5.4.6**), we can clearly see how the lesion is isointense to the rest of the liver parenchyma, reflecting their hepatocyte content. On DWI this focal liver lesion showed a moderate restriction (*arrows*), appearing hyperintense on both *b* 0 mm²/s (**5.4.7**) and *b* 1,000 mm²/s images (**5.4.8**). On the ADC map (**5.4.9**), the lesion appears moderately hypointense (*arrow*), with a mean ADC value of 1.5×10^{-3} mm²/s, remaining hyperintense the central scar, which did not demonstrate impeded water diffusion. The rest of the lesions seen on ultrasound correspond to liver hemangiomas (not shown).
Comments FNHs are lesions that typically contain hepatocytes, bile duct elements, Kupffer cells and fibrous tissue. They have a characteristic central scar in 10–49% of the cases. Their MRI appearance is slightly hypointense on T1-weighted and slightly hyperintense on T2-weighted sequences, typically presenting a central scar with high signal intensity on T2-weighted sequences. FNHs characteristically are hypervascular lesions, enhancing with an intense uniform blush on immediate postgadolinium images, having a quick washout and being nearly isointense to the liver parenchyma, typically at 1 min after contrast administration. On delayed hepatocellular phases, using hepatospecific contrast media, FNHs show enhancement in the same fashion or even higher than the rest of the liver parenchyma, because of their hepatocyte content. This last feature is important in the differentiation between FNHs and adenoma, as the latter may present similar MRI features to FNHs, especially in those without a central scar, but adenomas do not show enhancement in the hepatobiliary phase because of their lack of biliary ducts.On DWI, FNHs typically show restricted diffusion, with their ADC values in several series being intermediate between benign and malignant lesions (between 1.4 and 1.75×10^{-3} mm²/s). Overlap of the ADC values of FNH with those of malignant hepatocellular lesions has been reported. Adenomas behave similarly on DWI, which is not useful in their differential diagnosis

DWI is useful in the distinction between simple and hydatid cysts, as hydatid cysts most commonly remain as bright areas with high *b* values and show low ADC values (Fig. 5.5). Biliary cystoadenoma should be included in the same differential diagnosis.

Pyogenic hepatic abscesses show low ADC values because of their dense viscous content, demonstrating overlap with malignant lesions (Fig. 5.6). Therefore, as in other anatomic regions, hepatic abscesses are a potential pitfall for malignant disease. In the short number of reported cases of amebic abscesses using DWI, they have demonstrated higher ADC values than pyogenic ones. The ADC values of inflammatory lesions change over time depending on the phase of evolution. In the acute inflammatory phase, they show lower ADC values than later when liquefaction occurs.

5.6.4 Malignant Focal Liver Lesions

In most of the published series, metastases have demonstrated the lowest ADC values of all benign or malignant focal liver lesions (ADC values between

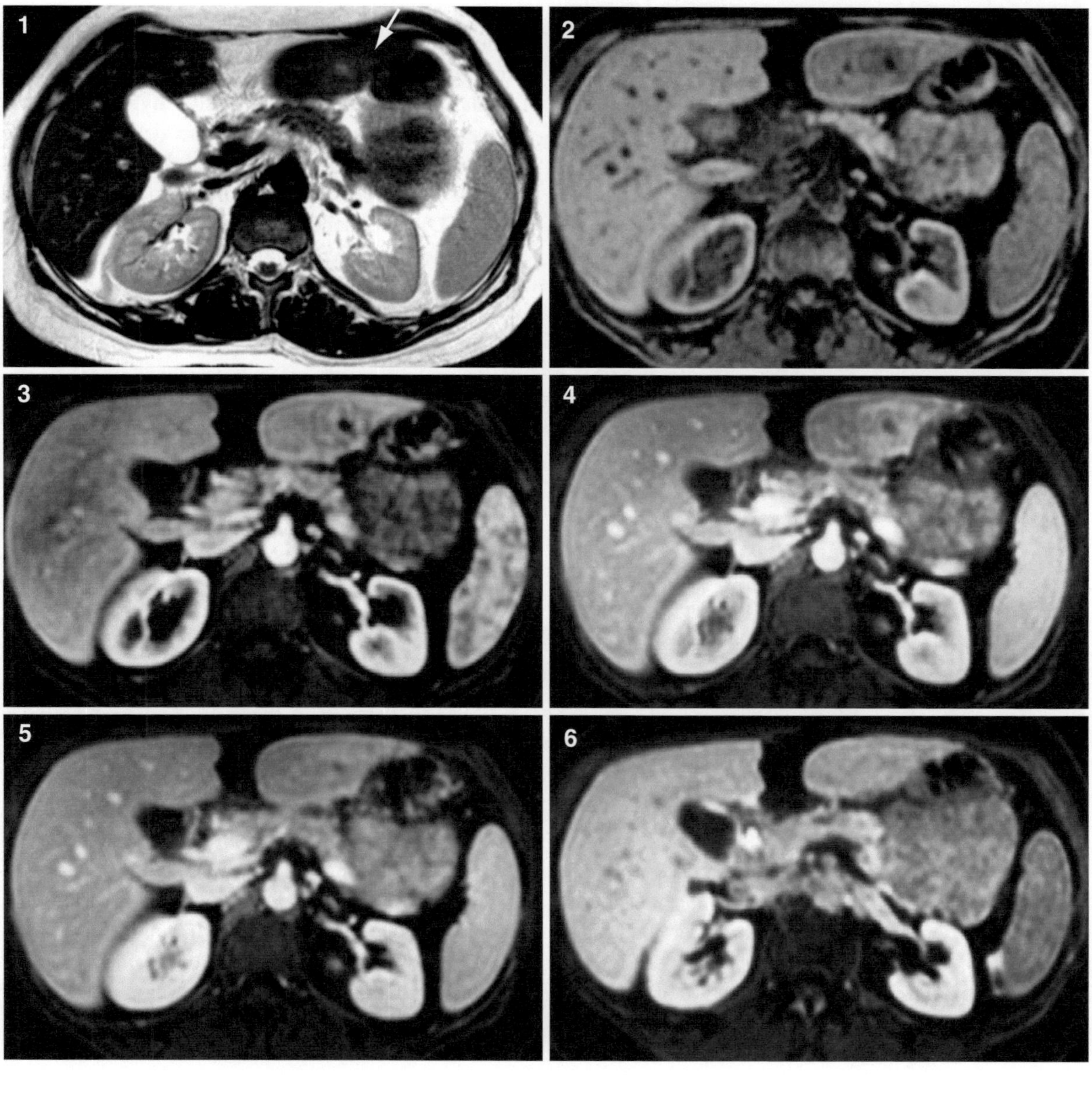

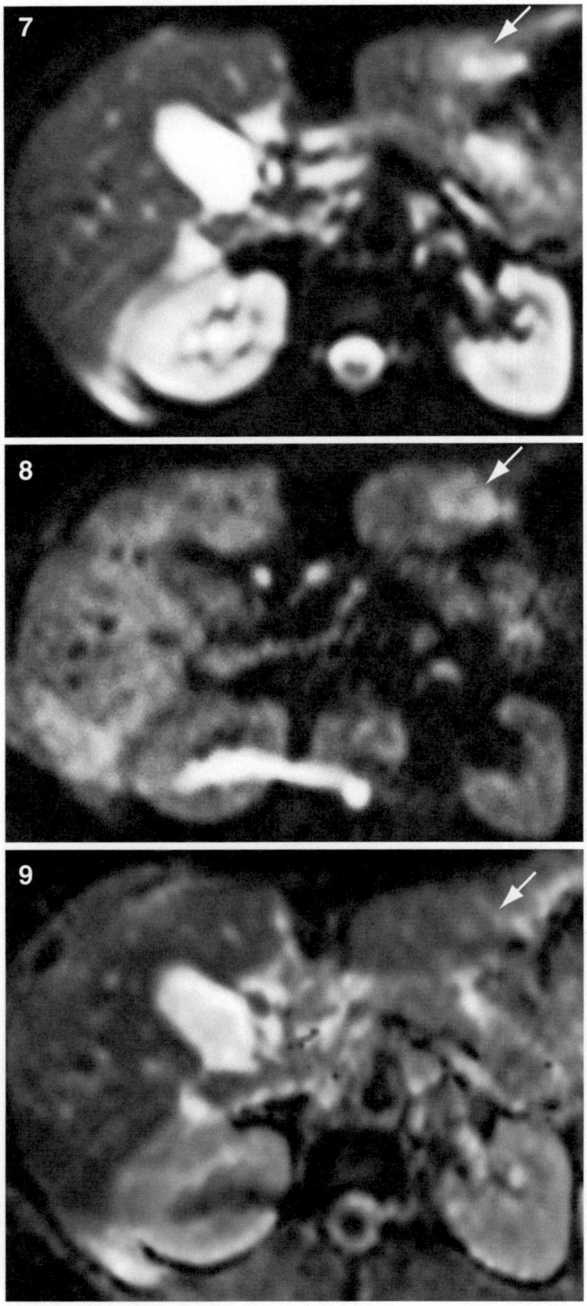

Fig. 5.4 (continued)

0.6 and 1.2×10^{-3} mm²/s). DWI improves detection of metastatic disease, which can be an important fact in presurgical counting of colorectal cancer metastases (Fig. 5.2).

Cholangiocarcinoma shows restriction of the diffusion in the hypercellular areas, although the central fibrous core usually does not show impeded diffusion in a significant manner. Mean ADC values of cholangiocarcinoma are slightly superior to those of HCC. In our experience, hepatic involvement by lymphoma also shows restricted diffusion because of marked cellularity.

5.6.5 Focal Liver Lesions in the Cirrhotic Liver

HCC shows restriction of water diffusion in a parallel manner to its grade of cellularity and undifferentiation. However, predicting the correct histopathologic grade of HCC on the basis of DWI findings is challenging because of the large overlap among histopathological grades (Fig. 5.7). Mean ADC values of HCC range from 0.90 to 1.55×10^{-3} mm^2/s in different series. Dysplastic nodules are usually hypointense on T2-weighted images, and they can demonstrate low ADC values because of increased cellularity and decreased perfusion. In a study by Muhi and colleagues using a DWI sequence with a high b value of 1000 s/mm^2, the mean ADC values of moderately poorly differentiated HCCs were significantly lower than those of well-differentiated HCCs and dysplastic nodules. Interestingly, all hypovascular tumors showing high signal intensity on high b value images corresponded to poorly differentiated HCCs, whereas lesions not visible on DW-MRI were low grade HCCs or dysplastic nodules. Conversely to previous published data, a recent series by Xu and colleagues described a promising role for DWI in the distinction between HCC and dysplastic nodules. With a high b value, HCCs showed high signal intensity in 97.5% of the cases, and dysplastic nodules demonstrated isointensity or low signal intensity compared to liver in 79% of the cases. Besides, ADC values of HCCs were significantly lower than those of dysplastic nodules. DWI has been proposed along with dynamic contrast-enhanced series to establish new diagnostic criteria increasing the sensitivity in the diagnosis of HCC.

Regenerative nodules are similar in cellularity and vascularity to normal liver, not showing alteration of signal on DWI. DWI can also help in the differential diagnosis of benign entities, which can mimic HCC in the cirrhotic liver as either focal confluent fibrosis or perfusion alterations such as arterioportal shunts (Fig. 5.8). These lesions will not show alteration of signal on high b value images.

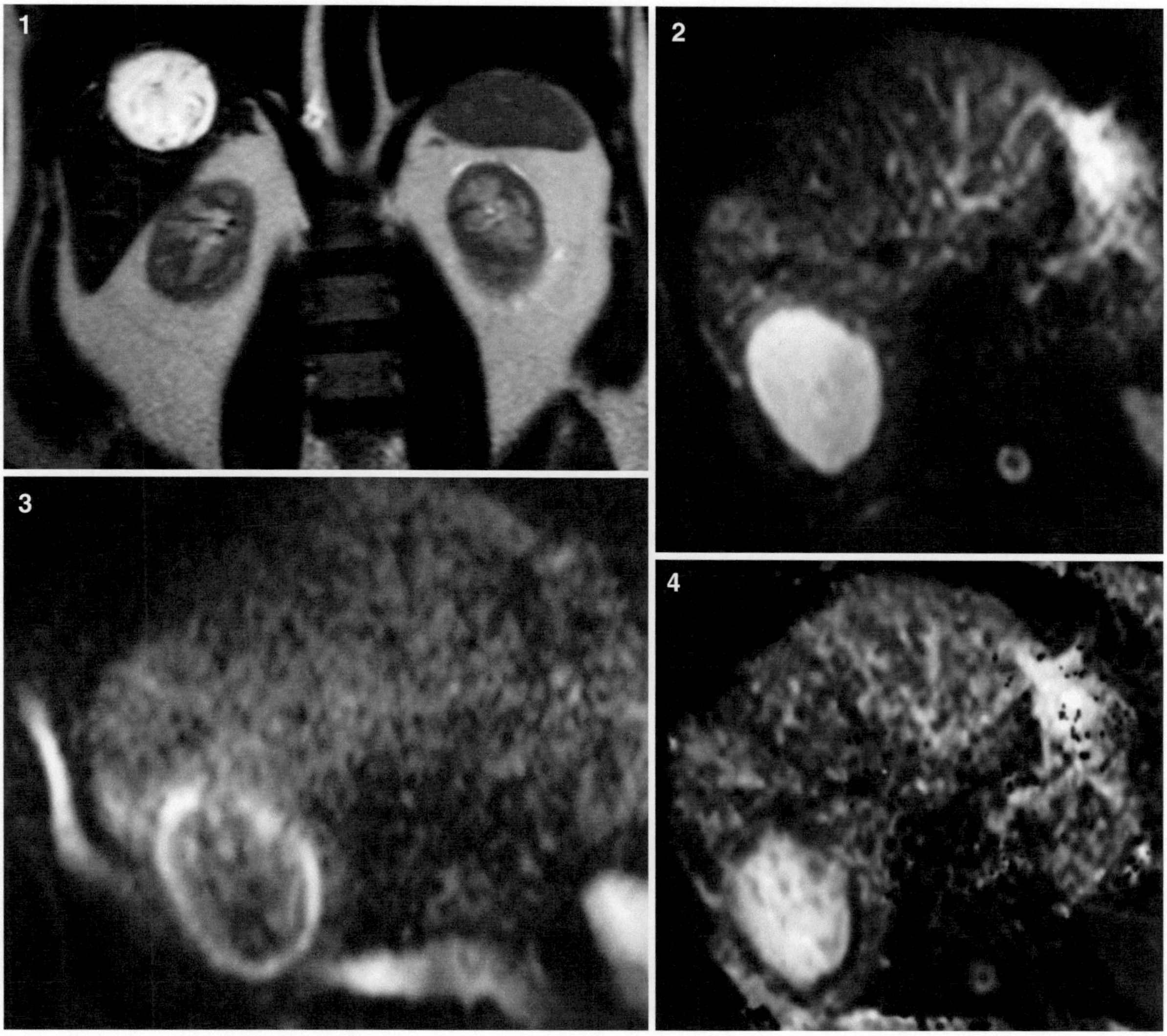

Fig. 5.5 Hydatic cyst. A 59-year-old female with abdominal pain incidentally presented a complex cystic lesion on a prior ultrasound exam. She was submitted to our department for a MRI study for characterization of this focal liver lesion.

Imaging Findings A hyperintense lesion is detected on coronal HASTE (**5.5.1**), containing linear hypointense structures inside, representing detached membranes of an hydatid cyst. On DWI, this lesion appears as a hyperintense lesion on b 0 s/mm^2 image (**5.5.2**), demonstrating a progressive loss of signal with a *b* value of 1,000 s/mm^2 (**5.5.3**), but containing tiny hyperintense areas inside the lesion, and also with hyperintensity of the capsule. On the ADC map (**5.5.4**), the mass appears mostly hyperintense, although there are tiny areas of hyperintensity on DWI with a high *b* value image, which are hypointense on ADC, representing the detached membranes of the cyst. The mean ADC value of this lesion was 2.4×10^{-3} mm^2/s.

Comments MRI has several advantages for the diagnosis of hydatid disease over other imaging modalities. MRI is useful in the characterization of the contents of the hydatid cyst matrix. MR cholangiography is an extremely helpful tool for the assessment of the potential communication between the hydatid cyst and the biliary tree. MR's lack of ionizing radiation permits the follow-up of non-specific appearing lesions in order to assess their growth pattern. Nevertheless, the major limitation of MRI in the evaluation of hydatid cysts is its inability to accurately detect calcifications. Daughter cysts, membranes and vesicles are typically identified as they appear as hypo- or isointense to mother cyst internal matrix on T1-weighted and T2-weighted images. Collapsed membranes are shown as linear serpentine hypointense structures on all pulse sequences. This is known as the snake sign. Daughter cysts can appear arranged at the periphery of the mother cyst, occupying the whole mother cyst (rosette or wheel-spoke appearance) or seen as solid masses, representing consolidated daughter cysts. DWI is useful in the distinction between simple and complicated or hydatid cysts, as the latter more commonly remain as bright areas with high *b* values and show lower ADC values than simple cysts. In the series by Inan and colleagues, 95% of hydatid cysts were hyperintense on DWI with a $b = 1{,}000$ s/mm^2. The ADC and cyst-to-liver ADC ratio of the hydatid cysts were significantly lower than those of simple cysts. Furthermore, Oruc and colleagues highlighted the role of DWI in the differentiation between abscesses and simple cysts from hydatid cysts, although this differentiation was not achieved based on ADC measurements alone in the concrete cases of unilocular non-complicated hydatid cysts from simple cysts and heterogeneous hydatid cysts without daughter vesicles from abscesses

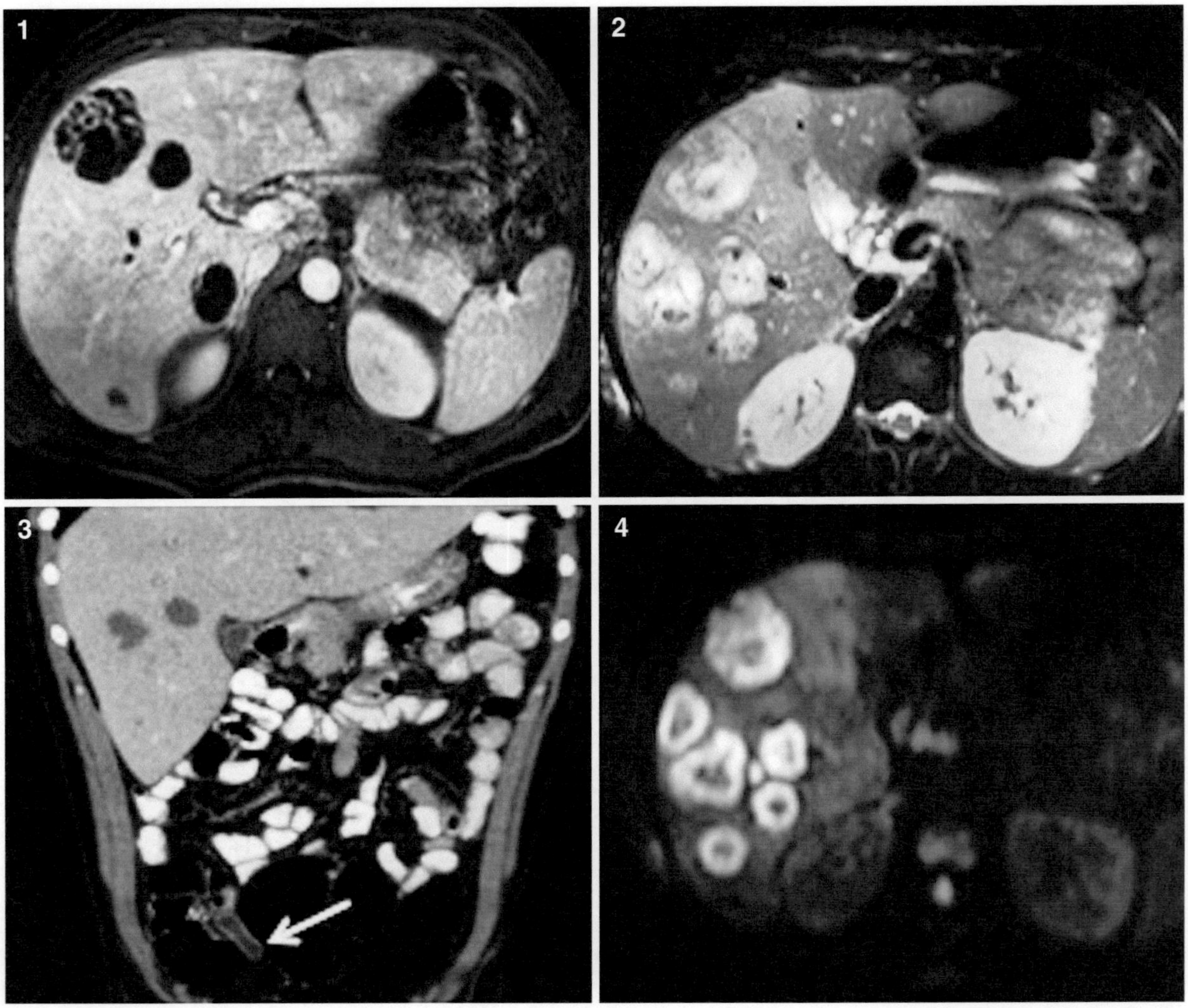

Fig. 5.6 **Hepatic abscesses secondary to appendicitis**. A 48-year-old male patient presented with acute right lower quadrant abdominal pain and fever. CT and MRI were performed for further assessment.

Imaging Findings (5.6.1) Axial contrast-enhanced T1 gradient echo image with fat saturation shows multiple round, focal hepatic lesions, which are hypointense and contain internal septations that enhance with gadolinium. (5.6.2) Axial T2-weighted image with fat saturation demonstrates focal lesions, which are heterogeneous in signal intensity, but predominantly hyperintense. (5.6.3) CT with MPR reconstruction in the coronal plane demonstrates a dilated and fluid-filled appendix (arrow). (5.6.4) DWI acquired with a b factor of 1,000 s/mm^2 shows the focal hepatic lesions with high signal intensity in the periphery, indicating restricted diffusion by hepatic abscesses.

Comments Acute appendicitis is the most common acute gastrointestinal disease that requires surgery in pregnant women and the general population. The usual clinical manifestations of appendicitis are leukocytosis, fever and right lower quadrant pain. MR imaging has high reported sensitivity (97–100%) and specificity (92–93%) for the diagnosis of acute appendicitis. The imaging criteria of non-perforated acute appendicitis are similar to those found with other cross-sectional modalities and include appendiceal diameter and wall thickness greater than 7 mm and 2 mm, respectively, and inflammatory changes in the peri-appendiceal fat. DWI demonstrates the inflamed appendix and surrounding fat as bright, secondary to restricted diffusion of water. Peri-appendiceal abscesses, septic portal thrombosis and hepatic abscesses can complicate acute appendicitis. Hepatic and peri-appendiceal abscesses demonstrate high signal intensity on and low signal on the respective ADC map, an indication of restricted diffusion. Liver abscesses can mimic necrotic liver metastases or hydatid cysts. DWI may aid in the differentiation between purulent abscesses and necrotic metastases. Pyogenic hepatic abscesses show low ADC values due to their dense viscous content, demonstrating overlap with malignant lesions. Furthermore, different characteristics of hepatic abscess have been described according to its age. Higher ADC values may be expected as the maturation process occurs. The small number of reported cases of amebic abscesses using DWI have demonstrated higher ADC values than pyogenic ones

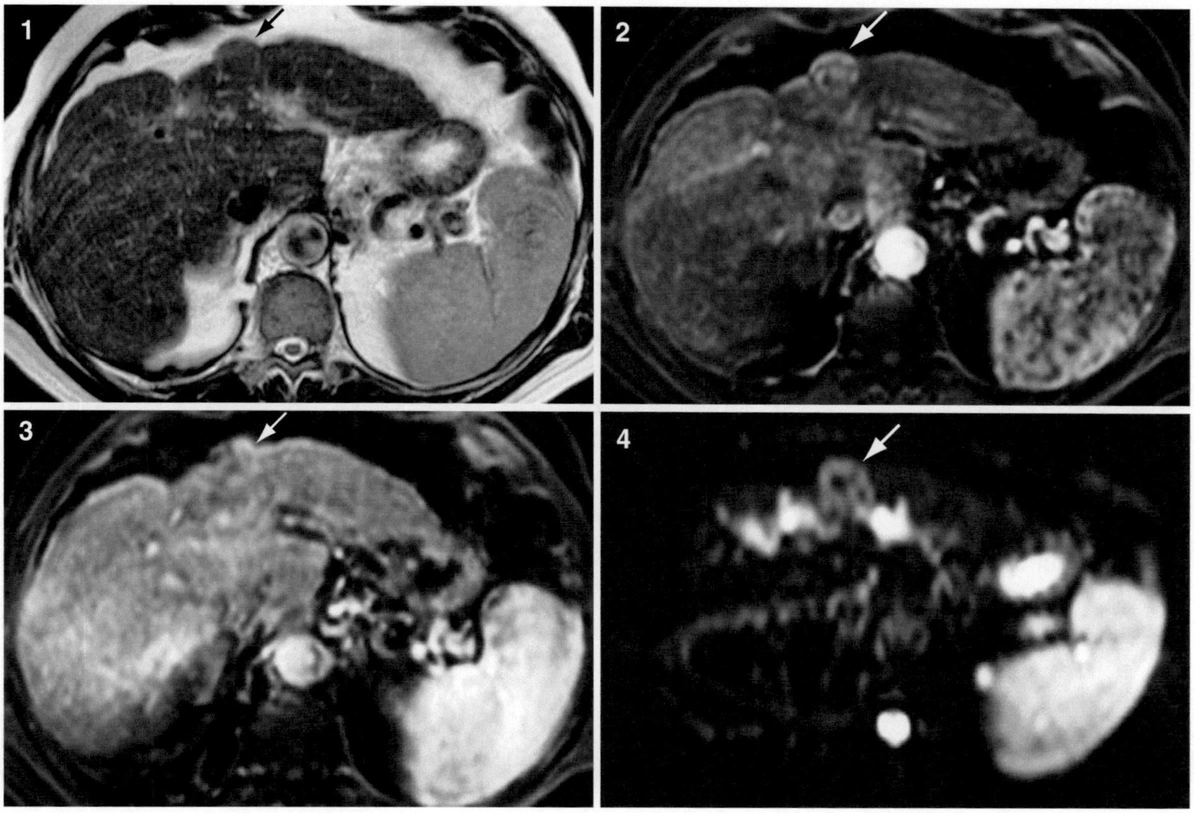

Fig. 5.7 Well-differentiated HCC. A 56-year-old with cirrhosis secondary to hepatitis C virus was submitted to our MRI unit for evaluation of a hypoechoic focal liver lesion of 2 cm in the left hepatic lobe on ultrasound.

Imaging Findings In this case we can see a cirrhotic liver with a slightly hyperintense nodule (arrow) on TSE T2-weighted images located in the anterior aspect of segment II (5.7.1). The nodule was hypervascular (arrow) in the arterial phase of the dynamic series (5.7.2). Posteriorly, in the postcontrast equilibrium phase, the nodule remained heterogeneously enhanced (arrow) compared to liver parenchyma (5.7.3). These findings in a cirrhotic liver may correspond either to a high grade dysplastic nodule or well-differentiated HCC. On DWI, the nodule showed high signal intensity (arrows) on both images with b values of 0 and 1,000 mm^2/s (5.7.4 and 5.7.5, respectively). The ADC map confirmed the moderate restriction of water diffusion of the lesion (ADC value: 1.1×10^{-3} mm^2/s) (arrow). After surgery, the nodule was confirmed to be a well-differentiated HCC.

Comments Any chronic liver disease leading to cirrhosis may be complicated by HCC. Neoplastic development in the liver can be seen as a multi-step process that is triggered by a variety of events. The multi-step development of HCC may be as follows: macro-regenerative nodule Þ low-grade dysplastic nodule Þ high-grade dysplastic nodule Þ well-differentiated HCC Þ undifferentiated HCC. Meanwhile, a nodule becomes undifferentiated, it progressively loses portal vascularization and increases the arterial perfusion. This is the reason why the more undifferentiated a nodule is, the more hypervascular in the arterial phase with faster wash-out in the portal phase it becomes. A reliable distinction between dysplastic nodules and well-differentiated hepatocarcinoma has not been demonstrated using any of the imaging techniques and is even challenging after nodulectomy for pathologists. Therefore, achieving this differentiation with a noninvasive method is critical for patient management. Like other novel imaging modalities, DWI is being evaluated for this purpose, although there is still no extensive experience. From the published data, some conclusions can be reached: (1) HCC shows restriction of water diffusion in a parallel manner to the grade of cellularity and undifferentiation; (2) the assessment of HCC differentiation only based on DWI behavior is not possible due to the large overlap in findings among histopathological grades; (3) dysplastic nodules, which are usually hypointense on T2-weighted images, usually show higher ADC values than HCC, although they can demonstrate low ADC values because of the increased cellularity and decreased perfusion; (4) DWI can be considered an adjunct tool to morphological and contrast-enhanced MRI sequences in the evaluation of hepatocarcinogenesis. In this sense, a recent series by Xu and colleagues presented optimistic data for the distinction between HCC and dysplastic nodules with DWI. In this series, HCCs showed high signal intensity in 97.5% of the cases and dysplastic nodules demonstrated isointensity or low signal intensity compared to liver in 79% of the cases in high b value images. Besides, ADC values of HCC were significantly lower than that of dysplastic nodules. Furthermore, DWI has been recently proposed along with dynamic contrast-enhanced series to establish new diagnostic criteria for HCC, increasing the sensitivity of its diagnosis

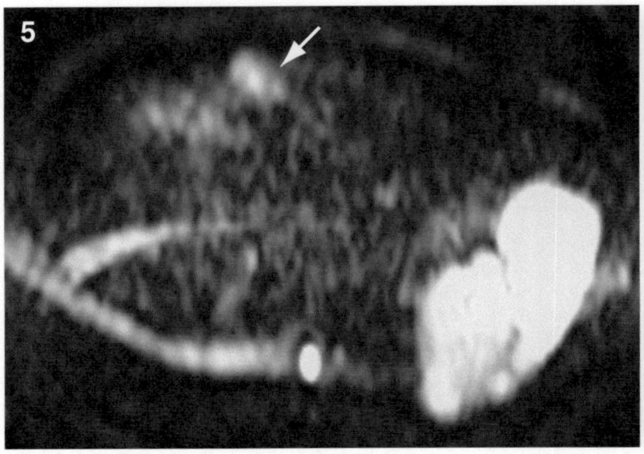

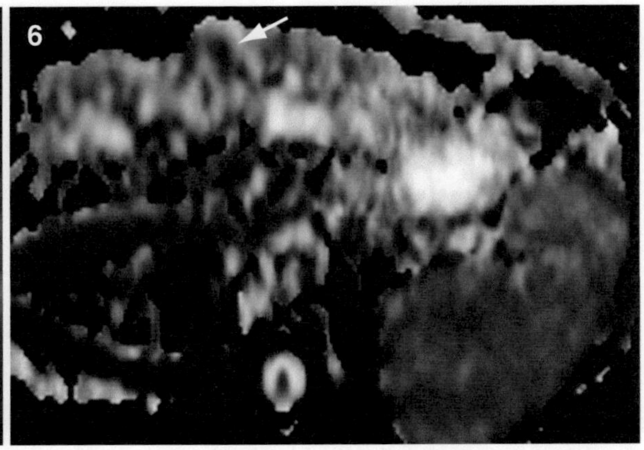

Fig. 5.7 (continued)

Portal vein thrombosis can be accurately depicted with DWI. Besides, Catalano and colleagues have recently reported promising results using DWI in the distinction between tumoral and bland portal thrombosis.

5.6.6 Monitoring Response to Treatment

DWI and ADC quantifications have been advocated as an early functional marker of tumor response to treatment. Several series have evaluated the role of DWI in the early response of HCC to transcatheter arterial chemoembolization (TACE). These studies have demonstrated measurable differences in ADC between viable and necrotic portions of HCCs before and after treatment. A fast and significant increase in the ADC value of the treated HCC, 2 or 3 days after TACE, has been related to good response. Anyhow, changes in HCC enhancement after TACE are faster and larger than ADC value changes, both being faster than variations in tumor size. Furthermore, DWI can be used to distinguish recurrent tumor from necrotic areas in HCC after TACE plus radiofrequency ablation. In patients submitted to TACE prior to liver transplantation, a significant correlation between ADC and necrosis has been achieved, as assessed with histopathology. In a series by Chung and colleagues, patients with HCC treated with TACE whose ADC increased from baseline by >15% immediately after TACE had a 100% rate of predicting a positive response at 1 month after therapy.

A significant increase during the first 3 months after treatment of the mean ADC value of HCC treated with Ytrium-90 radioembolization has also been related to adequate treatment response. DWI has not been shown to be a reliable predictor of local HCC recurrence after TACE as compared with enhanced MRI. In HCC treated with the antiangiogenic agent sorafenib, ADC first decreases and posteriorly increases, probably related to a reduction of extracellular space and vascular normalization (Fig. 5.9).

DWI and ADC measurements also have a role in pre- and posttreatment evaluation of hepatic metastases. In the prechemotherapy analysis of liver metastases from gastric and colorectal carcinoma, mean ADC values are lower in responding lesions in comparison with those of non-responding ones (Fig. 5.10). An early increase in ADC values in the first week after treatment is also typical of responding metastasis. There is not defined a threshold increase in ADC for considering a metastasis as responding or not.

5.6.7 Diffuse Liver Disease

DWI has been advocated to diagnose and stage liver fibrosis, in order to substitute the current gold standard, liver biopsy, which is associated with morbidity and sampling error. The mean ADC value of liver fibrosis patients is significantly lower than that of normal controls except for the initial grades of the disease (METAVIR stage 1). Therefore, DWI has been tested to distinguish moderate to severe hepatic fibrosis (F2 to F4) from mild grades (F0-F1), although, according to

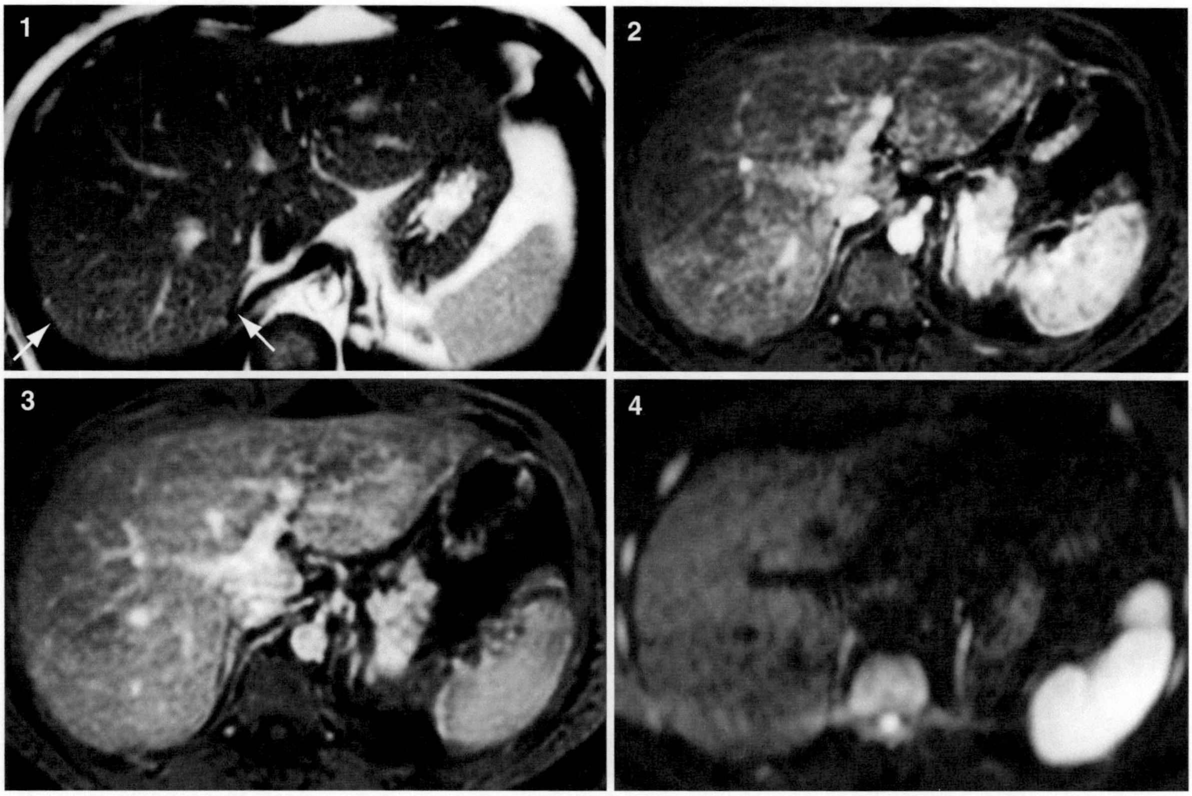

Fig. 5.8 Focal confluent fibrosis. A 53-year-old female with cirrhosis secondary to hepatitis C virus was submitted to our MRI unit for an abdominal MRI for further characterization of an ill-defined area of heterogeneous echogenicity in a recent ultrasound study.

Imaging Findings There was a peripheral ill-defined area of high signal intensity on T2-weighted sequences (5.8.1) located in the posterior aspect of segment VII (arrows). This area caused a slight retraction of the hepatic contour, representing areas of focal confluent fibrosis. The lesion showed hypervascularity on the postcontrast arterial phase (5.8.2), and it was predominantly isointense to liver parenchyma in the 2-min postcontrast delayed phase (5.8.3). On DWI, with a b value of 1,000 mm^2/s (5.8.4), the lesion showed no signal abnormality, being isointense to the liver.

Comments Focal confluent fibrosis represents large areas of confluent fibrotic masses in patients with advanced cirrhosis. Although its CT appearance is well known, there are limited reports describing their MR features. Their most common morphologic presentations are: total lobar or segmental involvement, and wedge-shaped or peripheral band-like lesions, usually associated with capsular retraction or volume loss. Their signal intensity varies in a similar manner to fibrotic tissue in other regions. In the acute phase, due to higher water content, they show high signal intensity on T2-weighted images and low signal intensity in chronic stages. On T1-weighted images, focal confluent fibrosis usually shows low-signal intensity. Enhancement of these lesions on a dynamic series is variable, although it is more intense on delayed phases. Their differential diagnosis includes tumors with high fibrotic components such as cholangiocarcinoma, hepatocarcinoma and fibrolamellar hepatocarcinoma. On DWI, focal confluent fibrosis typically does not show any restriction of water motion with high b values. Furthermore, in a recent series, the mean ADC value of focal confluent fibrosis ($2.07 \pm 0.39 \times 10^{-3}$ mm^2/s) was significantly greater than that of background cirrhotic liver parenchyma ($1.53 \pm 0.35 \times 10^{-3}$ mm^2/s), but it has been reported that in its earlier phase of fibrosis formation associated with cirrhosis, it may show restricted diffusion in relation to more cellular areas of fibrosis. DWI is an adjunct tool in the differential diagnosis of benign entities that can mimic HCC in the cirrhotic liver as either focal confluent fibrosis or perfusion alterations such as arterioportal shunts, because these lesions will not usually show alteration of signal on high b value images. Meanwhile, HCC usually shows high signal intensity on high b value images. Besides, regenerative nodules are similar in cellularity and vascularity to normal liver, not showing alteration of signal on DWI, with their accurate distinction from malignant lesions also being possible by means of DWI

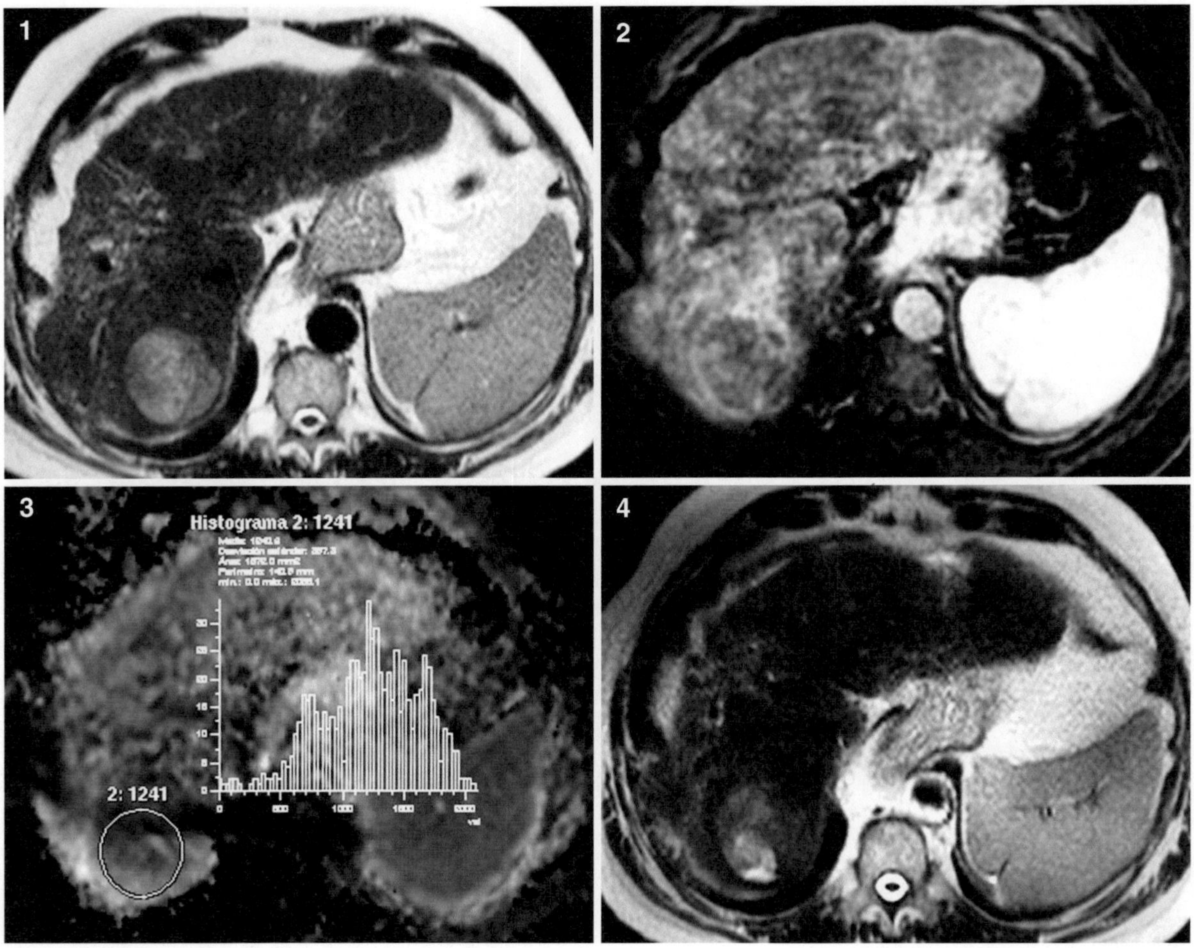

Fig. 5.9 Monitoring response to treatment of HCC. A 64-year-old male with antecedent of virus C hepatitis was submitted to our imaging center for a liver MRI for further characterization of a focal liver lesion in segment 7.

Imaging Findings Basal MRI showed a hyperintense nodule of 5 cm maximum diameter on T2-weighted sequence (5.9.1), with heterogeneous and poor enhancement on the arterial phase (5.9.2) and with moderate restriction of DWI as shown in the ADC map (mean ADC value of 1.24×10^{-3} mm^2/s) (5.9.3). A percutaneous biopsy could establish a diagnosis of poorly differentiated HCC. The patient was treated with tamoxifen and interferon due to concomitant systemic diseases that precluded surgery or other conservative treatments. Corresponding HASTE, postcontrast arterial phase THRIVE and ADC map of a follow-up MRI performed 5 months after the start of therapy (5.9.4–5.9.6, respectively) showed absence of growth of the tumor with areas of central necrosis and elevation of the ADC (mean ADC value of 1.42×10^{-3} mm^2/s), indicating theoretically partial response. However, the ADC histogram demonstrates a heterogeneus distribution of ADC values due to the presence of necrosis, which is increasing mean ADC. Therefore, mean ADC of viable HCC avoiding necrosis was that of 1.2 x 10^{-3} mm^2/s, similar to previous MRI. Corresponding HASTE, postcontrast arterial phase THRIVE and ADC map of another follow-up MRI study performed 18 months after the initial diagnosis (5.9.7–5.9.9, respectively) demonstrated a mild increase in the size of the tumor (maximum diameter 6 cm), heterogeneous increased arterial enhancement and reduction of ADC value compared to previous the MRI (ADC value of 1.21×10^{-3} mm^2/s), indicating persisting tumoral activity.

Comments HCC is a tumor with poor prognosis, and only 20% of patients will benefit from curative therapies (surgery, liver transplantation, percutaneous ablation). Systemic therapy with either a single drug or multidrugs is in effective, with a response rate of less than 20%. Immunotherapy, such as interferon or other cytokines, is not beneficial. Hormone therapy has not been promising, except for treatment with tamoxifen, which has been reported to show some beneficial effect. Gene therapy is still in its infancy. DWI has been proposed as a functional biomarker of treatment response to various types of treatment for HCC, such as TACE, Ytrium-90 radioembolization or antiangiogenic drugs. As a general rule, increases in ADC after treatment are related to partial or complete response. The exact mechanism of this process is unknown. Further research of the role of DWI in the therapeutic monitorization of HCC is necessary

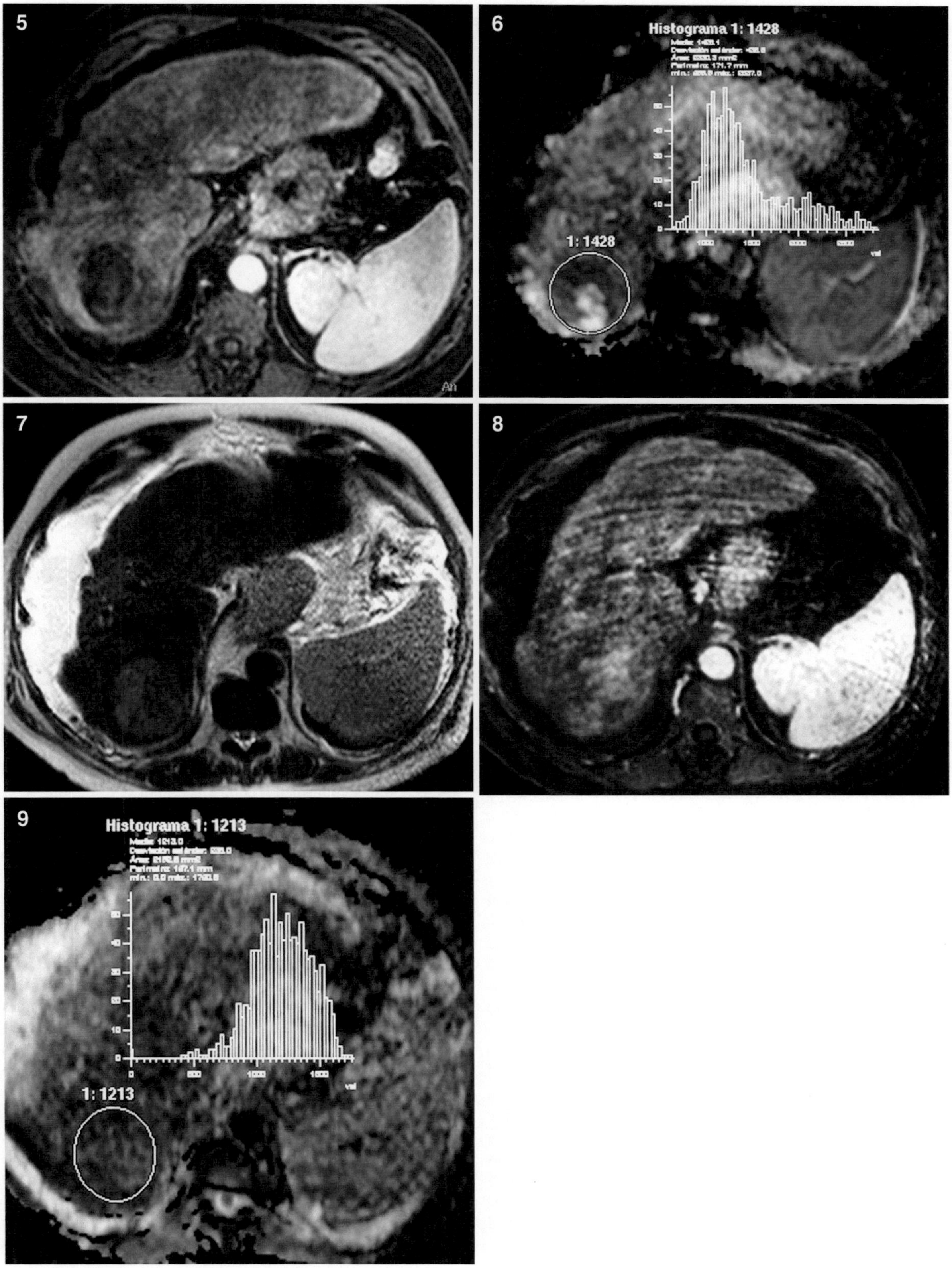

Fig. 5.9 (continued)

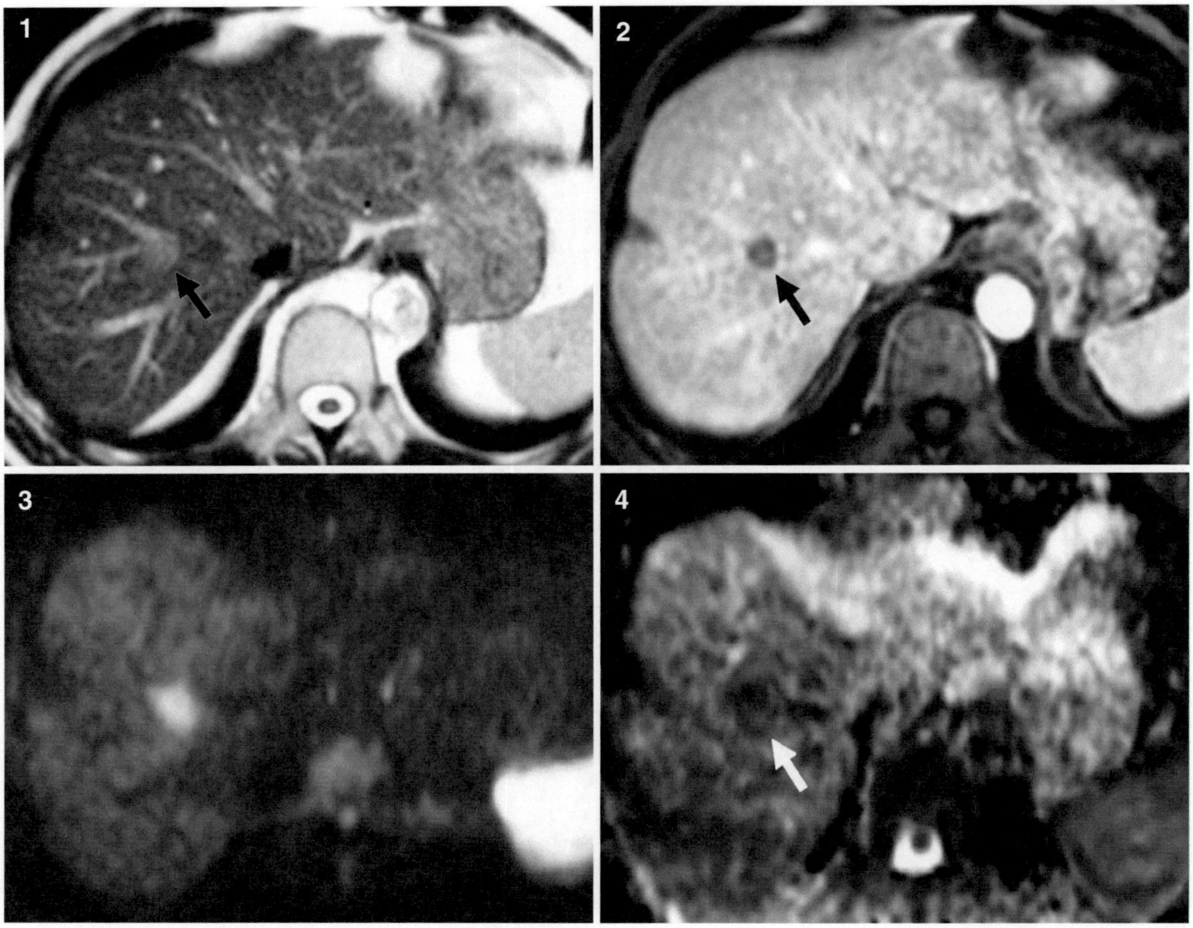

Fig. 5.10 Monitoring response to treatment of metastases. A 62-year-old male with clinical history of colorectal carcinoma was submitted to our department for follow-up hepatic imaging. Liver MRI demonstrated three liver metastases, which were treated with chemotherapy. Three months after the start of treatment, a new MRI was performed to assess response.

Imaging Findings In this case we identified three liver focal lesions before chemotherapy that were diagnosed as liver metastases from colorectal carcinoma. All of them presented similar behavior on MRI. Due to space limitations, only one of them will be presented. In the pretreatment MRI, a slightly hyperintense lesion on T2-weighted image was identified (*arrow*) in segment 8 (**5.10.1**), presenting typical peripheral enhancement (*arrow*) on postcontrast dynamic series (**5.10.2**). On DWI, this metastasis showed marked hyperintensity on *b* value image of 1,000 mm^2/s (**5.10.3**) and low signal (*arrow*) on the ADC map (**5.10.4**). The mean ADC value was 0.9×10^{-3} mm^2/s, predicting a good response to chemotherapy.In the follow-up MRI study performed 3 months after chemotherapy, the metastasis has completely disappeared (*arrows*), as can be seen in corresponding HASTE, postcontrast THRIVE, DWI with a *b* value of 1,000 mm^2/s and ADC map (**5.10.5–5.10.8**, respectively). The rest of the metastases were also not identified in this follow-up MRI. These findings confirmed a complete response to treatment, as was suggested, prior to chemotherapy because of the low ADC values of the lesions.

Comments DWI and ADC maps have been advocated as early functional markers of tumor response to treatment for several tumors, with the ability also to predict response to treatment. In a similar way, DWI and ADC measurements have a role in the prediction of response to treatment and posttreatment monitorization of hepatic metastases. Pretreatment low ADC values of liver metastasis from gastric and colorectal carcinoma have been described in responding lesions in comparison with non-responding lesions, which show higher ADC values. This fact suggests that metastases with higher pre-treatment ADC values present more necrosis and are probably more chemoresistant. DWI and ADC values are also useful in the control of response to treatment. In a recent report, an early increase in ADC values in the first week after treatment was described as typical in responding metastases. This ADC increase was not observed in lesions that showed either no change or disease progression in follow-up MRI

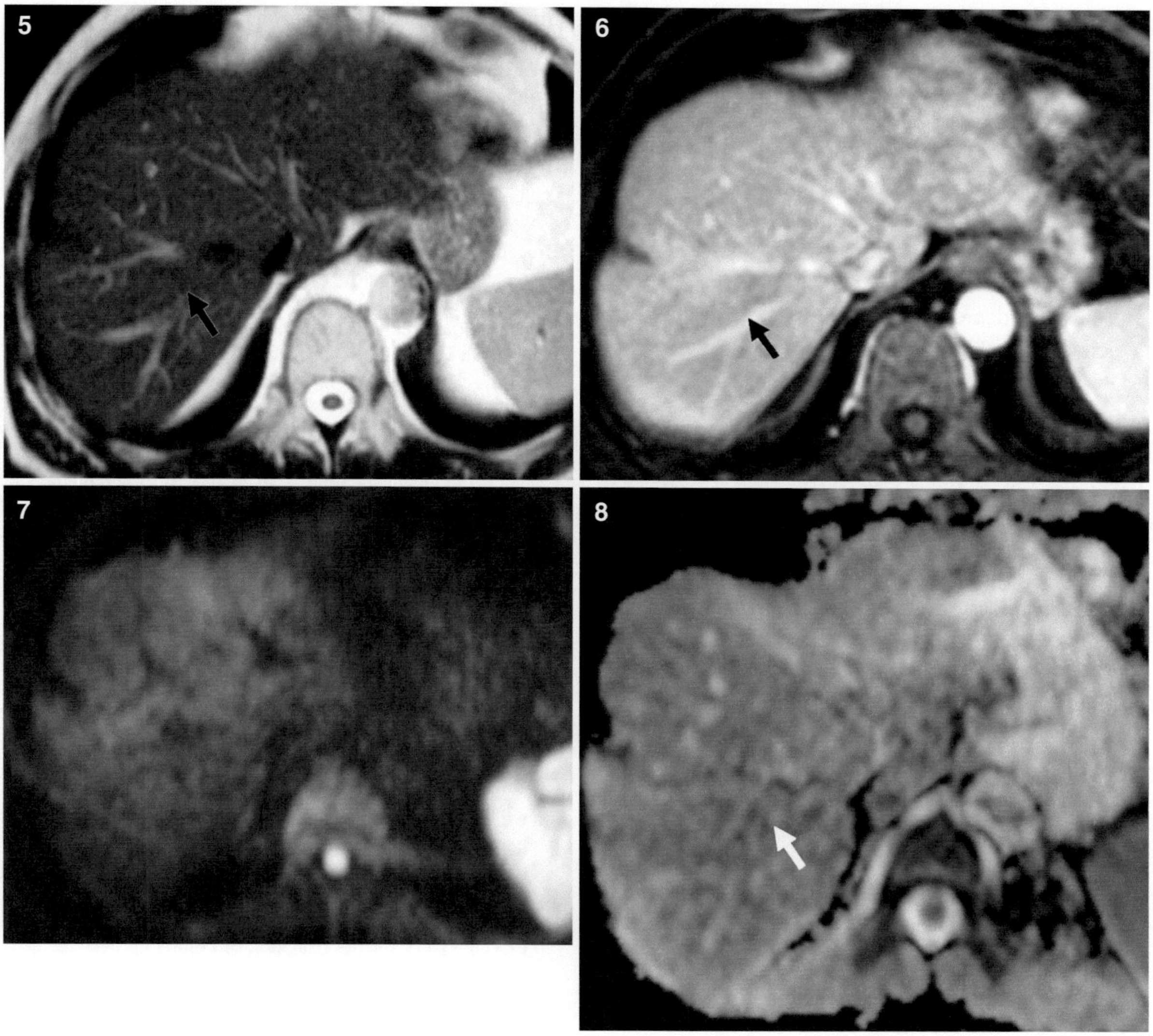

Fig. 5.10 (continued)

current data, it has not shown a clear capability to diagnose early stages of the disease. For example, Lewin and colleagues demonstrated lower ADC values in patients with moderate-to-severe fibrosis (F2–F4) than in those without or with mild fibrosis (F0–F1) and healthy volunteers. Using a threshold ADC value of 1.21×10^{-3} mm^2/s, they obtained an 87% sensitivity and specificity in the differentiation between fibrosis stage F3–F4 and F0 to F2. In the same discrimination, DWI using *b* values of 400–800 s/mm^2 showed an area under the curve equal to ultrasound elastography and better than blood tests. In two different recent series, DWI was shown to be a less reliable biomarker in the staging of liver fibrosis than MR elastography and gadoxetic acid-enhanced MRI.

Reported lower ADC values of fibrotic and cirrhotic livers compared to normal ones have been related to a decrease in capillary perfusion or restricted diffusion by extracellular fibrosis. Besides, Anderson et al. have reported in a murine model with ex-vivo analysis of hepatic ADC in an 11.7-T magnet that increasing degrees of steatosis result in decreased hepatic ADC values. Previous clinical studies have reported a range of sensitivities of 0.74–0.89 and specificities of

0.73–0.87 for ADC quantifications of the liver, in the detection of moderate fibrosis (stage F2 or higher). As in other areas, there is a lack of standardization in the definition of the most appropriate DWI approach to study fibrosis and cirrhosis. Prior reported mean ADCs for normal and cirrhotic livers are variable, depending on the type of sequence, combination of *b* values used and model of analysis of diffusion signal decay. The IVIM approach was shown to be able to detect the presence of decreased perfusion in cirrhotic livers, which is probably the main cause of the decreased ADC values of cirrhotic livers (Fig. 5.3). Taouli and colleagues proposed calculating the ADC value for this purpose, using a high *b* values of at least 500 s/mm^2, which showed a significant correlation with the liver fibrosis stage and the ADC value. In that series, a combination of *b* values of 0–1,000 s/mm^2 showed the highest significant correlation with fibrosis stage. Conversely, the same authors reported that a significant correlation was not achieved when using low *b* values for ADC quantification. Besides, entropy ADC and the normalization of liver ADC with spleen ADC have recently shown a greater correlation with the fibrosis stage than did mean ADC. Furthermore, the inflammatory activity grade, which shows a significant correlation with the pathological fibrosis stage, has been significantly related to a decrease in mean ADC and an increase in entropy ADC values.

5.7 Conclusions

DWI is a useful clinical tool in the evaluation of focal and diffuse liver pathology, with the technique being easy to perform and included in the state-of-the-art protocols of liver MRI. High detection of focal liver lesions is its most common clinical application, with its role in focal lesion characterization being of potential interest and its ability to stage liver fibrosis promising. Lack of standardization is the main limitation to a greater diffusion of using liver DWI in clinical practice.

Further Reading

Anderson SW, Soto JA, Milch HN et al (2011) Effect of disease progression on liver apparent diffusion coefficient values in a murine model of NASH at 11.7 Tesla MRI. J Magn Reson Imaging 33(4):882–888

Bittencourt LK, Matos C, Coutinho AC Jr (2011) Diffusion-weighted magnetic resonance imaging in the upper abdomen: technical issues and clinical applications. Magn Reson Imaging Clin N Am 19(1):111–131

Bonekamp S, Shen J, Salibi N et al (2011) Early response of hepatic malignancies to locoregional therapy-value of diffusion-weighted magnetic resonance imaging and proton magnetic resonance spectroscopy. J Comput Assist Tomogr 35(2):167–173

Bruegel M, Gaa J, Waldt S et al (2008) Diagnosis of hepatic metastasis: comparison of respiration-triggered diffusion-weighted echo-planar MRI and five T2-weighted turbo spin-echo sequences. Am J Roentgenol 191(5):1421–1429

Bruegel M, Holzapfel K, Gaa J et al (2008) Characterization of focal liver lesions by ADC measurements using a respiratory triggered diffusion-weighted single-shot echo-planar MR imaging technique. Eur Radiol 18(3):477–485; Epub Oct 25, 2007

Catalano OA, Choy G, Zhu A et al (2010) Differentiation of malignant thrombus from bland thrombus of the portal vein in patients with hepatocellular carcinoma: application of diffusion-weighted MR imaging. Radiology 254(1):154–162

Chiu FY, Jao JC, Chen CY et al (2005) Effect of intravenous gadolinium-DTPA on diffusion-weighted magnetic resonance images for evaluation of focal hepatic lesions. J Comput Assist Tomogr 29(2):176–180

Choi JS, Kim MJ, Choi JY et al (2010) Diffusion-weighted MR imaging of liver on 3.0-Tesla system: effect of intravenous administration of gadoxetic acid disodium. Eur Radiol 20(5):1052–1060

Chung JC, Naik NK, Lewandowski RJ et al (2010) Diffusion-weighted magnetic resonance imaging to predict response of hepatocellular carcinoma to chemoembolization. World J Gastroenterol 16(25):3161–3167

Coenegrachts K, De Geeter F, ter Beek L et al (2009) Comparison of MRI (including SS SE-EPI and SPIO-enhanced MRI) and FDG-PET/CT for the detection of colorectal liver metastases. Eur Radiol 19:370–379

Coenegrachts K, Delanote J, Ter Beek L et al (2009) Evaluation of true diffusion, perfusion factor, and apparent diffusion coefficient in non-necrotic liver metastases and uncomplicated liver hemangiomas using black-blood echo planar imaging. Eur J Radiol 69:131–138

Coenegrachts K, Orlent H, ter Beek L et al (2008) Improved focal liver lesion detection: comparison of single-shot spin-echo echo-planar and superparamagnetic iron oxide (SPIO)-enhanced MRI. J Magn Reson Imaging 27:117–124

Cui Y, Zhang XP, Sun YS, Tang L, Shen L (2008) Apparent diffusion coefficient: potential imaging biomarker for prediction and early detection of response to chemotherapy in hepatic metastases. Radiology 248(3):894–900

Dale BM, Braithwaite AC, Boll DT et al (2010) Field strength and diffusion encoding technique affect the apparent diffusion coefficient measurements in diffusion-weighted imaging of the abdomen. Invest Radiol 45(2):104–108

Do RK, Chandarana H, Felker E et al (2010) Diagnosis of liver fibrosis and cirrhosis with diffusion-weighted imaging: value of normalized apparent diffusion coefficient using the spleen as reference organ. Am J Roentgenol 195(3):671–676

Eiber M, Fingerle AA, Brügel M et al (2011) Detection and classification of focal liver lesions in patients with colorectal cancer: retrospective comparison of diffusion-weighted MR imaging and multi-slice CT. Eur J Radiol. Feb 11, 2011 [Epub ahead of print]

Erturk SM, Ichikawa T, Sano K et al (2008) Diffusion-weighted magnetic resonance imaging for characterization of focal liver masses: impact of parallel imaging (SENSE) and b value. J Comput Assist Tomogr 32(6):865–871

Fujimoto K, Tonan T, Azuma S et al (2011) Evaluation of the mean and entropy of apparent diffusion coefficient values in chronic hepatitis C: correlation with pathologic fibrosis stage and inflammatory activity grade. Radiology 258(3): 739–748

Girometti R, Furlan A, Esposito G et al (2008) Relevance of *b*-values in evaluating liver fi brosis: a study in healthy and cirrhotic subjects using two single-shot spin-echo echo-planar diffusion-weighted sequences. J Magn Reson Imaging 28(2):411–419

Goshima S, Kanematsu M, Kondo H et al (2008) Diffusion-weighted imaging of the liver: optimizing b value for the detection and characterization of benign and malignant hepatic lesions. J Magn Reson Imaging 28:691–697

Gourtsoyianni S, Papanikolaou N, Yarmenitis S et al (2008) Respiratory gated diffusion-weighted imaging of the liver: value of apparent diffusion coefficient measurements in the differentiation between most commonly encountered benign and malignant focal liver lesions. Eur Radiol 18(3):486–492

Hardie AD, Naik M, Hecht EM et al (2010) Diagnosis of liver metastases: value of diffusion-weighted MRI compared with gadolinium-enhanced MRI. Eur Radiol 20:1431–1441

Heo SH, Jeong YY, Shin SS et al (2010) Apparent diffusion coefficient value of diffusion-weighted imaging for hepatocellular carcinoma: correlation with the histologic differentiation and the expression of vascular endothelial growth factor. Korean J Radiol 11(3):295–303

Holzapfel K, Bruegel M, Eiber M et al (2010) Characterization of small (≤10 mm) focal liver lesions: value of respiratory-triggered echo-planar diffusion-weighted MR imaging. Eur J Radiol 76(1):89–95

Holzapfel K, Reiser-Erkan C, Fingerle AA et al (2011) Comparison of diffusion-weighted MR imaging and multidetector-row CT in the detection of liver metastases in patients operated for pancreatic cancer. Abdom Imaging 36(2):179–184

Hussain SM, De Becker J, Hop WC et al (2005) Can a single-shot black-blood T2-weighted spin-echo echo-planar imaging sequence with sensitivity encoding replace the respiratory-triggered turbo spin-echo sequence for the liver? An optimization and feasibility study. J Magn Reson Imaging 21:219–229

Inan N, Arslan A, Akansel G et al (2007) Diffusion-weighted imaging in the differential diagnosis of simple and hydatid cysts of the liver. Am J Roentgenol 189(5):1031–1036

Kandpal H, Sharma R, Madhusudhan KS et al (2009) Respiratory-triggered versus breath-hold diffusion-weighted MRI of liver lesions: comparison of image quality and apparent diffusion coefficient values. Am J Roentgenol 192:915–922

Kenis C, Deckers F, De Foer B et al (2011) Diagnosis of liver metastases: can diffusion-weighted imaging (DWI) be used as a stand alone sequence? Eur J Radiol. Mar 3, 2011 [Epub ahead of print]

Kim YK, Kim CS, Han YM et al (2011) Detection of liver malignancy with gadoxetic acid-enhanced MRI: is addition of diffusion-weighted MRI beneficial? Clin Radiol 66(6):489–496

Kim T, Murakami T, Takahashi S et al (1999) Diffusion-weighted single-shot echoplanar MR imaging for liver disease. Am J Roentgenol 173(2):393–398

Koh DM, Blackledge M, Collins DJ et al (2009) Reproducibility and changes in the apparent diffusion coefficients of solid tumours treated with combretastatin A4 phosphate and bevacizumab in a two-centre phase I clinical trial. Eur Radiol 19(11):2728–2738

Koh DM, Collins DJ (2007) Diffusion weighted MRI in the body: applications and challenges in oncology. Am J Roentgenol 188:1622–1635

Koh DM, Erica S, Collins D et al (2004) Diffusion coefficients and the perfusion fraction of colorectal hepatic metastases estimated using single-shot echo-planar sensitivity-encoded (SENSE) diffusion-weighted MR imaging. Proc Int Soc Magn Reson Med 11:908

Koh DM, Padhani AR (2010) Functional magnetic resonance imaging of the liver: parametric assessments beyond morphology. Magn Reson Imaging Clin N Am 18(3):565–585

Koh DM, Scurr E, Collins D et al (2007) Predicting response of colorectal hepatic metastasis: value of pretreatment apparent diffusion coefficients. Am J Roentgenol 188(4):1001–1008

Koike N, Cho A, Nasu K et al (2009) Role of diffusion-weighted magnetic resonance imaging in the differential diagnosis of focal hepatic lesions. World J Gastroenterol 15:5805–5812

Koinuma M, Ohashi I, Hanafusa K et al (2005) Apparent diffusion coefficient measurements with diffusion-weighted magnetic resonance imaging for evaluation of hepatic fibrosis. J Magn Reson Imaging 22(1):80–85

Kubota K, Yamanishi T, Itoh S et al (2010) Role of diffusion-weighted imaging in evaluating therapeutic efficacy after transcatheter arterial chemoembolization for hepatocellular carcinoma. Oncol Rep 24(3):727–732

Kwee TC, Takahara T (2011) Diffusion-weighted MRI for detecting liver metastases: importance of the b-value. Eur Radiol 21(1):150

Kwee TC, Takahara T, Koh DM et al (2008) Comparison and reproducibility of ADC measurements in breathhold, respiratory triggered, and free-breathing diffusion-weighted MR imaging of the liver. J Magn Reson Imaging 28(5): 1141–1148

Kwee TC, Takahara T, Niwa T et al (2009) Influence of cardiac motion on diffusion-weighted magnetic resonance imaging of the liver. Magn Reson Mater Phys 22:319–325

Le Bihan D, Breton E, Lallemand D et al (1986) MR imaging of intravoxel incoherent motions: application to diffusion and perfusion in neurologic disorders. Radiology 161(2):401–407

Le Bihan D, Breton E, Lallemand D et al (1988) Separation of diffusion and perfusion in intravoxel incoherent motion MR imaging. Radiology 168:497–505

Lewin M, Poujol-Robert A, Boëlle PY et al (2007) Diffusion-weighted magnetic resonance imaging for the assessment of fibrosis in chronic hepatitis C. Hepatology 46(3):658–665

Liu YB, Liang CH, Wang QS et al (2010) Clinical study of transcatheter arterial chemoembolization plus radiofrequency ablation in hepatocellular carcinoma by magnetic resonance imaging and functional diffusion-weighted imaging. Zhonghua Yi Xue Za Zhi 90(41):2922–2926

Low RN (2007) Abdominal MRI advances in the detection of liver tumours and characterisation. Lancet Oncol 8:525–535

Luciani A, Vignaud A, Cavet M et al (2008) Liver cirrhosis: intravoxel incoherent motion MR imaging-Pilot study. Radiology 249(3):891–899

Miller FH, Hammond N, Siddiqi AJ et al (2010) Utility of diffusion-weighted MRI in distinguishing benign and malignant hepatic lesions. J Magn Reson Imaging 32(1): 138–147

Moteki T, Horikoshi H (2011) Evaluation of noncirrhotic hepatic parenchyma with and without significant portal vein stenosis using diffusion-weighted echo-planar MR on the basis of multiple-perfusion-components theory. Magn Reson Imaging 29(1):64–73

Muhi A, Ichikawa T, Motosugi et al (2009) High-b-value diffusion-weighted MR imaging of hepatocellular lesions: estimation of grade of malignancy of hepatocellular carcinoma. J Magn Reson Imaging 30(5):1005–1011

Mwangi I, Hanna RF, Kased N et al (2010) Apparent diffusion coefficient of fibrosis and regenerative nodules in the cirrhotic liver at MRI. Am J Roentgenol 194(6):1515–1522

Nagayama M, Watanabe Y, Okumura A et al (2002) Blackblood T2-weighted SE-EPI imaging of the liver. Proc Int Soc Magn Reson Med 10:1963

Nasu K, Kuroki Y, Nawano S, Kuroki S, Tsukamoto T, Yamamoto S, Motoori K, Ueda T (2006) Hepatic metastases: diffusion-weighted sensitivity-encoding versus SPIO-enhanced MR imaging. Radiology 239(1):122–130

Nasu K, Kuroki Y, Tsukamoto T et al (2009) Diffusion-weighted imaging of surgically resected hepatocellular carcinoma: imaging characteristics and relationship among signal intensity, apparent diffusion coefficient, and histopathologic grade. Am J Roentgenol 193(2):438–444

Oruç E, Yıldırım N, Topal NB et al (2010) The role of diffusion-weighted MRI in the classification of liver hydatid cysts and differentiation of simple cysts and abscesses from hydatid cysts. Diagn Interv Radiol 16(4):279–287

Papanikolaou N, Gourtsoyianni S, Yarmenitis S et al (2010) Comparison between two-point and four-point methods for quantification of apparent diffusion coefficient of normal liver parenchyma and focal lesions. Value of normalization with spleen. Eur J Radiol 73(2):305–309

Parikh T, Drew SJ, Lee VS et al (2008) Focal liver lesion detection and characterization with diffusion-weighted MR imaging: comparison with standard breath-hold T2-weighted imaging. Radiology 246(3):812

Patel J, Sigmund EE, Rusinek H et al (2010) Diagnosis of cirrhosis with intravoxel incoherent motion diffusion MRI and dynamic contrast-enhanced MRI alone and in combination: preliminary experience. J Magn Reson Imaging 31(3): 589–600

Piana G, Trinquart L, Meskine N et al (2011) New MR imaging criteria with a diffusion-weighted sequence for the diagnosis of hepatocellular carcinoma in chronic liver diseases. J Hepatol 55(1):126–132

Sandrasegaran K, Akisik FM, Lin C et al (2009) Value of diffusion-weighted MRI for assessing liver fibrosis and cirrhosis. Am J Roentgenol 193(6):1556–1560

Sandrasegaran K, Akisik FM, Lin C et al (2009) The value of diffusion-weighted imaging in characterizing focal liver masses. Acad Radiol 16:1208–1214

Schraml C, Schwenzer NF, Martirosian P et al (2009) Diffusion-weighted MRI of advanced hepatocellular carcinoma during sorafenib treatment: initial results. Am J Roentgenol 193(4):301–307

Shimada K, Isoda H, Hirokawa Y et al (2010) Comparison of gadolinium-EOB-DTPA-enhanced and diffusion-weighted liver MRI for detection of small hepatic metastases. Eur Radiol 20(11):2690–2698

Sun XJ, Quan XY, Huang FH et al (2005) Quantitative evaluation of diffusion-weighted magnetic resonance imaging of focal hepatic lesions. World J Gastroenterol 11:6535–6537

Taouli B, Chouli M, Martin AJ et al (2008) Chronic hepatitis: role of diffusion-weighted imaging and diffusion tensor imaging for the diagnosis of liver fibrosis and inflammation. J Magn Reson Imaging 28(1):89–95

Taouli B, Koh DM (2010) Diffusion-weighted MR imaging of the liver. Radiology 254:47–66

Taouli B, Tolia AJ, Losada M et al (2007) Diffusion-weighted MRI for quantification of liver fibrosis: preliminary experience. Am J Roentgenol 189(4):799–806

Taouli B, Vilgrain V, Dumont E et al (2003) Evaluation of liver diffusion isotropy and characterization of focal hepatic lesions with two single-shot echo-planar MR imaging sequences: prospective study in 66 patients. Radiology 226:71–78

Turner R, Le Bihan D, Maier J et al (1990) Echo-planar imaging of intravoxel incoherent motion. Radiology 177(2): 407–414

Wang Y, Ganger DR, Levitsky J et al (2011) Assessment of chronic hepatitis and fibrosis: comparison of MR elastography and diffusion-weighted imaging. Am J Roentgenol 196(3):553–561

Wang H, Wang XY, Jiang XX et al (2010) Comparison of diffusion-weighted with T2-weighted Imaging for detection of small hepatocellular carcinoma in cirrhosis: preliminary quantitative study at 3-T. Acad Radiol 17(2):239–243

Watanabe H, Kanematsu M, Goshima S et al (2011) Staging hepatic fibrosis: comparison of gadoxetate disodium-enhanced and diffusion-weighted MR imaging – preliminary observations. Radiology 259(1):142–150

Xu PJ, Yan FH, Wang JH et al (2010) Contribution of diffusion-weighted magnetic resonance imaging in the characterization of hepatocellular carcinomas and dysplastic nodules in cirrhotic liver. J Comput Assist Tomogr 34(4):506–512

Yamada I, Aung W, Himeno Y et al (1999) Diffusion coefficients in abdominal organs and hepatic lesions: evaluation with intravoxel incoherent motion echo-planar MR imaging. Radiology 210(3):617–623

Zech CJ, Herrmann KA, Dietrich O et al (2008) Black-blood diffusion-weighted EPI acquisition of the liver with parallel imaging: comparison with a standard T2-weighted sequence for detection of focal liver lesions. Invest Radiol 43(4): 261–266

Diffusion-Weighted MR Imaging of the Pancreas

6

Jorge A. Soto, German A. Castrillon, Stephan Anderson, and Nagaraj Holalkere

6.1 Introduction

The DWI in the upper abdomen continues to grow and has expanded beyond the liver to other solid organs and hollow viscera as well. This growth in the clinical applications of DWI resulted mainly from improvements in MR technology, such as the development of stronger diffusion gradients and faster pulse sequences. Upper abdominal images with diffusion-weighting may be easily acquired within short breath-hold periods of 20 s or less, achievable by most patients. As in other parts of the body, contrast in DWI of the upper abdomen results mainly from differences in the movement of water molecules between the intra- and extracellular spaces and the vessels. In organs such as the pancreas, water motion is not random ("free") but, rather, it is limited by boundaries created by the various tissue and cellular compartments, organelles, and membranes. In the normal state, this limited motion of water is more or less predictable, but varies considerably between organs. Factors such as the cellularity and perfusion of the specific organ help determine the relative impedance to water diffusion. In general, tissues with low cellularity or containing cells with predominantly disrupted membranes tend to allow greater movement of water molecules than relatively hypercellular tissues. Sensitizing diffusion gradients can then be used to "activate" water molecules and the signal generated by motion of these molecules can be used for characterization of normal and abnormal tissues. Thus, the appearance of normal organs (in this case the pancreas) on DWI is relatively constant. However, organs affected by disease have a different appearance on DWI. Involvement with various pathological conditions, such as tumor, abscess, ischemia and fibrosis, affects water diffusion and the appearance of the organ on DWI. The extent to which water motion is affected by disease can be quantified with the generation of ADC maps from diffusion images obtained at various *b* values.

Publications exploring the use of DWI for evaluation of pancreatic disease are limited in number and scope. However, the value of DWI in various pancreatic conditions continues to be explored and available results suggest that there will likely be a niche for this technique in the clinic. Available studies have shown that the measured ADC values of the normal pancreatic glandular parenchyma on DWI vary considerably and are determined by factors such as age, the anatomic portion of the gland, and magnet field strength. For example, measured ADC of the pancreatic tail is lower than ADC of other parts of the pancreas, which is possibly caused by differences in surrounding tissues. As a person ages, the pancreas shows several age-related changes such as atrophy, fatty infiltration, and fibrosis, and pancreatic ADC may also change with age.

Jorge A. Soto (✉) • S. Anderson • N. Holalkere
Radiology Department,
Boston University School of Medicine,
Boston, MA, USA
e-mail: jorge.soto@bmc.org

G.A. Castrillon
Radiology Department, University of Antioquia,
Medellin, Colombia

A. Luna et al., *Diffusion MRI Outside the Brain*,
DOI 10.1007/978-3-642-21052-5_6, © Springer-Verlag Berlin Heidelberg 2012

6.2 Pancreatic Cancer

Oncologic applications of DWI in the pancreas have been of particular interest because lipophilic cell membranes in pancreatic ductal adenocarcinoma, typically a tumor with hypercellular tissue, serve as barriers to free diffusion in the intracellular and extracellular spaces. Thus, pancreatic tumors should demonstrate restricted diffusion relative to normal glandular parenchyma on DWI. There is data (albeit limited) to suggest that this hypothesis may in fact be true. Normal pancreas has significantly higher mean ADC than either pancreatic cancer or mass-forming pancreatitis, the two most commonly focal pancreatic lesions encountered in clinical practice. Furthermore, proper use of DWI may aid in the differentiation of focal pancreatitis from ductal adenocarcinoma. On DWI acquired with a $b=600$ s/mm^2, mass-forming focal pancreatitis is virtually indistinguishable from the remaining pancreas (Fig. 6.1), whereas pancreatic ductal adenocarcinoma tends to be hyperintense relative to the remaining pancreas (Fig. 6.2). The mean ADC value of pancreatic adenocarcinoma is significantly lower than normal pancreatic glandular parenchyma, whereas the ADC values of mass-forming focal pancreatitis and normal pancreas do not differ significantly.

In practice, DWI can be used in several ways in patients with suspected or known pancreatic cancer. First, as described above, diffusion images provide additional important data in the characterization of focal lesions demonstrated on CT or on traditional T1- or T2-weighted images and dynamic, contrast-enhanced images. A focal lesion exhibiting definite restricted diffusion is more likely to represent a malignancy and appropriate diagnostic or management procedures can be undertaken. Second, in patients with known tumors, the benefits of DWI include improved characterization of enlarged lymph nodes, detection of peritoneal carcinomatosis, and detection of distant (such as hepatic) metastases. It is also possible that ADC measurements can be used as a quantitative tool for predicting and monitoring tumor response (Fig. 4.7), as the free diffusion of water molecules increases as tumor cells respond to therapy and breakdown.

6.3 Cystic Masses

There is some data that supports the use of DWI for characterizing and determining the significance of pancreatic cystic lesions. The observed signal intensities of all cystic lesions are high on DWI with lower b values. However, when a *b* factor of 1,000 s/mm^2 is used, significant differences between the signal intensity ratios of various types of pancreatic cystic lesions can be detected. At this high *b* value, the contribution of the T2 shine-through to the signal intensity decreases, and tissue cellularity makes a greater contribution. At $b=1{,}000$ s/mm^2, the observed signals of simple cysts and pseudocysts are typically isointense to the pancreas (Figs. 6.3 and 6.4). In contrast, neoplastic cysts and abscesses remain hyperintense (Figs. 6.5–6.7). Therefore, the hyperintensity of abscesses and neoplastic cysts on $b = 1{,}000$ s/mm^2 images cannot be totally attributed to the T2 shine-through effect. ADC values, which by definition are not affected by the T2 shine-through effects, tend to be lower in neoplastic cysts (serous cystadenoma, mucinous cystadenoma/cystoadenocarcinoma) than in pseudocysts and simple cysts. Hence, the high signal on DWI is due to the reduced diffusion, which can be attributed to the differences in the internal contents of the cystic lesions. Because cystic tumors have a viscous content (mucin, hemorrhage, or high protein), they have decreased ADCs. Conversely, simple cysts and pseudocysts have a lower viscosity and, thus, a higher ADC.

6.4 Other Applications

As in other abdominal organs, the potential use of DWI and ADC values in the assessment of diffuse pancreatic disease has been given attention. In the acute setting, DWI allows the detection of pancreatitis in a similar fashion to enhanced-CT. Early data suggests that chronic pancreatitis affects mobility of water molecules in the pancreas, such that patients with the disease demonstrate high signal on DWI (Fig. 6.8). Furthermore, ADC values may correlate well with the severity of chronic pancreatitis, as assessed by the

Cambridge classification. Finally, abnormalities seen on secretin-enhanced DWI may serve as an early predictor of pancreatic exocrine dysfunction, as after secretin stimulation, the ADC values reveal either delayed peak or lower peak values in patients with early chronic pancreatitis.

Autoimmune pancreatitis (ALP) represents a distinct form of chronic pancreatitis which often presents as a pancreatic mass causing obstructive jaundice as well as pancreatic exocrine and endocrine insufficiency. It shows lower ADC values than chronic pancreatitis and pancreatic carcinoma. DWI is also useful to monitorize the effect of steroids during treatment.

6.5 Biliary Tract

As DWI has become an integral component of most abdominal MR protocols at many institutions, the experience with its application for evaluating patients with biliary tract disorders is growing accordingly. However, there is still very little published scientific data to support its use. Cross-sectional MR images, especially dynamic contrast-enhanced images with a delayed phase, and MR cholangiopancreatography are the preferred noninvasive imaging tests for diagnosis, staging, therapy planning, and follow-up of patients with cholangiocarcinoma. The characteristic appearance of hilar cholangiocarcinomas is well documented: The typically infiltrating lesion is isotense to slightly hyperintense on T2-weighted images and isotense to slightly hypointense on T1-weighted images. After contrast administration, the tumor lesion has a peripheral rim of enhancement and a characteristic retention of contrast on delayed phase images. On DWI, early experience suggests that the tumor exhibits diffusion restriction, which is helpful for separating the lesion from the surrounding hepatic parenchyma (Fig. 6.9). Regional extension of the tumor to porta hepatis lymph nodes can also be well depicted with DWI, since involved nodes may also demonstrate restricted diffusion. One potential application of DWI in biliary tract imaging is in the surveillance and early detection of cholangiocarcinoma in patients with primary sclerosing cholangitis. This, however, has not been convincingly proven yet. Recently, DWI has shown to be significantly more accurate in the detection of extrahepatic cholangiocarcinoma than MR cholangiopancreatography. The lesions were detected as areas of restricted diffusion with a mean ADC value of $1.31 \pm 0.29 \times 10^{-3}$ s/mm^2.

Neoplastic and inflammatory diseases of the gallbladder can also be evaluated with MR. Polypoid gallbladder tumors and acute inflammatory infiltration of the gallbladder wall also exhibit restricted diffusion on DWI (Fig. 6.10). This may be helpful for separating these diseases from other nonspecific, and less ominous, causes of gallbladder wall thickening such as chronic inflammation, hyperplastic cholecystosis (cholesterolosis, adenomyomatosis), and thickening secondary to liver disease or edematous states.

Case 6.1: Mass-Forming Focal Pancreatitis

A 55-year-old male who has history of chronic pancreatitis, now presenting with jaundice and abdominal pain.

Comments

Differentiation between mass-forming focal pancreatitis and pancreatic cancer can be difficult. Mass-forming focal pancreatitis is defined as a focal inflammatory process in the pancreas that may mimic pancreatic cancer. Standard cross-sectional imaging techniques including CT, MRI, and even histopathologic analysis of the biopsy material may be inconclusive to distinguish neoplasm from mass-forming focal pancreatitis. Recent studies have investigated the pattern of serial contrast enhancement as well as pancreatic and common bile duct changes on MRI and MRCP in patients with pancreatic cancer, as compared to those with mass-forming focal pancreatitis. Although the enhancement pattern and ductal changes are helpful in distinguishing these two entities, an overlap of findings on standard MRI and MRCP may exist. Masses due to pancreatic carcinoma and chronic pancreatitis show a pattern of contrast enhancement after dynamic infusion of gadopentetate dimeglumine that is altered when compared to that of normal pancreas. The similar gradual pattern of enhancement precludes distinction of the two entities on the basis of gadolinium-enhanced MR findings. Other dynamic MR imaging features may help distinguish the two pathologic entities.

Radiologists should recognize that radiologic differentiation between mass-forming focal pancreatitis and pancreatic carcinoma is important because, unlike pancreatic carcinoma, the mass-forming type of focal pancreatitis does not require any therapeutic surgical procedure. The majority of patients have spontaneous regression of the mass and any clinical symptoms, including obstructive jaundice. Therefore, the differentiation between both entities is of paramount importance. Early studies on DWI have produced preliminary results which indicate the diagnostic utility of DWI to achieve this goal. The mass-forming focal pancreatitis lesions have showed ADC values consistently indistinguishable from the remaining pancreas. DWI findings of pancreatic adenocarcinoma have been evaluated in various studies. ADC values of pancreatic adenocarcinoma tend to be lower than normal pancreas in most of the studies, although variations exist. Recently, the IVIM model has been explored in the pancreas and for differentiation between pancreatic cancer and chronic pancreatitis. IVIM-related mean perfusion fraction in chronic pancreatitis was around 16%, in pancreatic cancer 8%, and in healthy pancreatic tissue around 25%. DWI may be helpful as a complementary imaging method to distinguish between the two entities.

Imaging Findings

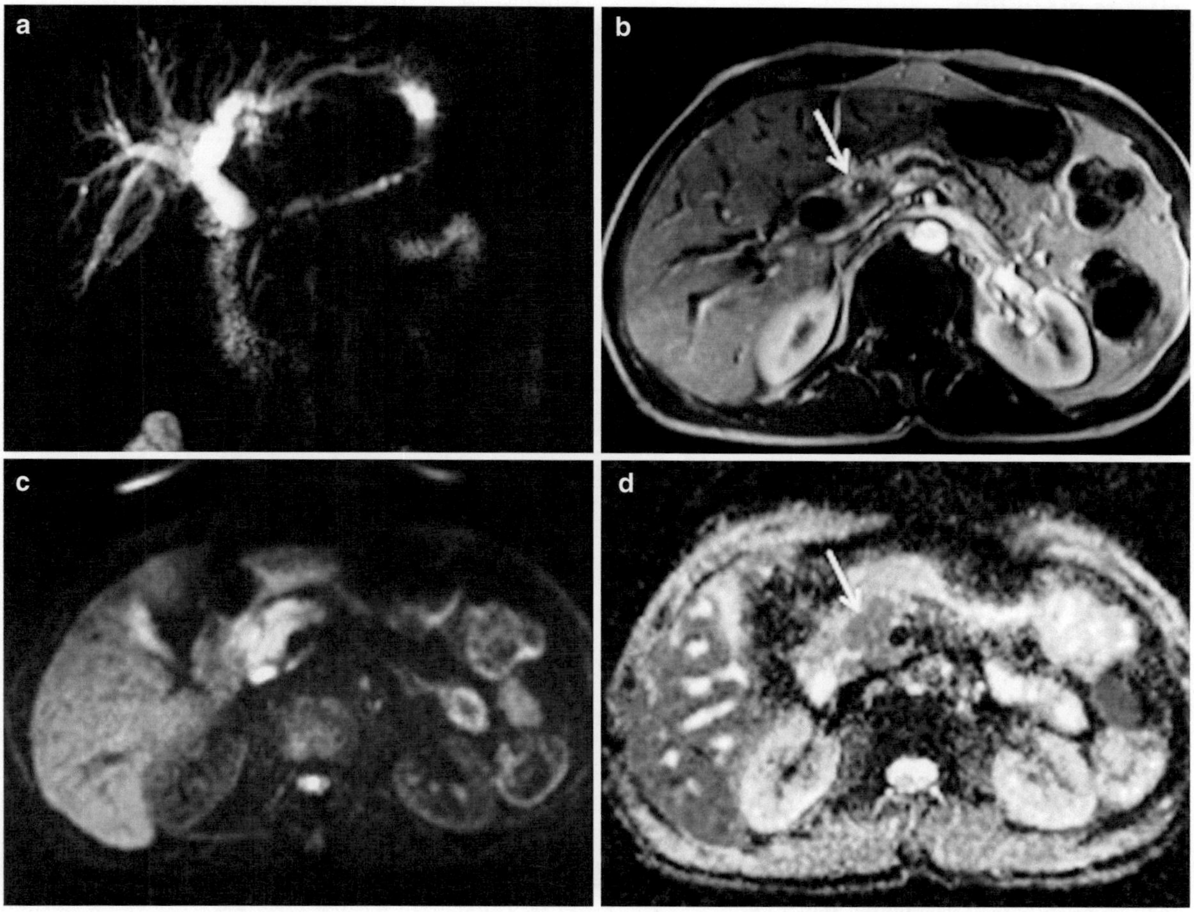

Fig. 6.1 (**a**) Coronal-oblique thick section single-shot MRCP image shows a stricture of the biliary and pancreatic ducts, with the "penetrating duct" sign in the pancreatic duct. (**b**) Axial postcontrast GE T1-weighted image with fat-suppression, obtained in the portal venous phase, shows a hypovascular mass in the head of the pancreas (*arrow*). (**c**) DWI acquired with a *b* factor of 600 s/mm^2 shows the lesion with signal intensity that is the same of the pancreatic gland. The lesion demonstrates the same signal intensity as the pancreatic gland on the corresponding ADC map (**d**, *arrow*). These findings suggest a mass-forming focal pancreatitis

Case 6.2: Pancreatic Ductal Adenocarcinoma

A 75-years-old male patient who presents with weight loss, jaundice, and abdominal pain.

Comments

Pancreatic ductal adenocarcinoma arises from the exocrine portion of the gland, accounts for 95% of malignant tumors of the pancreas, and is the fourth most common cause of cancer death in the United States. The lesion is more common in men and blacks and occurs most frequently in the eighth decade of the life. The tumor has a poor prognosis, with a 5-year survival rate of only 5%. Surgery remains as the sole curative treatment for patients with pancreatic carcinoma. Therefore, earlier detection of potentially resectable disease may result in improved patient survival. One study regarding prognostic factors after a Whipple procedure found that the 5-year survival rate was greater for patients with node-negative and small tumors than for those with node-positive and large tumors. Another study demonstrated a 5-year survival of 100% for patients with a tumor smaller than 1 cm when limited to the intraductal epithelium. Advances in MR imaging allow detection and characterization of focal pancreatic lesions smaller than 1 cm.

In general, diagnosis of pancreatic adenocarcinoma is made when the tumor is relatively large (approximately 5 cm) and has extended beyond the pancreas (85% of cases). Sixty percent to 70% of the lesions are located in the head, 15%, in the body, and 5% in the tail. Diffuse tumor infiltration is found in 10–20% of patients. The normal pancreatic parenchyma is high in signal intensity on non-contrast T1-weighted fat-suppressed images because of the presence of aqueous protein in the acini of the gland. After administration of intravenous gadolinium, the pancreas demonstrates a uniform capillary blush on immediate post-contrast images and fades to isointense signal to the liver on the interstitial phase. Conversely, pancreatic cancer appears as a low signal intensity mass on non-contrast T1-weighted fat-suppressed images and enhances to a lesser extent than the surrounding normal pancreatic tissue on immediate post-contrast images. These MR imaging features are related to their abundant fibrous stroma and relatively sparse tumor vascularity.

The appearance of pancreatic cancer on interstitial phase images is variable and reflects the volume of extracellular space and venous drainage of tumors compared with those of pancreatic tissue. Large pancreatic tumors tend to remain low in signal intensity on interstitial phase images, whereas the signal intensity of smaller tumors may range from hypointense to hyperintense on this phase. On T2-weighted images, tumors are usually minimally hypointense relative to the pancreas and are therefore difficult to visualize.

Although pancreatic adenocarcinoma usually appears as a focal low signal intensity mass that is relatively well demarcated from the adjacent normal pancreatic parenchyma on immediate post-contrast images, some tumors can be seen as poorly marginated lesions with decreased enhancement on immediate post-contrast images and slightly increased enhancement on interstitial phase images. This appearance is commonly observed in pancreatic cancer that has been treated with chemotherapy and radiation therapy, but may also be seen at initial presentation in up to 27% of patients, especially in the moderately differentiated histologic pattern.

DWI findings of pancreatic adenocarcinoma have been evaluated in various studies. Apparent diffusion coefficient values of pancreatic adenocarcinoma tend to be lower than normal pancreas in most of studies, although variations exist. In a recent study, ADC values of pancreatic adenocarcinomas were classified according to the histopathological composition of the tumors. When the tumor reveals loose fibrosis, that is, edematous fibrosis and loose collagen fibers that are more prevalent than the cellular component or mucin, the ADC values can be higher than the normal pancreas. When dense fibrosis and increased cellular elements are present, then the ADC values are lower than the normal pancreas. The detection of tumors on DWI with a high b value (1,000 s/mm^2) has been evaluated. The mean sensitivity and specificity for the detection of pancreatic adenocarcinoma were 96.2% and 98.6%, respectively, for the DWI with a high b value. The study showed that on DWI with a b value of 1,000 s/mm^2, pancreatic adenocarcinoma has restricted diffusion and is hyperintense compared with the rest of the gland.

Imaging Findings

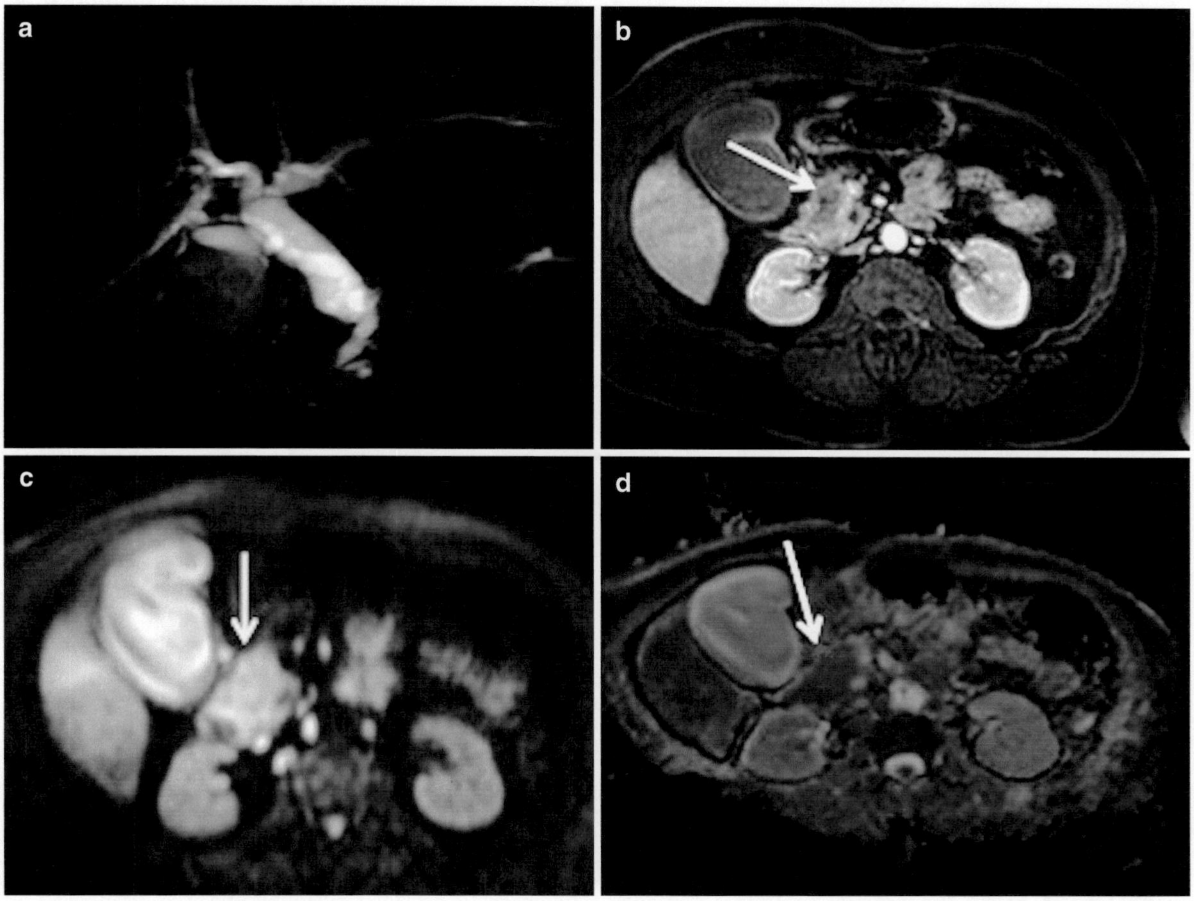

Fig. 6.2 (**a**) Coronal-oblique thick section single-shot MRCP image shows an abrupt stenosis of the distal common bile duct, with proximal upstream dilatation. The pancreatic duct is normal. (**b**) Axial postcontrast GE T1-weighted image with fat suppression acquired in a late arterial phase shows a hypovascular mass (*arrow*), which is causing the biliary ductal obstruction. DWI acquired with a *b* factor of 600 s/mm^2 (**c**) shows the mass with high signal intensity and low signal intensity on the corresponding ADC map (**d**, *arrows*). This finding is characteristic of a malignant lesion This case represents a histopathologically proven adenocarcinoma of the pancreas

Case 6.3: Serous Cystadenoma

A 65-year-old female patient with new onset of abdominal pain. Abdominal ultrasound (not shown) demonstrated a small cystic mass in head of the pancreas. MR was performed to further characterize the cystic lesion.

Comments

Pancreatic cystic neoplasms generally arise from the exocrine component of the gland. Although secondary cystic change can be seen in most types of pancreatic neoplasms, cystic pancreatic neoplasms are characterized by their dominant cystic configuration.

Cystic lesions of the pancreas include a variety of pathologic entities, as nonneoplastic cystic lesions (congenital simple cysts, pseudocysts, abscesses, hydatid cysts) and various neoplastic cysts (serous cystadenomas, mucinous cystadenomas, mucinous cystadenocarcinomas, cystic-degenerated adenocarcinomas, intraductal papillary mucinous neoplasm, and neuroendocrine tumors). Pseudocysts represent about 85–90% of all pancreatic cystic lesions. Because of the malignant potential of mucinous cystic neoplasms, cystic adenocarcinomas, and neuroendocrine tumors, careful consideration of the differential diagnosis is mandatory to select the optimal treatment for each patient. Cystic lesions with malignant potential are often managed surgically in appropriate candidates. However, asymptomatic simple cysts, pseudocysts, and serous cystadenomas are generally managed nonoperatively because they do not have malignant potential.

Serous cystadenoma (microcystic adenoma) is a benign neoplasm characterized by numerous tiny serous fluid–filled cysts. They are usually microcystic and multilocular and consist of multiple small cysts less than 1 cm in diameter. Rarely, serous cystadenomas can be macrocystic (cyst size between 1 and 8 cm) including multilocular, oligolocular, or unilocular subtypes. Microcystic serous cystadenomas are usually found in women older than 60 years with nonspecific complaints of abdominal pain or weight loss or, more commonly, as an incidental finding. Typical serous cystadenomas are composed of multiple cysts varying in size from 0.2 to 2.0 cm, and the size of the tumors ranges in greatest dimension from 1.4 to 27 cm. A central stellate scar is commonly present, often calcified. Internally, the cyst has a honeycomb appearance compatible with innumerable cysts. On MR images, the tumors are well defined and do not demonstrate invasion of fat or adjacent organs. On T2-weighted images, the small cysts and intervening septations may be well shown as a cluster of small grape-like high signal intensity cysts. Relatively thin uniform septations and absence of infiltration of adjacent organs and structures are features that distinguish serous cystadenomas from the very rare serous cystadenocarcinoma. Tumor septations usually enhance minimally with gadolinium on early and late post-contrast images, although moderate enhancement on early post-contrast images may occur as well. Delayed enhancement of the central scar may occasionally be observed and is more typical of large tumors. This enhancement pattern is typical of fibrous tissue in general.

Macrocystic or oligocystic serous cystadenoma is a variant of serous cystadenoma that is very difficult to differentiate from a mucinous cystadenoma. Location in the pancreatic head, lobulated contour, and lack of wall enhancement have been reported to be specific for macrocystic serous cystadenoma (as compared to mucinous cystic tumors).

There is some data that supports the use of DWI for characterizing and determining the significance of pancreatic cystic lesions. The observed signal intensities of all cystic lesions are high on diffusion-weighted images with lower *b* values. However, when a *b* factor of 1,000 s/mm^2 is used, significant differences between the signal intensity ratios of various types of pancreatic cystic lesions can be detected. At this high *b* value, the contribution of the T2 shine-through to the signal intensity decreases, and tissue cellularity and internal contents makes a greater contribution. Because cystic tumors have a viscous content (mucin, hemorrhage, or high protein), they have decreased ADCs. Conversely, simple cysts and pseudocysts have a lower viscosity and, thus, a higher ADC.

Imaging Findings

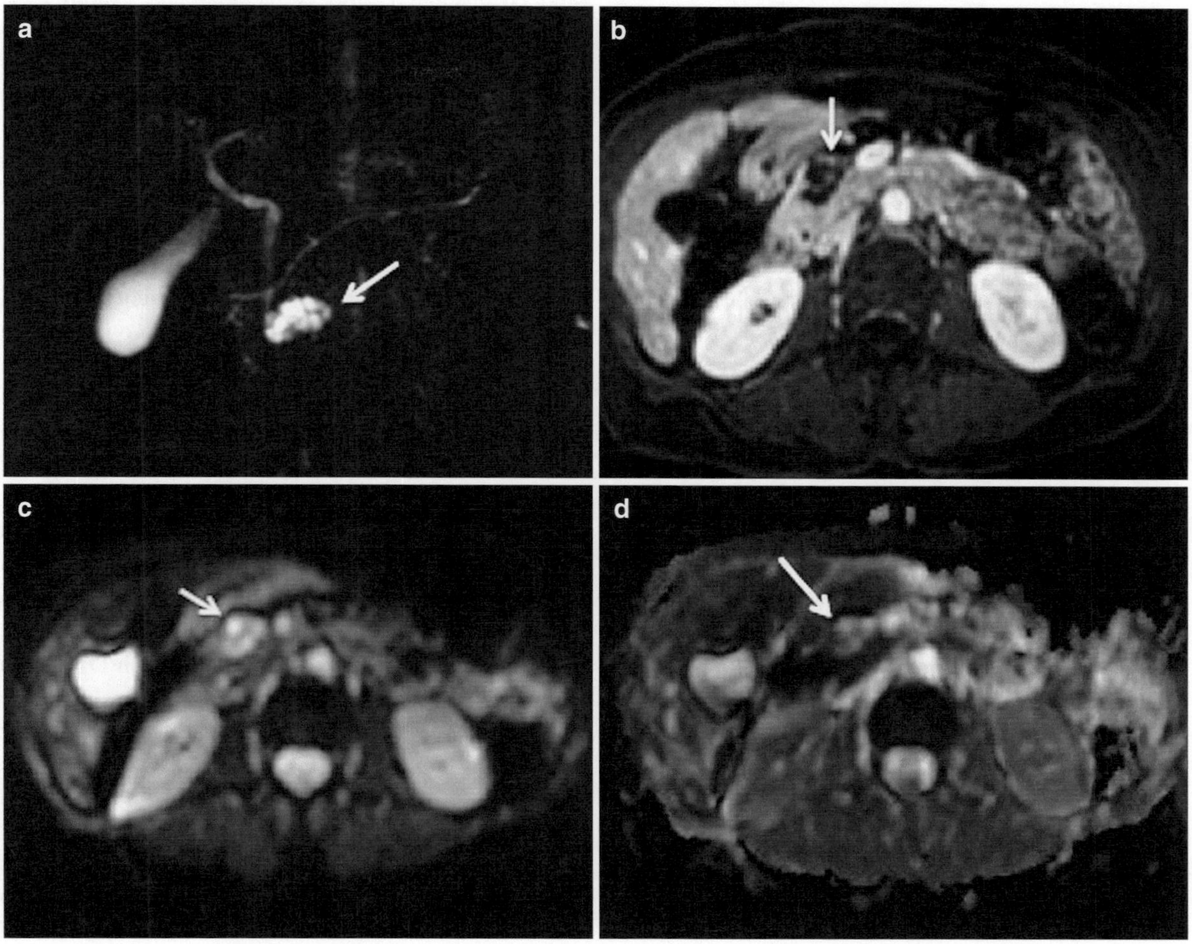

Fig. 6.3 (**a**) Coronal-oblique thick section single-shot MRCP image. (**b**) Axial contrast-enhanced GE T1-weighted sequence with fat suppression image. There is a multiloculated cystic lesion in the head of the pancreas, with thin internal septations, not communicating with the pancreatic duct. The high signal of the cystic lesion on both DWI with *b* factor of 600 s/mm^2 (**c**) and on the corresponding ADC map (**d**, *arrows*) indicates lack of restricted diffusion, characteristic of a benign lesion (serous cystadenoma). Note also findings of divisum pancreas on the MRCP image

Case 6.4: Pancreatic Pseudocyst

A 32-year-old pregnant woman with biliary pancreatitis who presents with a pancreatic pseudocyst as a complication. The MR examination was performed to follow the pseudocyst.

Comments

Complications of acute pancreatitis include hemorrhage, acute fluid collections, pseudocyst formation, and abscess. Pancreatic parenchymal hemorrhage and extrapancreatic hemorrhagic fluid collections are high in signal intensity on T1-weighted fat-suppressed images and low signal on T2-weighted images. Acute fluid collections may occur within the pancreatic gland or have an extrapancreatic location. When acute fluid collections contain serous fluid, they are low in signal intensity on non-contrast T1-weighted gradient-echo images with or without fat suppression and are relatively homogeneous and high in signal intensity on T2-weighted images. When acute fluid collections seal off and develop a wall, pseudocyst formation occurs. Uncomplicated pseudocysts are typically unilocular and encapsulated fluid collections that exhibit high signal intensity on T2-weighted and low signal intensity on T1-weighted sequences. Pseudocyst walls enhance minimally on early postgadolinium images and show progressively intense enhancement on 5-minute post-contrast images, consistent with the appearance of fibrous tissue. ERCP is usually required to reveal communication between a pseudocyst and the pancreatic duct, although sometimes it can be seen on MRI as well. Pseudocysts may contain debris, hemorrhage, or infected material and are heterogeneous in signal intensity on T2-weighted images. Debris can be present in the dependent portion of the lesion and represents proteinaceous material, which may appear as low signal intensity in T2 weighted images. At DWI with lower b values, all pancreatic cystic masses demonstrate a high signal intensity. At $b=1{,}000$, the observed signal in the pseudocyst is typically isointense to the pancreas, with higher signal intensity in the ADC map. This is in contrast with neoplastic cysts, which remain with high signal intensity in DWI with $b=1{,}000$ and demonstrate low signal intensity in the ADC maps.

Imaging Findings

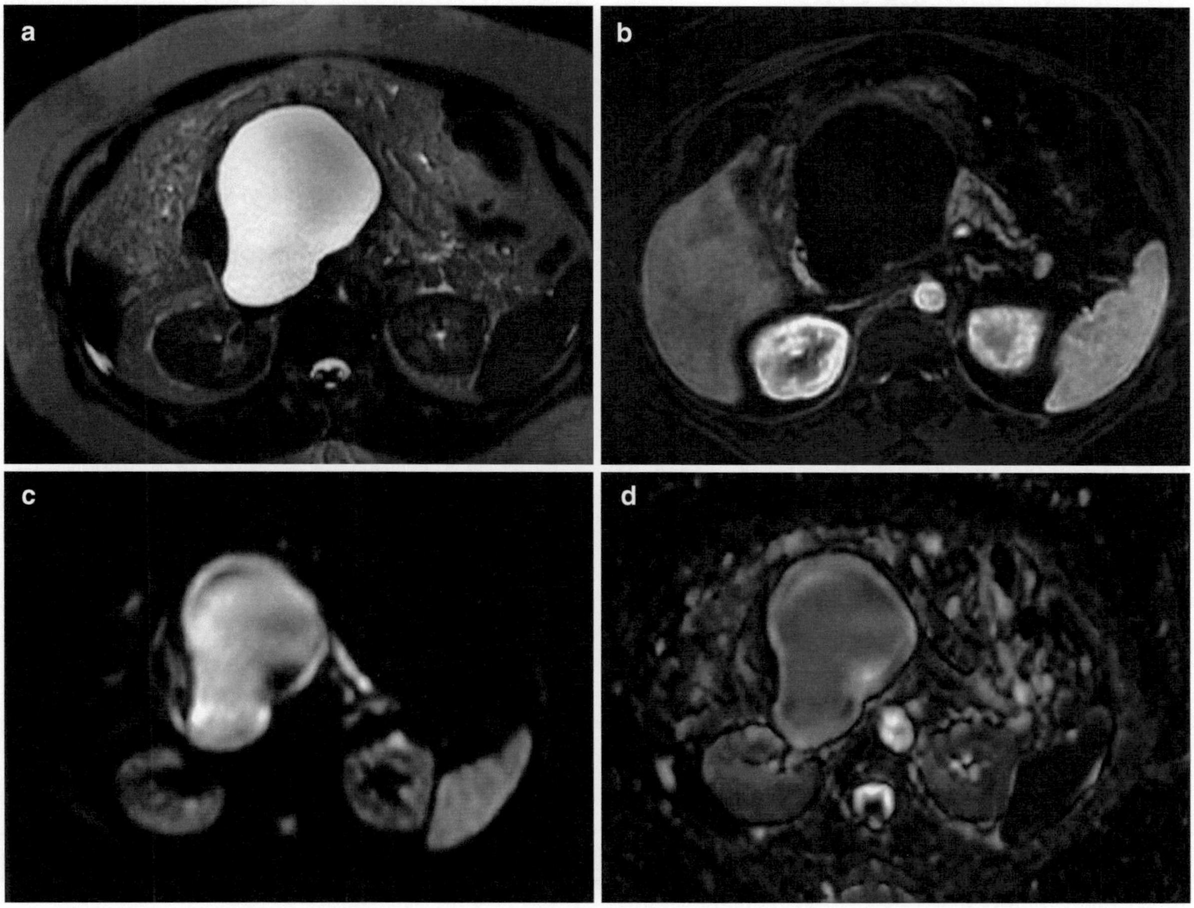

Fig. 6.4 (**a**) Axial FSE T2-weighted image with fat suppression and (**b**) axial contrast-enhanced GE T1-weighted sequence with fat suppression show a large unilocular cystic lesion in the neck of the pancreas. There is subtle enhancement of the wall of this cystic lesion. (**c**) The cystic lesion appears hyperintense compared with the pancreas in the DWI acquired with *b* factor of 600 s/mm^2, as well as in the corresponding ADC map (**d**). This finding is characteristic of a benign lesion

Case 6.5: Von Hippel Lindau Disease with Simple Pancreatic Cysts

A 25-year-old male with a personal history of Von Hippel Lindau disease who presents abdominal pain.

Comments

Von Hippel–Lindau (VHL) disease is a rare, inherited, multisystem disorder that is characterized by development of a variety of benign and malignant tumors. Inheritance is autosomal dominant with high penetrance and variable expression, and the condition is associated with inactivation of a tumor suppression gene located on chromosome 3p25.5. The prevalence is estimated to be between 1 in 31,000 and 1 in 53,000 individuals. The spectrum of clinical manifestations of the disease is broad. These include retinal and central nervous system (CNS) hemangioblastomas, endolymphatic sac tumors, renal cysts and tumors, pancreatic cysts and tumors, pheochromocytomas, and epididymal cystadenomas. The most common causes of death in patients with VHL disease are renal cell carcinoma and neurologic complications from cerebellar hemangioblastomas. According to the natural history of the disease, the median life expectancy is 50 years.

The diagnostic criteria for VHL disease include the following: (a) more than one CNS hemangioblastoma, (b) one CNS hemangioblastoma and visceral manifestations of VHL disease, and (c) any manifestation and a known family history of VHL disease.

Pancreatic involvement in VHL disease includes (in order of frequency): simple pancreatic cysts, serous (microcystic) adenomas, and, rarely, adenocarcinomas. Pancreatic neuroendocrine tumors also occur. Combined lesions occur, but neuroendocrine tumors and cystic lesions only rarely exist together. Mucinous macrocystic adenomas, which are regarded as premalignant, have so far not been described in VHL disease to our knowledge. The reported prevalence of pancreatic involvement in VHL disease varies from 0% in some family groups to 77% in others.

Pancreatic cysts are extremely rare in the general population; therefore, the presence of a single cyst in an individual undergoing VHL disease screening because of a family history makes it highly likely that the person has VHL disease.

On MR images, pancreatic simple cysts are well defined and do not demonstrate invasion of adjacent organs. On T2-weighted images, small cysts are seen as high signal intensity lesions. On T1-weighted images, these cysts are hypointense, with no enhancement with gadolinium. On DWI with lower b values, the cyst demonstrates a high signal intensity. At $b = 1,000$, the signal intensity is typically isointense to the pancreas, with higher signal intensity in the ADC map (T2 shine-through).

Imaging Findings

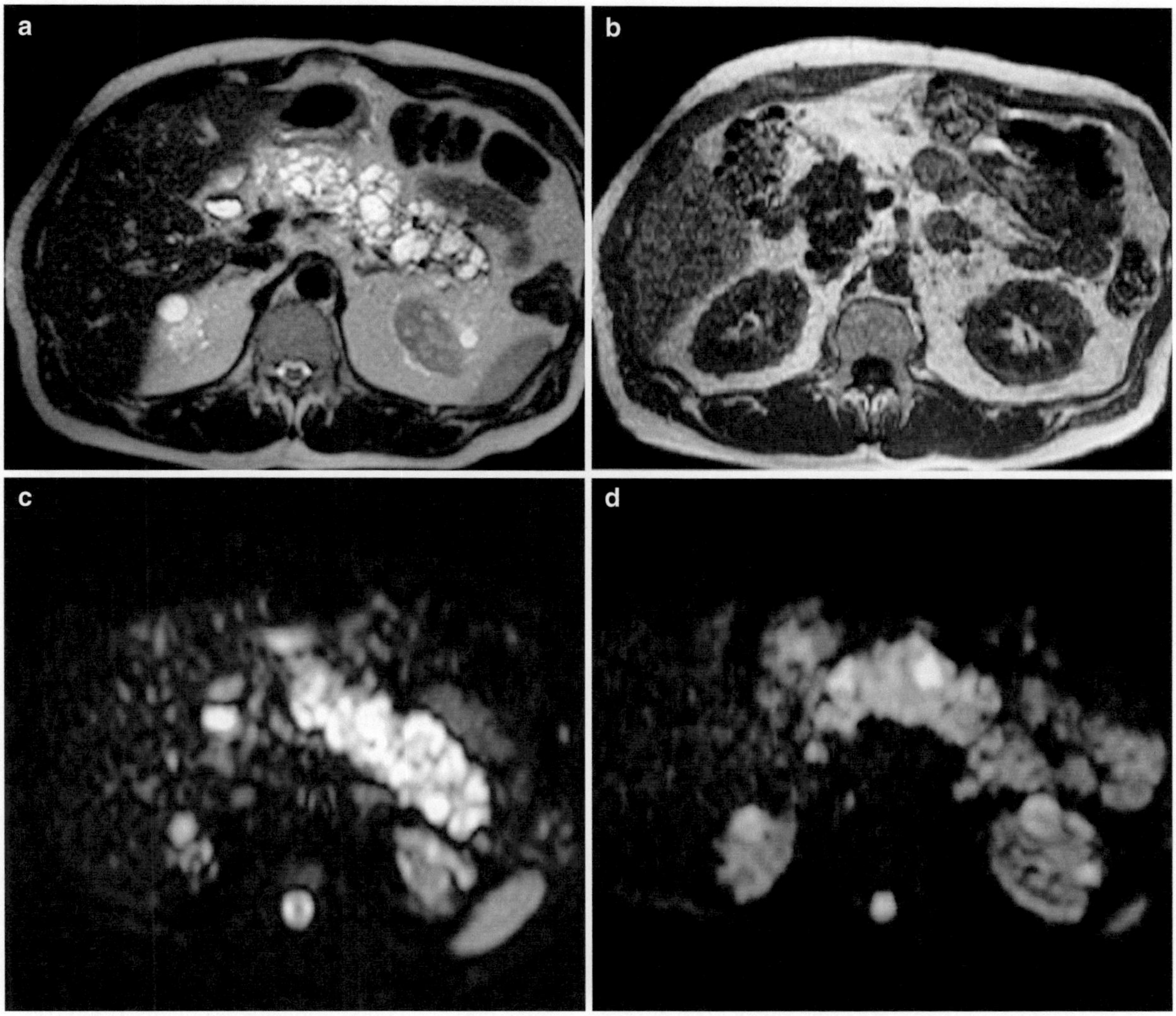

Fig. 6.5 (**a**) Axial FSE T2- weighted image and (**b**) axial non-enhanced in-phase GE T1-weighted images show multiple small cysts throughout the whole pancreas. The cysts appear hyperintense on both diffusion-weighted images acquired with *b* factors of 0 s/mm^2 (**c**) and 600 s/mm^2 (**d**)

Case 6.6: Mucinous Cystadenoma

A 65-year-old female who presents with abdominal pain. Abdominal CT showed a focal round mass in the pancreatic tail.

Comments

Pancreatic cystic neoplasms generally arise from the exocrine component of the gland. Although secondary cystic change can be seen in most types of pancreatic neoplasms, cystic pancreatic neoplasms are characterized by their dominant cystic configuration. Cystic lesions of the pancreas include a variety of pathological entities, such as nonneoplastic cysts (congenital simple cysts, pseudocysts, abscesses, hydatid cysts) and various neoplastic cysts (serous cystadenomas, mucinous cystadenomas, mucinous cystadenocarcinomas, cystic-degenerated adenocarcinomas, intraductal papillary mucinous neoplasm and cystic neuroendocrine tumors). Pseudocysts are the most common of all pancreatic cystic lesions. Because of the malignant potential of mucinous cystic neoplasms, cystic adenocarcinomas, and neuroendocrine tumors, careful consideration of the differential diagnosis is mandatory to choose the optimal treatment for each patient.

Mucinous cystic neoplasms are the most common cystic tumors of the pancreas. The large cystic spaces are lined by tall, mucin-producing columnar cells. Mucinous cystic neoplasms may be unilocular or multilocular and are commonly detected only after achieving a large size. Solid papillary excrescences sometimes protrude from the wall into the interior of these tumors. These tumors are divided into benign (mucinous cystadenoma), borderline, and malignant (mucinous cystadenocarcinoma) varieties.

However, at many institutions, all cases of mucinous cystic neoplasms are interpreted as mucinous cystadenocarcinomas of low-grade malignant potential to reinforce the need for complete surgical resection and close clinical follow-up. Mucinous cystic neoplasms occur more frequently in women between the ages of 40 and 60 years. These tumors usually are located in the body and tail of the pancreas. Of these tumors, 10% may have scattered calcifications. There is a great propensity for invasion of local organs and tissues.

On gadolinium-enhanced T1-weighted fat-suppressed images, large, irregular cystic spaces separated by septa are demonstrated. Cyst walls and septations are often thicker in mucinous cystadenocarcinomas than those of mucinous cystadenomas. Mucinous cystadenomas are well circumscribed, and they show no evidence of metastases or invasion of adjacent tissues. Mucinous cystadenomas described pathologically as having borderline malignant potential may be very large but may not show imaging or gross evidence of metastases or local invasion. Pathologically, these tumors show epithelial dysplasia.

Mucinous cystadenocarcinoma may be a very locally aggressive malignancy with extensive invasion of adjacent tissues and organs. The presence of solid components is suggestive of frank malignancy. Breathing-independent T2-weighted images are particularly effective at defining the cysts. Mucin produced by these tumors may result in high signal intensity on T1- and T2-weighted images of the primary tumor and liver metastases.

A DWI with a high *b* value (1,000 s/mm^2) can differentiate cystic lesions with clear fluid content from those with increased internal cellular elements or protein content. According to a recent study, congenital simple cysts and uncomplicated pseudocysts are isointense with background pancreas on images with a high *b* value, whereas abscesses, hydatid cysts, and neoplastic cysts such as mucinous cystadenomas and cystadenocarcinomas reveal a higher signal intensity than the pancreatic glandular parenchyma they arise from. Accordingly, the ADC values of simple cysts and pseudocysts are higher than the abscesses, hydatid cysts, and neoplastic cysts.

Imaging Findings

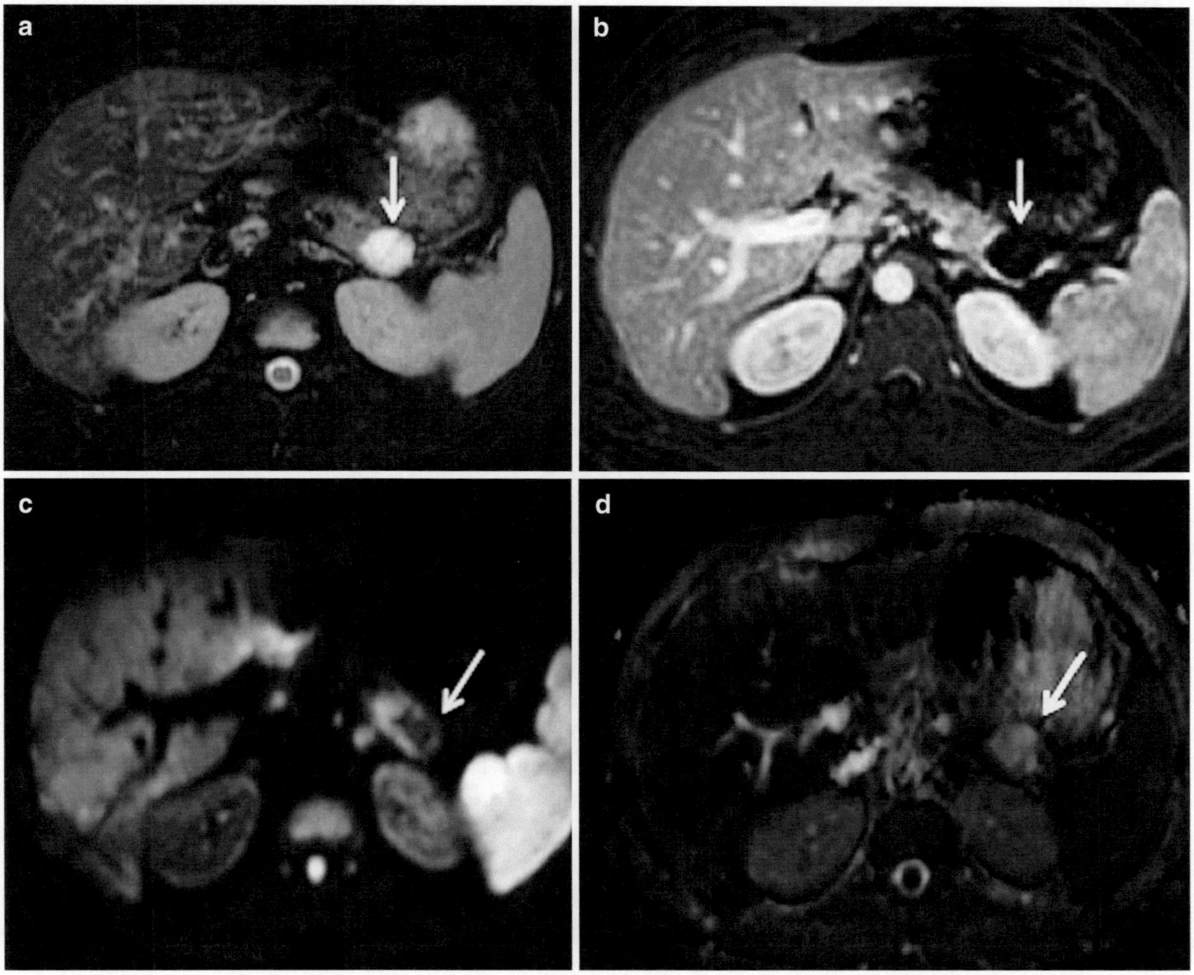

Fig. 6.6 (**a**) Axial FSE T2-weighted with fat suppression and (**b**) axial postcontrast fat suppressed GE T1-weighted images show a cyst with a single enhancing septum and capsule. The lesion shows low central signal intensity in the DWI with *b* value of 600 s/mm^2 (**c**) and intermediate signal intensity on the corresponding ADC map (**d**). The lesion was proven to be a mucinous cystadenoma at surgery, despite its slightly atypical appearance

Case 6.7: Intraductal Papillary Mucinous Neoplasm

A 55-year-old female who presents with nonspecific abdominal symptoms. Abdominal ultrasound showed a hypoechoic focal round mass in the pancreatic head. The MR examination was performed to characterize the mass.

Comments

Intraductal papillary mucinous neoplasms (IPMN) arise from the epithelial cells of the pancreatic duct. It has been increasingly diagnosed on various imaging modalities. Histologically, the lesions represent a wide spectrum of abnormalities, which include simple hyperplasia, adenoma, borderline lesions, and adenocarcinoma. This spectrum of abnormalities may coexist even within the same lesion. Benign lesions such as hyperplasia and adenoma may progress to carcinoma. The involved pancreatic duct is filled with mucinous gel-like material and results in varying degrees of ductal dilatation. Morphologically, IPMN can be classified as main duct, branch duct, or combined type, which shows features of both main duct and branch duct types. The main duct type of IPMN is characterized by a dilatation of main pancreatic duct of more than 1 cm in diameter, abundant mucin production, and papillary excrescences arising from ductal epithelium. Whereas diffuse tumors involve the entire or large portions of the main duct, segmental tumors involve one or more segments. In general, main duct IPMN is associated with a higher prevalence of carcinoma than the branch duct type. Given that these tumors produce large volumes of mucin, the main pancreatic duct becomes markedly dilated and direct visualization of this phenomenon on endoscopic retrograde cholangiopancreatography can confirm the diagnosis. With MRI, a prominently dilated main pancreatic duct is noted especially on T2-weighted and MRCP images. Frequently, papillary-growing mural nodules within a dilated main pancreatic duct are demonstrated on postgadolinium images. Surgical resection is the treatment of choice and a remnant margin histologically free of IPMN should be obtained.

The branch duct type of IPMN predominantly involves side branch ducts and appears as a pleomorphic cyst. This lesion consists of one or several cysts with variable morphology and is sometimes described as a "cluster of grapes" appearance. Typically, the branch duct type of IPMN occurs in the head of the pancreas. This type of IPMN shows an indolent benign course as compared with the main duct type. Direct communication of the lesion with the main pancreatic duct is another important feature that is suggestive of the branch duct type of IPMN. A branch duct type of IPMN that is less than 3 cm in diameter in asymptomatic patients is usually benign and grows very slowly. MR imaging is the modality of choice for characterizing IPMN and provides better depiction of ductal communication than CT. The location and type of an IPMN determine its MR imaging appearance. In tumors that involve the main pancreatic duct, ductal dilatation is a reliable feature and may be observed along the entire length of the duct or within a segment. Although chronic pancreatitis also causes diffuse ductal dilatation, there are associated parenchymal signal intensity changes, such as loss of T1 signal and delayed uptake of contrast material, which are indicative of chronic fibrosis. The most common MR finding in IPMN involving the pancreatic ductal side branches is dilatation of multiple side branches on T2-weighted images. The observed signal intensities of all cystic lesions are high on DWI acquired with lower *b* values. However, when a *b* factor of 1,000 s/mm^2 is applied, significant differences between the signal intensity ratios of various types of pancreatic cystic lesions can be detected: Neoplastic cysts and abscesses remain hyperintense while benign cysts show the same signal intensity that the pancreatic parenchyma shows. Hence, the high signal on DWI is due to the reduced diffusion, which can be attributed to the mucin content of the cystic lesions. Hence, IPMN exhibits ADC values which are lower than those of nonneoplastic cysts.

Imaging Findings

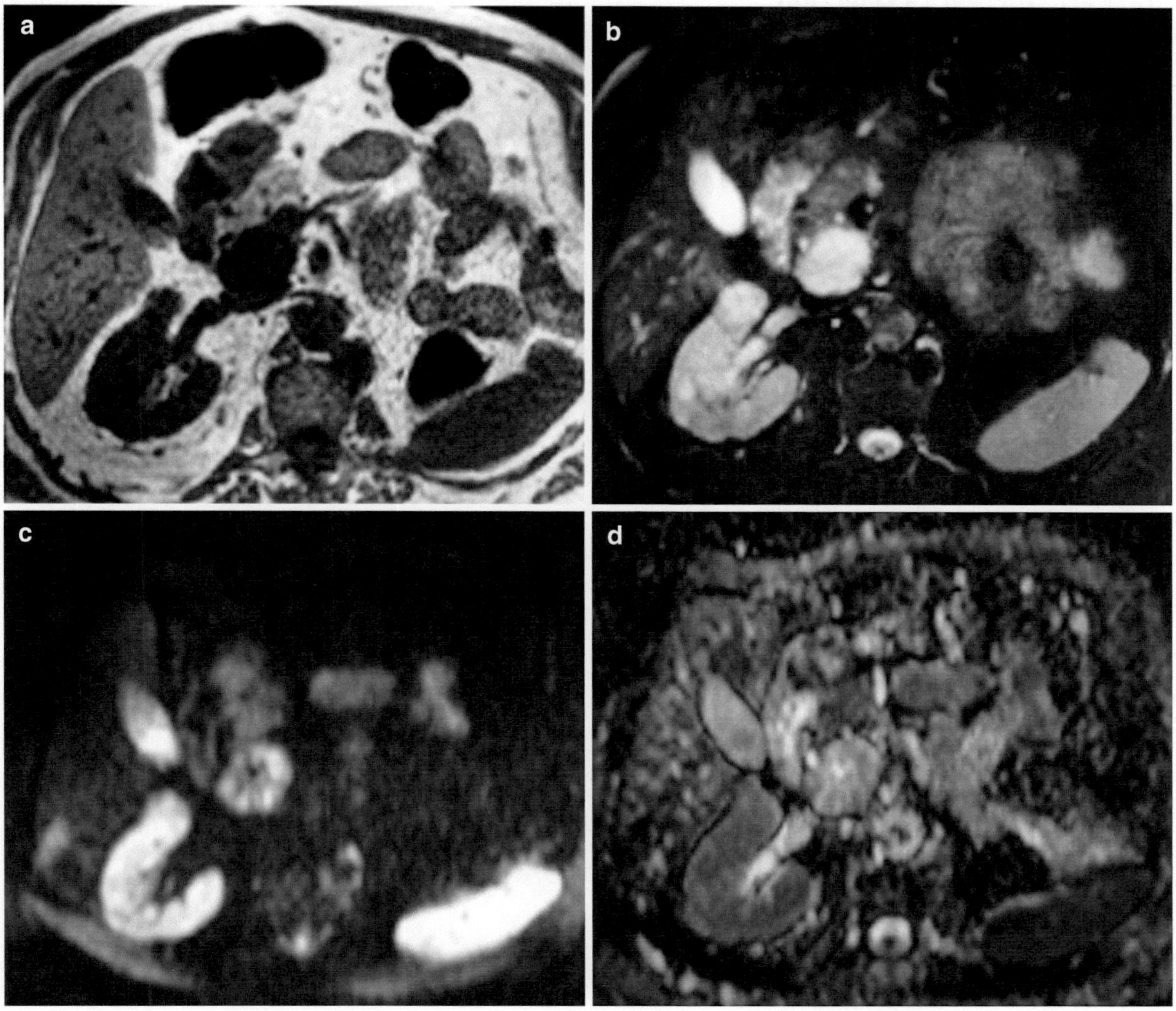

Fig. 6.7 (**a**) Axial non-enhanced GE T1-weighted image and (**b**) axial fat-supressed FSE T2-weighted image show a low and high (respectively) signal intensity mass in the uncinate process of the pancreas. (**c**) DWI acquired with a *b* factor of 800 s/mm^2 and (**d**) ADC map demonstrate the mass with high signal intensity in the DWI and low-to-intermediate signal intensity in the corresponding ADC map (restricted diffusion)

Case 6.8: Sclerosing Pancreatitis and Peripancreatic Collection

A 45-year-old male with diagnosis of primary sclerosing cholangitis, who presents to the emergency room with abdominal pain and fever.

Comments

Autoimmune pancreatitis is a subgroup of chronic pancreatitis with characteristic clinical, pathological, laboratory, and imaging findings. This form is associated with autoimmune disorders such as Sjogren's syndrome, primary biliary cirrhosis, and primary sclerosing cholangitis. Histopathological findings of chronic autoimmune pancreatitis show periductal chronic inflammation and fibrosis. This process may result in obstruction or destruction of ducts. Studies have described the MR appearance of autoimmune chronic pancreatitis that are characterized by an enlarged pancreas with moderately decreased signal intensity on T1-weighted images, moderately high signal intensity on T2-weighted images, and delayed enhancement of the pancreatic parenchyma after gadolinium administration. Additional findings that may be observed in autoimmune pancreatitis include: a capsule-like rim surrounding the diseased parenchyma that is hypointense on T2-weighted images and demonstrates delayed enhancement following gadolinium administration; absence of parenchymal atrophy; ductal dilatation proximal to the site of stenosis; and absence of extrapancreatic fluid. DWI has been used for the assessment of chronic pancreatitis. ADC values in patients with chronic pancreatitis are lower than normal pancreas, possibly because of the replacement of normal pancreatic parenchyma with fibrous tissue and/or the diminished exocrine function that may reduce diffusible tissue water and result in decreased ADC. Acute fluid collections may occur within the pancreatic gland or have an extrapancreatic location. When acute fluid collections contain serous fluid content, they are low in signal intensity on non-contrast T1-weighted gradient-echo images with or without fat suppression and are relatively homogeneous and high in signal intensity on T2-weighted images. At DWI with lower *b* values, all pancreatic cystic masses demonstrate high signal intensity. At $b = 1{,}000$, the observed signal in the noncomplicated collections is typically isointense to the pancreas with higher signal intensity in the ADC map.

Imaging Findings

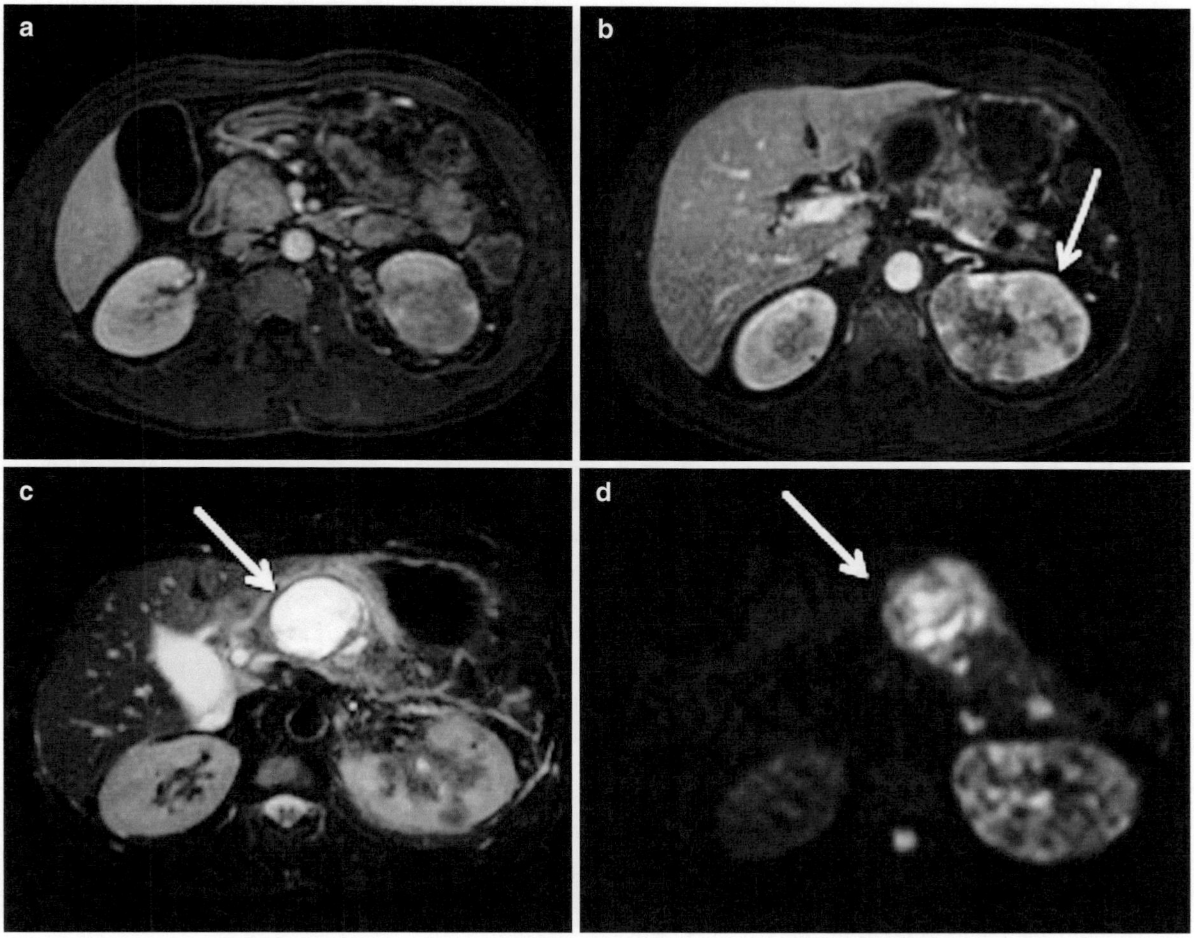

Fig. 6.8 (**a**, **b**) Axial contrast-enhanced GE T1-weighted image with fat suppression show an enlarged pancreas with heterogeneous enhancement and a peripancreatic fluid collection. The left kidney is enlarged and shows a striated pattern of enhancement and there are associated inflammatory changes in the perinephritic fat (*arrow*). (**c**) Axial FSE T2-weighted image with fat suppression shows a hyperintense peripancreatic collection (*arrow*). (**d**) DWI with a *b* value of 1,000 s/mm^2 shows high signal intensity in the peripancreatic collection (*arrow*), the left kidney, and, to a lesser degree, in the pancreas

Case 6.9: Hilar Cholangiocarcinoma

A 85-year-old male who presents with jaundice, weight loss, and abdominal pain. Ultrasonography showed a dilated biliary tract without evidence of a mass. The MRI was performed to establish the cause of obstruction.

Comments

Cholangiocarcinomas (CC) are malignant tumors originating from the epithelial cells lining the biliary tree and gallbladder. Intrahepatic CCs (ICC) arise within the liver and extrahepatic CCs (ECC) originate in the bile duct along the hepato-duodenal ligament. ICCs usually present as masses in the liver while jaundice is the most common presentation of ECCs. CCs are relatively rare tumors although their incidence is rising worldwide. The incidence of CC is rising in most countries and it is the second most common primary malignancy of the liver after hepatocellular carcinoma. The main risk factors for CC are: chronic inflammation, genetic predisposition, and congenital abnormalities of the biliary tree. The only curative treatment for CC is surgical resection with negative margins. Liver transplantation has been proposed only for selected patients with hilar CC that cannot be resected who have no metastatic disease after a period of neoadjuvant chemo-radiation therapy. US, MRI, MRCP, PET/CT, endoscopic US, and CT are the most frequently used modalities for diagnosis and tumor staging.

US is usually the initial imaging test performed to evaluate patients with suspected biliary obstruction. The sensitivity and accuracy of US for ECC diagnosis are 89% and 80–95%, respectively. Triple-phase CT scan is widely used to diagnose and stage CC as it provides valuable information regarding local spread, vascular invasion, lymph node involvement, and presence of distant metastases. On CT scans, ECC may be seen as a focal thickening of the ductal wall with various enhancement patterns. However, in many cases of ECC, visualization of the neoplasm is not definitive because they are too small to be detected. More recent studies have shown that modern contrast-enhanced MDCT is 78.6–92.3% accurate for the diagnosis of ECC, although there is a strong tendency to underestimate the longitudinal extension of the tumor, in comparison with the pathological results of the excised specimens. The overall accuracy of CT for determining resectability of CC is in the range of 60–85%. Recently, CT cholangiography has been shown to be a promising modality for delineating the biliary tree. MRI with concurrent MRCP can provide three-dimensional reconstructions of the biliary tree by using MR technology. Multiple studies have demonstrated the utility of MRCP in evaluating patients with CC. MRCP has diagnostic accuracy comparable to invasive cholangiographic techniques such as ERCP or percutaneous transhepatic cholangiography (PTC). A further advantage of MRCP over invasive cholangiography is that it does not require biliary instrumentation. Therefore, MRI along with MRCP is considered the imaging modality of choice for evaluating patients with suspected CC. MRCP/MRI allows definition of the anatomy and extent of CC within the hepatobiliary system, vascular invasion, local lymphadenopathy, and distant metastases. Ideally, MRCP should be performed before decompressing the biliary tree. On MRCP, ECC may appear as extrahepatic lesions which are hypointense on T1- and hyperintense on T2-weighted images with pooling of contrast within the tumor on delayed images. Regarding surrounding structures, MRI has been shown to have 66% accuracy for detection of lymph node metastases, 78% sensitivity and 91% specificity for portal vein invasion, and 58–73% sensitivity and 93% specificity for arterial invasion.

As DWI has become an integral component of most abdominal MR protocols at many institutions, the experience with its application for evaluating patients with biliary tract disorders is growing accordingly. However, there is still very little published scientific data to support its use. On DWI, early experience suggests that the tumor exhibits diffusion restriction, which is helpful for separating the lesion from the surrounding hepatic parenchyma. Regional extension of the tumor to porta hepatis lymph nodes can also be well depicted with DWI, since involved nodes may also demonstrate restricted diffusion. One potential application of DWI in biliary tract imaging is in the surveillance and early detection of cholangiocarcinoma in patients with primary sclerosing cholangitis. This, however, has not been convincingly proven yet. A recent study found that DWI has a greater sensitivity and specificity than MRCP in terms of detection of ECC.

ECC has an increased cell density, diminished extracellular space, and restricted movement of water molecules, all of which increase the signal. DWI possesses good background suppression effects; blood vessels, the bile ducts, and intra-abdominal fat, all exhibit low signal intensities. This increases tumor contrast with surrounding tissues, which improves lesion detection. However the use of DWI in cholangiocarcinoma is still undergoing testing and more research should be conducted to determine its value in clinical applications.

Imaging Findings

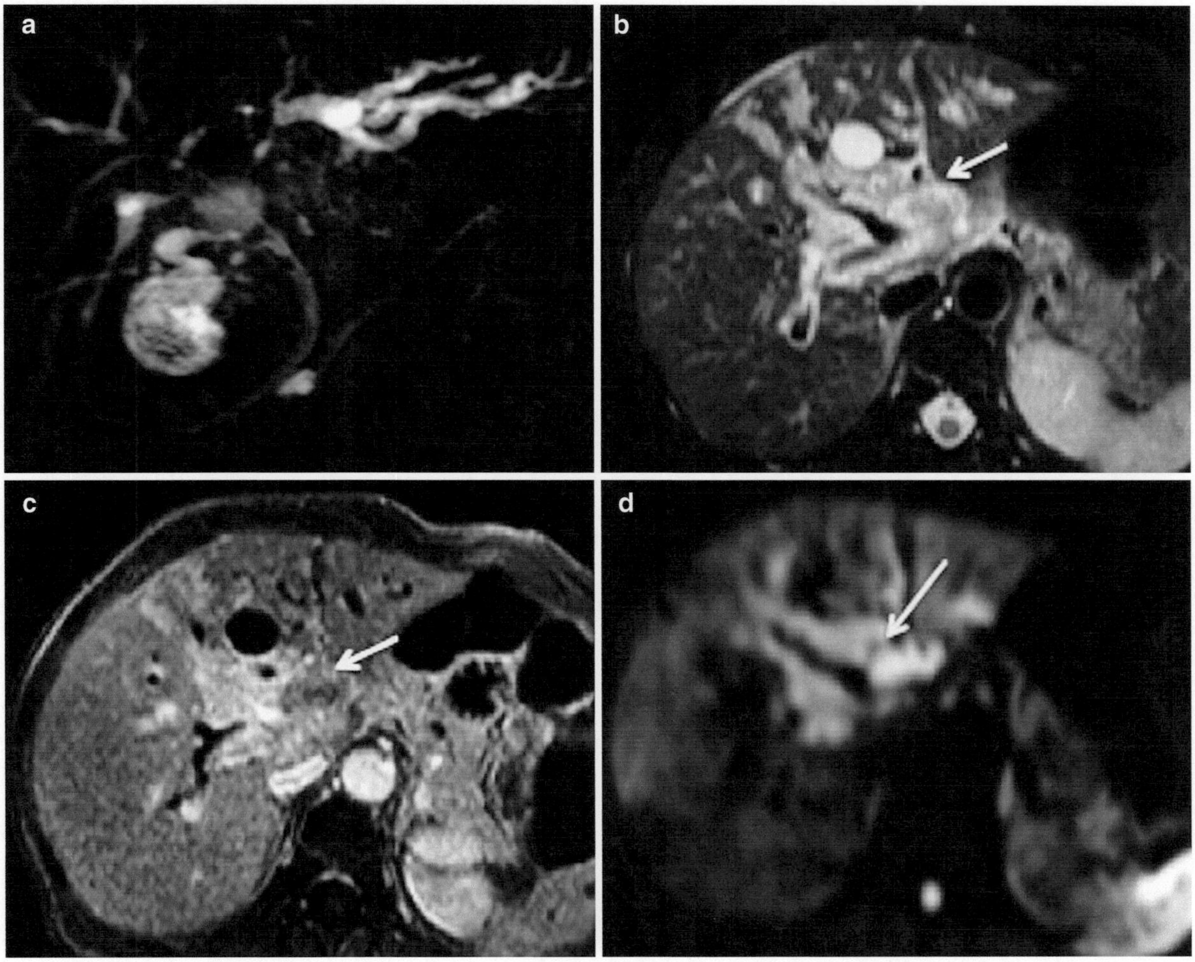

Fig. 6.9 (**a**) Coronal-oblique thick section single-shot MRCP image shows intrahepatic duct dilatation and obstruction at the porta hepatis (Bismuth IV); there is a biliary prosthesis in extrahepatic and right intrahepatic biliary ducts. (**b**) Axial FSE T2-weighted image with fat suppression shows excessive soft tissue at the porta hepatis with a hypointense mass (*arrow*). (**c**) Axial contrast-enhanced GE T1-weighted image with fat suppression acquired in a portal phase image shows a hypovascular mass (*arrow*), which is causing the biliary ductal obstruction. (**d**) DWI acquired with a *b* factor of 600 s/mm^2 shows the lesion with high signal intensity (*arrow*)

Case 6.10: Acute Cholecystitis

A 45-year-old female who visits the emergency room due to right upper quadrant tenderness, fever, and an increase in the white blood cell count. Abdominal ultrasound showed a thickened gallbladder wall without dilatation of the biliary tract.

Comments

Gallstones are the main cause of acute cholecystitis, for which an estimated 120,000 cholecystectomies are performed annually in the United States. The prevalence of acute cholecystitis is approximately 5% in patients who present with acute abdominal pain to the ED. Traditionally, the diagnosis has been based on the clinical trial of right upper quadrant tenderness, elevated body temperature, and elevated white blood cell count. The diagnostic criteria for acute cholecystitis are one local sign of inflammation (Murphy sign; mass, pain, and/or tenderness in right upper quadrant), one systemic sign of inflammation (fever, elevated C-reactive protein level, elevated white blood cell count), and confirmatory imaging findings.

Imaging findings are essential for making decisions regarding treatment for cholecystitis. Several imaging techniques are available for the evaluation of suspected acute cholecystitis. US is the most frequently performed modality for right upper quadrant pain and yields a sensitivity of 88% and a specificity of 80% in the diagnosis of acute cholecystitis. Features of cholecystitis include gallbladder wall thickening; enlarged tender, noncompressible gallbladder; and adjacent infiltration or fluid collection. According to the ACR appropriateness criteria, US is considered the most appropriate imaging modality for patients suspected of having acute calculous cholecystitis. In a highly select study sample, CT also showed good accuracy, with a sensitivity of 92% and a specificity of 99%. In patients with acute abdominal pain, CT has demonstrated accuracy comparable to that of US in the diagnosis of acute cholecystitis. Although US should be considered the primary imaging technique for patients clinically suspected of having acute cholecystitis, it is often difficult to demonstrate a stone impacted in the cystic duct or gallbladder neck. In these cases, MR imaging has a higher sensitivity than US for diagnosis of acute cholecystitis and therefore should be considered as an alternative imaging modality in problematic cases. MR imaging findings of acute uncomplicated cholecystitis include (a) gallstones, often impacted in the gallbladder neck or cystic duct; (b) gallbladder wall thickening (<3 mm); (c) gallbladder wall edema; (d) gallbladder distention.

A thickened gallbladder wall is observed in acute cholecystitis as well as other conditions such as chronic cholecystitis, adenomyomatosis, malignant neoplasm, and acute hepatitis. However, a thickened wall with a diffuse or patchy distribution of increased signal intensity on fat-suppressed T2-weighted images is suggestive of an acute inflammatory process. An acute inflammatory process extending into the adipose tissue surrounding the gallbladder also appears as a reticular or patchy hyperintense area on fat-suppressed T2-weighted images. On contrast-enhanced fat-suppressed T1-weighted images, increased contrast enhancement can be seen in the gallbladder wall, pericholecystic fat, and intrahepatic periportal tissues, findings that are supportive of acute cholecystitis.

Although there are no publications with a large number of patients confirming a role for DWI in the diagnosis of inflammatory gallbladder disease, it is expected that, as with other inflammatory conditions, findings would include high signal intensity and restricted diffusion.

Imaging Findings

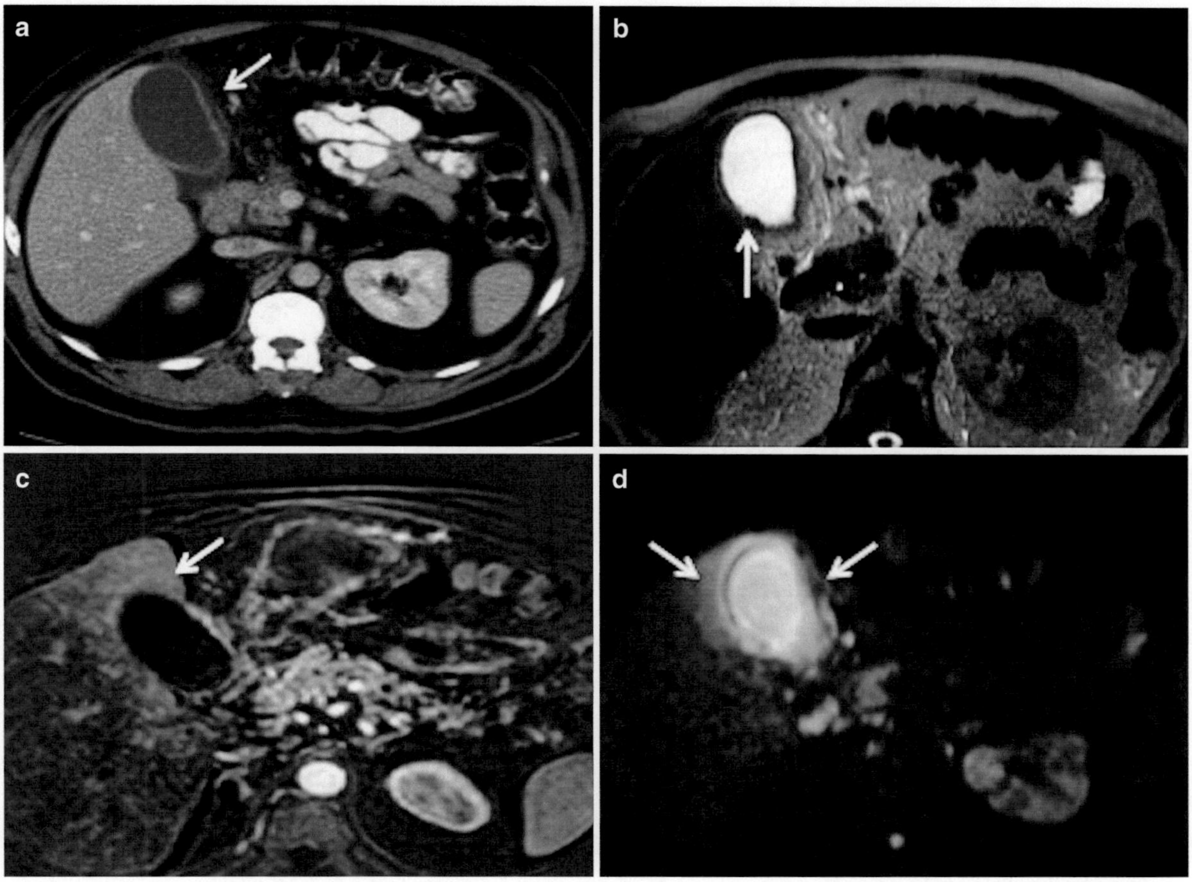

Fig. 6.10 (**a**) CT image acquired in the portal venous phase shows thickening and increased enhancement of the gallbladder wall with inflammatory findings in the adjacent fat (*arrow*). (**b**) Axial FSE T2-weighted image without fat suppression shows a thickened gallbladder wall and small dependent hypointense stones (*arrow*). (**c**) Axial contrast-enhanced GE T1-weighted image with fat suppression acquired in the arterial phase shows transient hyperemia (*arrow*) in the liver parenchyma adjacent to the gallbladder and wall hyperenhancement. (**d**) DWI acquired with a *b* factor of 600 s/mm^2 shows the high signal intensity in the gallbladder wall and the adjacent liver (*arrows*)

Further Reading

Balci NC, Perman WH, Saglam S et al (2009) Diffusion-weighted magnetic resonance imaging of the pancreas. Top Magn Reson Imaging 20(1):43–47

Cui XY, Chen HW (2010) Role of diffusion-weighted magnetic resonance imaging in the diagnosis of extrahepatic cholangiocarcinoma. World J Gastroenterol 16(25):3196–3201

Dale BM, Braithwaite AC, Boll DT et al (2010) Field strength and diffusion encoding technique affect the apparent diffusion coefficient measurements in diffusion-weighted imaging of the abdomen. Invest Radiol 45(2):104–108

Fattahi R, Balci NC, Perman WH et al (2009) Pancreatic diffusion-weighted imaging (DWI): comparison between mass-forming focal pancreatitis (FP), pancreatic cancer (PC), and normal pancreas. J Magn Reson Imaging 29(2):350–356

Grünberg K, Grenacher L, Klauß M (2011) Diffusion-weighted imaging of the pancreas. Radiologe 51(3):186–194

Inan N, Arslan A, Akansel G et al (2008) Diffusion-weighted imaging in the differential diagnosis of cystic lesions of the pancreas. Am J Roentgenol 191(4):1115–1121

Irie H, Honda H, Kuroiwa T et al (2002) Measurement of the apparent diffusion coefficient in intraductal mucin-producing tumor of the pancreas by diffusion-weighted echo-planar MR imaging. Abdom Imaging 27(1):82–87

Kamisawa T, Takuma K, Anjiki H et al (2010) Differentiation of autoimmune pancreatitis from pancreatic cancer by diffusion-weighted MRI. Am J Gastroenterol 105(8):1870–1875

Kartalis N, Lindholm TL, Aspelin P et al (2009) Diffusion-weighted magnetic resonance imaging of pancreas tumours. Eur Radiol 19:1981–1990

Klauss M, Lemke A, Grünberg K et al (2011) Intravoxel incoherent motion MRI for the differentiation between mass forming chronic pancreatitis and pancreatic carcinoma. Invest Radiol 46(1):57–63

Lee SS, Byun JH, Park BJ et al (2008) Quantitative analysis of diffusion-weighted magnetic resonance imaging of the pancreas: usefulness in characterizing solid pancreatic masses. J Magn Reson Imaging 28(4):928–936

Lemke A, Laun FB, Klau M et al (2009). Differentiation of pancreas carcinoma from healthy pancreatic tissue using multiple b-values: comparison of apparent diffusion coefficient and intravoxel incoherent motion derived parameters. Invest Radiol; Oct 15, 2009 [Epub ahead of print]

Masselli G, Manfredi R, Vecchioli A et al (2008) MR imaging and MR cholangiopancreatography in the preoperative evaluation of hilar cholangiocarcinoma: correlation with surgical and pathologic findings. Eur Radiol 18: 2213–2221

Matsuki M, Inada Y, Nakai G et al (2007) Diffusion-weighted MR imaging of pancreatic carcinoma. Abdom Imaging 32(4):481–483

Muraoka N, Uematsu H, Kimura H et al (2008) Apparent diffusion coefficient in pancreatic cancer: characterization and histopathological correlations. J Magn Reson Imaging 27(6):1302–1308

Park HS, Lee JM, Choi JY et al (2008) Preoperative evaluation of bile duct cancer: MRI combined with MR cholangiopancreatography versus MDCT with direct cholangiography. Am J Roentgenol 190:396–405

Shinya S, Sasaki T, Nakagawa Y et al (2009) The efficacy of diffusion-weighted imaging for the detection and evaluation of acute pancreatitis. Hepatogastroenterology 56(94–95): 1407–1410

Taniguchi T, Kobayashi H, Nishikawa K et al (2009) Diffusion-weighted magnetic resonance imaging in autoimmune pancreatitis. Jpn J Radiol 27(3):138–142

Yoshikawa T, Kawamitsu H, Mitchell DG et al (2006) ADC measurement of abdominal organs and lesions using parallel imaging technique. Am J Roentgenol 187(6):1521–1530

Diffusion-Weighted MR Imaging of the Renal and Adrenal Glands

7

Nagaraj Holalkere, Stephan Anderson,
and Jorge A. Soto

7.1 Introduction

DWI with ADC measurements potentially provides a noninvasive method for discriminating benign from malignant renal and adrenal lesions using molecular criteria. DWI was difficult to perform earlier in the body due to main-field inhomogeneity, local susceptibility gradients, chemical shift, and motion from respiration. Fortunately, recent advances in MRI techniques such as improvements in SS EPI parallel imaging, and the availability of arrays of multiple receiver coils that simultaneously sample the signal returning from more than one part of the body surface and then separate the encoded data provided by each element of the coil have resulted in significant improved image quality for advanced imaging such as DWI. The major advantage for routine clinical practice is that the benefits of DWI do not require the administration of intravenous contrast material and there is no risk of radiation as compared to other currently available functional techniques such as PET imaging or perfusion studies.

7.2 Technique

DWI of the upper abdomen, including renal and adrenal glands, is performed optimally on a high-field (1.5 T or above) system, using either conventional SE or stimulated echo, FSE, GE (e.g., SSFP), EPI, and line scan diffusion imaging. The degree of diffusion weighting is determined by the strength of the diffusion gradients, the duration of those gradients, and the time interval between the gradient pulses. Therefore, the use of high-field gradient systems with faster and more sensitive sequences makes diffusion weighting more feasible and resulting images are of better quality.

DWI of the renal and adrenal glands can be performed using either breath-hold or non-breath-hold (free breathing) or respiratory-triggered imaging sequences. However, respiratory-triggered imaging sequences offer the best image quality with very little degradation by motion artifact. The images retain very good anatomical detail and are usually only minimally degraded by volume averaging. On the other hand, breath-hold imaging allows a target volume to be rapidly assessed with thicker slices, at the expense of increased volume averaging. Accurate quantification of ADC and evaluation of small lesions is theoretically more precise on respiratory-triggered and breath-hold DWI than with a non-breath-hold technique. Respiratory triggering software for DWI is currently available only on some MR scanners.

The diffusion data can be presented as signal intensity or as an image map of the ADC. Calculation of the ADC requires two or more acquisitions with different diffusion weightings. A low ADC corresponds to high signal intensity (restricted diffusion), and a high ADC to low signal intensity on diffusion-weighted images. The signal intensity on DWI is influenced by spin density, T1 and T2 relaxation times, and TE and TR. Pure diffusion information can be obtained by eliminating these influences by calculating ADC maps. Hence, it is important to review both the DWI images and the

N. Holalkere (✉) • S. Anderson • J.A. Soto
Radiology Department, Boston University School of Medicine, Boston, MA, USA
e-mail: jorge.soto@bmc.org

A. Luna et al., *Diffusion MRI Outside the Brain*,
DOI 10.1007/978-3-642-21052-5_7, © Springer-Verlag Berlin Heidelberg 2012

corresponding area on ADC maps in order to eliminate possible false positives.

Authors prefer to use respiratory-triggered SS SE EPI with parameters of TE = minimum, TR = 3000–5000, NEX = 1, thickness/skip = 5–7/0 mm, *b* value = 0, 600 and 800 s/mm^2, matrix = 128 × 128, combined with parallel imaging (e.g., sensitivity encoding) and fat suppression for adrenal and renal imaging. Total image acquisition time is approximately 2–3 min. The disadvantages of this technique include a limited number of b-value images that can be acquired, poorer SNR compared with multiple averaging methods, and greater sensitivity to pulsatile and susceptibility artifacts. Some of these limitations can be overcome by using higher field scanners (3 T) in which the SNR is greater, and higher spatial resolution images can be achieved by using thinner (5 mm) slice thickness, as compared to 1.5-T scanners, which may be limited to a 7-mm slice thickness. Increased spatial resolution reduces partial volume artifacts and therefore increasing the precision of calculating the ADC value of neoplastic tissue.

7.3 Renal DWI

Accurate diagnosis of renal cell carcinoma (RCC) is important, as it enables early intervention and may result in an improved prognosis. The current established criteria have few limitations and DWI may overcome or provide additional information in renal lesion evaluation. The potential applications of DWI in the evaluation of focal renal masses are lesion characterization (Figs. 7.1, 7.2 and 7.3), lesion detection (Fig. 7.4), and alternative to contrast-enhanced MRI (Fig. 7.5), monitoring response to treatment (Fig. 7.6), and differentiation of simple hydronephrosis from pyonephrosis.

DWI of the kidneys is an area of growing interest. As in other organs, lack of standardization in the technique has limited the reproducibility of results. Furthermore, the monoexponential model of analysis of diffusion is the cause of the variability found in the ADC of healthy kidneys, and a biexponential model better fits to the diffusion characteristics of kidneys. The ADC value of the cortex is higher than the one of the renal medulla, and the FA value of the medulla higher than the one of the cortex. The different characteristics and microstructure of the different components of renal parenchyma have been explored with DTI (Figs. 3.6 and 3.7), allowing for accurate differentiation of renal cortex and medulla. There is evidence of reduced ADC values in cases of diffuse renal disease as acute and specially renal chronic failure, ischemia, infection, and inflammatory conditions. Furthermore, DWI allows to delineating the areas of involvement as areas with restricted diffusion.

With regard to focal renal lesions, malignant lesions tend to show lower ADC values than benign solid and cystic lesions. Furthermore, Taouli and colleagues demonstrated that DWI can be used to differentiate solid RCCs from oncocytomas and characterize the histologic subtypes of RCC. Besides, a significant difference between the diffusion properties of clear cell and nonclear cell RCCs has been achieved, which is important in the therapeutic management, as clear cell RCCs benefit from the use of antiangiogenic drugs. Very recently, Chandarana and colleagues have clinically explored the IVIM model in the differentiation of enhancing from nonenhancing renal lesions in 28 patients with 15 enhancing and 16 nonenhancing lesions, using a 1.5 T magnet. IVIM related parameters, such as perfusion fraction and tissue diffusivity, showed higher accuracy in this distinction than ADC derived from a monoexponential model. Furthermore, there was a good correlation between perfusion fraction and percent enhancement obtained from postcontrast series, allowing the assessment of lesion vascularity without the use of exogenous contrast agent.

An area under investigation is the role of DWI in the early evaluation of transplant kidneys. Significant lower ADC values obtained with different b values have been associated to patients with acute rejection compared to those without, as early as 2–3 weeks after transplantation. Furthermore, the IVIM approach has also been applied in this task with promising results, as DWI was able to determinate in a reliable manner diffusion and microcirculation in renal allografts. Marked reduction in perfusion fraction was related to acute rejection or acute tubular necrosis.

Finally, DWI has been proposed as a biomarker of renal fibrosis in murine models, as a decrease in ADC values was observed with fibrosis progression in the series by Togao et al. As decreased ADCs correlate with serum creatinine levels and the split glomerular filtration rate measured technetium 99m–diethylenetriaminepentaacetic acid scintigraphy and ADC decreases in a parallel manner to increases in cellularity, DWI is a potential noninvasive biomarker for evolution and response to treatment of renal fibrosis. These preliminary results must be validated in humans.

7.4 Adrenal DWI

Recent advances in imaging techniques and the widespread use of high-resolution thin slice CT imaging has led to an increased detection of adrenal lesions. It is essential to characterize all adrenal lesions in patients with known cancer elsewhere in the body because many tumors, particularly lung cancer, have a propensity to metastasize to the adrenal glands. DWI has the potential to characterize benign from malignant adrenal lesions by means of ADC measurements. Nevertheless, in the limited available series, there are contradictory results in the capabilities of DWI in the characterization of adrenal masses, with more data favoring the absence of a significant difference between the adenomas and malignant lesions. Furthermore, in the report by Miller et al., the median ADC of lipid-rich adenomas did not differ from that of the lipid-poor ones. Conversely, in the authors' experience, the diagnostic performance of DWI was comparable to chemical shift imaging in this task (Figs. 7.7 and 7.8). Besides, a difference in ADC values between pheochromocytomas and other types of adrenal lesions was established in the series by Tsushima et al, with higher ADC values for pheochromocytomas. As in other organs, susceptibility artifacts, necrosis, and hemorrhage may alter ADC values (Fig. 7.9). Therefore, at this moment, DWI may be considered as an adjunct tool in the MRI evaluation of adrenal lesions, and it should always be integrated with the information of the rest of MRI sequences including chemical shift imaging. Undoubtedly, more research is necessary in the evaluation of adrenal glands with DWI to clarify its role in the workup of both common and complex adrenal lesions (Fig. 7.10).

Case 7.1: Papillary Cell Carcinoma

A 46-year-old male with incidentally detected small left renal lesion on CT scan (not shown) was further evaluated with gadolinium-enhanced MRI including DWI.

Comments

The main criterion primarily used for *characterization* of a focal renal lesion as solid is the presence or absence of enhancement on contrast material–enhanced CT and MR images. When such enhancement is present, it generally indicates a diagnosis of RCC with small percentage of lesions being benign lipid-poor angiomyolipomas and oncocytomas. With MR imaging, enhancement can be assessed by measuring signal intensity changes or evaluated qualitatively by visually inspecting the images acquired with or without image subtraction. The hypothesis of restricted diffusion in malignant tissue has been proven in various experimental and brain tumor studies using DWI. Malignant tissues generally demonstrate decreased diffusion mainly due to hypercellularity from increased mitosis and cell death from apoptosis that results in decreased net space and surface, respectively, for diffusion of water molecules as compared to benign or normal tissues. Reduced or restricted diffusion of water molecules in a tissue can be effectively imaged and measured on DWI. In support of this hypothesis, a recent study by Taouli et al. on renal lesions has demonstrated that the DWI can be used to differentiate solid RCCs from oncocytomas and characterize the histologic subtypes of RCC. In their study, the mean ADC for RCCs ($1.41 \pm 0.61 \times 10^{-3}$ mm^2/s) was significantly lower ($P \leq 0.0001$) than that for benign renal lesions ($2.23 \pm 0.87 \times 10^{-3}$ mm^2/s).

Imaging Findings

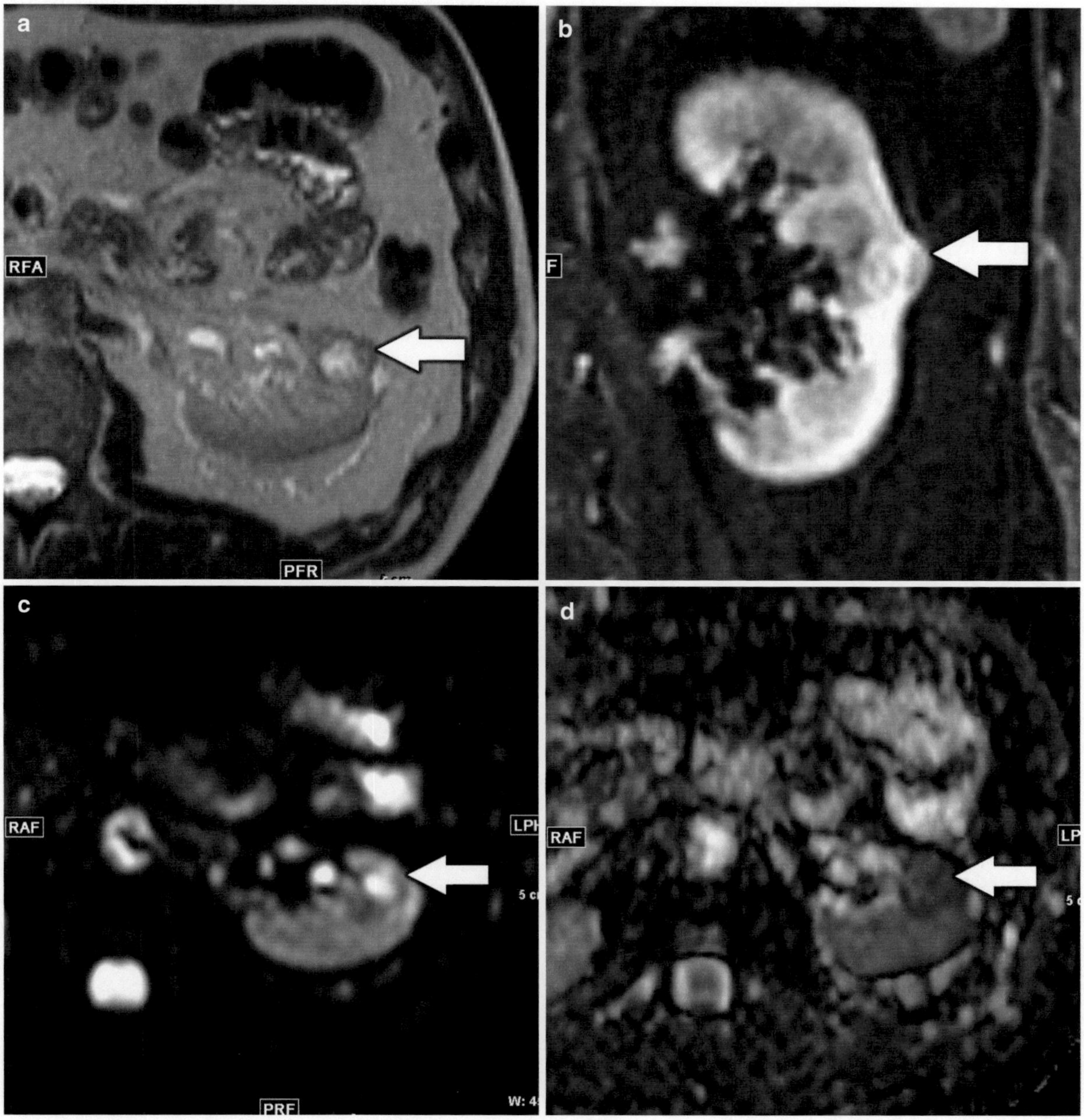

Fig. 7.1 (**a**) Axial TSE T2-weighted image, (**b**) coronal post-contrast GE T1-weighted image with fat-suppression, (**c**) axial DWI ($b=600$), and (**d**) corresponding axial ADC map at the level of interpolar region of the left kidney demonstrated a mildly T2 hyperintense renal lesion (*arrow*) with homogenous enhancement suspicious for RCC. The lesion was hyperintense on DWI and hypointense on ADC map relative to the background kidney suggestive of restricted diffusion and correlated with conventional MR findings. Patient subsequently underwent partial nephrectomy and histopathology was consistent with papillary cell carcinoma

Case 7.2: Cystic Clear Cell Carcinoma

A 57-year-old female with abnormal renal function and history of hematuria.

Comments

The characterization of complex cystic renal masses, such as T1 hyperintense lesions that include hemorrhagic or proteinaceous cysts and RCC can be challenging for the determination of presence or absence of enhancement owing to the similarly high signal intensity on precontrast images. Image subtraction has been shown to be superior to measurement of the enhancement ratio in the characterization of such lesions; however, it has inherent limitations, such as misregistration artifacts, owing to the variability of patient breath holding.

A recent study by Taouli et al. has shown that papillary RCCs had lower ADCs than nonpapillary RCCs. However, in another recent study, Kim et al. have shown that the performance of DWI is equivalent to that of contrast-enhanced MRI in the characterization of T1 hyperintense renal lesions, with both methods having lower sensitivity. The low sensitivity for T1 hyperintense renal lesions is probably related to multiple factors, including T2-blackout effects and restricted diffusion in hemorrhage or high-protein components, as described in patients with brain hematomas. The T2-blackout effect has been described in patients with T2 hypointense brain hematomas which is a corollary of the T2 shine-through effect in markedly T2 hyperintense lesions and is related to T2 contamination of DWI.

Imaging Findings

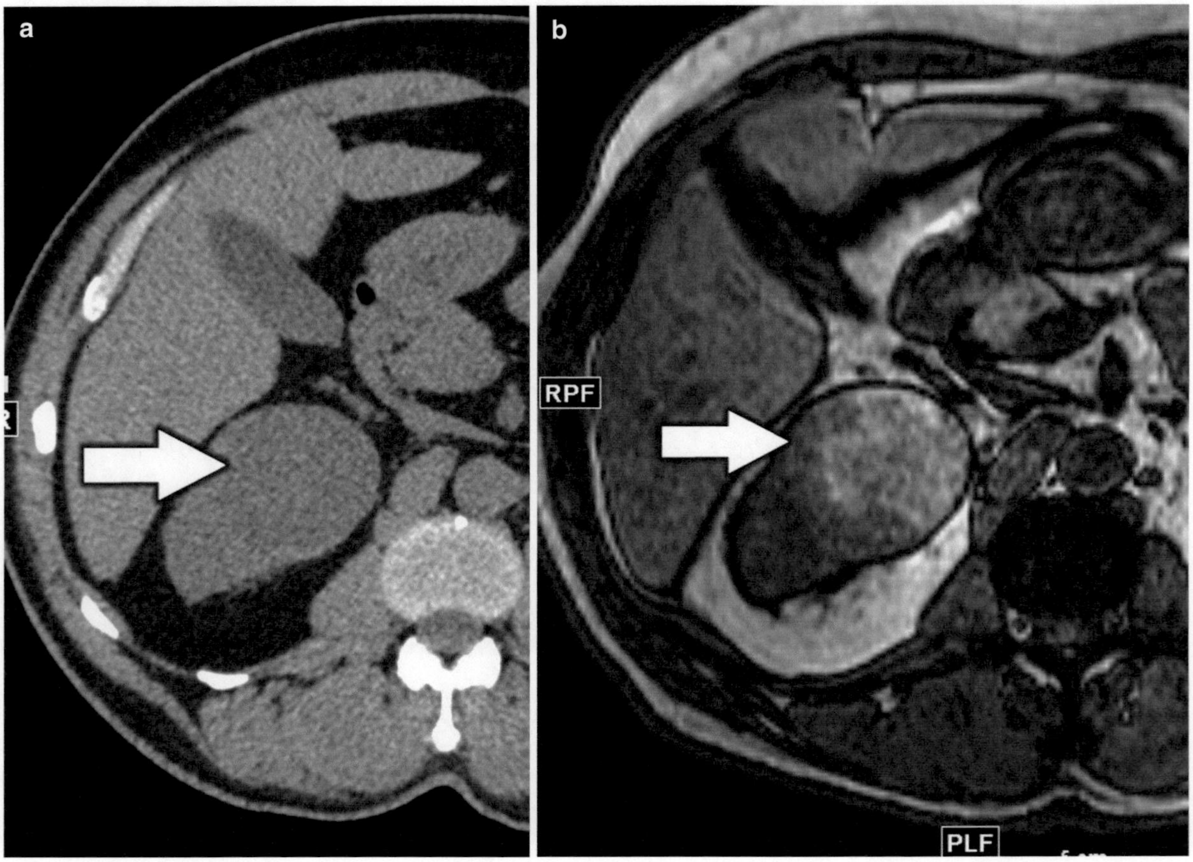

Fig. 7.2 Initial non-enhanced CT (**a**) demonstrated a heterogeneous cystic lesion in the right kidney that was followed up with MRI including axial, (**b**) axial out-of-phase GE T1-weighted image, (**c**) axial HASTE, (**d**) DWI ($b=600$), and (**e**) ADC map. The lesion on MRI depicted a crescent shaped (*arrow*) peripheral T1 hypointensity and T2 hyperintensity with corresponding hyperintensity on both DWI and ADC map suggestive of lack of restricted diffusion or T2-shine-through, that is typically seen in benign cysts. However, the remaining lesion demonstrated T1 and T2 hyperintensity that corresponds to hyperintensity on DWI and hypointensity to isointensity on ADC map relative to the background kidney suggestive of restricted diffusion and malignancy. Patient subsequently underwent nephrectomy, and histopathology was consistent with cystic clear cell carcinoma

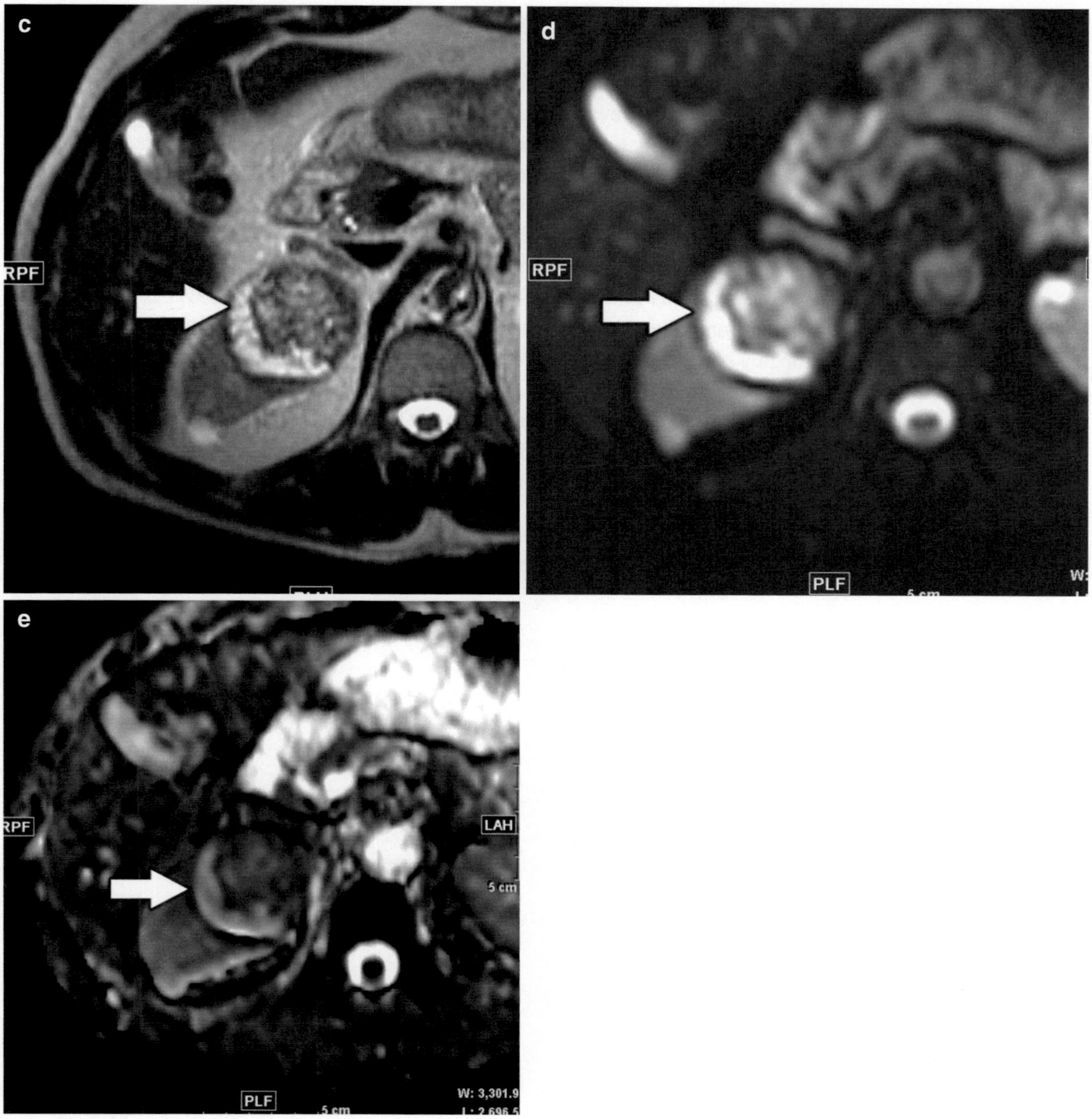

Fig. 7.2 (continued)

Case 7.3: Hemorrhagic Renal Cyst

A 60-year-old female with questionable enhancing lesion in the left kidney on CT scan was further evaluated with MRI.

Comments

Reliable differentiation of simple cyst versus infected/hemorrhagic cyst or abscess and normal kidney versus medical renal disease or nephropathy is sometimes challenging and DWI may provide an added role when performed together with other conventional T1, T2, and postcontrast MRI images. The hypothesis in these conditions is that in the presence of infection, hemorrhage, or chronic renal disease, the ADC values decrease due to reduced diffusion and DWI helps to differentiate these specific disease entities. However, these studies were conducted in small population of patients and there is a need to evaluate DWI further, before it can be utilized in routine clinical practice for these applications. Presence of hemorrhage in a benign lesion may demonstrate restriction of diffusion and results in false-positive results on DWI for malignancy. Awareness of this limitation on DWI is important for accurate characterization. In addition, this limitation of DWI also highlights the importance of correlating DWI with routine conventional sequences while interpretation of DWI to prevent false-positive results, since hemorrhagic cyst will be nonenhancing and T1 hyperintense on conventional sequences.

Imaging Findings

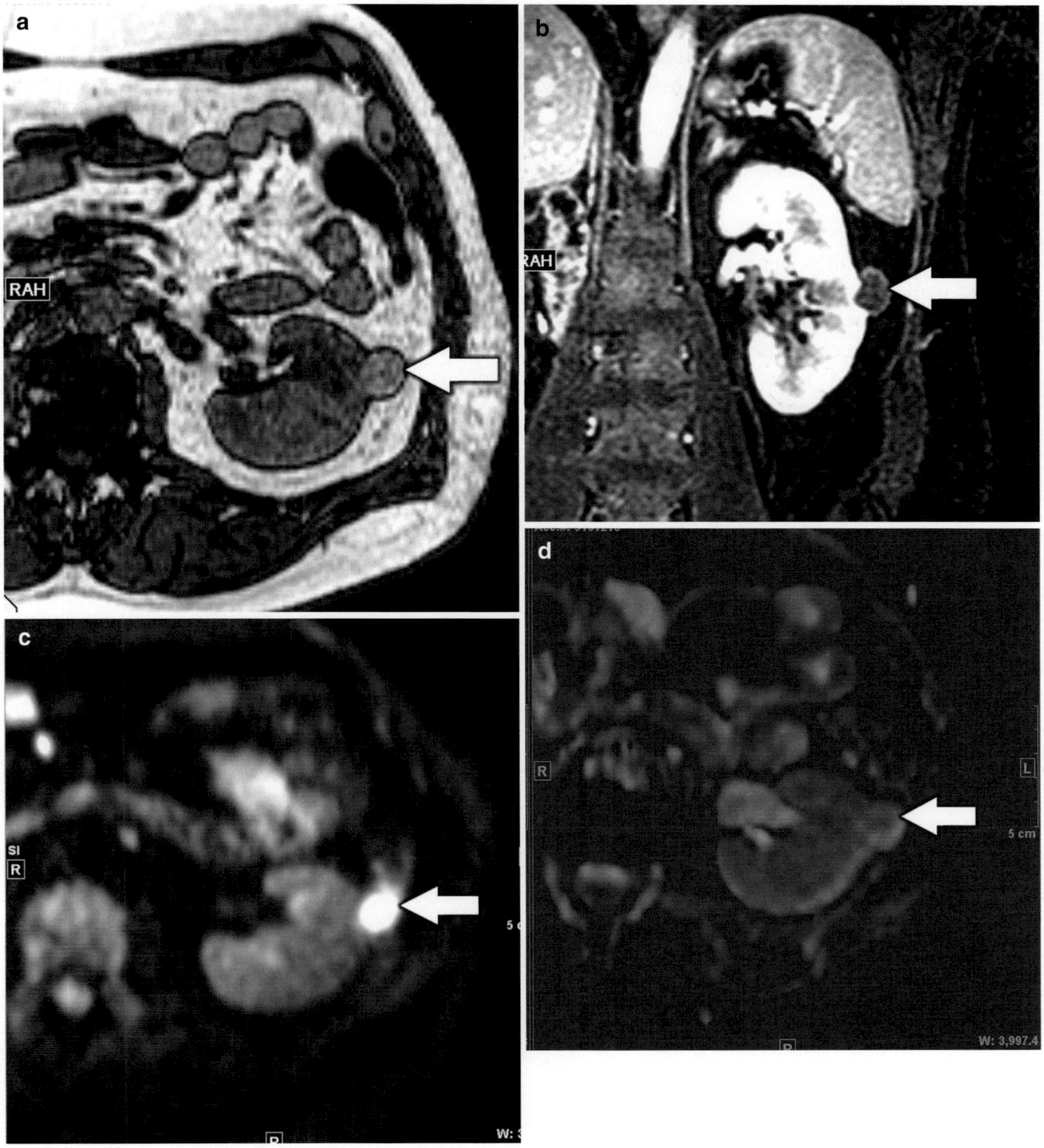

Fig. 7.3 The (**a**) axial out-of-phase GE T1-weighted image (**b**) coronal postcontrast GE T1-weighted image with fat-suppression (**c**) DWI ($b=600$) and (**d**) ADC map demonstrated the lesion to be hyperintense on T1W sequence with no enhancement suggestive of hemorrhagic cyst. The lesion was hyperintense on both DWI and ADC maps as compared to adjacent kidney suggestive of lack of restriction and benign lesion. Here the DWI findings were correlative to conventional MRI sequence

Case 7.4: Lymph Node Metastasis

A 55-year-old male with RCC in the left kidney (not shown) with a borderline enlarged left retroperitoneal lymph node on CT was submitted to MRI for further evaluation.

Comments

DWI provides very high signal intensity in the presence of malignancy and good contrast resolution between the lesion and the remaining structures which helps to detect smaller and more lesions. It has been shown in liver that DWI alone can detect more lesions. Local spread as well as distant metastasis can be detected with high sensitivity on DWI. However, there are many false-positive results due to T2-shine-through and T2-blackout effects. Recently, Takenaka et al concluded on their study on non-small cell lung cancer that assessment of bone metastases on whole body MRI with DWI is as accurate as bone scintigraphy and or PET/CT. The same principle can potentially be extrapolated to RCC detection and staging, but this remains to be proven. Besides, recent available data have shown the potential role of DWI in the characterization and differentiation between benign and malignant lymph nodes in several types of pelvic cancers such as rectal, prostate, cervical, and uterine ones. There are also similar data in the characterization of mediastinal lymph nodes.

Imaging Findings

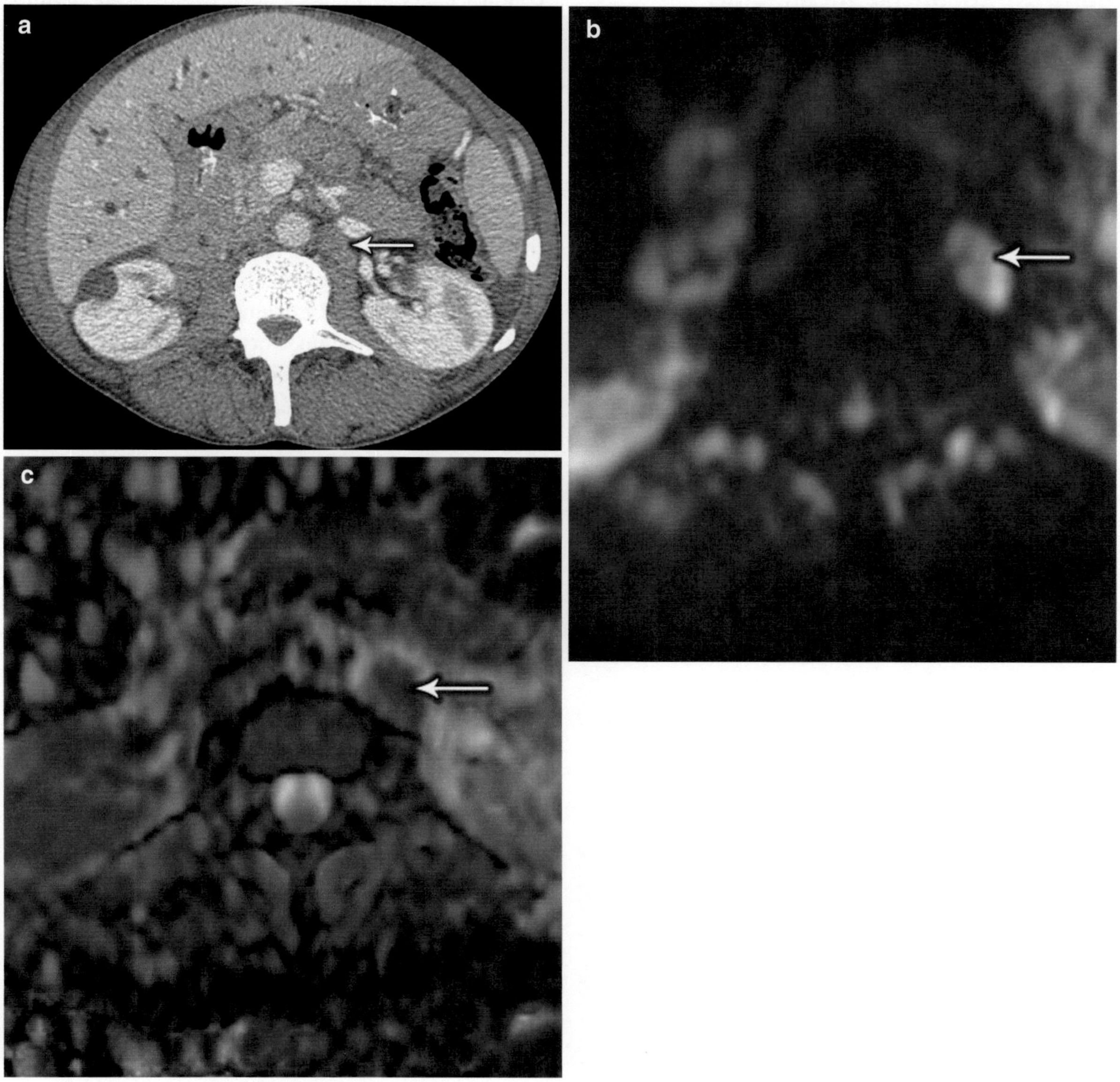

Fig. 7.4 CT (**a**) demonstrated a left retroperitoneal lymph node which showed restricted diffusion on axial DWI with a *b* value of 600 s/mm^2 (**b**) and corresponding ADC map (**c**) consistent with metastatic lymphadenopathy. Subsequently the patient underwent radical nephrectomy and lymph node dissection. The lymph node was proven to be metastatic on histopathology

Case 7.5: Alternative to Contrast-Enhanced MR Imaging

A 66-year-old-female with history of diabetes and chronic renal failure incidentally found to have an indeterminate renal lesion on a non-enhanced CT (not shown). Unenhanced MRI including DWI was performed for further characterization.

Comments

In view of recently reported concerns regarding the development of nephrogenic systemic fibrosis in patients with renal insufficiency that undergo contrast-enhanced MR imaging, and given the risk of iodinated contrast material–induced nephropathy with contrast-enhanced CT in the same population, there is increasing interest in assessing the efficacy of non-enhanced imaging modalities that might be useful for characterizing renal lesions. DWI provides qualitative and quantitative tissue characterization without the need for intravenous contrast material administration. DWI sequences can easily be added to a routine renal MR imaging protocol and this approach has been shown to be equally accurate for renal lesion characterization as contrast-enhanced MR imaging. Thus, DWI could represent a potential adjunct or alternative criterion for renal lesion characterization in patients at risk of developing nephrogenic systemic fibrosis.

Imaging Findings

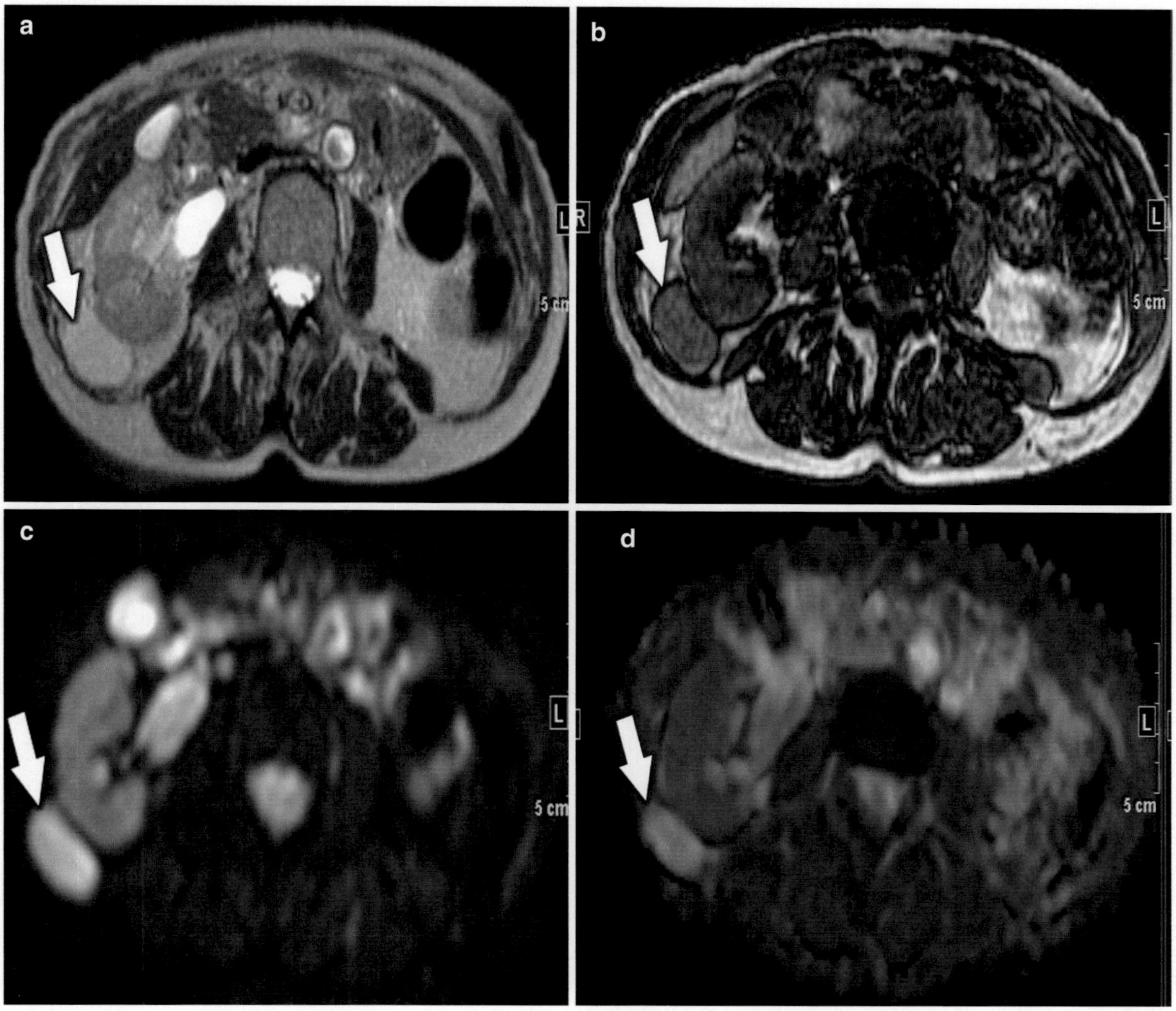

Fig. 7.5 A 66-year-old-female with history of diabetes and chronic renal failure incidentally found to have an indeterminate renal lesion on a non-enhanced CT (not shown). The conventional T1- and T2-weighted images (**a**, **b**) fail to offer additional information due to lack of postgadolinium images (*arrow*). The lesion was hyperintense (*arrow*) on both DWI (**c**) and ADC maps (**d**) consistent with lack of restricted diffusion and a possible diagnosis of benign lesion was made. On follow-up imaging over 2 years (not shown), the lesion remained stable suggestive of a benign cyst

Case 7.6: Recurrent Renal Cancer

Status post total left nephrectomy and chemotherapy in a 68-year-old female with advanced clear cell cancer on follow-up MRI.

Comments

Various options are available for treatment of renal cancer based on the stage and other coexiting conditions. Early stages of cancer can be treated with minimally invasive image-guided ablation procedures using radiofrequency, cryotherapy, laser, or microwave and nephron-sparing laparoscopic nephrectomy. Advanced stages can be treated with newer adjuvant therapies. DWI provides both subjective and quantitative parameters and can be used potentially for the evaluation of the effectiveness of treatment to detect residual disease or asymptomatic recurrence, to identify treatment or cancer related-complications, and for dose adjustments and patient reassurance.

Imaging Findings

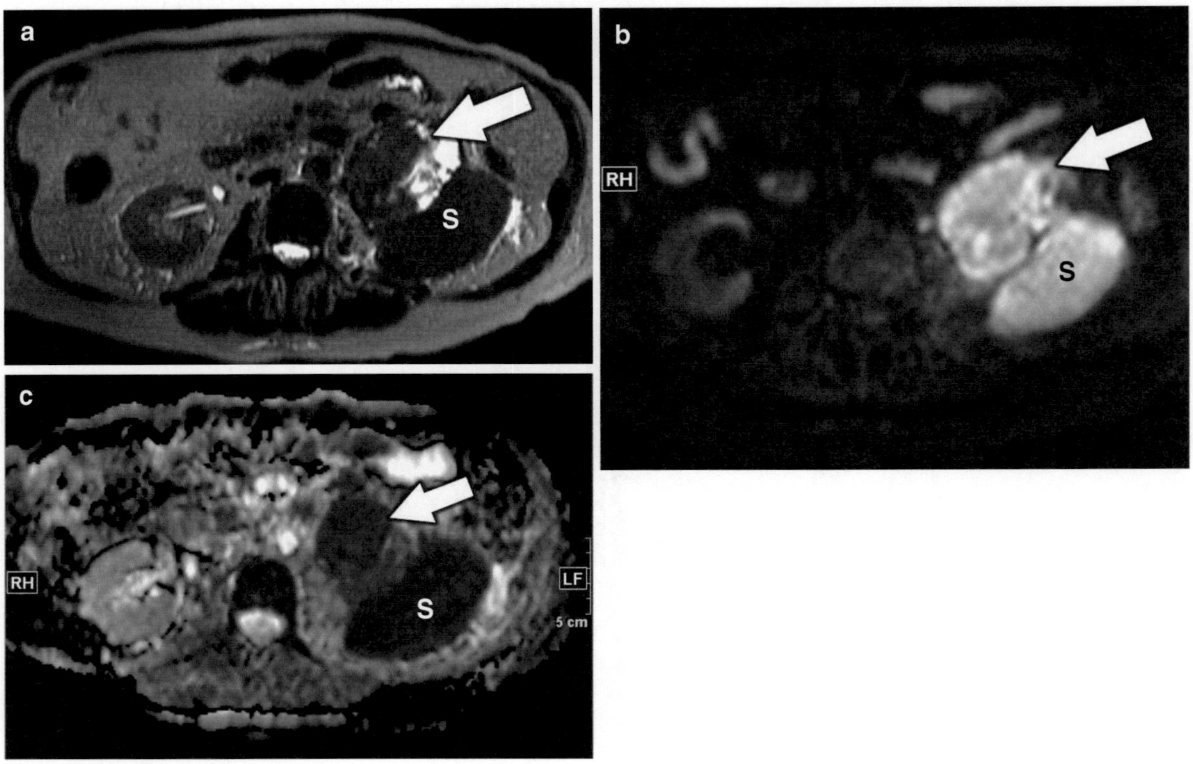

Fig. 7.6 MRI included axial (**a**) axial TSE T2-weighted image, (**b**) DWI, and (**c**) ADC map at 6 months interval demonstrates a large heterogeneous lesion (*arrow*) in the nephrectomy bed on T2WI with corresponding hyperintensity on DWI and hypointensity on ADC map, similar to adjacent spleen (S) that always shows restricted diffusion suggestive of recurrent cancer

Case 7.7: Adrenal Metastatic Lesion

Patient with known lung cancer is submitted to perform a MRI as part of the imaging workup.

Comments

The majority of adrenal lesions are still benign cortical adenomas and only 26–36% of adrenal lesions in patients with a known cancer are metastatic. Nonetheless, it is critical to differentiate benign from malignant lesions because the presence of metastasis might contraindicate a curative surgery or radiotherapy and may have significant impact on life expectancy. Conventional imaging techniques with measurements of attenuation (Hounsfield units) on non-enhanced CT, washout characteristics on CT, and drop in signal intensity on out-of-phase chemical shift MR imaging help to characterize the majority of these adrenal lesions. However, still a sizable percentage of adrenal lesions require either biopsy or surgery or interval imaging follow-up to determine the type of lesion. Recent advances in image acquisition and postprocessing techniques on both CT and MR are helping to expand the research tools available for adrenal imaging. DWI can provide an insight into water composition within a tumor. Benign tumors tend to have proportionate increase of cells as well as intercellular space whereas malignant tumors usually have a disproportionate increase of cells (mitotic activity) as compared to interstitial tissue as well as disrupted cell membranes. These properties of malignancies result in selective restriction of diffusion of water molecules that may provide strong evidence for malignancy in an adrenal lesion.

Imaging Findings

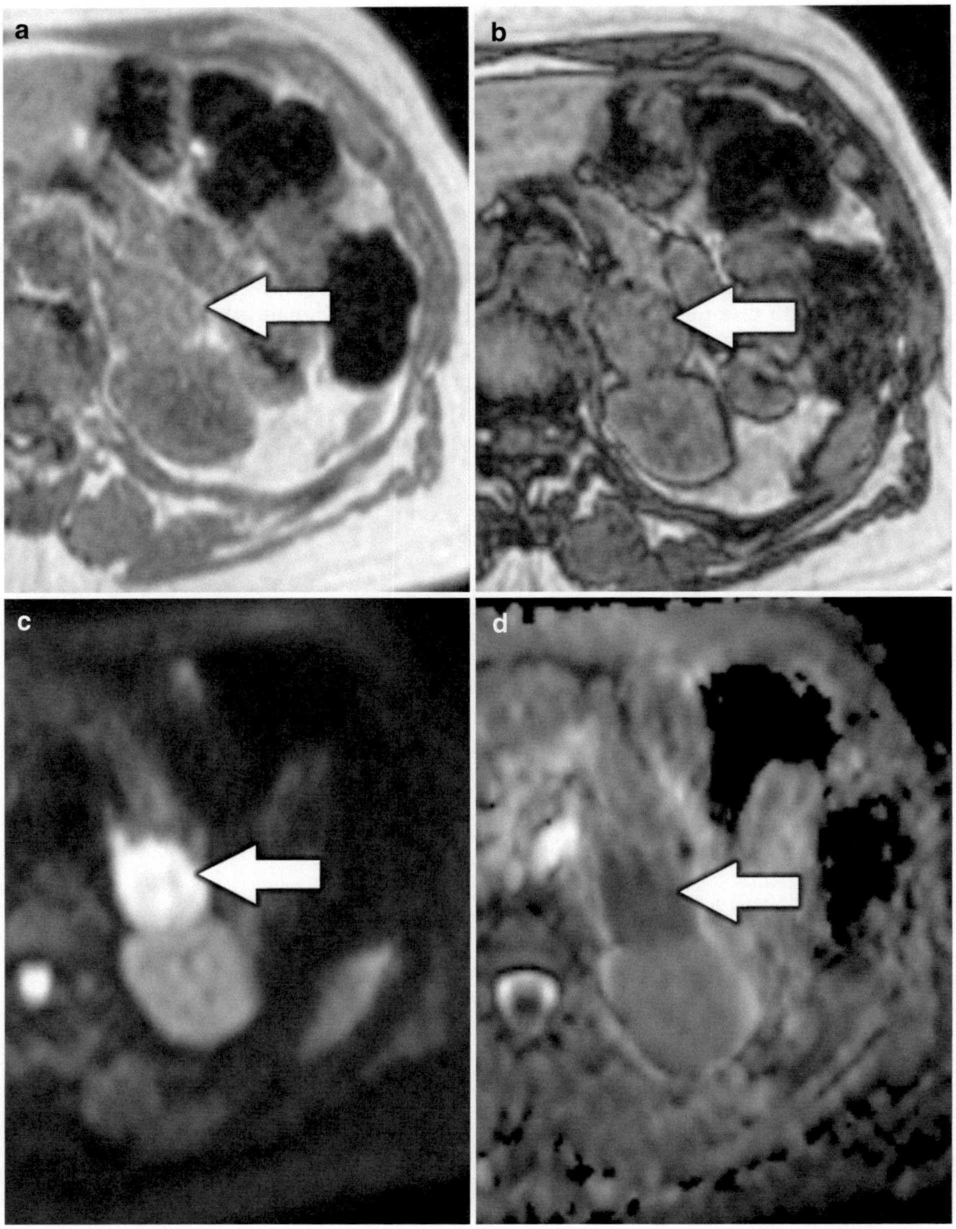

Fig. 7.7 The left adrenal lesion (*arrow*) demonstrates lack of drop in signal on axial (**b**) out-of-phase as compared to (**a**) in-phase images consistent with metastatic lesion. These findings were correlated on DWI (**c**) with ADC map (**d**) that showed restricted diffusion.

Case 7.8: Lipid Rich Adrenal Adenoma

A 72-year-old male with upper esophageal cancer and a right adrenal indeterminate lesion on CT (not shown) was followed up with MRI.

Comments

The lack of restricted diffusion may correlate with a benign or borderline neoplastic tumor. This information, if sufficiently validated, would have significant implications on the management of patients with adrenal lesions. For example, a benign-appearing adrenal lesion on the DWI exam would be managed conservatively, whereas a malignant appearance would guide appropriate treatment. To date, there are limited studies on the utility of DWI and ADC maps in characterization of adrenal lesions. Uhl et al. have demonstrated restricted diffusion in 7/7 (100%) neuroblastoma cases including two in the adrenal gland. At our institution, we have compared the performance of DWI and chemical shift MR for adrenal lesion characterization. Our initial results indicate that the quantitative DWI technique performed considerably better than the conventional chemical shift imaging. A high sensitivity and accuracy were achieved with a comparable specificity on DWI. The ADC of benign (1.7 ± 0.6) and malignant (1.1 ± 0.3) lesions were statistically different ($p = 0.01$). Although the quantitative ADC values were different among benign and malignant lesions, the diagnostic performance of DWI was comparable to chemical shift imaging. More work is necessary in this area and, undoubtedly, additional data will be available in the near future.

Imaging Findings

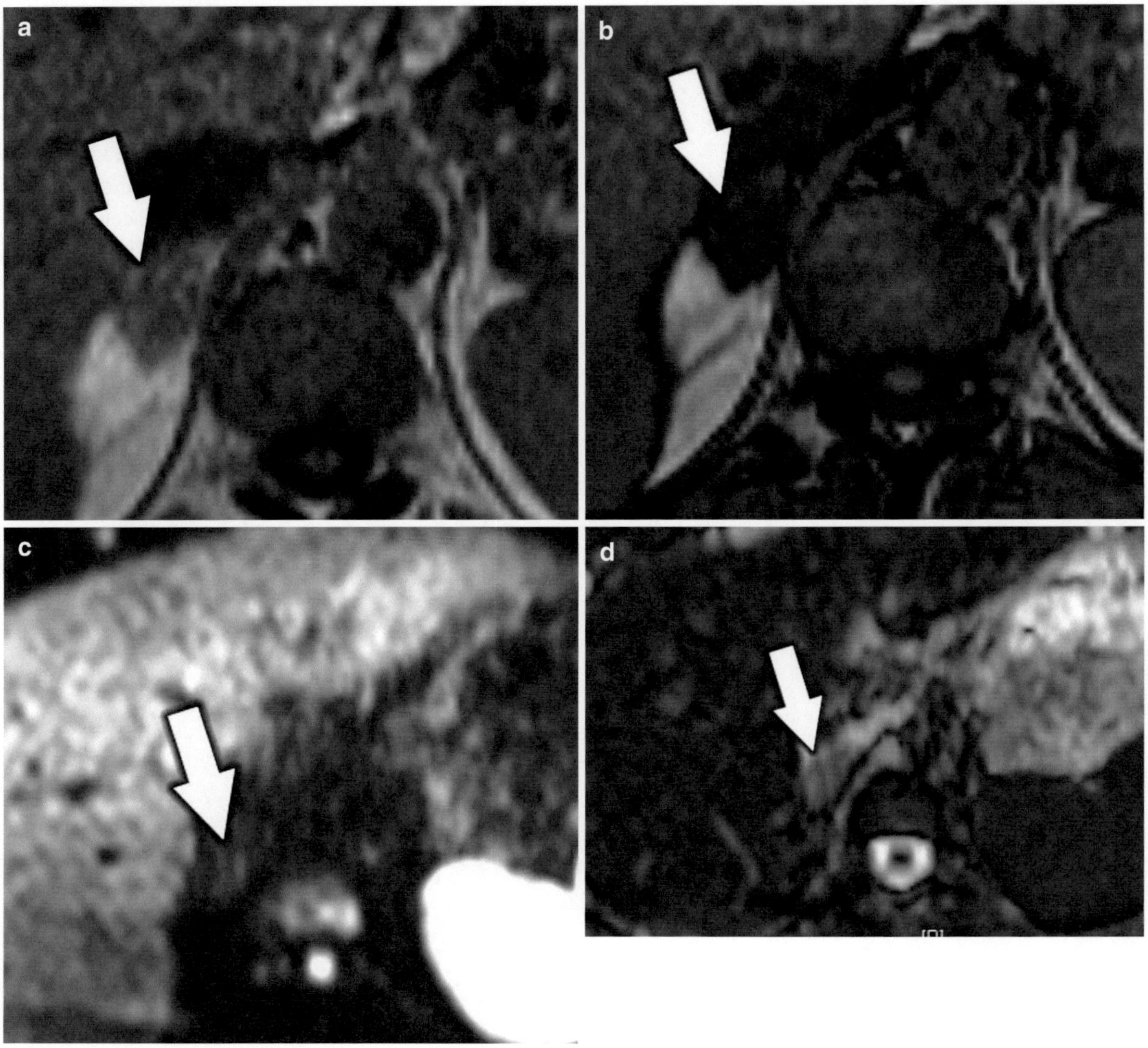

Fig. 7.8 MRI confirms the right adrenal lesion, using axial (**a**) in-phase, (**b**) out-of-phase, (**c**) DWI and (**d**) ADC map. The lesion showed significant drop in signal on out-of-phase as compared to in-phase suggestive of lipid-rich adenoma. On DWI, the lesion was hypointense with corresponding hyperintensity on ADC map as compared to spleen consistent with lack of restricted diffusion and benign lesion

Case 7.9: Adrenal Hematoma

A 60-year-old woman with a history of lung cancer is submitted to our center to perform a MRI for characterization of an adrenal gland lesion.

Comments

Adrenal hematomas generally result from trauma, sepsis, hypotension, or anticoagulation therapy. The appearance of adrenal hematoma on CT and ultrasound is nonspecific and varies considerably with hematoma age. The appearance on MRI also varies with the age of the blood products. Acute hemorrhage will have intermediate or high T1 signal. Chronic hematoma has nonspecific low T1/high T2 or low T1 and T2 signal intensity. Accurate differentiation from benign hematoma from hemorrhagic malignancy is difficult even on conventional MRI. DWI may play an important role in differentiation of adrenal hemorrhage from hemorrhagic tumor if the lesion demonstrates lack of restricted diffusion. However, hemorrhage can also sometime show restriction on DWI due to increased viscosity of the hematoma which results in false-positive results. Any restricted diffusion should be evaluated with suspicion and correlated further with all the available imaging sequences.

Imaging Findings

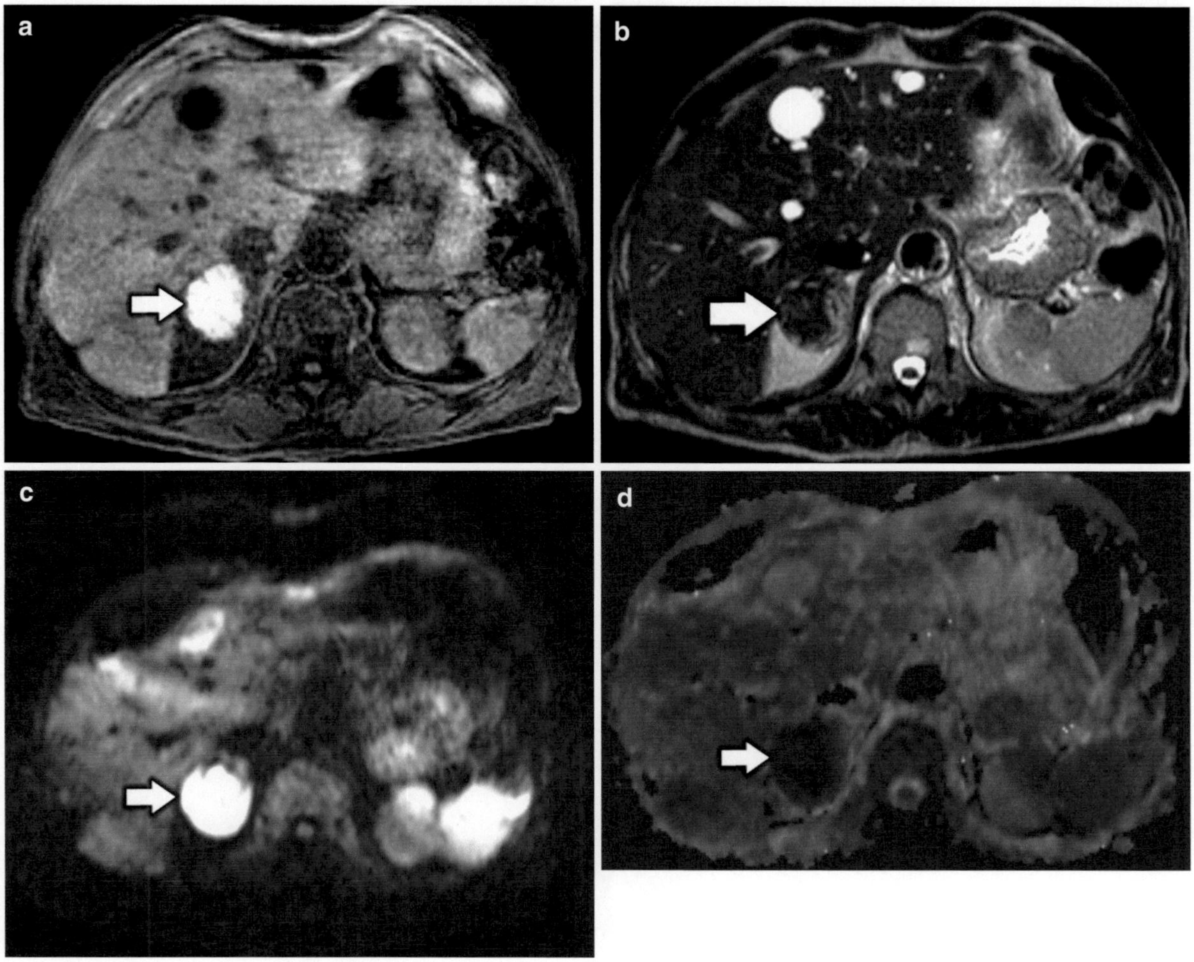

Fig. 7.9 MRI shows a right adrenal lesion on an axial GE T1-weighed image with fat saturation (**a**), axial T2-weighted image (**b**), axial DWI (**c**), and ADC map (**d**). The lesion is hyperintense on T1 with corresponding T2 heterogeneity (*arrows*), suggestive of the hematoma. However, reliable exclusion of hemorrhagic metastasis from benign adrenal hemorrhage was not possible even on DWI and ADC maps where the lesion is hyperintense and hypointense respectively suggestive of restricted diffusion. Here a final diagnosis of adrenal hematoma was made since there was no lesion in the right adrenal in a 3-month earlier CT, and additional laboratory findings were suggestive of above therapeutic levels of INR from anticoagulation. The lesion was followed up by CT 3-, 6-month and 1-year interval (not shown) where the reduction in size was consistent with hematoma

Case 7.10: Collision Tumor

A 65-year-old man presented with a known history of lung cancer and adrenal adenoma in the left adrenal gland. MRI is performed for follow-up.

Comments

Collision tumors represent an admixture of two different cell types in the tumor or at the junction of the tumor. The two tumors may be malignant, or both may be benign, or one may be benign and the other malignant. Adrenal collision tumors are rare, and their prevalence is unknown. The most common cause for adrenal collision tumors is due to metastasis at the margin of a preexisting adrenal adenoma. Adenoma/metastasis collision tumors should be suspected on chemical shift MR images when there is only focal decrease in the signal intensity of the mass on opposed-phase images or significant interval change in the morphology of the preexisting adrenal lesion as compared with prior imaging studies. However, hemorrhage or necrosis in a preexisting lesion may also mimic a collision tumor. Many adrenal collision tumors are not diagnosed by biopsy because of sampling error or a significant difference in the size of the two components, making it more likely that only the larger component will be examined at pathologic analysis. DWI may help to identify the metastatic portion within a benign adenoma by demonstration of restricted diffusion.

Imaging Findings

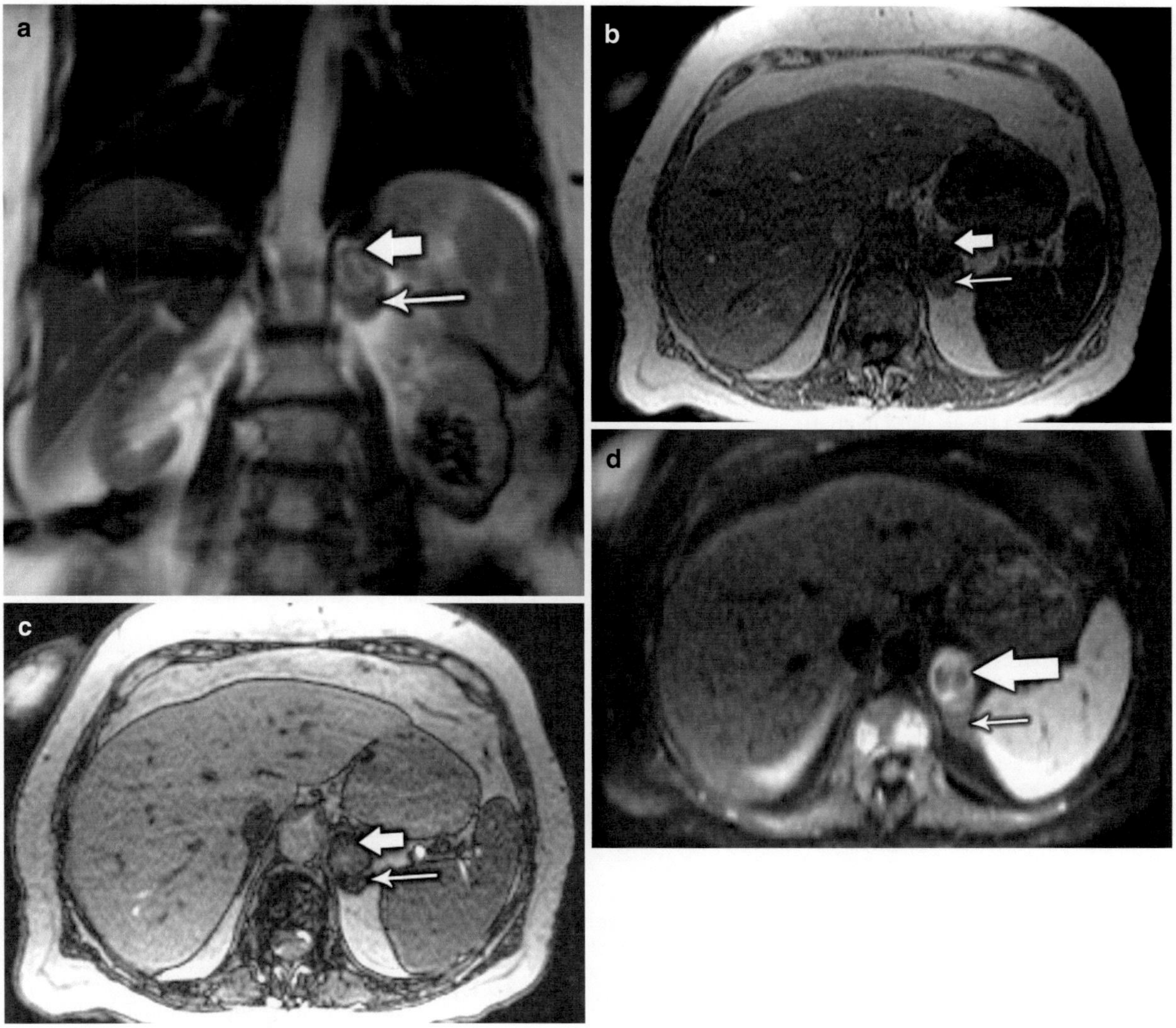

Fig. 7.10 Note typical features of metastasis (*arrow*) and adrenal adenoma (*small arrow*) in a collision tumor on (**a**) coronal T2W MR image, where the metastasis in the upper portion of the adenoma is slightly more hyperintense than the adenoma, and on (**b**) in-phase T1W and (**c**) out-off phase T1W the adenoma (*small arrow*) demonstrated signal drop of out-off phase image consistent with microscopic fat, where there was a drop of signal in the metastasis. The metastasis demonstrated restricted diffusion on (**d**) DWI (*arrow*) whereas there was no restriction in the adenoma portion of the lesion (*small arrow*)

Further Reading

Bittencourt LK, Matos C, Coutinho AC Jr (2011) Diffusion-weighted magnetic resonance imaging in the upper abdomen: technical issues and clinical applications. Magn Reson Imaging Clin N Am 19(1):111–31

Chandarana H, Lee VS, Hecht E et al (2011) Comparison of biexponential and monoexponential model of diffusion weighted imaging in evaluation of renal lesions: preliminary experience. Invest Radiol 46:285–291

Eisenberger U, Thoeny HC, Binser T et al (2010) Evaluation of renal allograft function early after transplantation with diffusion-weighted MR imaging. Eur Radiol 20(6):1374–83

Gurses B, Kilickesmez O, Tasdelen N et al. Diffusion tensor imaging of the kidney at 3 Tesla: normative values and repeatability of measurements in healthy volunteers. Diagn Interv Radiol; Nov 25, 2010. doi: 10.4261/1305-3825.DIR.3892-10.1 [Epub ahead of print]

Holalkere NS Belludi C, Gupta A et al (2009) Diffusion-weighted imaging (DWI) versus chemical shift imaging (CSI): a comparative study on MRI characterization of adrenal lesions using receiver operating characteristic curve (ROC) analysis. In: RSNA: 2009; CODE: SSE10-05, Session: Genitourinary (adrenal Glands), Chicago, IL

Karadeli E, Ulu EM, Yildirim E et al (2010) Diffusion-weighted MR imaging of kidneys in patients with systemic lupus erythematosus: initial experience. Rheumatol Int 30(9): 1177–81

Karadeli E, Ulu EM, Yilmaz S et al (2009) Diffusion-weighted MRI of the kidneys in patients with familial Mediterranean fever: initial experience. Diagn Interv Radiol 15(4):252–5

Kataoka M, Kido A, Yamamoto A et al (2009) Diffusion tensor imaging of kidneys with respiratory triggering: optimization of parameters to demonstrate anisotropic structures on fraction anisotropy maps. J Magn Reson Imaging 29(3): 736–44

Kido A, Kataoka M, Yamamoto A et al (2010) Diffusion tensor MRI of the kidney at 3.0 and 1.5 Tesla. Acta Radiol 51(9):1059–63

Kilickesmez O, Inci E, Atilla S et al (2009) Diffusion-weighted imaging of the renal and adrenal lesions. J Comput Assist Tomogr 33(6):828–33

Kim S, Jain M, Harris AB et al (2009) T1 hyperintense renal lesions: characterization with diffusion-weighted MR imaging versus contrast-enhanced MR imaging. Radiology 251(3):796–807

Miller FH, Wang Y, McCarthy RJ et al (2010) Utility of diffusion-weighted MRI in characterization of adrenal lesions. Am J Roentgenol 194(2):179–85

Notohamiprodjo M, Reiser MF, Sourbron SP (2010) Diffusion and perfusion of the kidney. Eur J Radiol 76(3):337–47

Paudyal B, Paudyal P, Tsushima Y et al (2010) The role of the ADC value in the characterisation of renal carcinoma by diffusion-weighted MRI. Br J Radiol 83(988):336–43

Rosenkrantz AB, Niver BE, Fitzgerald EF et al (2010) Utility of the apparent diffusion coefficient for distinguishing clear cell renal cell carcinoma of low and high nuclear grade. Am J Roentgenol 195(5):W344–51

Sandrasegaran K, Sundaram CP, Ramaswamy R et al (2010) Usefulness of diffusion-weighted imaging in the evaluation of renal masses. Am J Roentgenol 194(2):438–45

Takenaka D, Ohno Y, Matsumoto K et al (2009) Detection of bone metastases in non-small cell lung cancer patients: comparison of whole-body diffusion-weighted imaging (DWI), whole-body MR imaging without and with DWI, whole-body FDG-PET/CT, and bone scintigraphy. J Magn Reson Imaging 30(2):298–308

Taouli B, Thakur RK, Mannelli L et al (2009) Renal lesions: characterization with diffusion-weighted imaging versus contrast-enhanced MR imaging. Radiology 251(2):398–407

Thoeny HC, Binser T, Roth B et al (2009) Noninvasive assessment of acute ureteral obstruction with diffusion-weighted MR imaging: a prospective study. Radiology 252(3):721–8

Thoeny HC, Grenier N (2010) Science to practice: can diffusion-weighted MR imaging findings be used as biomarkers to monitor the progression of renal fibrosis? Radiology 255(3):667–8

Togao O, Doi S, Kuro-o M et al (2010) Assessment of renal fibrosis with diffusion-weighted MR imaging: study with murine model of unilateral ureteral obstruction. Radiology 255(3):772–80

Tsushima Y, Takahashi-Taketomi A et al (2009) Diagnostic utility of diffusion-weighted MR imaging and apparent diffusion coefficient value for the diagnosis of adrenal tumors. J Magn Reson Imaging 29(1):112–7

Uhl M, Altehoefer C, Kontny U et al (2002) MRI-diffusion imaging of neuroblastomas: first results and correlation to histology. Eur Radiol 12(9):2335–2338

Wang H, Cheng L, Zhang X et al (2010) Renal cell carcinoma: diffusion-weighted MR imaging for subtype differentiation at 3.0 T. Radiology 257(1):135–43

Xu X, Fang W, Ling H et al (2010) Diffusion-weighted MR imaging of kidneys in patients with chronic kidney disease: initial study. Eur Radiol 20(4):978–83

Xu Y, Wang X, Jiang X (2007) Relationship between the renal apparent diffusion coefficient and glomerular filtration rate: preliminary experience. J Magn Reson Imaging 26(3): 678–681

Xu JJ, Xiao WB, Zhang L et al (2010) [Value of diffusion-weighted MR imaging in diagnosis of acute rejection after renal transplantation]. Zhejiang Da Xue Xue Bao Yi Xue Ban 39(2):163–167

Diffusion-Weighted Imaging of Prostate, Bladder, and Retroperitoneum

8

Joan C. Vilanova, Roberto García-Figueiras, Joaquim Barceló, and Antonio Luna

8.1 DWI of Prostate

8.1.1 Biophysical Basis

The diffusion property in the tissue is determined by the distribution of water molecules between extracellular and intracellular spaces. Extracellular water has a greater range of diffusion than intracellular water because diffusion of water is more restricted by membranes or other cellular structures in the intracellular space. The prostate is an organ containing abundant glandular tissue with extracellular spaces. In contrast, prostate cancer shows decreased diffusion since it has abundant inter- and intracellular membranes, a high cell density, substantial cellular edema, and elevating interstitial pressure due to the loss of ATP-dependent sodium-potassium pumps. These histological characteristics result in different diffusion properties when comparing normal gland to cancer tissue in the prostate.

J.C. Vilanova • J. Barceló (✉)
Department of Radiology,
Clínica Girona-Hospital Sta. Caterina,
University of Girona, Girona, Spain
e-mail: jbarcelo@cetir.es; kvilanova@comg.cat

R. García-Figueiras
Department of Radiology,
Complexo Hospitalario Universitario de Santiago de Compostela,
Santiago de Compostela, Spain
e-mail: elhabibi.xray@gmail.com

A. Luna
Chief of MRI, Health Time Group,
Jaén, Spain
e-mail: aluna70@sercosa.com

8.1.2 Technical Adjustments

Prostatic MRI is usually performed 6–8 weeks after biopsy, as hemorrhage may hamper cancer detection and staging with morphological sequences and spectroscopy. Although hemorrhage increases susceptibility artifacts and may decrease ADC values of normal tissue, according to different researchers and our own experience, the effect of postbiopsy hemorrhage in DWI is trivial, even at 3 T magnets. Therefore, it is not necessary to wait a long time after biopsy to perform DWI of the prostate. Recent recommendations refer a delay of 2 or 3 weeks after biopsy to avoid the chance of T2 black-out effect.

Best results are obtained using a pelvic phase-array coil. The use of antiperistaltic agents is recommended. To avoid susceptibility artifact from the rectal air content, it is also useful to fill in the rectum with ultrasound gel. Optimum in-plane resolution may vary from 1.5×1.5 to 2×2 mm.

To minimize the influence of bulk motion as a distorting factor and minimizing T2 shine-through, typically a TE as short as possible is chosen. Typical sequence parameters for the prostate include *b* values of 0, and at least a high *b* value between 800 and 1,000 s/mm^2 in three orthogonal directions with parallel imaging if it is possible.

ADC quantification via monoexponential fitting is highly recommended for lesion characterization and cancer grading. To our knowledge, a bicompartmental model, using multiple *b* values and allowing separating true diffusion without perfusion contamination (*D*) and the perfusion fraction, has not been fully explored in the prostate. Preliminary reports have demonstrated that low and fast diffusion components are present in

A. Luna et al., *Diffusion MRI Outside the Brain*,
DOI 10.1007/978-3-642-21052-5_8, © Springer-Verlag Berlin Heidelberg 2012

the prostate as previously reported in the brain. Fast diffusion dominates the signal at low *b* values and low diffusion at high *b* values. With low *b* values, the signal decay is due to the perfusion effect over diffusion, and with higher *b* values over 100 s/mm^2, the true diffusion signal decay may be calculated. Furthermore, the biexponential model provided a statistically better fit over the monoexponential model on the peripheral zone, transitional zone, and prostate cancer. The fast and slow ADCs of cancer were significantly lower than those of transitional zone and peripheral zone, and the apparent fraction of the fast diffusion component was significantly smaller in cancer than in peripheral zone. In another series by Döpfert and colleagues using a biexponential approach of DWI in a 3 T magnet, the perfusion fraction of cancer was significantly decreased compared to healthy tissue and the ADC values were found to be increased by perfusion effects (Fig. 8.1).

8.1.3 DWI of the Prostate at 3 T

Improved SNR at 3 T may be of benefit for DWI, which shows improvement in spatial resolution for zonal and tumor delineation. It also allows improved ability to compare ADC mapping with whole-mount sectioned prostatectomy specimens for research purposes. Although 3 T magnets are prone to susceptibility artifacts which are enhanced with the use of EPI sequences, the use of an endorectal coil in conjunction with surface coil and parallel imaging improves image quality of DWI at 3 T. Furthermore, DWI is very susceptible to motion artifacts, but at 3 T, shorter imaging time and the use of lower TE is possible, improving image quality. This may result in improved overall performance of DWI in the localization, characterization, and depiction of prostate carcinoma compared to 1.5 T magnets. Limitations of DWI in prostate carcinoma remain in its low spatial resolution, which can be overcome by using this approach in combination with conventional T2-weighted imaging at 3 T and by projecting the ADC maps as color overlay images on T2-weighted images.

It must be noticed that differences between cancer and normal and peripheral zones have also been confirmed at 3 T. A report by Kim and colleagues at 3 T found that an ADC cutoff value of 1.67×10^{-3} mm^2/s had 0.97 area under the curve (AUC) in peripheral zone cancer prediction and an ADC cutoff value of 1.61×10^{-3} mm^2/s showed 0.92 AUC for the prediction of transitional zone cancer.

8.1.4 Benign Conditions

The correct interpretation of diffusion and ADC images relies on good knowledge of the diffusion characteristics of the different anatomic zones of the prostate and of benign prostatic conditions compared with prostate cancer.

Benign prostatic hyperplasia (BPH) is characterized by nodular adenomas in the transition zone. The peripheral zone is usually not affected by BPH, retaining its own histologic characteristics. Nodular hyperplasia gives rise to inhomogeneous diffusion patterns and because tubular structures often remain in place, the increased cellular density of hyperplasia, which is far less predominant than in prostate carcinoma, might explain the observed reduction in ADC levels of the central gland on DWI, because of decreased ratio of extracellular to intracellular volume. However, an increase in ADC also has been observed, due to the inhomogeneous diffusion characteristics of BPH. Stromal hyperplasia tends to show significant reduced ADC values compared to glandular hyperplasia, as this one shows prominent glandular-luminal extracellular space.

Prostatitis almost always originates in the peripheral zone. Chronic prostatitis might mimic BPH, often associated with elevated prostate-specific antigen levels, raising the suspicion of prostate cancer. Histologically, chronic prostatitis is characterized by extracellular edema surrounding the involved prostatic cells with lymphocytes, plasma cells, macrophages, and neutrophils in the prostatic stroma. This abundance in cells as compared with normal prostatic tissue may lead to an ADC decrease because of decreased extracellular to intracellular fluid volume ratio, but probably not as low as prostate cancer (Fig. 8.2). To our knowledge, there is only a series available on the DWI characteristics of chronic prostatitis compared to prostatic cancer using a 3 T magnet, which demonstrated significant lower ADC values for cancerous tissue (mean ADC value: 1.39 ± 0.22 mm^2/s) compared to the ADC values of prostatitis (1.57 ± 0.12 mm^2/s) and normal prostate tissue (1.62 ± 0.12 mm^2/s). Besides, there was no significant difference between the ADC values of prostatitis and normal prostate tissue.

8.1.5 Cancer Detection

Morphological T2-weighted sequences allow for limited detection of cancer, mainly in the transitional zone in patients with benign prostatic hyperplasia. Native DWI images are limited for cancer detection due to the long T2-relaxation time of peripheral zone, causing T2 shine-through in the peripheral zone even with *b* values of 1,000 s/mm^2. Several reports have confirmed that the combination of DWI with a *b* value of 1,000 s/mm^2 and T2-weighted sequences has shown higher diagnostic accuracy than T2-weighted sequences alone in lesion-based analyses. Furthermore, the use of ADC maps has been proposed as more adequate than native DWI, even for visual detection of prostatic carcinoma. Recent technological advances in gradients and parallel imaging allowed using ultrahigh *b* values up to 3,000 s/mm^2 for pelvic DWI (Fig. 4.9). In a recent series using visual assessment on a 1.5 T magnet, a *b* value of 2,000 s/mm^2 in addition to T2-weighted sequences improved the diagnostic accuracy, sensitivity, and specificity of prostate cancer detection in both peripheral and transitional zone in comparison to T2-weighted sequence alone or in combination with a *b* value of 1,000 s/mm^2. The use of these ultrahigh *b* values allows to clearly depict the tumor against a totally suppressed background, improving tumor delineation (Fig. 8.1). Conversely, Kim et al. found lesser sensitivity in ADC maps obtained with *b* values of 0 and 2,000 s/mm^2 compared to the ones obtained with *b* values of 0 and 1,000 s/mm^2 in the detection of localized prostate cancer using a 3 T magnet. In a similar manner, Kitajima et al. found little diagnostic advantage in measuring ADC using a high *b* value (2,000 s/mm^2) over the standard *b* value (1,000 s/mm^2) to discriminate malignant from normal prostate tissue. It must be noticed that ADC maps calculated with ultrahigh *b* values will show decreased SNR being critical to maintain TE as short as possible to increase SNR.

DWI is only able to differentiate areas of high density cancer cells (tumor exceeding 50% of tumor volume) from normal prostatic tissue, which is a limitation of DWI in prostate cancer detection. Recent reports have established the role of DWI using ADC measurements in the differentiation between cancer and normal prostatic tissue in the peripheral zone. Despite the tendency to show different ADC values of both prostate cancer and non-cancerous tissue, several studies have also shown a significant overlap of the ADC values between prostate cancer and non-cancerous tissue, which is attributed to the fact that the ADC varies widely in both prostate cancer and non-cancerous tissue. This overlap seems to be more prominent between both prostate cancer and non-cancerous transitional zone tissue, because it has a lower ADC than peripheral zone tissue. Besides, a recent paper by Otto and colleagues demonstrated significant differences in ADC value between central gland cancer, stromal and glandular hyperplasia with average ADC values of 1.05×10^{-3} mm^2/s, 1.27×10^{-3} mm^2/s, and 1.73×10^{-3} mm^2/s, respectively. These findings open a new field of research in the detection of central gland cancer with DWI (Fig. 8.3).

Several series have demonstrated that multiparametric MRI including T2-weighted, dynamic contrast-enhanced, diffusion-weighted sequences, and spectroscopy in combination depicts the greater number of cancers compared to any other combination of these data (Fig. 8.4).

Postbiopsy hemorrhage is known to decrease the detection accuracy of prostate cancer on T2-weighted sequences and functional techniques such as dynamic contrast-enhanced series and spectroscopy. In a similar manner, DWI decreases its sensitivity in areas of hemorrhage, although according to reported data, it performs superiorly in cancer detection compared to T2-weighted sequences and in a significant manner over dynamic contrast-enhanced MRI.

8.1.6 Cancer Localization

Clinical applications of DWI on prostate cancer rely on diagnosis, staging, and treatment follow-up. Several studies have shown that prostate carcinoma displays significantly lower ADC values compared with benign prostatic tissue making it a potential useful measurement for the localization of prostate carcinoma. In various reports, mean ADC values range between 1 and 1.35×10^{-3} mm^2/s for malignant prostate tissue and 1.60 and 1.96×10^{-3} mm^2/s for benign tissue, including peripheral zone and central gland. These results suggest the potential role of DWI, especially in combination with T2-weighted imaging, as DWI alone lacks high spatial resolution. Improvement of prostate cancer localization has been recently demonstrated combining conventional T2-weighted imaging with functional sequences such as DWI, spectroscopy, and dynamic contrast enhancement MRI. Besides, in a recent report elaborated in the European Consensus meeting evaluating the role of MRI in prostatic cancer imaging, DWI was considered as the only functional MRI sequence that was able to clinically exclude alone significant disease, as defined by a lesion size of $\geq 0.2\ cm^3$ (approximately 7 mm of transverse diameter) in the peripheral zone or to exclude clinically significant cancer according to the definition of a lesion of $\geq 0.5\ cm^3$ and/or Gleason $\geq 4+3$ in the peripheral zone.

8.1.7 Tumoral Grading and Local Staging (T-Staging)

DWI has also potential for grading prostate carcinoma because increased cellular density and loss of tubular structures implicate a higher Gleason score and also seriously hamper self-diffusion in the involved tissue leading to lower ADC levels on DWI. Furthermore, ADC values have confirmed an inverse relationship to Gleason grades in peripheral zone prostate cancer. Higher ADC values are associated with lower Gleason grades in the peripheral zone prostate cancers (Fig. 8.4). This relationship has not been demonstrated for central gland cancer with the available data. Furthermore, DWI has confirmed a high discriminatory performance in the differentiation of low-, intermediate-, and high-grade cancer. Besides, significant differences in tumor ADC values have been reported between patients with low-risk and those with higher-risk localized prostate cancer. In the same European Consensus Meeting referred above, DWI was considered the only adequate sequence to evaluate in isolation the Gleason grade of lesions in the peripheral zone between both morphological and functional sequences.

Currently, prostate MRI, including T2-weighted sequences, stands as the best technique to predict seminal vesicles invasion by prostate cancer. One of the benefits to use DWI sequence within the protocol of MRI for prostate cancer imaging is the improvement in the detection of the possible invasion of the seminal vesicles (Fig. 8.5). A recent study reported that 3 T DWI used in conjunction with T2-weighted imaging improved the prediction of seminal vesicles invasion in prostate cancer compared with T2-weighted imaging alone.

8.1.8 N and M Staging

Noninvasive nodal staging of prostate carcinoma is challenging. CT and MRI have been demonstrated to be inaccurate in this regard. Novel functional techniques are under evaluation. Preliminary results reported by Eiber et al., showed the role of DWI in the differentiation between benign and malignant lymph nodes in 36 patients with prostate cancer. In this series, a highly significant difference between the mean ADC-value of malignant ($1.07 \pm 0.23 \times 10^{-3}\ mm^2/s$) versus benign ($1.54 \pm 0.25 \times 10^{-3}\ mm^2/s$) lymph nodes was achieved, even in subgroup analysis for lymph nodes smaller versus larger than 10 mm (Fig. 8.6). Conversely, in the series by Budiharto and colleagues, DWI showed a better sensitivity than (11)C-Choline PET-CT in the detection of nodal metastases in 36 patients with histologically proven prostate cancer and high risk of lymph node metastases, which were not demonstrated on contrast-enhanced CT before retropubic radical prostatectomy with extended pelvic lymph node dissection. Sensitivity, specificity, PPV, NPV, and the number of correctly recognized cases at DWI were 18.8%, 97.6%, 46.2%, 91.7%, and 15.8%, respectively. These data reflect the inaccuracy of DWI for pretreatment detection of occult lymph node metastases.

Ultrasmall superparamagnetic iron oxide particles (USPIO), which are also taken up in normal lymph nodes, have shown to improve the performance of MR in nodal staging, although it is not yet widely available. Furthermore, specificity of USPIO increases with the addition of DWI by suppressing signal from normal but not pathologic nodes, also allowing an earlier acquisition of the images compared to conventional USPIO approach without DWI.

Moreover, whole body DWI has shown superiority to bone scintigraphy in detecting osseous metastases, and it should be considered a first row staging tool in the M-staging of prostate cancer (Fig. 16.3).

8.1.9 Posttreatment Monitorization, Detection of Recurrence, and Prediction of Response to Treatment

DWI has been shown to have the potential benefit in monitoring treatment response after hormonotherapy, cryotherapy, or radiation, for differentiating posttherapeutic changes from residual active tumor, and for detecting recurrent cancer after prostatectomy.

Posttreatment imaging is usually performed in patients with rising PSA levels, positive digital rectal examination, or clinical symptoms of recurrence or metastasis. DWI has shown increasing applications to detect recurrent tumor and to follow the changes in normal prostatic tissues and cancer after treatment. Responding prostate cancers after radiotherapy show a significant early increase in mean ADC value and both peripheral and transitional zones show a decrease in ADC measurements (Fig. 8.7). Conversely, nonresponding tumors demonstrate no change or even decrease in ADC values. Besides, DWI along with T2-weighted sequences improves significantly the results of T2-weighted sequences alone in the detection of recurrent cancer, with a sensitivity and specificity of 62% and 91% for both techniques compared to 25% and 57% for T2-weighted sequences alone.

In a similar manner, ADC measurements of subcutaneous tumor xenografts of human prostate cancer cells implanted in nude mice have demonstrated to increase as early as 24 h after the beginning of photodynamic therapy, suggesting a potential role for DWI as a noninvasive imaging marker for early monitoring of tumor response. Furthermore, DWI in combination with T2-weighted sequences allowed to detect prostate cancer recurrence after high focused ultrasonic ablation in a series by Kim and colleagues. In this report, DWI in combination with T2-weighted sequence was more specific and less sensitive than dynamic contrast-enhanced MRI.

Therefore, a recent series by Giles and colleagues has revealed a potential role for DWI in patients with prostate cancer in active surveillance, as ADC values were significantly lower in tumors that were subsequently upgraded on histology. Besides, both tumor volume and the slow ADC (obtained with *b* values lower than 300 s/mm^2) were significant but independent predictors of histologic progression.

All these data suggest that ADC values may be a useful imaging biomarker for monitoring the therapeutic response of prostate cancer to different types of treatment (Fig. 8.8), although larger series are needed to correlate the results with clinical endpoints.

A recent report by Kim and colleagues opens a new area of research for DWI in treated prostate cancer. These investigators demonstrated that pretreatment mean ADC of prostate cancer with biochemical recurrence after radical prostatectomy was significantly lower than those of tumors without signs of recurrence. Univariate analysis revealed that several parameters as tumor ADC, Gleason score at biopsy and surgical specimen, serum PSA, greatest percentage of cancer in biopsy core, percentage of positive cores in all biopsy cores and tumor volume were all significantly related to biochemical recurrence. However, multivariate analysis identified tumor ADC as the only independently predictive factor. Therefore, as previously demonstrated for other tumors as rectal cancer, DWI with ADC measurements may be used as a predictor of tumoral response following radical prostatectomy.

8.1.10 Diffusion Tensor Imaging (DTI)

DTI of the prostate is feasible at both 1.5 and 3 T magnets. Different diffusion and anisotropy properties have been demonstrated for peripheral and central gland. The central gland shows different components, such as stroma, smooth muscle fibers, and organized ductal structures, which causes diffusion anisotropy. Besides, the less structured peripheral zone shows less anisotropy. DTI is able to detect these microstructural differences by means of the fractional anisotropy (FA) value, as the diffusion properties of the tissues are studied in at least six different gradient directions.

Contradictory results have been reported in the currently limited series about the role of DTI and FA measurements in the detection and characterization of prostate cancer. With the available data, a significant difference between prostate cancer and normal peripheral zone can be assumed (Fig. 4.5). Furthermore, in most of these series, prostate cancer shows higher FA values than normal prostatic tissue. Recently, a significant difference in the FA values of chronic prostatitis and cancer has also been reported. If FA values have an additional role to ADC measurements in prostate cancer management has still to be fully explored, although FA is more sensitive to noise, which limits its clinical applicability as a repeatable marker compared to ADC.

8.2 Applications of DWI in Bladder Cancer

There are limited series evaluating the role of DWI in bladder cancer. As in cancer of other organs, bladder cancer tends to show high signal on native DWI images and an ADC value lower than that of normal bladder wall, prostate, and seminal vesicles (Fig. 8.9). Available data support that DWI outperforms conventional T2-weighted and dynamic contrast-enhanced MRI in the T-staging of bladder cancer, which is critical for patient management. T1 bladder carcinoma is treated with transurethral resection (TUR) and tumors of stage T2 or greater are managed by partial or total cystectomy or by adjuvant therapies, because TUR for invasive tumors often results in local tumor recurrence and in a poor prognosis. Furthermore, the combination of all dynamic contrast-enhanced MRI with DWI and TSE T2-weighted images improves the local staging compared to any other combination of MRI techniques, with an overall staging accuracy over 90%. Less overstaging has also been reported using DWI than dynamic contrast-enhanced MRI in the T-staging of bladder cancer. Correlation between histologic grade and ADC values has also been achieved, as mean ADC of G3 tumors has been significantly lower than that of G1 and G2 tumors

DWI also improves the detection of pelvic lymph nodes, with a promising role in the distinction of metastatic and inflammatory lymph nodes.

In a study assessing therapeutic response to induction chemoradiotherapy in muscular invasive bladder cancer, DWI was significantly superior in specificity and accuracy to T2-weighed and dynamic contrast-enhanced MRI, despite comparable sensitivity. DWI was also useful to accurately predict pathologic complete response.

8.3 Assessment of the Retroperitoneum with DWI

There is scarce reports evaluating the role of DWI in the detection and characterization of retroperitoneal masses. As in other locations, DWI may increase the detection of small retroperitoneal lymph nodes. Furthermore, DWI has demonstrated potential in their characterization in several anatomic locations. With regard to retroperitoneal tumors, a series by Nakayama and colleagues evaluated the usefulness of EPI DWI using a maximum *b* factor of 1,100 s/mm^2 in the characterization of 50 patients with known retroperitoneal masses. The ADC value of malignant lymphoma was significantly lower than that of malignant mesenchymal lesions and benign ones. Furthermore, malignant epithelial tumors showed a significant difference in the restriction of diffusion compared to benign mesenchymal lesions (Fig. 8.10). Therefore, DWI may help in the differentiation between lymphoma and benign and malignant retroperitoneal masses, although further research is still needed to confirm these limited data.

Case 8.1: Evaluation of Prostatic Cancer with DWI at 3 T Magnet

A 66-year-old male with confirmed prostatic cancer in the right prostatic lobe, Gleason score of 3+4, and PSA level of 6.3 ng/mL. Digital examination was unremarkable, MRI was performed for further staging.

Comments

In several series, DWI at 3 T magnet of prostate gland has demonstrated to be feasible with advantage over 1.5 T magnets in SNR. As in 1.5T magnets, DWI at 3 T permits to differentiate with ADC quantification prostatic cancer from normal tissue. ADC quantification via monoexponential fitting has demonstrated its accuracy for lesion characterization and cancer grading. The use of multiple *b* values allows for the use of a bicompartmental analysis of DWI. This model has shown a statistically better fit over the monoexponential model on the peripheral zone, transitional zone, and prostate cancer. Preliminary reports have demonstrated that low and fast diffusion components are present in the prostate as previously reported in the brain, which may be separated using this approach. Fast diffusion dominates the signal at low *b* values and low diffusion at high *b* values. In the limited series available, the fast and slow ADCs of cancer were significantly lower than those of transitional zone and peripheral zone, and the apparent fraction of the fast diffusion component was significantly smaller in cancer than in peripheral zone. In another series by Döpfert and colleagues using a biexponential approach of DWI in a 3 T magnet, the perfusion fraction of cancer was significantly decreased compared to healthy tissue and the ADC was found to be increased by perfusion effects. As shown in this case, monoexponential analysis of the DWI is useful in the clinical setting, although a bicompartmental model is more accurate.

Imaging Findings

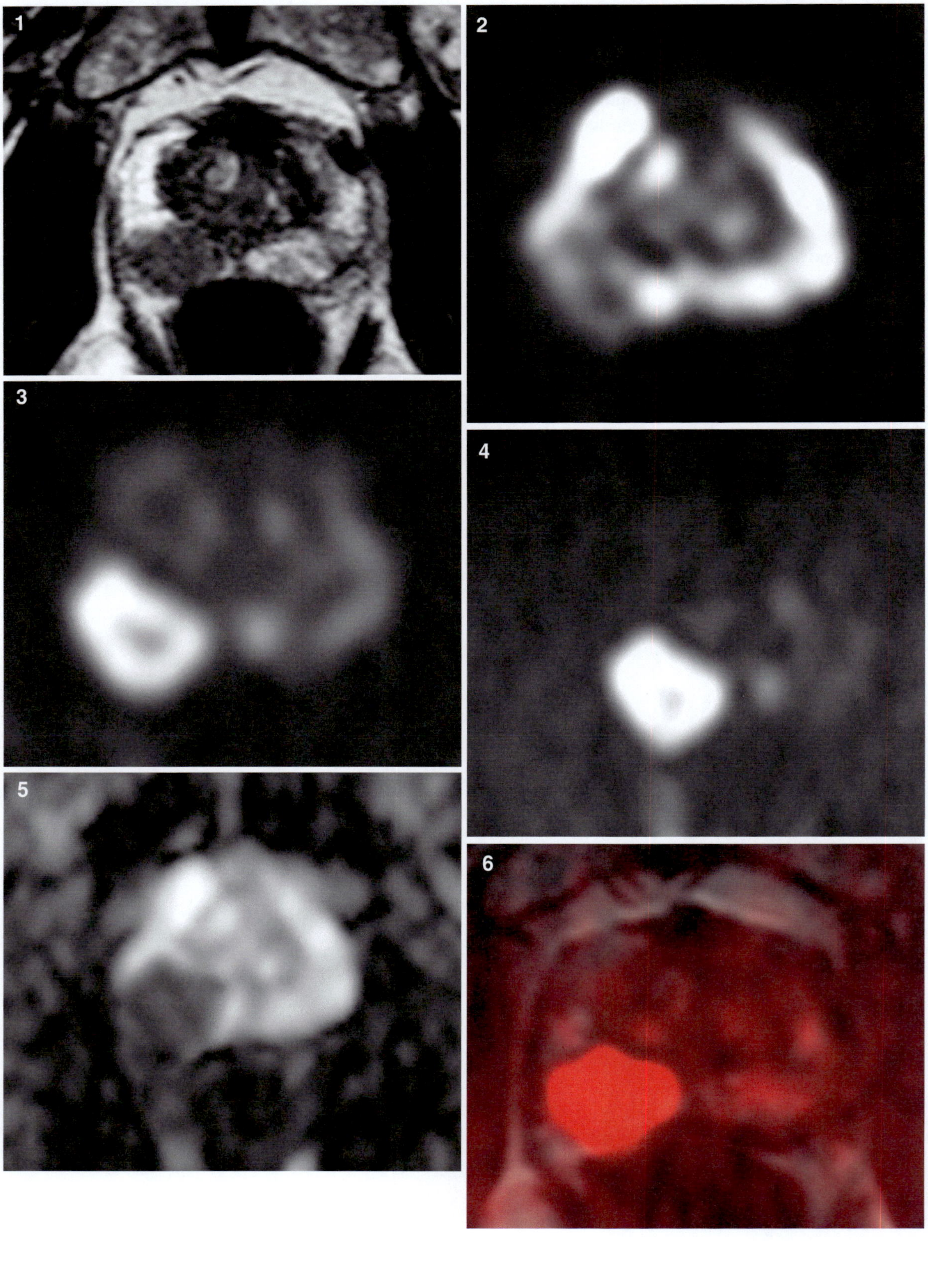

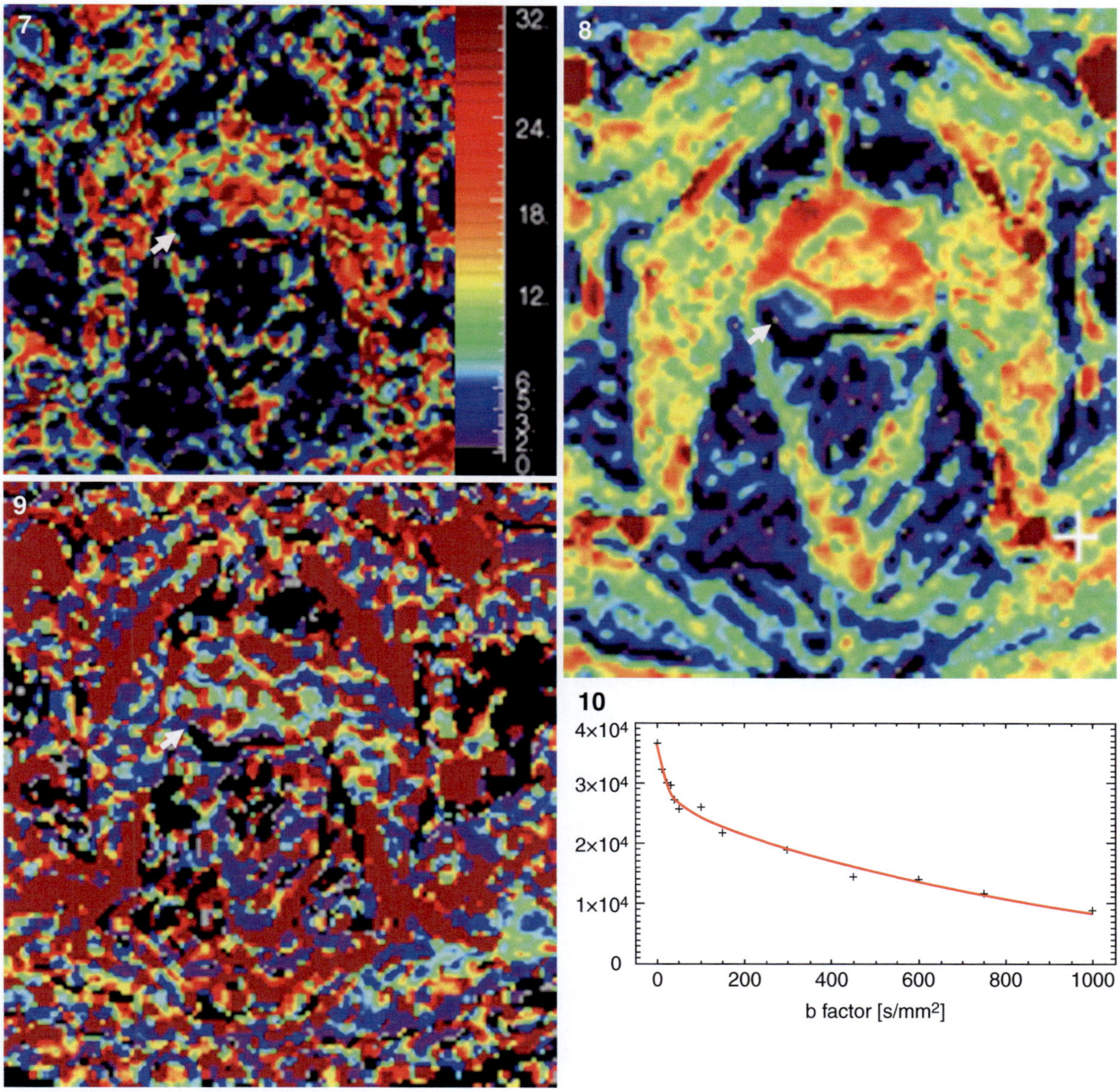

Fig. 8.1 The tumor was clearly depicted on TSE T2-weighted image (**8.1.1**). DWI was performed using a SS EPI sequence with 6 *b* values between 0 and 100 s/mm^2 and another 6 *b* values between 100 and 2,500 s/mm^2. DWI with *b* values of 0, 1,000 and 2,500 are shown in Figs. **8.1.2–8.1.4**, respectively. When increasing the *b* value, the tumor is better identified in spite of decrease in SNR. The tumor does not show sign of extracapsular spread neither on T2-weighted nor DWI sequences, consistent with T2-stage. Corresponding ADC map, using a monocompartimental approach in the analysis of the diffusion, shows the tumor as a hypointense nodule (**8.1.5**), with a *b* value of 0.87×10^{-3} mm^2/s. Fusion imaging of T2-weighted and DWI with a *b* value of 2,500 mm^2/s nicely depicts the tumor (**8.1.6**). A bicompartmental model of the diffusion (IVIM approach) allows for calculation of f (*perfusion fraction*), *D* (*real diffusion of H20 molecules*), and *D** (*perfusion contribution to signal decay*) parametric maps, which are shown in Figs. **8.1.7–8.1.9**, respectively. The signal decay of DWI within the tumor shows a first fast component of signal decay with *b* values lower than 100 s/mm^2, due to the contribution of perfusion to diffusion and a second slow component with higher *b* values, corresponding to the true diffusion (**8.1.10**). *D* value was 0.72×10^{-3} mm^2/s. The difference between ADC and *D* values is probably related to the microvascular perfusion within the tumor

Case 8.2: Chronic Prostatitis

A 45-year-old male with dysuria, malaise, and intermittent fever of unknown origin for several weeks revealed a PSA level of 17 ng/mL. A repeated analytic examination showed a similar PSA value.

Comments

Chronic prostatitis is one of the diagnostic challenges on MRI imaging. Either conventional T2-weighted MRI or MR spectroscopy might show similar findings as prostate cancer. On T2-weighted sequences, prostatitis might show also low signal intensity within the normal high signal of the peripheral zone. Nevertheless, prostatitis might usually show either diffuse low signal intensity or a patchy pattern with regular margins which could differentiate the nodular irregular pattern of prostate cancer. There is much overlap with the metabolic ratio on spectroscopy with prostatitis and prostate cancer as both conditions might show elevated CC/Ci ratio (choline plus creatine/citrate).

Histologically, chronic prostatitis is characterized by extracellular edema surrounding the involved prostatic cells with lymphocytes, plasma cells, macrophages, and neutrophils in the prostatic stroma. This abundance in cells as compared with normal prostatic tissue may lead to an ADC decrease because of decreased extracellular to intracellular fluid volume ratio, but probably not as low as prostate cancer. To our knowledge, there is only a series available on the DWI characteristics of chronic prostatitis compared to prostatic cancer using a 3 T magnet, which demonstrated significant lower ADC values for cancerous tissue (mean ADC value: 1.39 ± 0.22 mm^2/s) compared to the ADC values of prostatitis (1.57 ± 0.12 mm^2/s) and normal prostate tissue (1.62 ± 0.12 mm^2/s). Therefore, DWI sequence with the ADC map might help to differentiate prostatitis and prostate cancer combining also the information of T2-weighted images. Either spectroscopy or dynamic contrast MR imaging might show similar findings in chronic inflammatory and neoplastic disease; for this reason, DWI might improve the negative predictive value of functional MRI on patients with high level PSA due to either chronic prostatitis or benign prostatic hyperplasia.

Imaging Findings

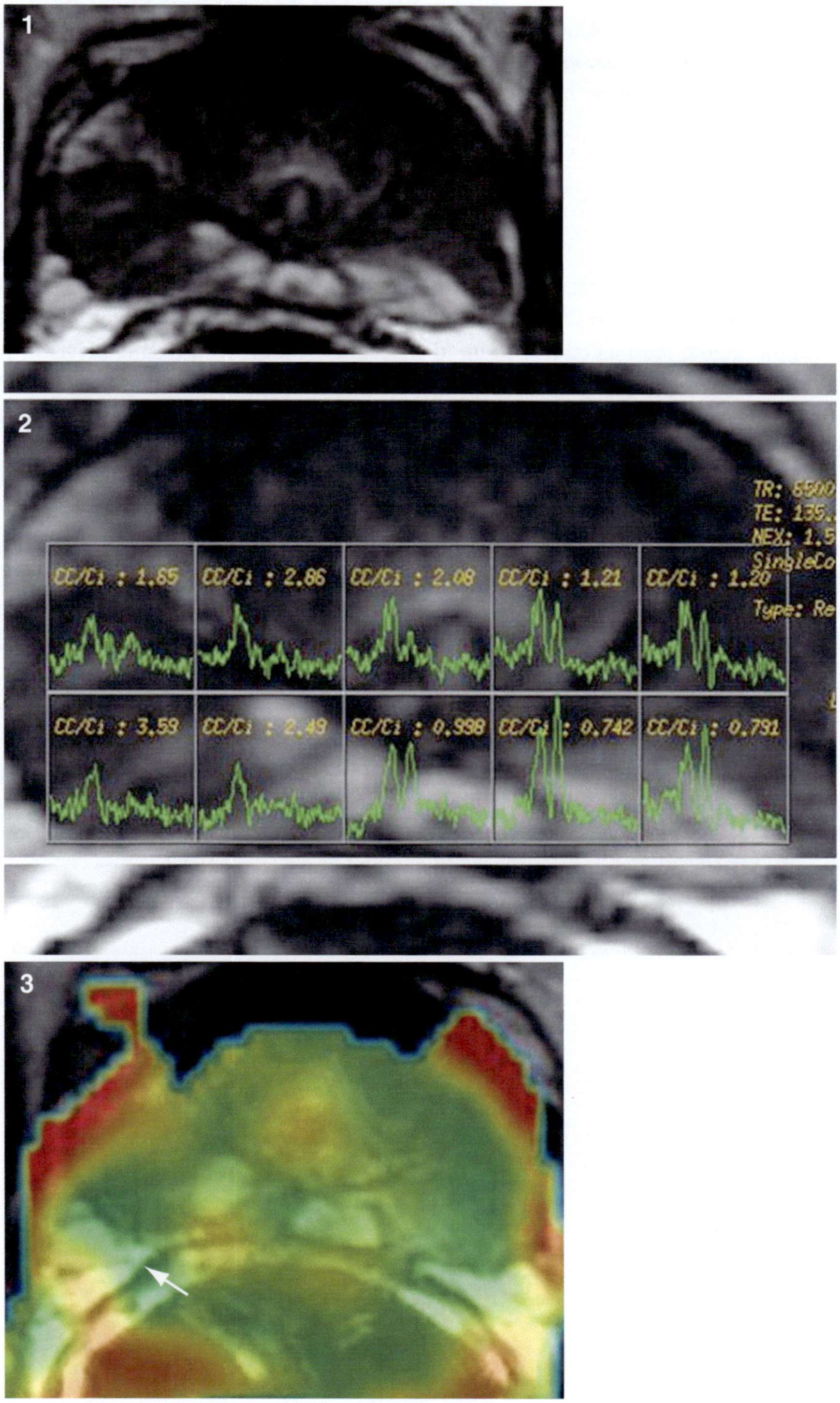

Fig. 8.2 Axial FSE T2-weighted MRI (**8.2.1**) shows bilateral low signal intensity focus, although with regular edges suspicious for malignancy. The corresponding three-dimensional 1H MR spectroscopic imaging data (**8.2.2**) shows an elevated CC/Ci ratio (*choline plus creatine/citrate*) on both sides suspicious for cancer. The ADC map (**8.2.3**) shows neither areas of restriction of diffusion nor low ADC values, which are represented by *blue color* (*arrow*)

Case 8.3: Central Gland Prostate Cancer

A 67-year-old male with four previous negative biopsies for prostate cancer. PSA level shows progressive rising from 6.70 ng/mL to currently 16.57 ng/mL. Free-to-total PSA ratio:14.40%

Comments

Prostate cancer occurs in the peripheral zone in 75–85% of cases; however, it has been shown that the transition zone, central gland, harbors cancer in up to 25% of radical prostatectomy specimens. Cancers located in the transition zone show some pathologic and clinical features that are different from the features shown by cancers located in the peripheral zone. It is important to accurately distinguish transition zone cancers with imaging to guide biopsy, plan disease-targeting therapies, and avoid positive anterior surgical margins at radical prostatectomy. Moreover, it is important to detect central gland prostate cancer in order to avoid repeated overlooked blinded biopsies Biopsying the target lesion detected by MRI, especially using DWI, is more accurate than the current blind biopsy method, and the indication for biopsy could be more efficient than with current methods based on DRE and PSA values. Thus, performing prostate biopsy with MRI/DWI data available could improve the biopsy detection rate of prostate cancer. Despite the tendency of different ADC values in prostate cancer and non-cancerous tissue, studies have also shown a significant overlap of the ADC values between prostate cancer and non-cancerous tissue, which is attributed to the fact that the ADC varies widely in both prostate cancer and non-cancerous tissue. This overlap of the ADC limits the accuracy of DWI in cancer detection. This overlap seems to be prominent between both prostate cancer and non-cancerous transitional zone tissue because it has a lower ADC than peripheral zone tissue. Therefore, a higher diagnostic accuracy based on a ROI analysis in previous studies might be exaggerated, and the actual diagnostic accuracy for cancer detection may not be as satisfactory as expected in clinical practice. Nevertheless, ADC values of prostate cancer seem to show lower values than those of central gland tissue. Besides, a recent paper by Otto and colleagues demonstrated significant differences in ADC value between central gland cancer, stromal and glandular hyperplasia with average ADC values of 1.05×10^{-3} mm^2/s, 1.27×10^{-3} mm^2/s, and 1.73×10^{-3} mm^2/s, respectively.

One of the advantages of MRI is the possibility to combine conventional T2-weighted sequences with functional techniques such as DWI, spectroscopy, or dynamic contrast enhancement sequences. The diagnostic power for prostate cancer increases using combined functional MRI.

Imaging Findings

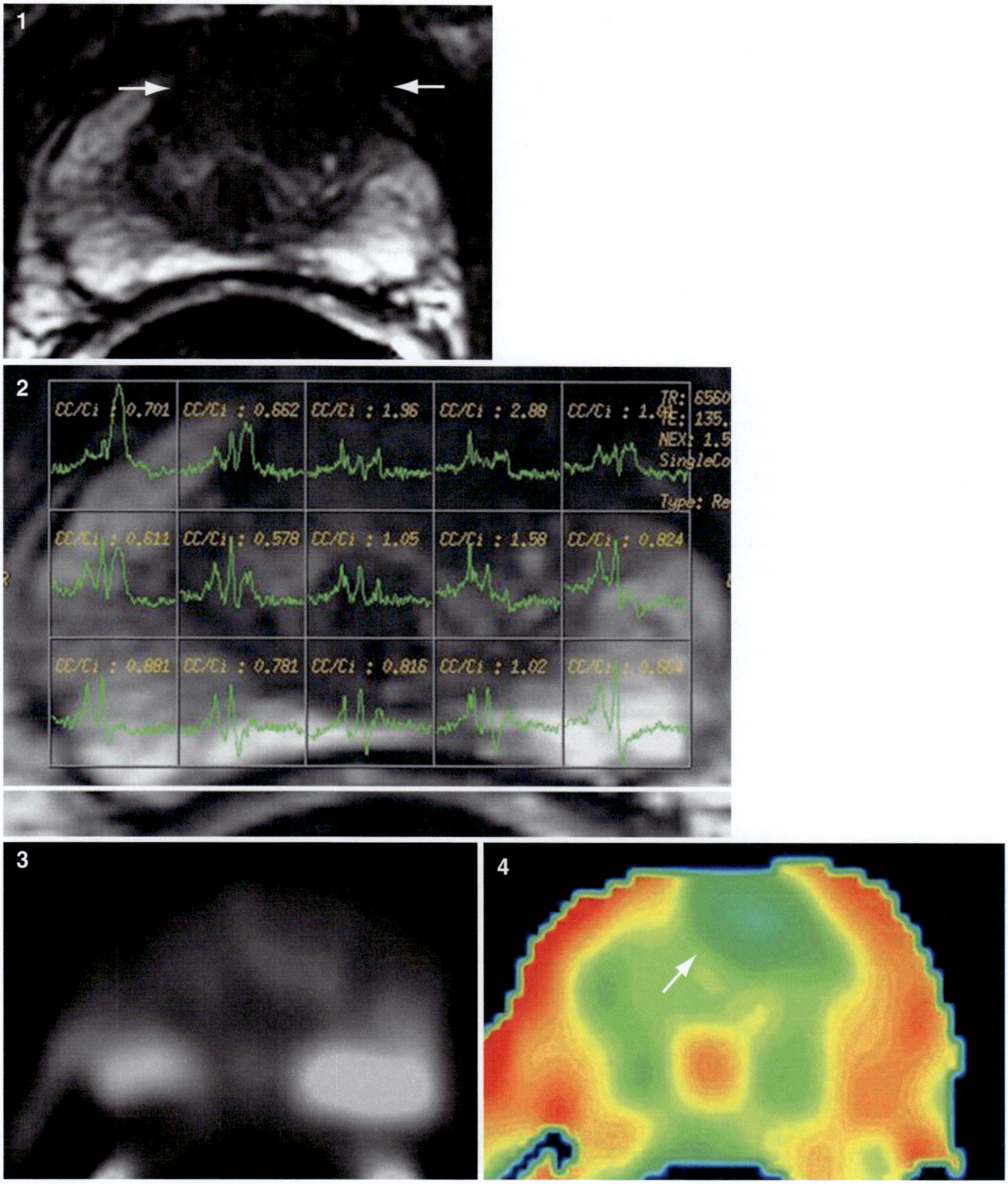

Fig. 8.3 Axial FSE T2-weighted image reveals a low signal intensity nodular lesion in the central anterior left gland (*arrows*) (**8.3.1**). Combined spectroscopy curves show higher level of choline related to citrate corresponding to prostate cancer profile (**8.3.2**). Axial DWI at $b=1{,}000$ s/mm^2 shows slight higher signal intensity on the left side of the central gland but not in a significant manner (**8.3.3**). The same image on the ADC color parametric map shows the significant low ADC value demonstrated as *blue color* (*arrow*) (**8.3.4**). It is necessary to perform the ADC map to display accurate data from the DWI sequence and minimize the T2 shine-through effect

Case 8.4: Bilateral Peripheral Prostate Cancer

A 58-year-old male presents with a PSA level of 3.90 ng/mL and a free-to-total PSA ratio of 7%. Before a biopsy is performed, the urologist requests an MRI study to rule out prostate cancer. Due to the MRI findings, a targeted biopsy was performed with the final result of bilateral peripheral prostate cancer, Gleason 6 (3+3) on the right side, and Gleason 7 (4+3) on the left side.

Comments

Tumor detection on standard T2-weighted MRI in the evaluation of prostate cancer is recognized as a focus of low signal intensity relative to the surrounding signal intensity of the peripheral zone, in a similar manner to the appearance of other benign conditions such as prostatitis or hyperplasia. But the accuracy of T2-weighted MRI in the detection of prostate cancer is approximately 65–77% using a high-resolution endorectal technique.

Advanced functional imaging techniques, such as DWI, spectroscopy (MRSI), and dynamic contrast enhance technique (DCE), significantly increase the sensitivity of MRI in the detection and staging of prostate cancer. MRSI, DW-MRI, and DCE-MRI, all deliver additional information to morphologic changes depicted on T2-weighted MR images. It is important to carefully tailor MRI examination protocols to individual patient clinical history; if applied to appropiately selected patients, each of the three techniques will help better characterize, stage, and grade potential malignancy of the prostate. Although experience with DWI is still relatively limited, interest is growing in this technique as an adjunct to T2-weighted imaging. DWI might have potential for grading of prostate carcinoma. The histopathologic Gleason score remains one of the most important prognostic factors for progression-free and disease-specific survival in prostate cancer. Previous reports have found that higher Gleason grades were associated with lower tumor-muscle signal intensity ratios on T2-weighted imaging. Hypothetically, DWI has far more potential than any other MR imaging sequence in grading of prostate carcinoma, because increased cellular density and loss of tubular structures implicate a higher Gleason score and also seriously hamper self-diffusion in the involved tissue leading to lower ADC levels on DWI.

Fig. 8.4 Axial T2-weighted images (**8.4.1**) show bilateral low signal intensity in the peripheral gland, with a higher size on the left side. MR spectroscopy curves reveal no significant increase of choline levels on both side lesions although coline was slightly higher on the left side lesion (**8.4.1**). Parametric ADC color map (**8.4.2**) shows a significant lower value on the left side lesion demonstrated as a *blue color* (*arrow*). The lesion of the right side does not show restricted diffusion on the ADC map (**8.4.2**). The dynamic contrast-enhanced sequence reveals a significant wash-in with delayed wash-out curve of the left side lesion (ROI number 3) and a moderate wash-in with a plateau curve on the right side lesion (ROI number 4) compared to normal peripheral zone (ROIs number 5 and 6) (**8.4.3**)

Imaging Findings

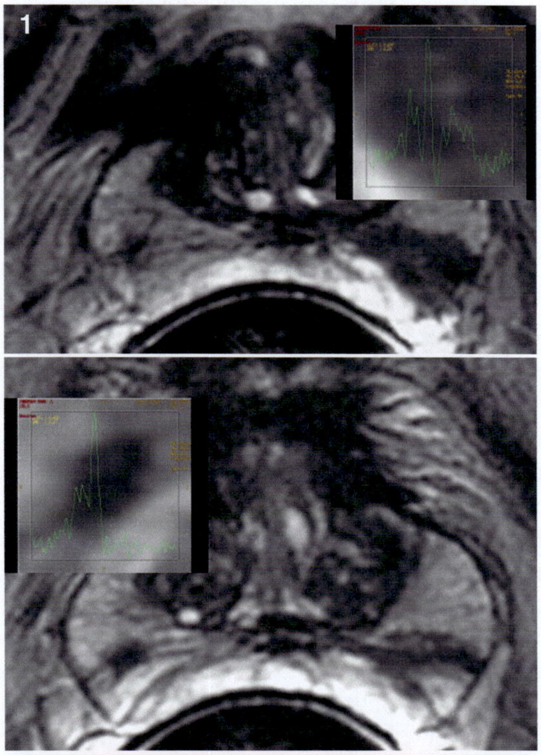

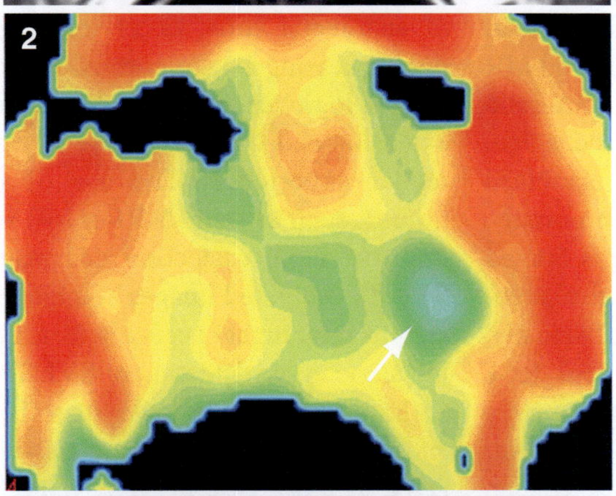

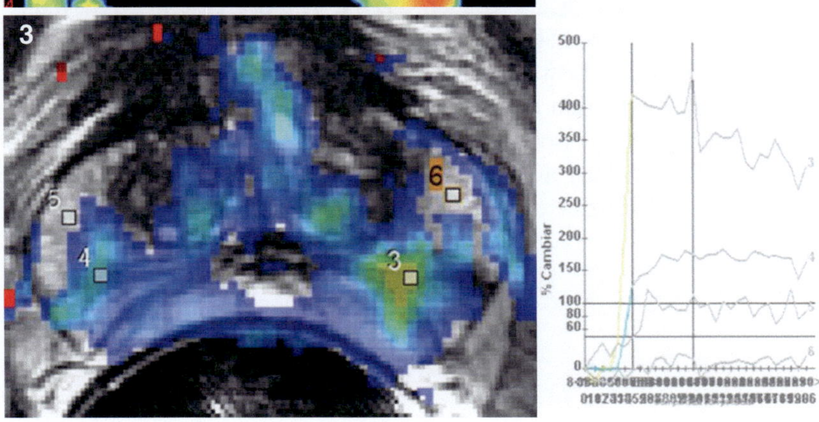

Case 8.5: Seminal Vesicles Infiltration

A 67-year-old male without a previous biopsy presented with a PSA level of 6.7 ng/mL and free-to-total PSA ratio (% fPSA) of 8%. Digital rectal examination (DRE) was unremarkable. The urologist requested an MRI previously to perform a biopsy.

Comments

The methods most commonly used to detect prostate cancer (PC) are DRE and serum PSA levels. Both methods provide suboptimal accuracy for PC diagnosis. The specificity of PSA levels is poor for PSA level below 10 ng/mL. A high percentage of biopsy-proven PCs manifest with PSA level of less than 4 ng/mL, and many patients with PSA level greater than 4 ng/mL do not have PC. Thus, these patients undergo unnecessary biopsy. There have been attempts to improve the specificity of PSA levels. Recently, measurements of molecular isoforms of PSA in the serum are used. In men with a total PSA level between 3 and 10 ng/mL, the %fPSA ratio is better to distinguish prostate cancer from benign disease than the measurement of total PSA alone. Vilanova et al. reported that MR and MR spectroscopy combined with free-to-total PSA ratio improves the predictive value for PC detection. Therefore, %fPSA could be a useful tool combined with imaging for prostate cancer detection. Currently, the threshold for pretreatment MRI staging is limited to high-risk, localized PC, although some also advocate men with intermediate-risk disease. Actually, some authors think that it may be time to consider a role for MRI before prostate biopsy. The latter strategy could avoid biopsy, and hence unnecessary treatment, in those with no disease or insignificant cancer. Improved staging is crucial to determine risk and prognosis, especially when differentiating between organ-confined PC and extracapsular extension or seminal vesicle invasion (SVI). Clinical factors associated with an increased incidence of SVI include a high PSA level, a high Gleason grade, the presence of tumor at the base of the prostate gland, and lymph node metastases. MRI is superior to DRE, transrectal ultrasound, and CT in predicting prostate-confined cancer.

SVI may result from direct tumor spread in a contiguous fashion, or tumor infiltration following the course of the ejaculatory ducts or urethra. MRI is useful in demonstrating SVI in patients with PC. SVI is associated with microscopic lymph node metastases, and increased risk of recurrence after prostatectomy. Tumor in the SV appears as a low signal area in the high signal fluid on T2-weighted images and as a low signal area on T1-weighted images. Other findings, such as loss of the normal architecture of the SV, asymmetry, loss of the fat plane between the base of the bladder and the inferior aspect of the SV, focal or diffuse wall thickening, obliteration of the angle between the prostate and the SV, or direct tumor extension from the base of the prostate into and around the SV, may represent SVI. There is a great variation of MRI sensitivity of SVI between different published series but the accuracy of MRI in local staging has increased with time, most likely because of the maturation of MRI technology (3 T, faster imaging sequences, more powerful gradients, the use of endorectal coils, faster imaging sequences, and postprocessing image correction), refinement of the morphologic criteria for diagnosing extracapsular extension and seminal vesicle invasion, and growing reader experience. The use of functional techniques, such as DCE-MRI or MR spectroscopy, can improve tumor detection and staging. Concerning SVs, T2-weighted images combined with DWI show significantly higher accuracy than T2-weighted imaging alone in the detection of SVI. The ADC values of SVI are significantly lower than those of normal SV and cases of SVI exhibit high signal intensity on DWI. The decrease in ADC values in SVI is attributed to histopathological characteristics of malignant tissue, and no significant difference between the ADC values of PC foci and SVI can be detected. On the contrary, normal SV usually show low signal on DWI and high ADC values due to the fast molecular translation of water.

Imaging Findings

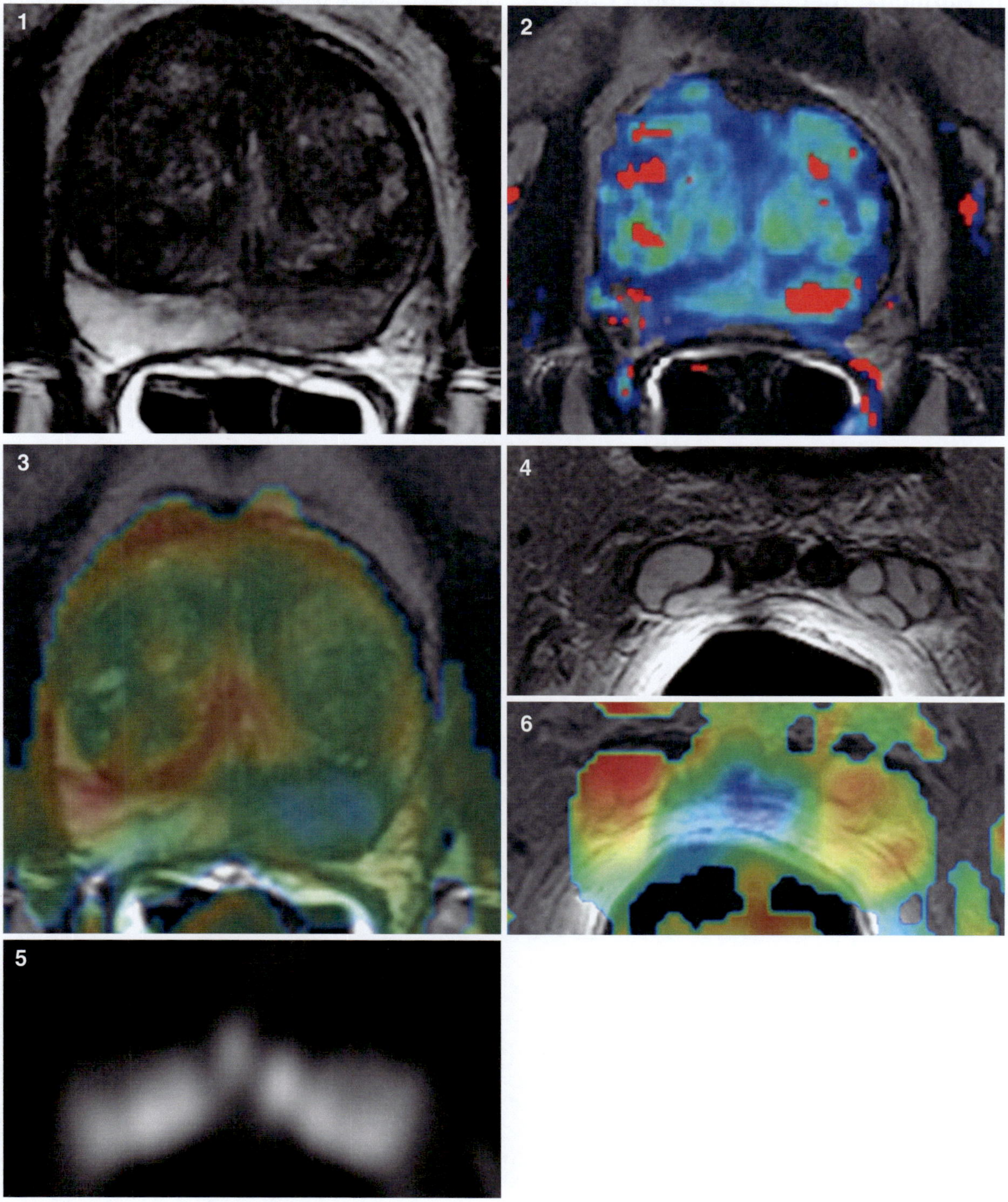

Fig. 8.5 Axial FSE T2-weighted (**8.5.1**) shows diffuse low signal in left peripheral gland; DCE-MR (**8.5.2**) demonstrates a focal area of increased wash-in rate (*red area*). Combined FSE T2-weighted image plus ADC parametric map (**8.5.3**) demonstrates low ADC values (*blue color*) in the left peripheral gland. Axial FSE T2-weighted (**8.5.4**), DWI (**8.5.5**) and combined T2-weighted plus ADC parametric map (**8.5.6**), at the level of SVs, confirm the SVI demonstrating hypointense signal on T2-weighted image and high signal on DWI with high be value (although non discernible of the rest of SV). SVI is better depited on ADC map as an area with low ADC value (*blue color*) in the seminal vesicles

Case 8.6: Monitorization of Response to Hormonal Therapy in a Patient with Prostate Cancer and Metastatic Pelvic Lymph Nodes

A 60-year-old male patient was referred to our MRI unit for prostate cancer staging. A year later, after hormone treatment, a follow-up study was performed.

Comments

Prostate cancer is one of the most common malignancies in elderly men. In recent years, there has been an important development of the MRI applications in its diagnosis, staging and assessment of local recurrence of prostate cancer. Functional techniques as diffusion-weighted sequences, perfusion techniques and H1 proton spectroscopy have increased the MRI applications in prostate cancer management. However, for metastatic nodal depiction, morphological criteria are still used, as size or signal intensity on T2-weighted sequences to discriminate between metastatic nodes and reactive ones.

In our knowledge, very few studies have focused on the characterization on DWI sequences of lymph nodes. Series using USPIO (specific reticuloendothelial contrast) have shown promising results in detecting pelvic lymph node tumor infiltration. However, this type of contrast has not yet been approved by the FDA for habitual clinical use.

Eiber et al. have recently published a feasibility study of the characterization of lymph nodes in patients with prostate cancer using DWI and ADC measurements. In this study, a significant difference between mean ADC value of malignant ($1.07 \pm 0.23 \times 10^{-3}$ mm^2/s) versus benign nodes ($1.54 \pm 0.25 \times 10^{-3}$ mm^2/s) was observed, using a threshold value of 1.3×10^{-3} mm^2/s.

The characterization of metastatic prostatic nodes using ADC values is a promising method due to its ability to detect metastatic nodes, even in very small ones (<6 mm). The ADC values could be also used to assess the response to treatment, as hormonal therapy. A rising in ADC values, due to necrosis, will become a sign of adequate response to treatment.

The detection of pathological nodes may be improved by using fusion images DWI and T2-weighted sequences that allows an adequate correlation between morphological and functional images.

Imaging Findings

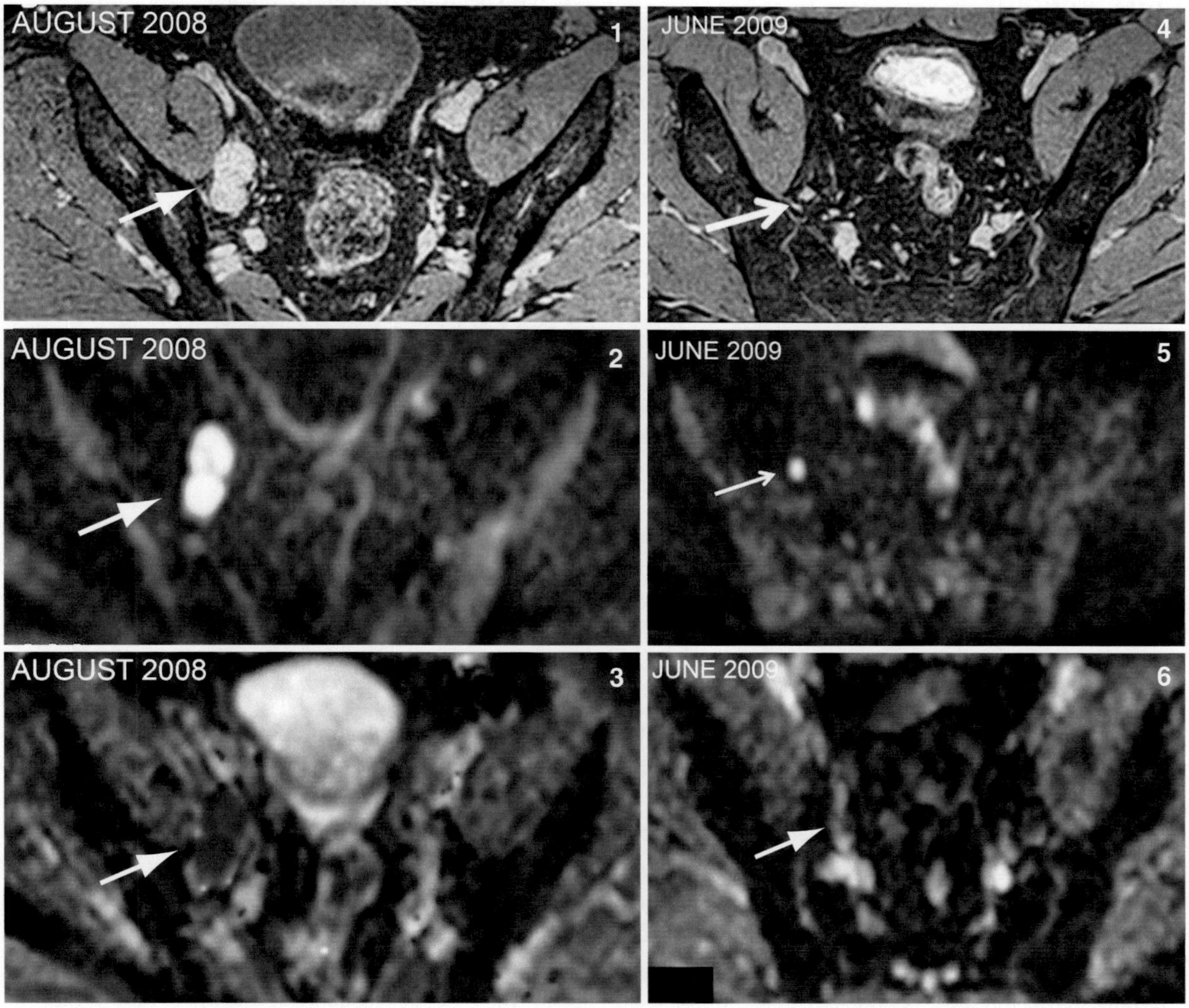

Fig. 8.6 Postcontrast axial THRIVE (**8.6.1**), DWI with a *b* value of 1000 s/mm^2 (**8.6.2**) and ADC map (**8.6.3**) performed in August 2008 showed right iliac lymph nodes (*arrows*) with restricted diffusion and low mean ADC value (0.8×10^{-3} mm^2/s). Staging of prostate cancer was that of T3 N2. Corresponding sequences in the follow-up MRI performed in June 2009 after hormonal therapy showed a marked decrease in size of metastatic nodes (**8.6.4**), which also present an increase in diffusivity (**8.6.5**) and higher ADC mean value than in previous study (1.5×10^{-3} mm^2/s) due to necrosis (**8.6.6**) in relation to appropriated response to treatment (*arrows*)

Case 8.7: Local Recurrence After Brachytherapy

A 60-year-old male with clinical history of prostate cancer (pT2N0, Gleason 3+3 and PSA 5.5 ng/mL) was treated with brachytherapy (BT) 4 years ago. Two years later, PSA value was 0.6 ng/mL. Currently, the patient presents high serum PSA level: 4 ng/mL.

Comments

In recent years, there have been significant improvements in the management of localized prostate cancer but the optimal treatment remains undefined. BT is an effective option for prostate cancer treatment in selected patients. The indications for prostate BT are very similar to those for any form of radical treatment for prostate cancer; it is a treatment for organ-confined, early stage disease. Prostate BT delivers a high dose of radiation to a very small target volume. Hence, there is very little unnecessary irradiation of adjacent bowel loops and bladder.

After BT, serum PSA levels decrease slowly with a nadir observed at 2–4 years, but a temporary increase of PSA levels followed by a further decrease can occur. This temporary increase is named PSA bounce. Follow-up after BT is performed clinically and imaging has a limited role for direct patient management. Unfortunately, there is no consensus definition of biochemical failure following BT. ASTRO criteria and Phoenix definition have been used. Based upon sensitivity and specificity profiles, as well as regression analysis, a serum PSA level of the nadir + 2 appears to be the best value for defining a biochemical failure.

Imaging usually has a limited role for detecting local recurrence after BT. In practice, exclusion of metastatic relapse with CT and bone scanning will be used as indirect evidence of local failure in patients with biochemical failure. Local recurrence after BT is difficult to detect. MRI of the post-treatment gland can be difficult to evaluate. Areas of low signal may represent recurrent/residual disease, or merely be part of the spectrum of therapy change. Additionally, BT seeds result in metallic susceptibility artifacts, which obscure fine detail and can impair interpretation of certain MRI sequences, such as DWI or MR spectroscopy, within the prostate. At MRI, "normal" post-BT prostate shows diffuse low signal intensity on T1-weighted and T2-weighted images and little or no enhancement on dynamic contrast-enhanced images. MRSI shows a metabolic atrophy. Recurrences may be depicted on DCE-MRI due to their early enhancement, but interpreting post-BT DCE images is difficult, because the decrease of prostate vascularization is not homogeneous. Beside this, there is a short experience using MRSI in patients with BF after BT and its role is not clear. Increased metabolic activity within the implanted prostate may indicate local recurrence but this is still an area of research.

DWI has its own limitations. False positive results can occur in the setting of hemorrhage, infection or artifact from implanted metal. But, DWI may be a powerful adjunct to the detection of residual or recurrent prostate carcinoma. Highly cellular tumor tissue will demonstrate significantly restricted diffusion, compared with nonspecific hypointense areas on T2-weighted imaging and it will exhibit high signal intensity on the high b value images with a low ADC value, consistent with restricted diffusion. Occasionally, discordant results between techniques are found; for example, DCE-MRI might not depict suspicious areas but DWI could be indicative for active tumor. This may occur because of intrinsic tumor biology (with high cellularity but low perfusion) and it illustrates the importance of using a multiparametric MRI approach to assess the pelvis, when a recurrent prostate cancer is suspected.

Salvage treatment options are limited in recurrence. New therapeutic procedures such as high-intensity focused ultrasound (HIFU) or cryotherapy are currently under evaluation. MRI may detect and localize local recurrences early and it might be used in the future to define HIFU or high-dose-rate BT target areas.

Imaging Findings

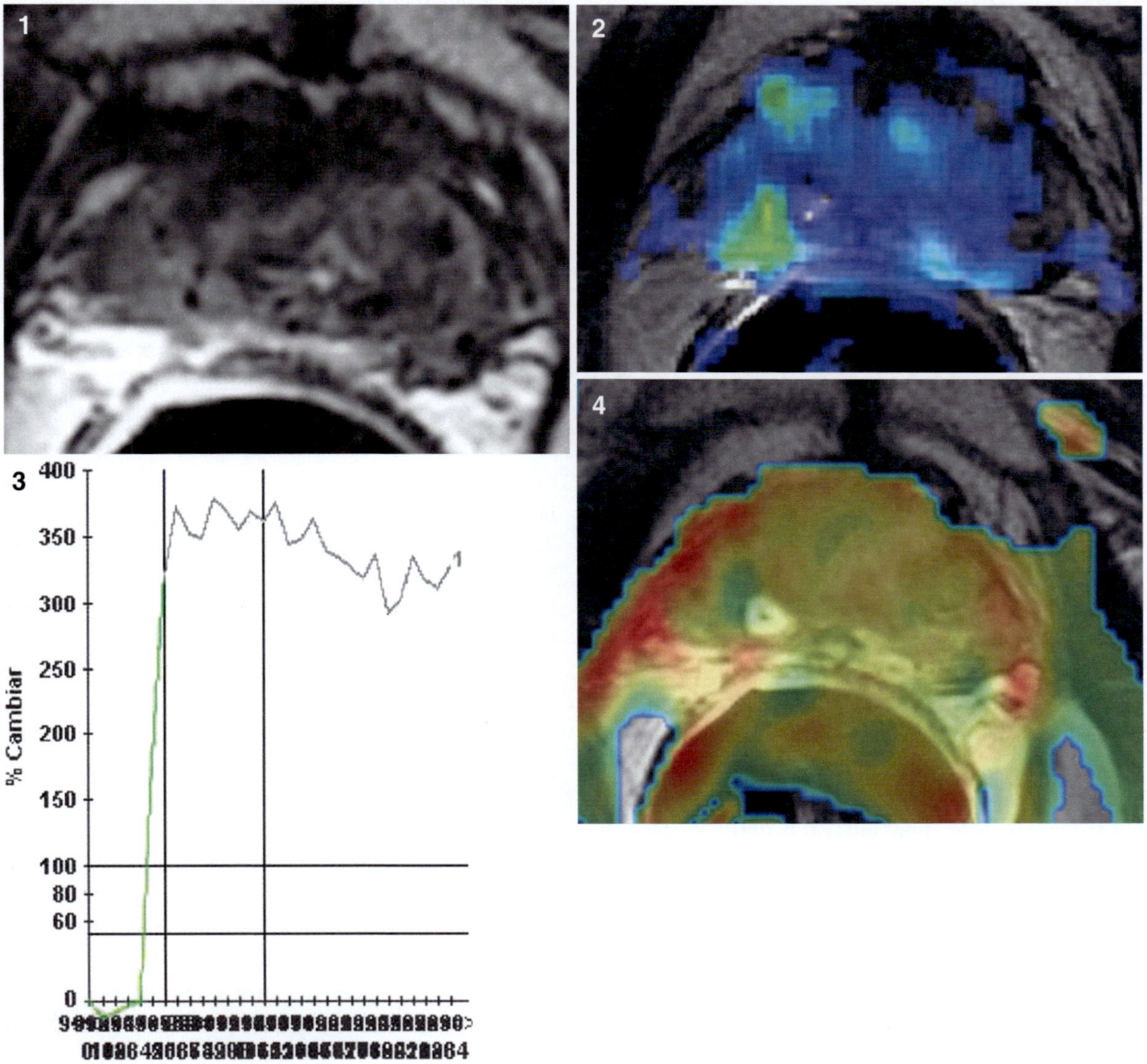

Fig. 8.7 Axial FSE T2-weighted image (**8.7.1**) shows a diffuse low signal intensity secondary to brachytherapy. Several brachytherapy seeds can be depicted. The recurrent cancer is not visible on this sequence. Parametric map from DCE-MRI (**8.7.2**) shows increased wash-in rate in the right peripheral gland (*green area*) corresponding to the recurrent cancer. Semi-quantitative analysis of this area (**8.7.3**) demonstrates a type III curve that shows a wash-in/wash-out pattern. Combined image of FSE T2-weighted image and ADC parametric map (**8.7.4**) clearly depicts an area with low ADC value (*green*) at the same level of anomalous dynamic pattern on DCE-MRI

Case 8.8: Local Recurrence After Radical Prostatectomy

A 68-year-old male presented with clinical history of radical prostatectomy (RP) 1 year ago for prostate cancer (pT2c, Gleason 6, PSA 6.45 ng/mL). Currently, the patient presents fast rising serum PSA level, increasing from 2.36 to 2.60 ng/mL during the last 3 months.

Comments

After definitive RP, serum PSA should fall to undetectable levels (less than 0.1 ng/mL). A rise in serum PSA is usually the first indication of cancer recurrence. The reported incidence of BF following radical prostatectomy ranges from 15% to 53%, and it often precedes detectable recurrence by years. The definition of BF varies in the literature from 0.2 to 0.5 ng/mL, but a PSA level of 0.2 ng/mL is considered indicative of BF. A PSA level of 0.4 ng/mL or greater is associated most strongly to local or disease progression. Clinically, we can consider four main categories of recurrence: PSA-only relapse, local recurrence in the prostatectomy bed, metastatic disease, and combined local and distance recurrence. Different nomograms based on the combination of pathologic stage and tumor grade at diagnosis, PSA doubling time, time interval between surgery and PSA relapse, and others help to distinguish among these four situations in order to decide patient's treatment.

Local recurrence after RP is frequently not detectable by rectal examination. Accurate information on local patterns of failure has frequently used to improve target volume definition for adjuvant radiotherapy. MRI may be a basic tool in the evaluation of the postsurgical pelvis to define the site of local recurrence in the tumor bed region after surgery.

It must be addressed that it is not infrequent to observe small amounts of residual benign prostatic tissue responsible for persistent mild elevation of PSA levels. Tumoral relapse is more frequently demonstrated in the perianastomotic area (from the bladder neck to the penile bulb). At MRI, normal postsurgical perianastomotic fibrosis appears hypointense on T1-weighted and T2-weighted images and with small or no enhancement on dynamic contrast-enhanced DCE images. Incomplete resection of the SVs after RP is not an infrequent finding and patients may fail within these retained remnants. The retained SVs are easily diagnosed when they keep their characteristic morphology and high signal intensity on T2-weighted images. They can also appear as distorted low signal intensity nodules or linear structures suggesting residual fibrotic SV tips. Recurrences present as lobulated masses with intermediate signal intensity on T2-weighted images and they enhance early on DCE-MRI and show restricted diffusion. MRI can detect and localize local recurrences early, in patients with low PSA levels and it might be used in the future to define and reduce the radiotherapy clinical target volume to the suspicious area.

The role of MRSI in patients with BF after prostatectomy remains controversial. MRSI is a demanding technique. It is limited by its poor spatial resolution and it shows high sensitivity to field inhomogeneities induced by surgical clips. Besides, diagnostic criteria using MRSI are still unclear, since normal citrate is in theory undetectable after RP and thus the classic choline-to-citrate ratio might not be accurate.

The best treatment for local recurrence is salvage external beam radiotherapy. Its outcome is more favorable in patients at PSA levels <1–1.5 ng/mL. New therapeutic procedures such as HIFU or cryotherapy are currently under evaluation.

Imaging Findings

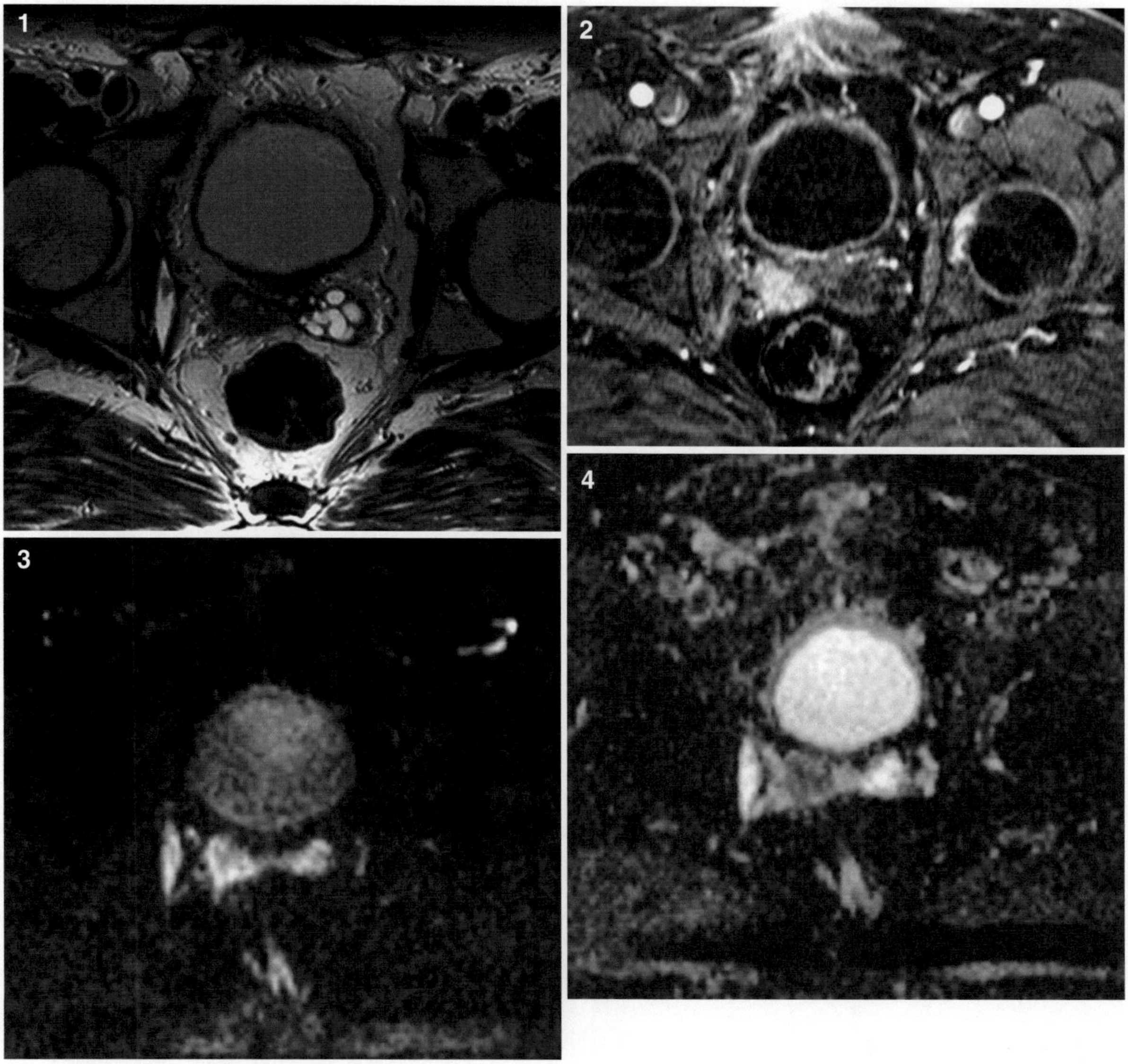

Fig. 8.8 Axial TSE T2-weighted (**8.8.1**), DCE (**8.8.2**), and DWI with a *b* value of 800 s/mm^2 (**8.8.3**) images and ADC map (**8.8.4**) demonstrate retained seminal vesicles. Tumoral invasion can be clearly depicted on the right side with low signal on T2-weighted imaging, early enhancement on DCE-MRI, high signal on DWI, and low ADC value. Axial (**8.8.5**) and coronal T2-weighted TSE images (**8.8.6**) in a different case of post-prostatectomy recurrence shows a tumoral mass with intermediate signal situated posterolateral to the perianastomotic area and invading the bladder. DWI with a *b* value of 1,000 s/mm^2 (**8.8.7**) images shows high signal intensity on the high *b* value image with a low ADC value, in the corresponding ADC map, consistent with restricted diffusion (**8.8.8**)

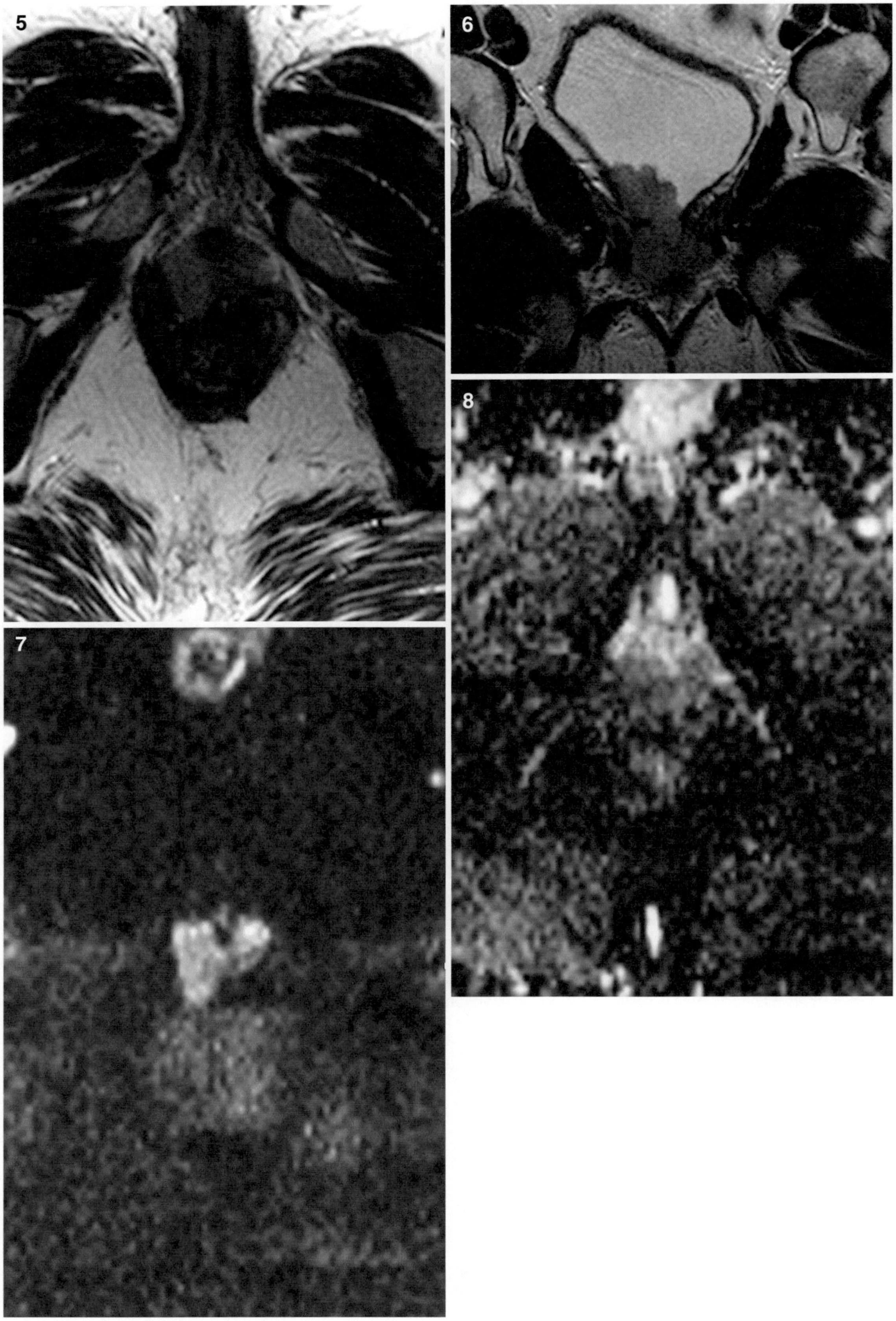

Fig. 8.8 (continued)

Case 8.9: Bladder Carcinoma

A 67-year-old female presented hematuria. Ultrasound revealed a bladder mass and right ureteral obstruction. MRI was performed for further assessment.

Comments

In cases of gross hematuria, DWI is a powerful tool to investigate its origin. In a series by Abou-El-Ghar and colleagues, DWI showed a sensitivity and positive predictive value of 98.5% and 100%, respectively, for determining the cause of hematuria, with a consensus diagnostic performance for identification of bladder tumors of: sensitivity, 98.1% specificity, 92.3%; and accuracy 97.0% (128 of 132). Two cases were falsely negative on T2-weighted MR images in this series but were correctly diagnosed by using DWI.

Although, there are limited data evaluating the role of DWI in bladder cancer, this technique may have a role in locoregional staging, histological grading and assessment and prediction of response to treatment. As in cancer of other organs, bladder cancer tends to show high signal on native DWI images and an ADC value lower than that of normal bladder wall, prostate, and seminal vesicles. Lower ADC values have been related to more aggressive tumor of greater histological grade. Available data support that DWI outperforms conventional T2-weighted and dynamic contrast-enhanced MRI in the T-staging of bladder cancer, which is critical for patient management. DWI also improves the detection of pelvic lymph nodes, with a promising role in the distinction of metastatic and inflammatory lymph nodes. Assessment of response to treatment is possible with DWI, which in a recent series was significantly superior in specificity and accuracy to T2-weighed and dynamic contrast-enhanced MRI, despite comparable sensitivity. In the same report, DWI was also useful to accurately predict pathologic complete response.

Imaging Findings

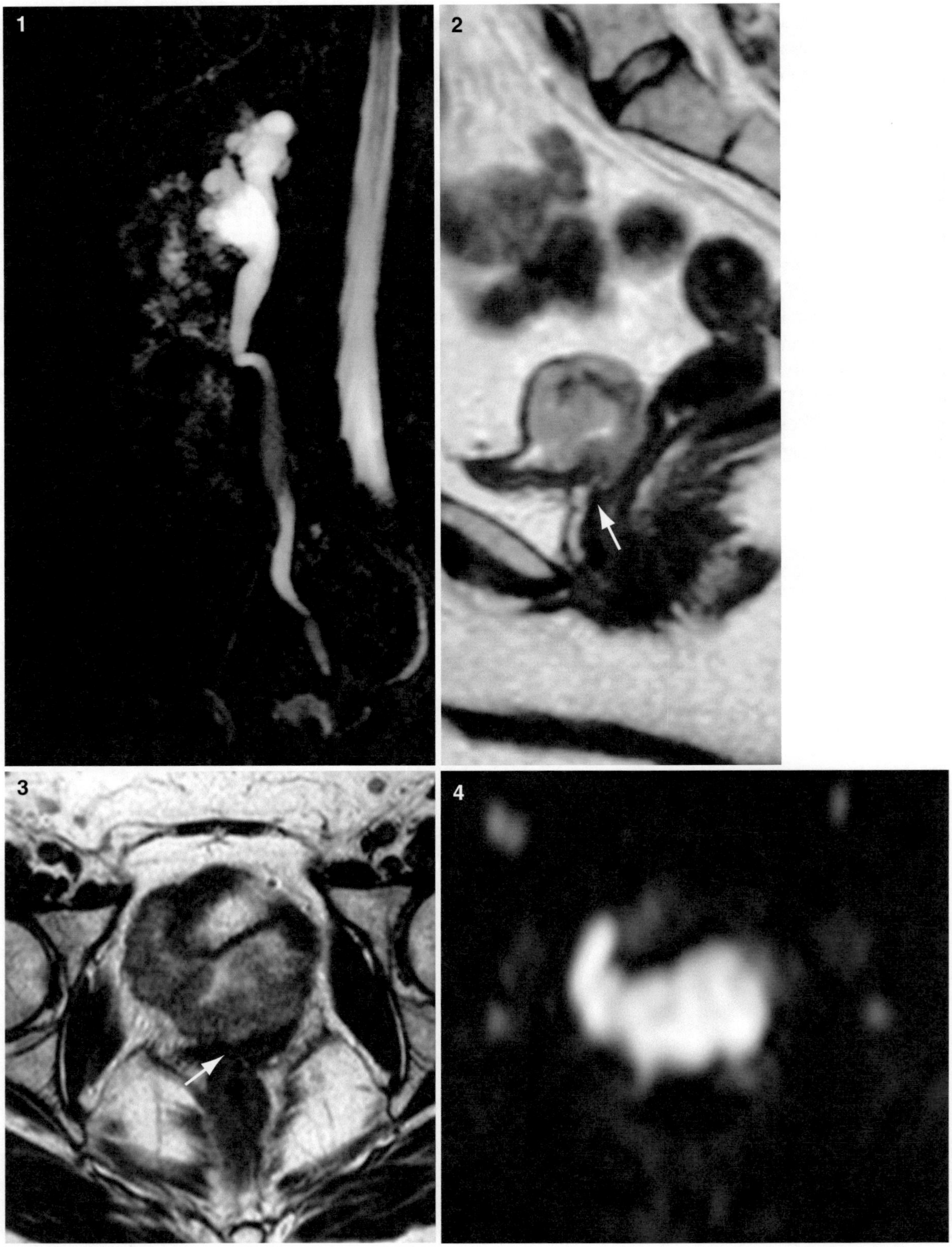

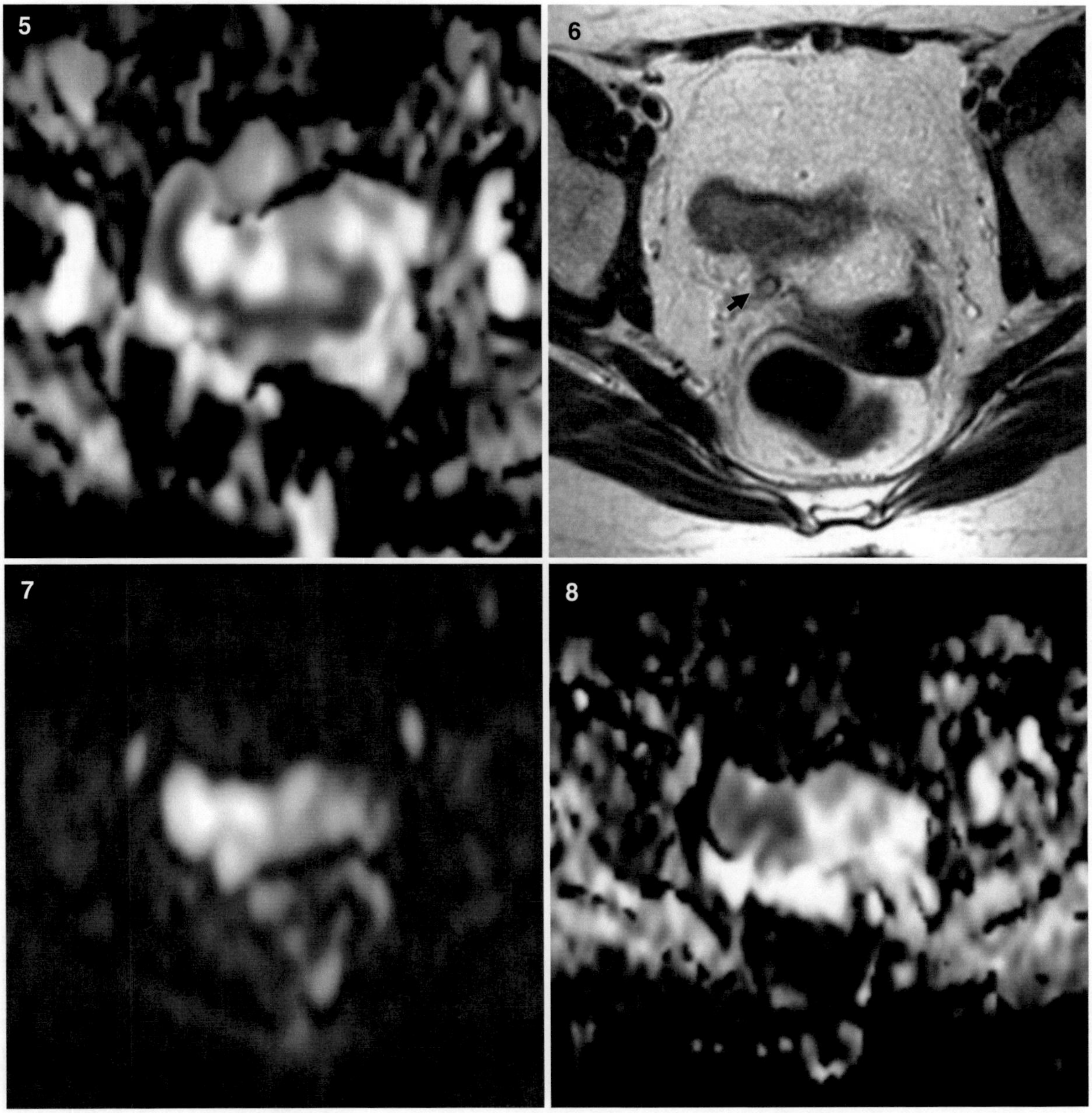

Fig. 8.9 (continued)

Fig. 8.9 Thick slice 2D SS TSE MR urography shows dilatation and distal obstruction of right ureter (**8.9.1**). A huge mass in the posterior aspect of the bladder is revealed on sagittal TSE T2-weighted image (**8.9.2**), which infiltrates the anterior aspect of the vagina (*arrow*). The vaginal infiltration is confirmed on axial TSE T2-weighted image (*arrow*) (**8.9.3**) Its aggressive biological nature is confirmed on DWI with a *b* value of 800 s/mm^2 (**8.9.4**) and its corresponding ADC map (**8.9.5**), as the lesion shows restricted diffusion. Notice how ADC map better depicts the real extension of the tumor and its irregular margins as a low signal mass. At a superior level, TSE T2-weighted (**8.9.6**), DWI with a *b* value of 800 s/mm^2 (**8.9.7**), and ADC map (**8.9.8**) demonstrate the infiltration of right ureter (*arrow*)

Case 8.10: Recurrent Retroperitoneal Leiomyosarcoma

A 72-year-old female, with antecedent of resected pelvic retroperitoneal leiomyosarcoma in complete clinical remission, presented with long-standing lumbar pain of 3 months of evolution. Previous lumbar spine MRI was unremarkable. MRI of abdomen and pelvis was performed for further investigation.

Comments

DWI may be useful to characterize the histological behavior of retroperitoneal tumors, as in other locations. A series by Nakayama and colleagues evaluated the usefulness of EPI DWI using a maximum *b* factor of 1,000–1,100 s/mm² in the characterization of 50 patients with known retroperitoneal masses. The lowest ADC value was demonstrated by malignant lymphoma, with a mean ADC value of $0.66 \pm 0.26 \times 10^{-3}$ mm²/s . Malignant epithelial neoplasms demonstrated a significant lower ADC value than mesenchymal malignant ones, ADC values of $0.90 \pm 0.20 \times 10^{-3}$ mm²/s and 1.26 $\pm 0.500.90 \pm 0.20 \times 10^{-3}$ mm²/s, respectively. Besides, ADC value of benign mesenchymal tumors was that of $1.87 \pm 0.48 \times 10^{-3}$ mm²/s. The ADC value of malignant lymphoma was significantly lower than that of malignant mesenchymal lesions and benign ones. Furthermore, both malignant epithelial and mesenchymal tumors showed a significant difference with benign mesenchymal lesions. Therefore, DWI may help in the differentiation between lymphoma and benign and malignant retroperitoneal masses, although further research is still needed to confirm these limited data.

Imaging Findings

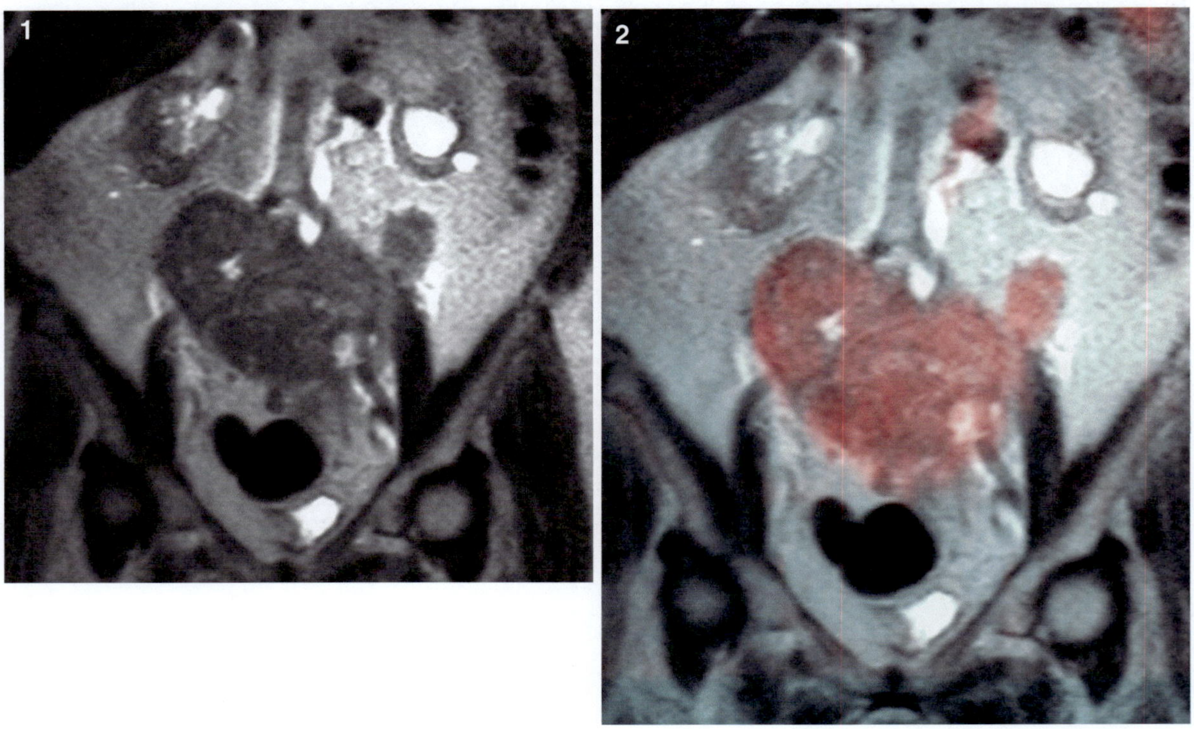

Fig. 8.10 Coronal HASTE (**8.10.1**) depicts a huge retroperitoneal mass, causing left ureteral obstruction. The mass is highly aggressive as demonstrated in the fusion image of HASTE and high *b* value DWI sequence (**8.10.2**). The mass shows high signal intensity on axial DWI (**8.10.3**) and a homogeneous low mean ADC value of 0.79×10^{-3} mm²/s, as demonstrated in the histogram analysis of the lesional ADC (**8.10.4**). Tumoral volume may be calculated using either MIP (**8.10.5**) or volume rendering (**8.10.6**) reconstructions

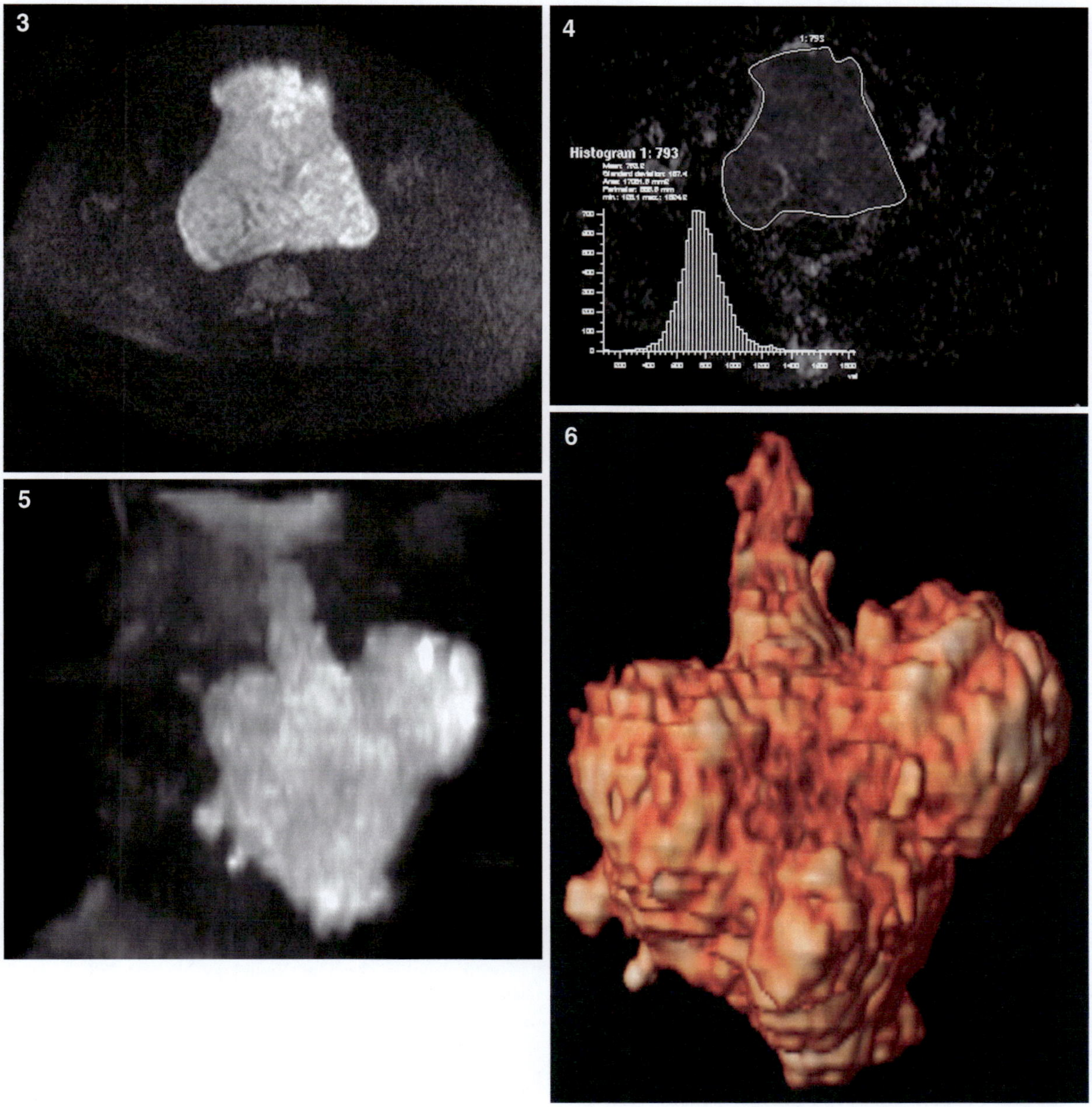

Fig. 8.10 (continued)

Further Reading

Abou-El-Ghar ME, El-Assmy A, Refaie HF et al (2009) Bladder cancer: diagnosis with diffusion-weighted MR imaging in patients with gross hematuria. Radiology 251(2):415–421

Budiharto T, Joniau S, Lerut E et al (2011) Prospective evaluation of (11)C-choline positron emission tomography/computed tomography and diffusion-weighted magnetic resonance imaging for the nodal staging of prostate cancer with a high risk of lymph node metastases. Eur Urol; Jan 18, 2011 [Epub ahead of print]

Candefjord S, Ramser K, Lindahl OA (2009) Technologies for localization and diagnosis of prostate cancer. J Med Eng Technol 31:1–19

Choi YJ, Kim JK, Kim N et al (2007) Functional MR imaging of prostate cancer. Radiographics 27:63–75

De Visschere PJ, De Meerleer GO, Fütterer JJ et al (2010) Role of MRI in follow-up after focal therapy for prostate carcinoma. Am J Roentgenol 194(6):1427–1433

deSouza NM, Riches SF, Vanas NJ et al (2008) Diffusion-weighted magnetic resonance imaging: a potential non-invasive marker of tumour aggressiveness in localized prostate cancer. Clin Radiol 63:774–782

Eiber M, Beer AJ, Holzapfel K et al (2010) Preliminary results for characterization of pelvic lymph nodes in patients with prostate cancer by diffusion-weighted MR-imaging. Invest Radiol 45(1):15–23

El-Assmy A, Abou-El-Ghar ME, Mosbah A et al (2009) Bladder tumour staging: comparison of diffusion- and T2-weighted MR imaging. Eur Radiol 19(7):1575–1581

Franiel T, Stephan C, Erbersdobler A et al (2011) Areas suspicious for prostate cancer: MR-guided biopsy in patients with at least one transrectal US-guided biopsy with a negative finding – multiparametric MR imaging for detection and biopsy planning. Radiology 259:162–172

Gibbs P, Tozer DJ, Liney GP et al (2001) Comparison of quantitative T2 mapping and diffusion-weighted imaging in the normal and pathologic prostate. Magn Reson Med 46: 1054–1058

Gibbs P, Liney GP, Pickles MD et al (2009) Correlation of ADC and T2 measurements with cell density in prostate cancer at 3.0 Tesla. Invest Radiol 44:572–576

Giles SL, Morgan VA, Riches SF et al (2011) Apparent diffusion coefficient as a predictive biomarker of prostate cancer progression: value of fast and slow diffusion components. Am J Roentgenol 196(3):586–591

Gurses B, Tasdelen N, Yencilek F et al (2010) Diagnostic utility of DTI in prostate cancer. Eur J Radiol; [Epub ahead of print]

Haider MA, van der Kwast TH, Tanguay J et al (2007) Combined T2-weighted and diffusion-weighted MRI for localization of prostate cancer. Am J Roentgenol 189:323–328

Hambrock T, Somford DM, Huisman HJ et al (2011) Relationship between apparent diffusion coefficients at 3.0-T MR imaging and gleason grade in peripheral zone prostate cancer. Radiology; Mar 15, 2011 [Epub ahead of print]

Jacobs MA, Ouwerkerk R, Petrowski K et al (2008) Diffusion-weighted imaging with apparent diffusion coefficient mapping and spectroscopy in prostate cancer. Top Magn Reson Imaging 19:261–272

Kelloff GJ, Choyke P, Coffey DS (2009) Challenges in clinical prostate cancer: role of imaging. Am J Roentgenol 192: 1455–1470

Kiliçkesmez O, Cimilli T, Inci E et al (2009) Diffusion-weighted MRI of urinary bladder and prostate cancers. Diagn Interv Radiol 15(2):104–110

Kim CK, Park BK, Lee HM et al (2008) MRI techniques for prediction of local tumor progression after high-intensity focused ultrasonic ablation of prostate cancer. Am J Roentgenol 190(5):1180–1186

Kim CK, Park BK, Kim B (2010) Diffusion-weighted MRI at 3 T for the evaluation of prostate cancer. Am J Roentgenol 194(6):1461–1469

Kim JK, Jang YJ, Cho G (2009) Multidisciplinary functional MR imaging for prostate cancer. Korean J Radiol 10: 535–551

Kitajima K, Kaji Y, Kuroda K et al (2008) High b-value diffusion-weighted imaging in normal and malignant PZ tissue of the prostate: effect of signal-to-noise ratio. Magn Reson Med Sci 7:93–99

Kozlowski P, Chang SD, Meng R et al (2010) Combined prostate diffusion tensor imaging and dynamic contrast enhanced MRI at 3 T – quantitative correlation with biopsy. Magn Reson Imaging 28(5):621–628

Langer DL, van der Kwast TH, Evans AJ et al (2008) Intermixed normal tissue within prostate cancer: effect on MR imaging measurements of apparent diffusion coefficient and T2 – sparse versus dense cancers. Radiology 249(3):900–908

Langer DL, van der Kwast TH, Evans AJ et al (2009) Prostate cancer detection with multi-parametric MRI: logistic regression analysis of quantitative T2, diffusion-weighted imaging, and dynamic contrast-enhanced MRI. J Magn Reson Imaging 30:327–334

Lim HK, Kim JK, Kim KA et al (2009) Prostate cancer: apparent diffusion coefficient map with T2-weighted images for detection – a multireader study. Radiology 250:145–151

Mazaheri Y, Shukla-Dave A, Hricak H et al (2008) Prostate cancer: identification with combined diffusion-weighted MR imaging and 3D 1 H MR spectroscopic imaging – correlation with pathologic findings. Radiology 246:480–488

Mazaheri Y, Hricak H, Fine SW et al (2009) Prostate tumor volume measurement with combined T2-weighted imaging and diffusion-weighted MR: correlation with pathologic tumor volume. Radiology 252:449–457

Nakanishi K, Kobayashi M, Nakaguchi K et al (2007) Whole-body MRI for detecting metastatic bone tumor: diagnostic value of diffusion-weighted images. Magn Reson Med Sci 6(3):147–155

Nakayama T, Yoshimitsu K, Irie H et al (2004) Usefulness of the calculated apparent diffusion coefficient value in the differential diagnosis of retroperitoneal masses. J Magn Reson Imaging 20(4):735–742

Noworolski SM, Vigneron DB, Chen AP et al (2008) Dynamic contrast-enhanced MRI and MR diffusion imaging to distinguish between glandular and stromal prostatic tissues. Magn Reson Imaging 26(8):1071–1080

Oto A, Kayhan A, Jiang Y et al (2010) Prostate cancer: differentiation of central gland cancer from benign prostatic hyperplasia by using diffusion-weighted and dynamic contrast-enhanced MR imaging. Radiology 257(3):715–723

Park SY, Kim CK, Park BK et al (2010) Prediction of biochemical recurrence following radical prostatectomy in men with prostate cancer by diffusion-weighted magnetic resonance imaging: initial results. Eur Radiol; Nov 3, 2010 [Epub ahead of print]

Petralia G, Thoeny HC (2010) DW-MRI of the urogenital tract: applications in oncology. Cancer Imaging 10(Spec no A):S112–S123

Ravizzini G, Turkbey B, Kurdziel K et al (2009) New horizons in prostate cancer imaging. Eur J Radiol 70:212–226

Reischauer C, Wilm BJ, Froehlich JM et al (2010) High-resolution diffusion tensor imaging of prostate cancer using a reduced FOV technique. Eur J Radiol; Jul 15, 2010 [Epub ahead of print]

Ren J, Huan Y, Li F et al (2009) Combined T2-weighted and diffusion-weighted MRI for diagnosis of urinary bladder invasion in patients with prostate carcinoma. J Magn Reson Imaging 30:351–356

Ren J, Huan Y, Wang H et al (2009) Seminal vesicle invasion in prostate cancer: prediction with combined T2-weighted and diffusion-weighted MR imaging. Eur Radiol 19:2481–2486

Scherr MK, Seitz M, Müller-Lisse UG et al (2010) MR-perfusion (MRP) and diffusion-weighted imaging (DWI) in prostate cancer: quantitative and model-based gadobenate dimeglumine MRP parameters in detection of prostate cancer. Eur J Radiol 76(3):359–366

Seitz M, Shukla-Dave A, Bjartell A et al (2009) Functional magnetic resonance imaging in prostate cancer. Eur Urol 55(4):801–814

Somford DM, Futterer JJ, Hambrock T et al (2008) Diffusion and perfusion MR imaging of the prostate. Magn Reson Imaging Clin N Am 16:685–695, ix

Song I, Kim CK, Park BK et al (2010) Assessment of response to radiotherapy for prostate cancer: value of diffusion-weighted MRI at 3 T. Am J Roentgenol 194(6):477–482

Takayama Y, Kishimoto R, Hanaoka S et al (2008) ADC value and diffusion tensor imaging of prostate cancer: changes in carbon-ion radiotherapy. J Magn Reson Imaging 27:1331–1335

Takeuchi M, Sasaki S, Ito M et al (2009) Urinary bladder cancer: diffusion-weighted MR imaging – accuracy for diagnosing T stage and estimating histologic grade. Radiology 251(1): 112–121

Tamada T, Sone T, Jo Y et al (2008) Prostate cancer: relationships between postbiopsy hemorrhage and tumor detectability at MR diagnosis. Radiology 248(2):531–539

Tan CH, Wang J, Kundra V (2011) Diffusion weighted imaging in prostate cancer. Eur Radiol 21(3):593–603

Tanimoto A, Nakashima J, Kohno H et al (2007) Prostate cancer screening: the clinical value of diffusion-weighted imaging and dynamic MR imaging in combination with T2-weighted imaging. J Magn Reson Imaging 25:146–152

Thoeny HC, Triantafyllou M, Birkhaeuser FD et al (2009) Combined ultrasmall superparamagnetic particles of iron oxide-enhanced and diffusion-weighted magnetic resonance imaging reliably detect pelvic lymph node metastases in normal-sized nodes of bladder and prostate cancer patients. Eur Urol 55(4):761–769

van As NJ, de Souza NM, Riches SF et al (2009) A study of diffusion-weighted magnetic resonance imaging in men with untreated localised prostate cancer on active surveillance. Eur Urol 56(6):981–987

Verma S, Rajesh A, Morales H et al (2011) Assessment of aggressiveness of prostate cancer: correlation of apparent diffusion coefficient with histologic grade after radical prostatectomy. Am J Roentgenol 196(2):374–381

Wang H, Fei B (2010) Diffusion-weighted MRI for monitoring tumor response to photodynamic therapy. J Magn Reson Imaging 32(2):409–417

Watanabe H, Kanematsu M, Kondo H et al (2009) Preoperative T staging of urinary bladder cancer: does diffusion-weighted MRI have supplementary value? Am J Roentgenol 192(5):1361–1366

Yamamura J, Salomon G, Buchert R et al (2011) Magnetic resonance imaging of prostate cancer: diffusion-weighted imaging in comparison with sextant biopsy. J Comput Assist Tomogr 35(2):223–228

Yoshida S, Koga F, Kawakami S et al (2010) Initial experience of diffusion-weighted magnetic resonance imaging to assess therapeutic response to induction chemoradiotherapy against muscle-invasive bladder cancer. Urology 75(2):387–391

9 Use of DWI in Female Pelvis

German A. Castrillon, Stephan Anderson, Nagaraj Holalkere, and Jorge A. Soto

9.1 Introduction

Improvements in MR scanner hardware and the development of new imaging techniques, such as parallel imaging, and of novel methods for rapid data with minimal image degradation by artifacts acquisition (such as SS EPI sequences) have resulted in a significant improvement in image quality in body MR applications. Not surprisingly, investigators have explored the potential beneficial role of DWI in the evaluation of various diseases outside of the central nervous system. The pelvis is no exception. Multiple applications of DWI in the pelvis have been described, and some have demonstrated to be of considerable practical utility, such that they are now acquired routinely as part of the MR imaging protocol of specific subgroups of patients at many institutions. Other applications are still the focus of extensive research. In this chapter, we review the methods most commonly used for acquiring DWI of the female pelvis and discuss and illustrate with examples the most relevant clinical applications of this method in patients with various gynecologic diseases.

G.A. Castrillon
Department of Radiology,
University of Antioquia,
Medellin, Colombia

S. Anderson • N. Holalkere • J.A. Soto (✉)
Radiology Department,
Boston University School of Medicine,
Boston, MA, USA
e-mail: jorge.soto@bmc.org

9.2 Normal Appearance of Uterus and Cervix on DWI

The uterus is divided anatomically into corpus, isthmus, and cervix. In the corpus, the myometrium and endometrium are hyperintense on T2-weighted images and separated by the junctional zone, which is characteristically seen as a low-signal-intensity stripe located between the myometrium and the endometrium. It is hypothesized that the junctional zone corresponds to the inner myometrium. There are many theories to explain the low signal intensity of the junctional zone: The inner myometrium has lower concentration of water and the junctional zone is composed mainly of compact smooth muscle fiber and little extracellular matrix. Since DWI demonstrates the restriction of water diffusion, tissues with a high cellular density would show high signal intensity, especially on images acquired with higher *b* values. On DWI, the normal endometrium has the highest signal intensity in the uterus, the cervix has higher signal intensity than the myometrium, and the junctional zone has the lowest signal intensity. On the ADC maps, the cervix shows a significantly higher value than cervical carcinoma. The ADC values of normal endometrial tissue are higher than the ADC values of endometrial carcinoma. Endometrial polyps show almost the same signal intensity as the normal endometrial tissue. When the junctional zone is affected by adenomyosis, the ADC values are significantly higher than those of the normal junctional zone and lower than those of normal myometrium. The normal myometrial tissue shows higher mean ADC values than leiomyomas; however, the cause of this lower ADC value in leiomyomas remains unknown.

A. Luna et al., *Diffusion MRI Outside the Brain*,
DOI 10.1007/978-3-642-21052-5_9, © Springer-Verlag Berlin Heidelberg 2012

9.3 Clinical Applications

9.3.1 Cervical Carcinoma

Cervical carcinoma is the second most common female malignancy and has a high mortality rate. It occurs predominantly in middle age women. Due to its superior tissue contrast resolution, MR has gained acceptance as the most effective imaging modality for detecting and staging cervical carcinoma, as well as for establishing a therapeutic strategy. In addition to T1- and T2- weighted sequences in multiple planes, other techniques are used to extract metabolic and physiological information. Studies have found that the mean ADC values can be used to differentiate between normal and cancerous tissues in the uterine cervix, with little overlap. Squamous cell carcinoma tends to have lower ADC values than adenocarcinoma and normal tissue has higher ADC values than both primary malignancies: cervical carcinoma $0.88–1.11 \times 10–3$ mm^2/s vs. normal tissue $1.5–1.8 \times 10–3$ mm^2/s, according to several series. ADC values can also provide information about the histology of the tumor. Tumors with higher cellular density and higher histologic grade show a tendency toward lower ADC values compared with those of tumors with lower histologic grade and lower cellular density, which have higher ADC values. Even in cases of stage 1 cervical cancer, DWI has demonstrated a significant difference in ADC values between well/moderately and poorly differentiated tumors. This suggests that DWI and ADC values of uterine cervical cancer may indirectly characterize the cellular density of the tumor.

According to several investigators, the ADC values in uterine cervical cancer increase after chemotherapy and/or radiation therapy and, therefore, following the ADC values through the course of treatment may add to the value of MRI for monitoring response to therapy (Fig. 9.1). After chemotherapy, ADC values increase as a result of cellular apoptosis, which occurs earlier than changes in tumoral perfusion, that can be assessed by means of dynamic contrast MRI. ADC may also increase soon after radiotherapy as a consequence of hyperemia. After therapy, the treated cervical area shows lower values than normal nontreated cervical tissue. Furthermore, these ADC values could be useful in the delineation of tumor boundaries and in providing information for planning therapy and determining the eligibility for surgical resection. DWI and ADC quantifications have also demonstrated to be an early (2 weeks to 1 month after the beginning of therapy) and reproducible response indicator in advanced cervical cancer treated with chemoradiation. In a series by Liu et al., ADCs after 15 days of treatment increased significantly compared to pretreatment ones, without significant changes in tumor size. The percentage of ADC change after 1 month of chemoradiation correlated positively with percentage size reduction after 2 months of therapy. In patients with squamous cell carcinoma, Mc Veigh et al. found a difference in the ADC values between responders and non-responders to chemoradiation therapy. The ADC values were lower in responders than non-responders ($p < 0.05$). However, this evidence must be considered preliminary at this point in time. Long-term studies are necessary to determine the true clinical utility.

DWI increases the conspicuity of pelvic nodes, as high-intensity lesions against a suppressed background. This is of special interest in lymph nodes adjacent to structures such as vessels or small bowel loops. Besides, DWI has recently demonstrated its capacity to distinguish between metastatic and hyperplastic lymph nodes using ADC quantifications, with significant lower ADC values for metastatic lymph nodes. Furthermore, the signal intensity of malignant lymph nodes is often comparable to that of the primary tumor or other metastatic sites on high-*b*-value images.

9.3.2 Endometrial Cancer

Endometrial carcinoma is the most common uterine malignancy in developed countries, and occurs mainly in postmenopausal women. Various factors influence the prognosis of endometrial cancer, including the histological subtype and grade and the tumor stage, especially the presence and depth of myometrial invasion. MRI is an excellent modality to determine the local stage of endometrial carcinoma, including presence of myometrial and cervical invasion. Usually, the endometrial tumor is demonstrated as a thickened endometrium on T2-weighted images. However, the signal intensity of the tumor itself is variable and, therefore, it may be difficult to differentiate from normal endometrium and adjacent myometrium. Consequently, the qualitative assessment of endometrial cancer vs. the normal endometrium on the basis of signal intensity on T2-weighted images alone is subjective and can be influenced by adjustment of the window level and width. Dynamic contrast-enhanced sequences are usually necessary for proper evaluation of endometrial carcinoma with MR, as the diagnostic accuracy is higher than that of T2-weighted images alone.

Data are accumulating to support the use of DWI as a tool to detect endometrial carcinoma and to differentiate benign from malignant lesions (Fig. 9.2). Tamai et al. found an increased signal intensity on DWI acquired with *b* values of 1,000 s/mm^2 of all endometrial carcinoma compared to normal endometrium. However, it is difficult to differentiate between normal and cancerous tissue based solely on the signal intensity on DWI. For this reason, the quantitative evaluation provided by the ADC values calculated from diffusion-weighted images is very useful. Several studies have demonstrated that the ADC values of endometrial carcinoma are lower than the ADC values of endometrial polyps, submucosal leiomyomas, and normal endometrial tissue. Causes of false-positive cases on DWI are secretory and hyperplastic endometrium. False-negative findings are most commonly caused by well-differentiated adenocarcinomas with low cellularity and necrotic poorly differentiated tumors, since necrosis associated with poor differentiation increases the ADC values. Recently, in a series by Wang et al., DWI at a 3 T magnet demonstrated the potential to quantitatively differentiate stage IA endometrial carcinoma from normal endometrium and benign diseases of the endometrium, without any overlap in ADC values.

The prognosis of endometrial cancer (as assessed by 5-year survival rates) varies with the histological tumor grade and the depth of myometrial invasion, which also correlate strongly with the risk of lymph node metastases. Investigators have attempted to correlate histological tumor grade with measured ADC values and found higher ADC values in lower grade cancers and decreased ADC values in higher grade cancers. However, there is considerable overlap, which currently limits a precise estimation of histological grade based on ADC values alone. Dynamic contrast-enhanced fat-suppressed GE T1-weighted images have traditionally been used to determine the depth of myometrial invasion on MR images, especially in postmenopausal women or in patients with a thinned endometrium. These dynamic sequences are helpful for showing the hypovascular tumor in a background of hypervascular myometrium. Unfortunately, some tumors are either iso- or hypervascular relative to the hypervascular myometrium. Appearance on DWI is independent of differences in vascularity. Hyperintensity of tumors on DWI improves the visualization of depth of tumor invasion (Fig. 9.3). Inada et al. showed an improved performance for establishing the depth of myometrial invasion when findings on T2-weighted and DWI were combined. Furthermore, Takeuchi and colleagues demonstrated a better performance of DWI than gadolinium-enhanced T1-weighted images in the assessment of myometrial invasion by endometrial cancer. Contrarily, Shen et al. found postcontrast T1-weighted images superior to DWI in the same task.

9.3.3 Myometrium

The value of MRI for evaluating uterine diseases such as fibroids and adenomyosis is well established. This is derived from the excellent tissue contrast that allows differentiation of normal from diseased myometrium. DWI may be an additional tool to characterize uterine lesions such as adenomyosis (Fig. 9.4) or leiomyomas. The ADC values of leiomyomas are lower than those of normal myometrial tissue. However, the cause of these decreased ADC values in this lesion is unknown. Ordinary leiomyomas tend to contain hyalinized collagen and this may explain in part the low signal intensity of ordinary leiomyomas on DWI. Another explanation is the "T2 blackout effect," in which the low signal on DWI is caused by a low signal on T2-weighted images (Figs. 3.2 and 9.5). Since DWI images are inherently T2-weighted, changes in tissue T2 relaxation properties can influence the appearance on DWI, independently of tissue diffusibility.

Tamai et al. found that the ADC values were useful for differentiation of degenerated leiomyomas and normal myometrium from the rare malignant uterine sarcomas. However, there was overlap in the low ADC values of sarcomas, ordinary leiomyomas, and cellular leiomyomas. In this circumstance, ADC value measurements have a limited clinical role. In that same study, all but one uterine sarcoma exhibited high signal intensity on DWI. According to these results, the authors suggest that all hyperintense myometrial tumors on DWI must be evaluated further for any findings suggestive of malignancy, such as the presence of intratumoral necrosis or signs of an infiltrative nature of the lesion. Similar results were obtained by Namimotoa and colleagues using a 3 T magnet, although a combination of ADC and the tumor-myometrium contrast ratio on T2-weighted sequence achieved a 100% in sensitivity and specificity in the distinction between uterine sarcomas and benign leiomyomas, without any overlap. However, Takeuchi et al. showed a significant difference in the ADC values of uterine sarcomas and benign leiomyomas. Furthermore, cellular leiomyomas demonstrated significantly lower ADC values than degenerated leiomyomas.

DWI has also showed its potential as an adjunct for assessing treatment of uterine fibroids. Although, changes in ADC values following tumor embolization are often not seen until several days after treatment, treated lesions demonstrate lower ADC values than untreated ones, and myometrial ADC values do not significantly change after therapy. DWI has also demonstrated a heterogeneous increase in signal intensity in treated fibroid regions using MRI-guided, high-intensity focused ultrasound surgery (HIFU).

9.3.4 Characterization of Ovarian Masses

The use of DWI in ovarian tumors has not been studied thoroughly. There are only a few reports describing the clinical utility of DWI for characterization of ovarian tumors as benign or malignant, but results are conflicting and the technique is not universally accepted for this clinical application. Although ovarian masses with low intensity on DWI and high ADC values suggest a benign lesion, it is difficult to differentiate benign and malignant lesion only on the basis of DWI. The ADC values of malignant ovarian tumors vary widely, a phenomenon that is attributable to their heterogeneous histology and morphology. Endometriomas (Figs. 4.8 and 9.6), thecomas (Fig. 9.7), and malignant cystic ovarian tumors exhibit lower ADC values than other benign, non-hemorrhagic, ovarian cysts and benign cystic tumors.

The ADC values calculated from the DWI may add useful information to the differential diagnosis of ovarian cystic masses in limited populations, such as those with mature cystic teratomas with a small amount of fat (Fig. 9.8). Detecting the keratinoid substance by means of DWI and the calculated ADC values may be useful and serve as an adjunctive tool to ensure the accuracy of the diagnosis, particularly in patients with "fat-poor" (or "fat-less") mature cystic teratomas. Currently, there is only weak evidence to suggest a utility of DWI and ADC for evaluation of solid ovarian tumors (Fig. 9.9).

9.3.5 Assessment of Peritoneal Spread of Ovarian Carcinoma

Morphological CT and MRI perform in a limited manner to detect malignant peritoneal metastasis, mainly when the size of the deposits is less than 1 cm. DWI has demonstrated high sensitivity in the detection of these small deposits due to high CNR, even in challenging anatomical areas such as right subdiaphragmatic space, omentum, root of the mesentery, and serosal surface of the small bowel (Figs. 11.10). Preliminary results have demonstrated lower ADC values for peritoneal deposits than in primary ovarian tumors and omental cake, reflecting the heterogeneous diffusivity according to the anatomical site and biological properties of disease.

9.3.6 Vagina and Vulva

Although to our knowledge, there is no reported series evaluating the value of DWI in vulvar and vaginal pathology, its role may be similar to that described for endometrial and cervical cancer (Fig. 9.10).

Case 9.1: Residual Cervical Carcinoma

A 36-year-old female patient with diagnosis of cervical adenosquamous carcinoma, currently undergoing chemotherapy and radiation therapy. MRI and PET/CT of the pelvis were performed for surveillance following therapy.

Comments

Cervical carcinoma is the second most common malignancy in women, and is an important cause of morbidity and mortality. Accurate staging and follow-up of the tumor are essential for optimal treatment planning. Cervical carcinoma is staged by clinical examination according to system proposed by the International Federation of Gynecology and Obstetrics (FIGO). However, clinical staging has inherent limitations in evaluating several parameters that are critical for treatment planning. Nowadays, MRI has an important role to play in staging and following these tumors. MRI can provide objective measurements of tumor size with a high negative predictive value for determining presence of parametrial invasion and stage IVA disease. Additionally, MRI and PET/CT play key roles in identifying recurrent disease.

PET/CT is also useful in detecting nodal and distant metastases and in helping to properly plan radiation therapy. The use of FDG-PET is now well established in cervical cancer since most cervical tumors are FDG-avid. Adenocarcinomas, which usually have a low FDG uptake, are an exception. FDG-PET/CT can be used at the time of presentation for staging and to monitor response, to detect recurrence, and to plan radiotherapy. However, FDG is not entirely specific for malignancy, and there are a number of pitfalls when using this radiotracer.

Proper technique and adequate patient preparation are critical to ensure obtaining high-quality diagnostic images with MR. The patient should fast for at least 4 h prior to the study in order to limit artifacts arising from small bowel peristalsis. An antiperistaltic agent should be administered to the patient to further reduce peristalsis. It helps if the bladder is partially full at the time of the scan. Patients are imaged in the supine position using a surface phased-array coil. This provides higher signal-to-noise ratio, with increased spatial resolution and reduced imaging time. The initial image is acquired before contrast, with subsequent dynamic images after contrast administration. Small tumors enhance avidly in the early dynamic phase, compared with the mild enhancement of the cervical epithelium and stroma. This may help in distinguishing recurrent tumors from radiation fibrosis. T2-weighted images in the axial, sagittal, and oblique coronal planes are useful to determine tumor size, presence of lymphadenopathy, involvement of the pelvic sidewall, and parametrial invasion.

DWI is an emerging imaging technique that is being evaluated for the detection of primary tumor and recurrent disease and in the assessment of treatment response. DWI, which is now readily used in the pelvis, achieves high image contrast by evaluating the random motion of water molecules within tissues. It yields information on tissue cellularity, microcirculation, and cell membrane integrity. DWI appears to be of value in both identifying and in characterizing abnormal tissue. The images generated should be looked at in conjunction with ADC maps and the T2-weighted images. DWI requires only short scan times and intravenous contrast is not necessary. Although, there is scarce experience, DWI may be helpful in detection of residual tumor or suspicious lymph nodes after chemoradiotherapy, and might be competitive with PET, as reflected in the 2010 guidelines for staging of uterine cervical cancer with MRI of the European Society of Urogenital Radiology (ESUR)

Imaging Findings

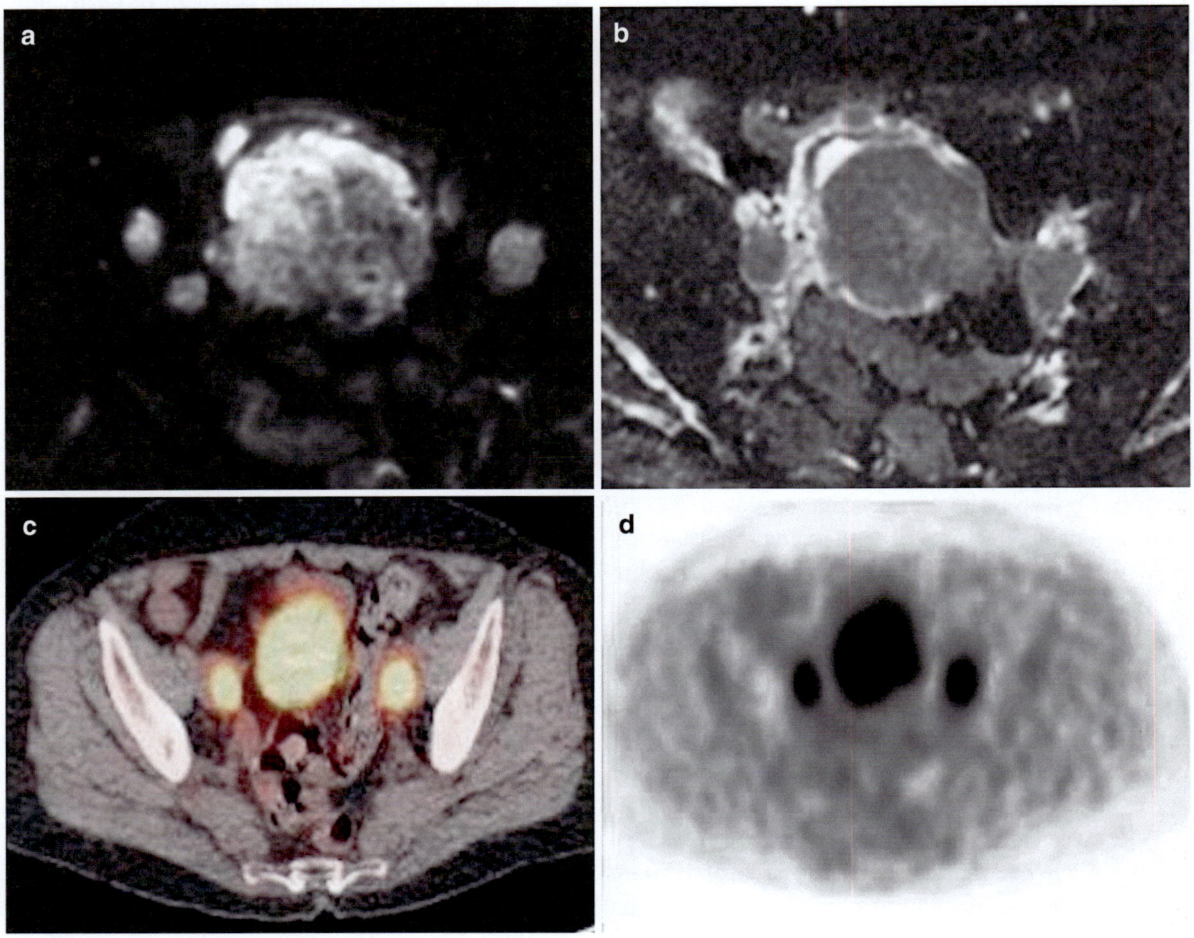

Fig. 9.1 (**a**) DWI acquired with a *b* factor of 800 s/mm^2 demonstrates a large cervical mass and enlarged iliac nodes with high signal intensity. (**b**) ADC map at the same level of A shows the mass and nodes with low signal intensity, indicating restricted diffusion. PET-CT (**c**) and PET (**d**) images demonstrate the mass and iliac nodes with tumoral hypermetabolism, which is typical of cervical malignancies

Case 9.2: Characterization of Endometrial Adenocarcinoma

A 59-year-old female with new onset of vaginal bleeding. Transvaginal ultrasound (not shown) demonstrated an enlarged uterus and a possible mass. MRI of the pelvis was performed for further characterization of the mass.

Comments

Endometrial carcinoma is the fourth most common cancer in women and the most common malignancy of the female reproductive tract. Five-year survival rates vary between 96% for stage I disease and 26% for stage IV disease. The disease occurs most frequently in white women, with a peak incidence between ages 55 and 65, and usually presents clinically as postmenopausal bleeding. Risk factors include unopposed estrogen intake, nulliparity, obesity, diabetes, and polycystic ovary syndrome. The prognosis of endometrial carcinoma depends on a number of factors, including stage, depth of myometrial invasion, lymphovascular invasion, nodal status, and histological grade. Determination of the depth of myometrial invasion is important, since it correlates with the incidence of lymph node metastases. Preoperative evaluation of prognostic factors helps in decision making and treatment planning. Endometrial cancer primarily presents at stage I (80% of cases), and the standard treatment is total abdominal hysterectomy and bilateral salpingo-oophorectomy.

Endometrial carcinomas are usually diagnosed at endometrial biopsy or dilatation and curettage, with imaging being reserved to determine extent of disease. Dynamic contrast-enhanced MRI offers a "one-stop" examination, with the highest efficacy for pretreatment evaluation in patients with endometrial cancer. On unenhanced T1-weighted images, endometrial carcinoma is isointense with the normal endometrium. Although endometrial cancer may demonstrate high signal intensity on T2-weighted sequences, it is more typically heterogeneous, and may even be of low signal intensity. Routine use of dynamic intravenous contrast enhancement is necessary for evaluation of endometrial carcinoma. Following intravenous contrast administration, there is early enhancement of endometrial cancer relative to the normal endometrium, allowing identification of small tumors, even those contained within the endometrium. In the later phases of enhancement, i.e., equilibrium phase, the tumor appears hypointense relative to the myometrium. MRI is significantly superior to CT and US in the evaluation of both tumor extension into the cervix and myometrial invasion. The overall staging accuracy of MRI has been reported to be between 85% and 93%.

Results of recent publications support the use of DWI in the detection of endometrial carcinoma. Endometrial cancer shows high signal intensity on DWI and low signal intensity on the ADC maps. In the example illustrated in the figure, DWI clearly established the malignant nature of the uterine tumor mass and, more importantly, demonstrated restricted diffusion in the iliac lymph nodes, which were proven to be involved with tumor.

Imaging Findings

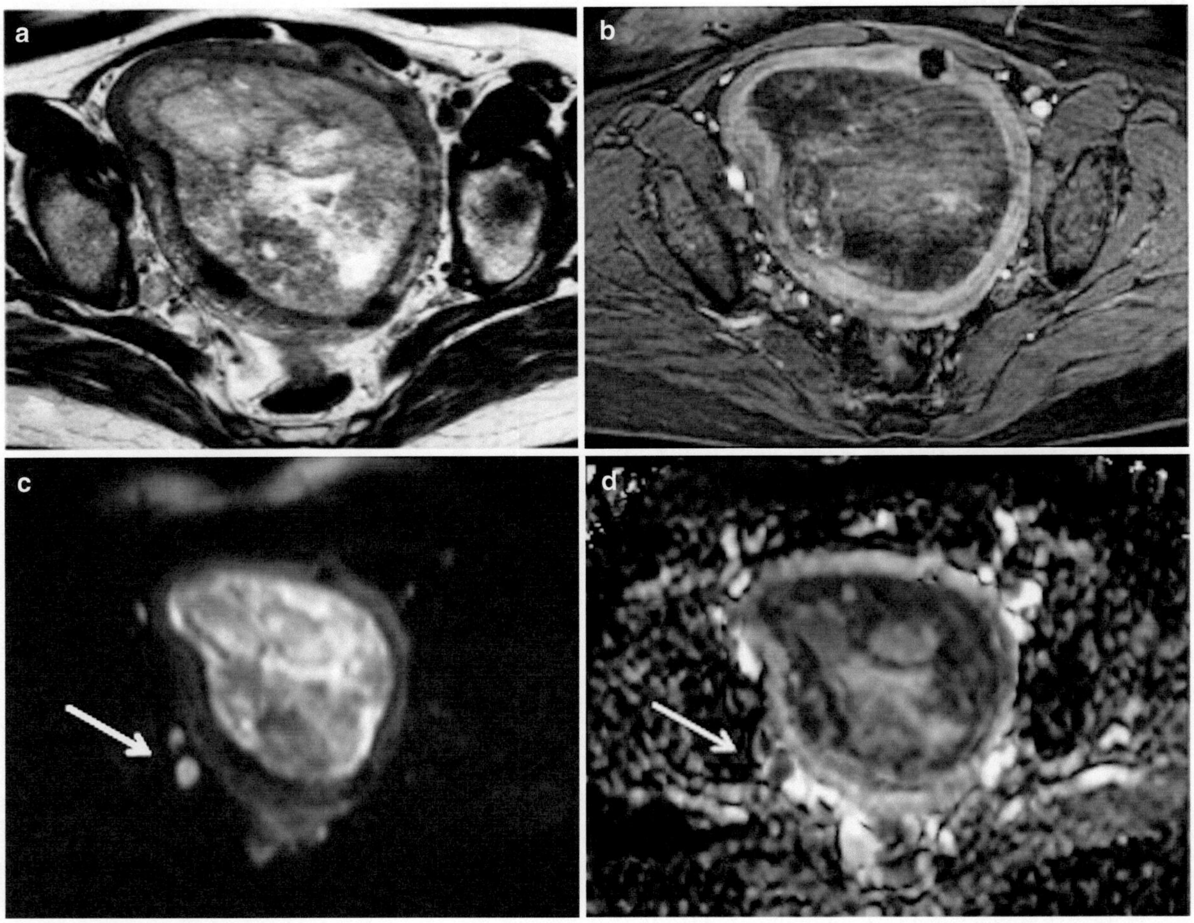

Fig. 9.2 (**a**) Axial FSE T2-weighted image shows a mass with heterogeneous signal intensity (but predominantly hyperintense) filling and expanding the endometrial cavity, as well as two enlarged internal iliac lymph nodes. (**b**) Contrast-enhanced axial T1-weighted GE image with fat suppression shows heterogeneous enhancement of the mass. (**c**, **d**), DWI with *b* factor of 800 s/mm^2 (**c**) and ADC map (**d**) images show predominantly high-signal-intensity mass in the endometrial cavity and the enlarged internal iliac nodes (*arrows*) and low signal intensity in the ADC map (**d**). This indicates that there is restricted diffusion in the endometrial mass, which was subsequently proven to be a stage IIIC carcinoma, with nodal involvement

Case 9.3: Early Endometrial Adenocarcinoma

A 50-year-old postmenopausal female with vaginal bleeding. Transvaginal ultrasound (not shown) was unremarkable. Curettage and biopsy showed endometrial adenocarcinoma. MRI of the pelvis was indicated to stage the carcinoma.

Comments

Imaging criteria for staging of endometrial cancer are based on the TNM/FIGO classification. MRI is superior to ultrasound (US) and CT in the evaluation of both tumor extension into the cervix and myometrial invasion. The overall staging accuracy of MRI has been reported to vary between 85% and 93%.

Stage I endometrial cancers include tumors confined to the corpus. Stage IA tumors (limited to endometrium) appear as a normal or widened (focal or diffuse) endometrium. An intact junctional zone and a smooth band of early subendometrial enhancement exclude deep myometrial invasion. Regardless of the pulse sequence, the tumor–myometrium interface is smooth and sharp. In stage IB disease, the tumor extends less than 50% into the myometrium, with associated disruption or irregularity of the junctional zone and abnormal subendometrial enhancement. Stage IB tumor is suggested by an irregular tumor–myometrium interface. Presence of low-signal-intensity tumor within the outer myometrium or beyond indicates deep myometrial invasion (a finding of stage IC disease). Erroneous MRI assessment of the depth of myometrial invasion may occur if there is a large polypoid endometrial carcinoma, which distends the uterus so that the thin rim of myometrium is stretched over it rather than deeply infiltrated. Other causes of inaccuracies include the presence of leiomyomas, congenital anomalies, and indistinct zonal anatomy (e.g., in the presence of adenomyosis). Stage II includes tumors that extend beyond the uterine corpus into the cervix. In stage IIA, invasion of the endocervix appears as widening of the internal os and endocervical canal with preservation of the normal low-signal-intensity fibrocervical stroma on T2-weighted images. Findings of stage IIB include disruption of the fibrocervical stroma by high-signal-intensity tumor on T2-weighted images along with interruption of normal enhancement of the cervical mucosa by low-signal-intensity tumor on late dynamic contrast-enhanced images. In Stage III disease, the tumor extends beyond the uterus but remains confined within the true pelvis. In stage IIIA, there is parametrial involvement, which appears as disruption of the serosa with direct extension into the surrounding parametrial fat. In stage IIIB disease, the tumor extends into the upper vagina, and there is segmental loss of the low-signal-intensity vaginal wall. Presence of lymphadenopathy is an indication of stage IIIC disease. Stage IV disease exists when tumor extends beyond the true pelvis or invades the bladder or rectum. Loss of low signal intensity of the bladder or rectal wall indicates stage IVA disease. In stage IVB disease, distant metastases, malignant ascites, or peritoneal carcinomatosis is present.

The prognosis of endometrial cancer varies with the histological tumor grade and the depth of myometrial invasion, which correlate strongly with the risk of lymph node metastases. Investigators have attempted to correlate histological tumor grade with measured ADC values and found higher ADC values in lower grade cancers and decreased ADC values in higher grade cancers. However, there is considerable overlap, which currently limits a precise estimation of histological grade based on ADC values alone. Hyperintensity of tumors on DWI improves the visualization of depth of tumor invasion especially when the evaluation is combined with the T2-weighted images. In this case, the DWI was important to detect and stage the endometrial carcinoma.

Imaging Findings

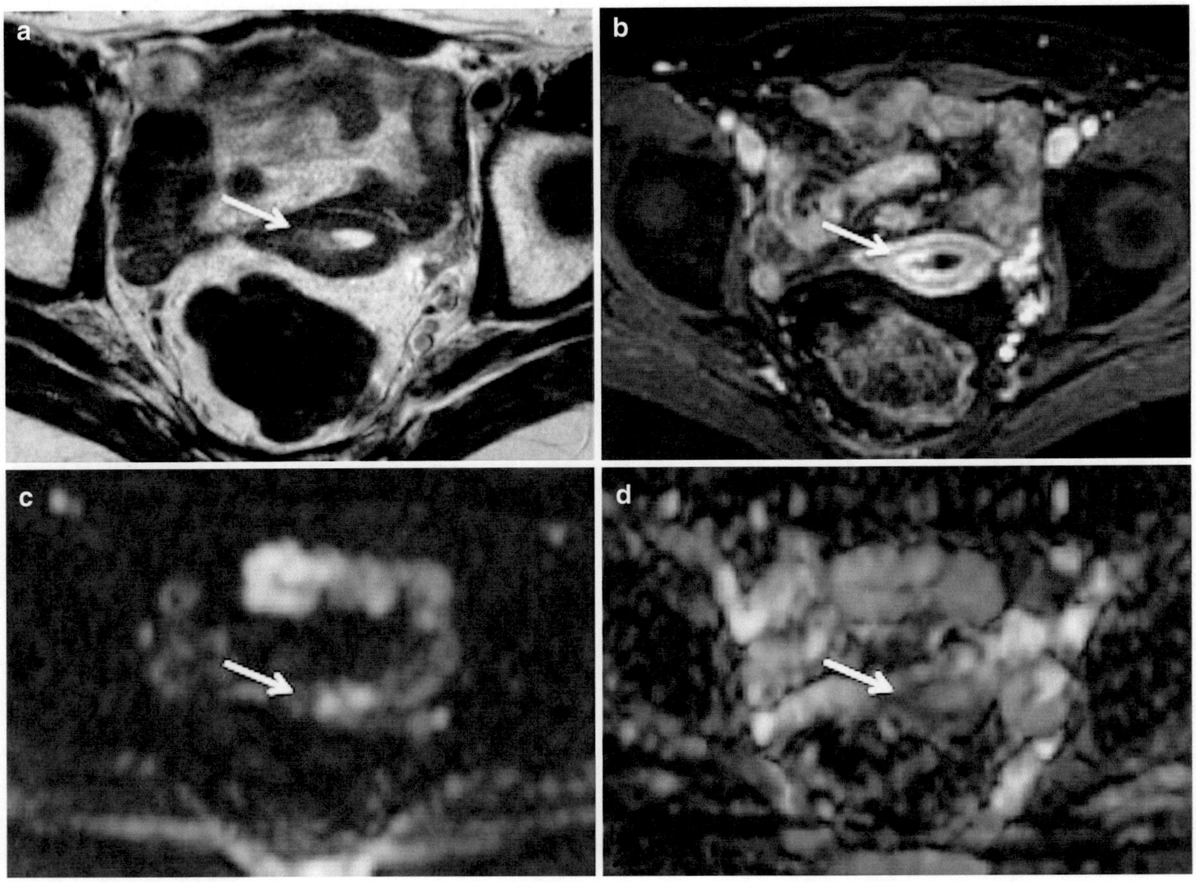

Fig. 9.3 (**a**) Axial FSE T2-weighted image shows a subtle high signal intensity focus in the endometrium (*arrow*), with loss of the junctional zone. (**b**) Axial contrast-enhanced T1-weighted GE image with fat saturation shows a small area of irregular subendometrial hyperenhancement (*arrow*). (**c**, **d**) DWI with *b* factor of 800 s/mm^2 shows a corresponding area of high signal intensity in the endometrium (**c**) with low signal intensity in the ADC map (**d**). There was no evidence of extra-uterine spread in the MR examination. At hysterectomy and histopathological examination, the tumor was determined to be a stage IB

Case 9.4: Adenomyosis

A 32-year-old patient who presents with pelvic pain, abnormal uterine bleeding, dysmenorrhea, menorrhagia, and dyspareunia. Transvaginal sonography (not shown) demonstrated an enlarged uterus with a heterogeneous myometrium.

Comments

Adenomyosis is a common gynecologic condition that affects menstruating women. The diagnosis based on clinical findings alone is difficult due to the fact that symptoms are usually nonspecific and often there are other, coexisting, diseases. Adenomyosis is a non-neoplastic condition, characterized pathologically by benign invasion of ectopic endometrium into the myometrium, with adjacent smooth muscle hyperplasia.

Trans-abdominal or transvaginal ultrasonography is commonly used as the initial imaging modality in patients with symptoms referable to the gynecologic tract. Unfortunately, sonography does not usually allow a reliable diagnosis of adenomyosis or consistent differentiation from leiomyomas because of its limited spatial and contrast resolution. MR imaging is the most accurate noninvasive modality for diagnosing adenomyosis and is more helpful than sonography in distinguishing adenomyosis from leiomyomas, which is perhaps the most clinically important distinction.

Nowadays, the diagnosis is based on high-resolution imaging techniques, especially MRI. MRI is an accurate, noninvasive modality for diagnosing adenomyosis with a high sensitivity (78–88%) and specificity (67–93%). MR is also more helpful than sonography for delineating the location and extent of adenomyosis and in monitoring the evolution of disease in patients receiving hormonal therapy. Adenomyosis appears as either diffuse or focal thickening of the junctional zone, forming ill-defined areas of low signal intensity, occasionally with embedded bright foci on T2-weighted images. Histologically, the areas of low signal intensity correspond to smooth muscle hyperplasia, and the bright foci on T2-weighted images correspond to islands of ectopic endometrial tissue and cystic dilatation of glands. As illustrated with this case, the ectopic endometrial tissue can be associated with restricted diffusion on DWI. This helps to confirm the diagnosis in questionable or difficult cases.

Imaging Findings

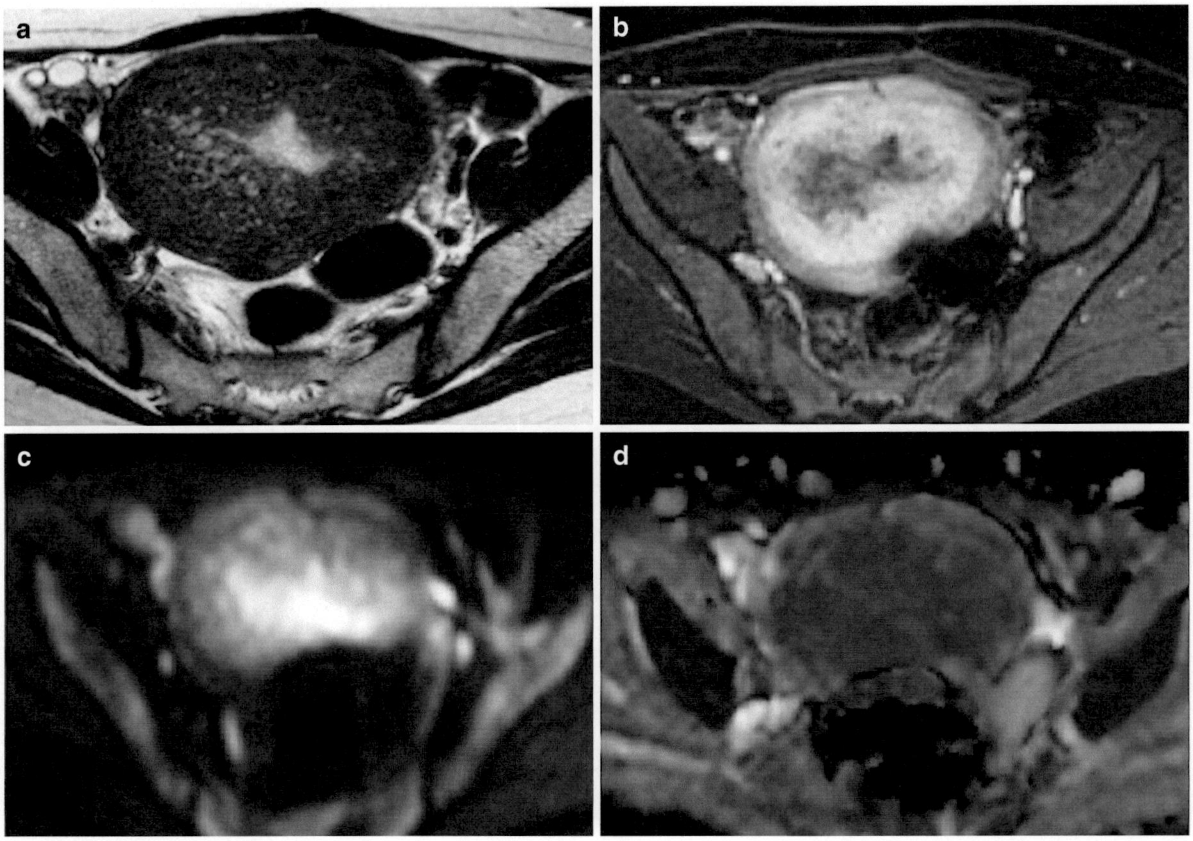

Fig. 9.4 (**a**) Axial FSE T2-weighted image shows a markedly enlarged uterus with a markedly thickened junctional zone and multiple foci of high signal intensity within the deep myometrium. (**b**) Axial contrast-enhanced T1-weighted GE image acquired with fat suppression shows diffuse hyperenhancement of the deep myometrium. (**c**, **d**) DWI acquired with a *b* factor of 800 s/mm^2 (**c**) and corresponding ADC map image (**d**) show scattered foci of high signal intensity in the deep myometrium in the DWI (**c**) and corresponding low signal intensity in the ADC map (**d**), an indication of restricted diffusion

Case 9.5: Uterine Leiomyoma

A 40-year-old patient who presents with increased urinary frequency, thought to be secondary to bladder compression. A large palpable pelvic mass was found on physical examination.

Comments

Leiomyomas (fibroids) are the most common uterine neoplasm and are composed of smooth muscle with varying amounts of fibrous connective tissue. As they enlarge, fibroids may outgrow their blood supply, resulting in various types of degeneration: hyaline or myxoid degeneration, calcification, cystic degeneration, and hemorrhagic ("red") degeneration. Leiomyomas are classified as submucosal, intramural, or subserosal; the latter may be pedunculated and simulate ovarian neoplasms. Although most leiomyomas are asymptomatic, patients may present with abnormal uterine bleeding, pressure on adjacent organs, pain, infertility, or a palpable abdomino-pelvic mass. Histopathologically, leiomyomas are benign tumors composed predominantly of smooth muscle cells separated by variable amounts of fibrous connective tissue. Although there is no true capsule, these tumors are well circumscribed and surrounded by a pseudocapsule. The size of uterine leiomyomas is variable, ranging from microscopic to large tumors that fill the abdomen. Leiomyomas may be single or, more frequently, multiple.

MRI is the most accurate imaging technique for detection and localization of leiomyomas. On T2-weighted images, nondegenerated leiomyomas appear as well-circumscribed masses of decreased signal intensity; however, cellular leiomyomas can have relatively higher signal intensity on T2-weighted images and demonstrate enhancement on contrast material–enhanced images. Degenerated leiomyomas have variable appearances on T2-weighted and contrast-enhanced images. The differential diagnosis of leiomyomas includes adenomyosis, solid adnexal mass, focal myometrial contraction, and uterine leiomyosarcoma. For patients with symptoms, medical or surgical treatment may be indicated. MRI also has a role in treatment of leiomyomas by assisting in surgical planning and monitoring the response to medical therapy. DWI has emerged as a tool which allows characterization and differentiation of various uterine lesions. Leiomyomas show low signal intensity o DW images and demonstrate lower ADC values than those of normal myometrial tissue. This is likely explained by the higher content of hyalinized tissue in leiomyomas, as illustrated by the example shown in this particular case.

DWI with ADC values has demonstrated utility for differentiation of degenerated leiomyomas from the rare malignant uterine sarcomas. All hyperintense myometrial tumors on DW images must be evaluated further for any findings suggestive of malignancy, such as the presence of intratumoral necrosis or signs of an infiltrative nature of the lesion.

Imaging Findings

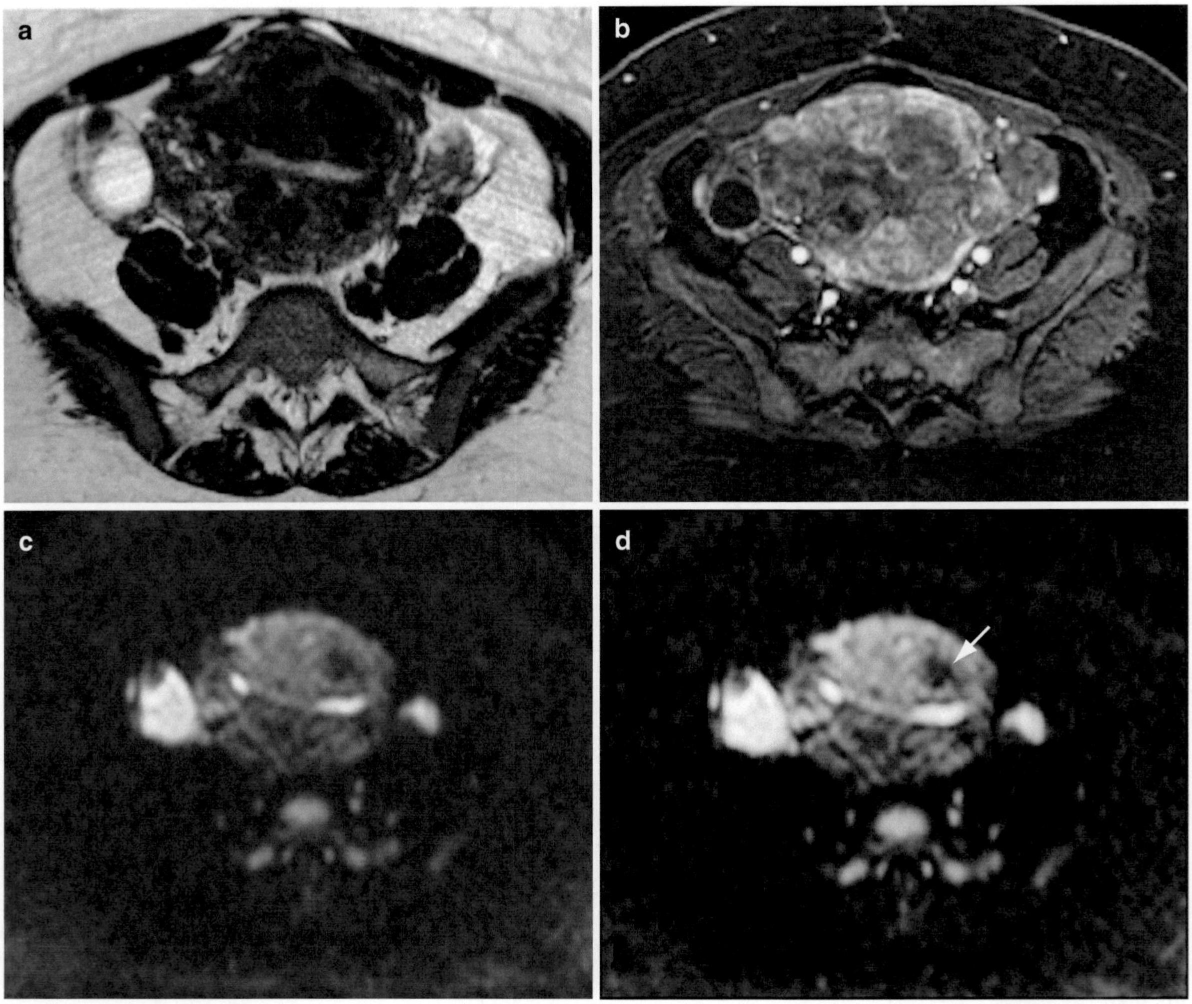

Fig. 9.5 (**a**) Axial FSE T2-weighted image shows intramural round masses with low signal intensity and a small right ovarian simple cyst. (**b**) Contrast-enhanced axial GE T1-weighted image with fat suppression shows heterogeneous enhancement of the myometrial masses. (**c**, **d**) DWI acquired with *b* factors of 500 and 800 s/mm^2, respectively, show the low signal intensity in the masses (**d**, *arrow*), as shown on the T2-weighted sequence as well. This is the "T2 blackout" effect

Case 9.6: Adnexal Endometrioma

A 28-year-old patient with pelvic pain, dysmenorrhea, dyspareunia, and back pain. Transvaginal US (not shown) demonstrated a cystic mass with low-level internal echoes adjacent to the right ovary; the MRI examination was performed to further characterize the mass.

Comments

Endometriosis is defined as the presence of functional endometrial glands and stroma outside the uterine cavity (ectopic as opposed to normally located). In older literature, endometriosis was classified as endometriosis interna and endometriosis externa. Endometriosis interna referred to endometrial tissue within the uterine musculature, and endometriosis externa referred to endometrial tissue in all other sites. Currently, the term "adenomyosis" has replaced endometriosis interna. Adenomyosis is considered a distinct and different clinical entity because its pathogenesis, symptoms, and epidemiology differ from those of endometriosis externa which nowadays is only known as endometriosis.

Endometriosis is a common and important clinical problem in women, predominantly those in the reproductive age group. At pathological analysis, the disease can vary from microscopic foci to large, grossly visible endometriotic cysts (endometriomas). Endometriosis is found predominantly in women of childbearing age. The mean age at diagnosis is 25–29 years, but women who present with infertility and pelvic pain are often older. Endometriosis is not uncommon among adolescents. About 5% of endometriosis cases are seen in postmenopausal women, and exogenous estrogen replacement therapy is suggested to play a role. Radiologists are involved in the diagnosis of the disease in two ways: They are asked to exclude endometriosis in a woman with pelvic pain or infertility or when clinicians are considering endometriomas in the differential diagnosis of an adnexal mass.

Laparoscopy is the standard of reference for the diagnosis of endometriosis. Although histologic analysis of biopsy specimens to confirm the diagnosis is desirable, it is not always necessary. Staging of the disease can also be done at laparoscopy. Endometriotic implants, endometriomas, and adhesions are the typical findings. Implants may measure from a few millimeters to a few centimeters and may be superficial or deep. The confident US differentiation of endometriotic cyst from other adnexal masses may be difficult at times. MRI has been shown to have greater specificity for the diagnosis of endometriomas than other noninvasive imaging techniques. Therefore, MR imaging can be a helpful adjunct for evaluation of adnexal masses. Endometriomas have a relatively homogeneous high signal intensity (similar to or greater than that of fat) on T1-weighted images and are better depicted with fat saturation sequences. Administration of gadolinium is not mandatory for the diagnosis of endometriomas. When used, the cyst wall demonstrates a nonspecific, variable enhancement pattern that does not differentiate it from other benign and malignant processes. Use of gadolinium should be reserved for those cases in which there is a genuine concern for ovarian carcinoma.

The most problematic lesions to differentiate from endometriomas are hemorrhagic corpus luteum cysts, which can have a near-identical MRI appearance. Hemorrhagic cysts are usually unilocular, as opposed to endometriomas, which are frequently multilocular and bilateral. In addition, hemorrhagic cysts do not exhibit "shading" (i.e., dependent loss of signal within the lesion on T2-weighted images) and usually resolve over time. A follow-up examination (which can be done with US) can help establish the diagnosis.

The use of DWI in the characterization of ovarian masses has not been well studied. There are only a few reports describing the clinical utility of DWI for characterization of ovarian tumors as benign or malignant, but results are conflicting and the technique is not universally accepted for this clinical application. The ADC values of malignant ovarian tumors vary widely, a phenomenon that is attributable to their heterogeneous histology and morphology. Endometriomas and malignant cystic ovarian tumors tend to exhibit lower ADC values (as is demonstrated in this case) than other benign, non-hemorrhagic, ovarian cysts and benign cystic tumors. Currently, there is only weak evidence to suggest a utility of DWI and ADC for evaluation of ovarian tumors.

Imaging Findings

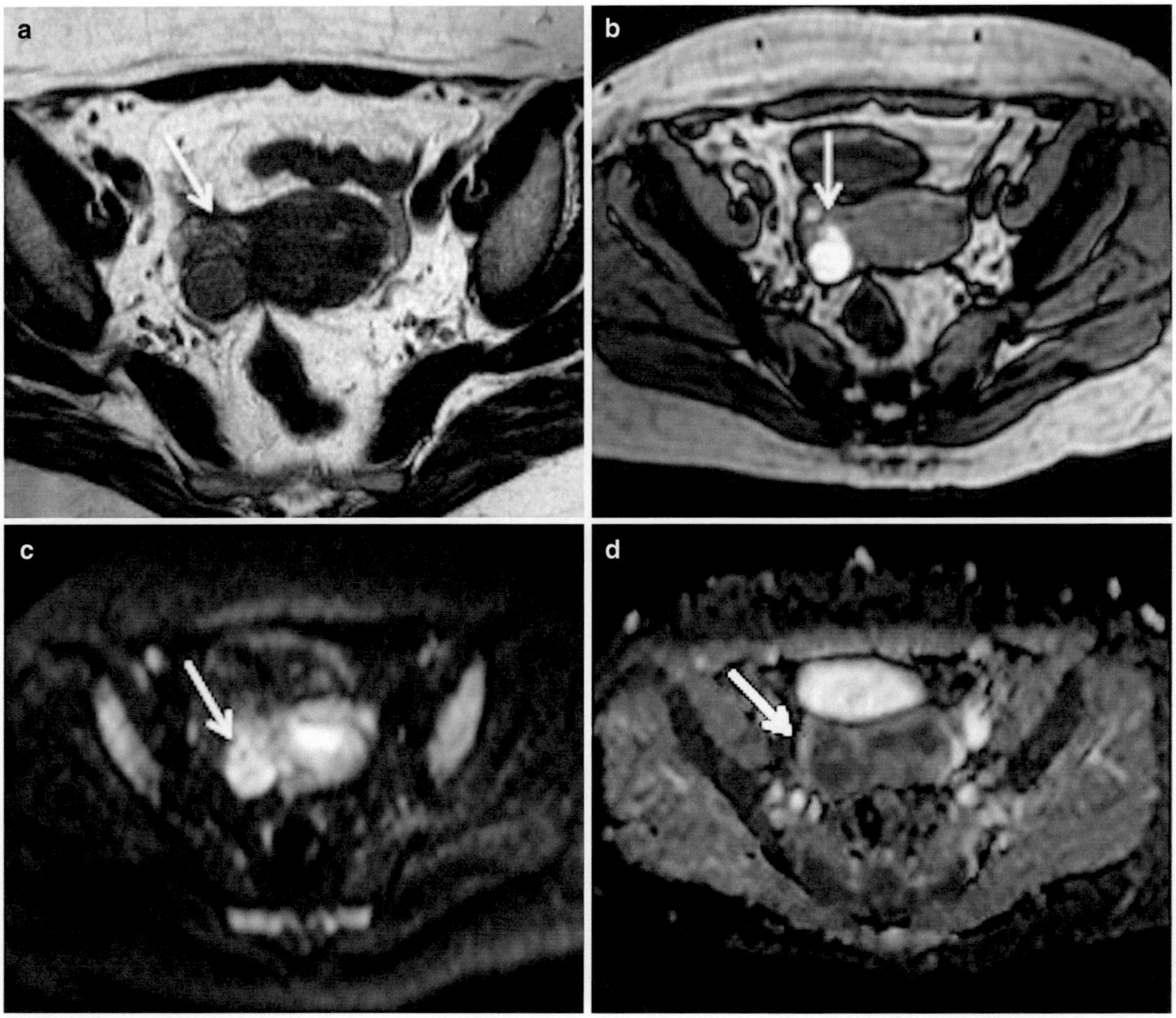

Fig. 9.6 (**a**) Axial FSE T2-weighted image shows a low-to-intermediate signal intensity cystic lesion in the region of the right ovary (*arrow*). (**b**) Axial GE T1-weighted image shows a homogeneous high-signal-intensity mass (*arrow*). (**c**) DWI acquired with a *b* factor of 800 s/mm^2 shows high signal intensity in the cystic mass (*arrow*). (**d**) ADC map demonstrates low signal intensity in the cystic mass, indicating restricted diffusion (*arrow*)

Case 9.7: Ovarian Fibroma

A 40-year-old patient with pelvic pain and a palpable mass in whom a transvaginal US demonstrated a solid lesion in the left ovary. MRI was indicated to characterize the lesion.

Comments

Fibroma, fibrothecoma, and thecoma form a spectrum of benign tumors of the ovary. These tumors constitute approximately 4% of all ovarian neoplasms and occur in both premenopausal and postmenopausal women. Fibroma is the most common sex cord tumor. Although fibroma arising from nonfunctioning stroma shows no estrogenic activity, lipid-rich thecomas can show estrogenic activity. Fibromas can be associated with Meigs' syndrome (ascites, ovarian tumor, and right-sided pleural effusion).

Fibromas have abundant collagen and fibrous content, and therefore, these tumors show relatively characteristic imaging findings. The mass appears as a homogeneous solid tumor with delayed enhancement on CT and as a hypointense mass on T1-weighted MR images with very low signal intensity on T2-weighted images. Scattered high-signal-intensity areas in the mass indicate edema or cystic degeneration. Dense calcifications are often seen on CT.

Fibromas can be the underlying cause of adnexal torsion. CT and MRI findings in adnexal torsion with fibroma include tube thickening, ascites, deviation of the uterus to the torsed side, hemorrhage in the thickened tube, and a torsion "knot." It is difficult to diagnose associated hemorrhagic infarction after adnexal torsion because the fibroma is a solid tumor. The finding of a high-signal-intensity area in the periphery of the mass on T1-weighted images is helpful in the MRI diagnosis of hemorrhagic infarction of a fibroma-containing ovary. Recently, the use of DWI has demonstrated a capacity to characterize tissue, especially in the differentiation of benign from malignant tissue. DWI provides information about tissue cellularity, microcirculation, and cell membrane integrity; all of these are altered in malignant tissue. In this particular case, the DWI permits us establish the possibility of malignancy characterizing the abnormal tissue, which demonstrates restriction of the tissular diffusion.

Imaging Findings

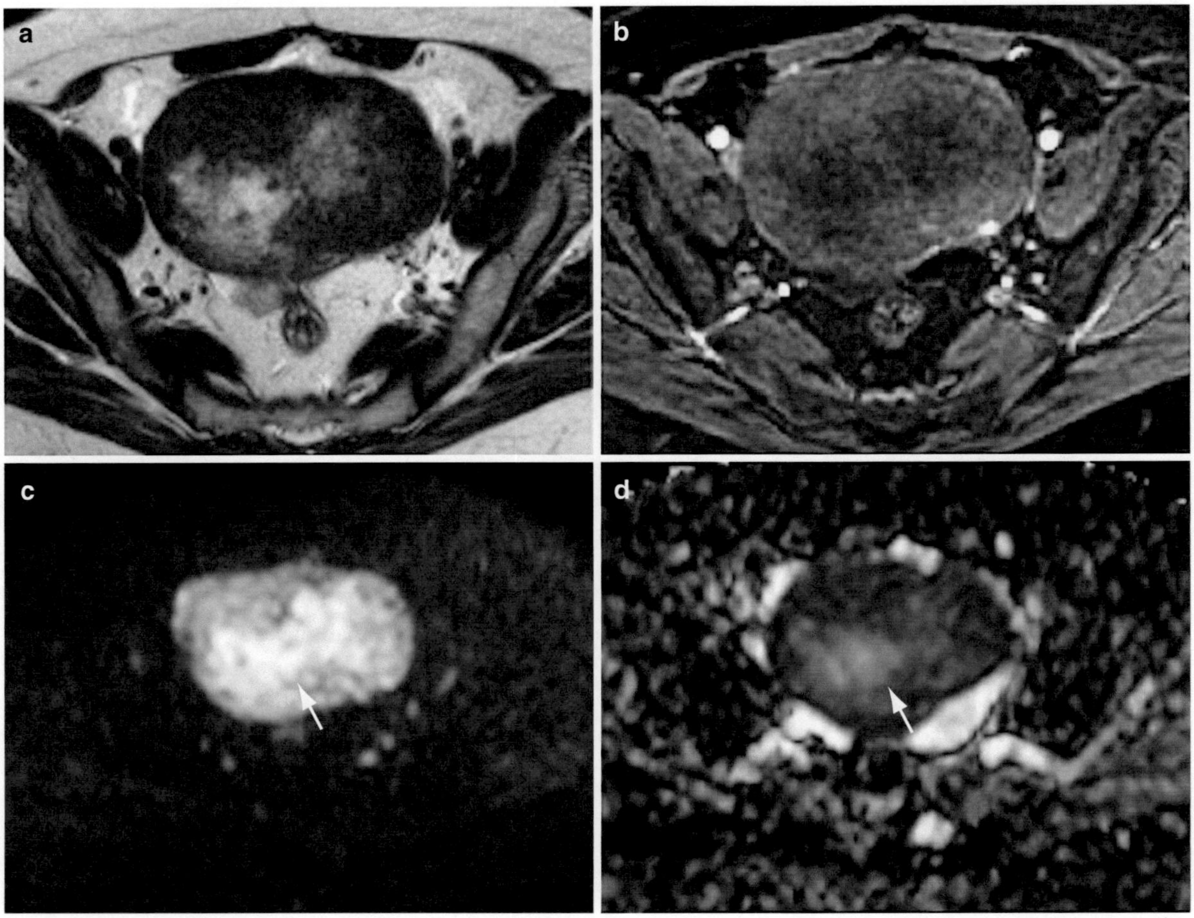

Fig. 9.7 (**a**) Axial FSE T2-weighted image shows a heterogeneous but predominantly hypointense signal intensity mass with a hyperintense central area. (**b**) Axial contrast-enhanced GE T1-weighted image with fat suppression shows the mass with heterogeneous enhancement, especially in the hypointense area on the T2-weighted image. (**c**, **d**) DWI acquired with a *b* factor of 800 s/mm^2 (**c**) and corresponding ADC map image (**d**) show the predominantly hyperintense mass on DWI and hypointense mass on ADC map images, respectively, indicating restriction of diffusion. The central area of the mass is hyperintense on both images ("T2 shine-through" effect), possibly secondary to lesion necrosis (*arrow*)

Case 9.8: Didelphus Uterus and Ovarian Dermoid Tumor

A 32-year-old patient with pelvic pain. Transvaginal US (not shown) demonstrated an echogenic mass in the left ovary and an abnormal appearance of the uterus, possibly due to a didelphus uterus. The MRI was performed to characterize the mass and the uterine anomaly.

Comments

The female reproductive system develops from the Müllerian ducts, two ducts that originate from the embryonal mesoderm, lateral to each Wolffian duct. The paired Müllerian ducts grow in medial and caudal directions. The most cephalad parts of the ducts remain separate and form the fallopian tubes. The lower parts of the ducts fuse (lateral fusion). The midline septum disappears, leaving a single canal: the uterus and upper two-thirds of the vagina. The lower third of the vagina is formed from the ascending sinovaginal bulb, which fuses with the lower Müllerian system (vertical fusion). The entirely separate origin of the ovaries from the gonadal ridge explains the infrequent association of uterovaginal anomalies with ovarian anomalies. The close developmental relationship of the Müllerian and Wolffian ducts explains the frequent association of anomalies of the female genital system and urinary tract. Renal anomalies associated with uterovaginal anomalies include renal agenesis, ectopic kidney, cystic dysplasia, and a duplicated collecting system.

The best diagnostic imaging modality to evaluate Mullerian duct anomalies is MRI, especially the T2-weighted sequences in the coronal, oblique coronal, sagittal and axial planes. In a didelphus uterus, there are two uterine bodies and two cervices. The uterine horns are widely splayed with a deep fundal cleft, and the intercornual angle is greater than 60°. The endometrial and myometrial zonal widths are preserved. Vaginal septa are most commonly associated with this type of uterine anomaly.

Mature cystic teratomas, also known as "dermoid cysts," are cystic tumors composed of well-differentiated derivatives from at least two of the three germ cell layers (ectoderm, mesoderm, and endoderm). They affect a younger age group (mean patient age, 30 years) than epithelial ovarian neoplasms. Mature cystic teratoma is the most common germ cell neoplasm and, in some series, the most common ovarian neoplasm removed at surgery. It is the most common ovarian mass in young girls. Most mature cystic teratomas are asymptomatic. Mature cystic teratomas requiring removal can be treated with simple cystectomy, thus sparing the ovaries. The tumors are bilateral in about 10% of cases. Many teratomas can be confidently diagnosed at US; however, the presence of tissue components results in a variety of appearances at US. The most specific appearance is a cystic lesion with a densely echogenic nodule (Rokitansky nodule) projecting into the lumen of the cyst. The second manifestation is a diffusely or partially echogenic mass with the echogenic area usually demonstrating attenuation of sound waves, secondary to the sebaceous material and hair commonly found within the cyst cavity. The third manifestation consists of multiple thin, echogenic bands caused by hair in the cyst cavity. The best diagnostic modalities to diagnose mature cystic teratomas with certainty are MRI and CT due to their high sensitivity for detecting fat. At MRI the sebaceous component of dermoid cysts in the T1-weighted sequences with and without fat suppression follows the signal intensity of retroperitoneal fat. The signal intensity on T2-weighted images is more variable and depends on the relative content of fat and hemorrhagic elements. The use of DWI has not been studied specifically in ovary teratoma; however, it appears to be of value in both identifying and in characterizing abnormal tissue. Therefore, DWI could be a useful tool in patients with "fat-less" mature ovarian cystic teratomas, especially with the calculated ADC values which may help differentiate benign from malignant tumors.

Imaging Findings

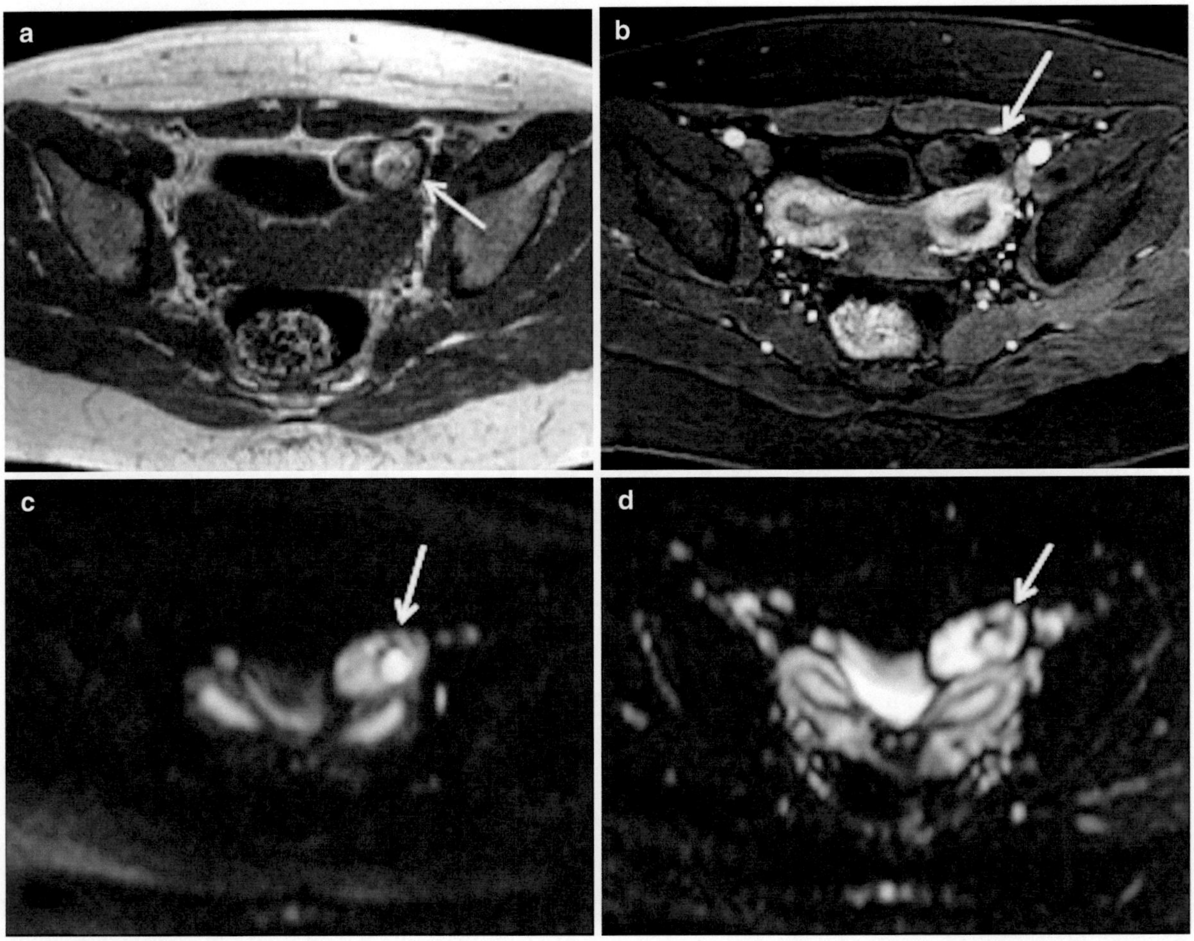

Fig. 9.8 (**a**) Non-enhanced axial GE T1-weighted image without fat suppression shows two uterine horns and a high-signal-intensity tumor in the left ovary (*arrow*). (**b**) Contrast-enhanced axial GE T1-weighted image with fat suppression shows loss of signal intensity in the left ovarian tumor (*arrow*), indicating macroscopic fat content and two well-defined uterine horns. (**c, d**) DWI acquired with *b* values of 800 and 500 s/mm^2, respectively, show high signal intensity in the left ovarian mass (*arrows*)

Case 9.9: Ovarian Carcinoma

A 45-year-old asymptomatic patient in whom a routine transvaginal US disclosed a small solid lesion in the left ovary. MRI was performed to characterize the lesion.

Comments

Tumors arising from the surface epithelium account for 90% of ovarian cancers and are pathologically designated as serous, mucinous, clear cell, endometrioid, or Brenner (transitional) tumors based on the cell type. Each histologic type is further classified as benign, borderline malignant (tumors of low malignant potential), or malignant, reflecting differences in clinical behavior. Borderline tumors are more frequently diagnosed in young women, and management decisions require that the relatively low risk of tumor-related mortality be balanced against considerations of operative risks, fertility preservation, and long-term morbidity of premature menopause if a complete cancer operation is required.

Several studies have evaluated the additional value of a second test for an indeterminate adnexal mass detected on US, and these have determined that MRI with IV contrast administration is the most appropriate modality, as compared to CT, Doppler US, or non-enhanced MRI. When used for evaluation of an indeterminate mass detected on US, contrast-enhanced MRI has high sensitivity and specificity in the diagnosis of malignancy. Although MRI can be helpful in cancer detection, the main contribution of MRI in adnexal mass evaluation is its specificity because it provides a confident diagnosis of many common benign adnexal lesions. MRI better characterizes indeterminate adnexal lesions seen on US, especially if an extraovarian cystic lesion is suspected but a normal ipsilateral ovary is not seen or if a predominantly solid lesion requires more tissue-specific characterization for diagnosis. Extraovarian cystic lesions include peritoneal inclusion cysts, paratubal cysts, hydrosalpinx, and endometrioma. Solid-appearing adnexal lesions include dermoids, exophytic uterine, and broad ligament fibroids and ovarian fibrothecomas.

The use of DWI in ovarian tumors has not been studied thoroughly. There are only a few reports describing the clinical utility of DWI for characterization of ovarian tumors as benign or malignant. The results of these studies are conflicting and the technique is not universally accepted for this clinical application. However, DWI allows detection and characterization of abnormal tissue and, therefore, could become a useful tool that adds information in complex cases, especially when using the ADC values as demonstrated in this case. The low ADC values of this mass helped to characterize it as malignant.

Imaging Findings

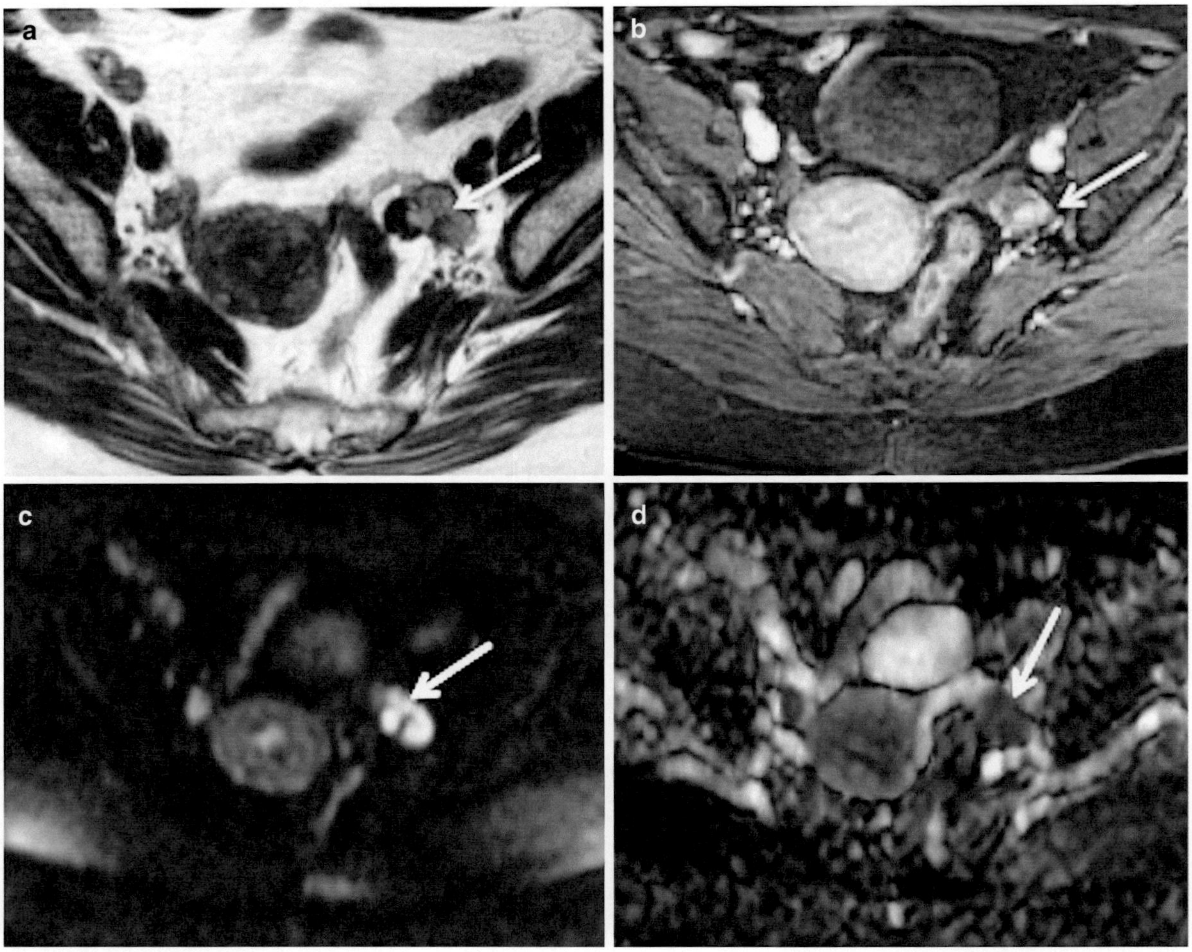

Fig. 9.9 (**a**) Axial TSE T2-weighted image demonstrates a small high-signal-intensity mass in the left ovary (*arrow*). (**b**) Contrast-enhanced axial GE T1-weighted image with fat suppression acquired at the same level as A shows the mass with nodular enhancement (*arrow*). (**c**, **d**) DWI acquired with a *b* factor of 800 s/mm^2 (**c**) and corresponding ADC map (**d**) image demonstrate the mass with high signal intensity in the DWI and low signal intensity in the ADC map, indicating restricted diffusion (*arrows*)

Case 9.10: Vulvar Sarcoma

A 17-year-old-female with painful mass in left major labia. US demonstrated a lobulated hypoechoic mass. MRI was requested to characterize the mass.

Comments

Rhabdomyosarcoma is the most common soft-tissue sarcoma in children and adolescents. Rather than representing primary sarcomas of striated muscle per se, rhabdomyosarcomas are thought to originate from primitive mesenchymal tissue that has the capacity to form rhabdomyoblasts. Many of these pelvic malignancies originate in or secondarily invade the uterus, vagina, and vulva. MRI has been recommended as the optimal imaging modality both for initial detection and for posttreatment follow-up of these aggressive neoplasms. Signs of poor prognosis that can be evaluated with imaging studies include large size (5 cm), regional lymphadenopathy, and local organ invasion. The findings on MRI include high signal intensity on T2-weighted images, low signal intensity on T1-weighted images, and enhancement with after administration of intravenous gadolinium. On DWI, the tumor shows restriction in the diffusion with high signal intensity on DWI and low signal in the corresponding ADC maps, as demonstrated in this case.

Imaging Findings

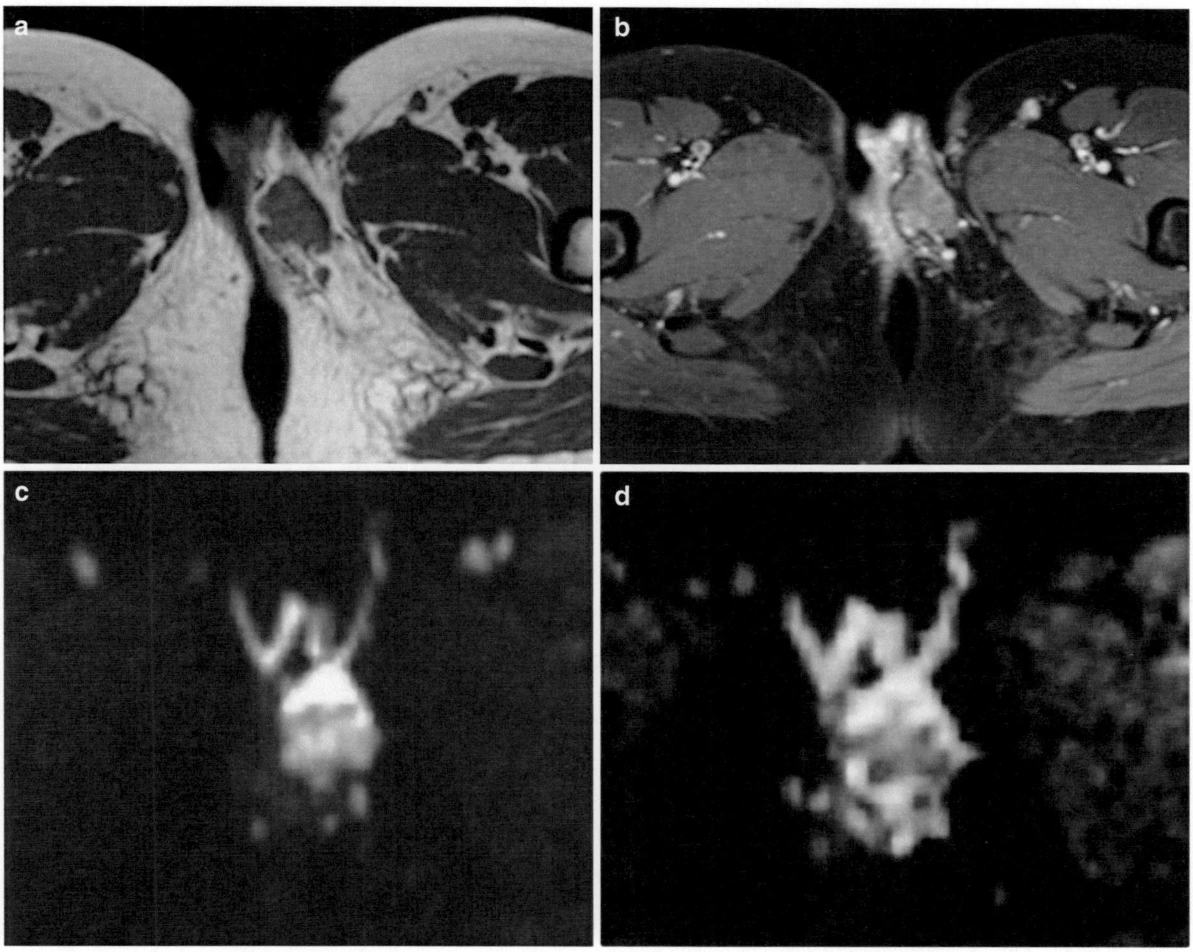

Fig. 9.10 (**a**) Non-enhanced T1-weighted image shows a lobulated mass with low signal intensity in the left major labia. (**b**) Contrast-enhanced axial GE T1-weighted image with fat-suppression shows enhancement of the mass. (**c, d**) DWI and ADC map demonstrate restricted diffusion of the mass with high signal intensity on the DWI acquired with a *b* factor of 800 s/mm^2 and low signal intensity on the corresponding ADC map

Further Reading

Balleyguier C, Sala E, Da Cunha T et al (2011) Staging of uterine cervical cancer with MRI: guidelines of the European Society of Urogenital Radiology. Eur Radiol 21(5):1102–1110; Epub Nov 10, 2010

Boronow RC, Morrow CP, Creasman WT et al (1984) Surgical staging in endometrial cancer: clinical-pathologic findings of a prospective study. Obstet Gynecol 63(6):825–832

Charles-Edwards EM, Messiou C, Morgan VA et al (2008) Diffusion-weighted imaging in cervical cancer with an endovaginal technique: potential value for improving tumor detection in stage Ia and Ib1 disease. Radiology 249(2): 541–550

Chen J, Zhang Y, Liang B et al (2010) The utility of diffusion-weighted MR imaging in cervical cancer. Eur J Radiol 74(3):101–106

Chen YB, Hu CM, Chen GL et al (2010) Staging of uterine cervical carcinoma: whole-body diffusion-weighted magnetic resonance imaging. Abdom Imaging; Aug 21, 2010 [Epub ahead of print]

Fujii S, Kakite S, Nishihara K et al (2008) Diagnostic accuracy of diffusion-weighted imaging in differentiating benign from malignant ovarian lesions. J Magn Reson Imaging 28(5):1149–1156

Fujii S, Matsusue E, Kigawa J et al (2008) Diagnostic accuracy of the apparent diffusion coefficient in differentiating benign from malignant uterine endometrial cavity lesions: initial results. Eur Radiol 18(2):384–389

Harry VN, Semple SI, Gilbert FJ et al (2008) Diffusion-weighted magnetic resonance imaging in the early detection of response to chemoradiation in cervical cancer. Gynecol Oncol 111(2):213–220

Hiwatashi A, Kinoshita T, Moritani T et al (2003) Hypointensity on diffusion-weighted MRI of the brain related to T2 short- ening and susceptibility effects. Am J Roentgenol 181:1705–1709

Inada Y, Matsuki M, Nakai G et al (2009) Body diffusion-weighted MR imaging of uterine endometrial cancer: is it helpful in the detection of cancer in nonenhanced MR imaging? Eur J Radiol 70(1):122–127

Jacobs MA, Gultekin DH, Kim HS (2010) Comparison between diffusion-weighted imaging, T2-weighted, and postcontrast T1-weighted imaging after MR-guided, high intensity, focused ultrasound treatment of uterine leiomyomata: preliminary results. Med Phys 37(9):4768–4776

Jacobs MA, Ibrahim TS, Ouwerkerk R (2007) AAPM/RSNA physics tutorials for residents: MR imaging: brief overview and emerging applications. Radiographics 27:1213–1229

Katayama M, Masui T, Kobayashi S et al (2002) Diffusion-weighted echo planar imaging of ovarian tumors: is it useful to measure apparent diffusion coefficients? J Comput Assist Tomogr 26:250–256

Kilickesmez O, Bayramoglu S, Inci E et al (2009) Quantitative diffusion-weighted magnetic resonance imaging of normal and diseased uterine zones. Acta Radiol 50(3):340–347

Kinkel K (2006) Pitfalls in staging uterine neoplasm with imaging: a review. Abdom Imaging 31:164–173

Kyriazi S, Collins DJ, Morgan VA et al (2010) Diffusion-weighted imaging of peritoneal disease for noninvasive staging of advanced ovarian cancer. Radiographics 30(5):1269–1285

Le Bihan D (1990) Diffusion/perfusion MR imaging of the brain: from structure to function. Radiology 177:328–329

Liapi E, Kamel IR, Bluemke DA et al (2005) Assessment of response of uterine fibroids and myometrium to embolization using diffusion-weighted echoplanar MR imaging. J Comput Assist Tomogr 29(1):83–86

Lin G, Ho KC, Wang JJ et al (2008) Detection of lymph node metastasis in cervical and uterine cancers by diffusion-weighted magnetic resonance imaging at 3 T. J Magn Reson Imaging 28(1):128–135

Lin G, Ng KK, Chang CJ, Wang JJ et al (2009) Myometrial invasion in endometrial cancer: diagnostic accuracy of diffusion-weighted 3.0-T MR imaging – initial experience. Radiology 250(3):784–792

Liu Y, Bai R, Sun H et al (2009) Diffusion-weighted magnetic resonance imaging of uterine cervical cancer. J Comput Assist Tomogr 33(6):858–862

Liu Y, Bai R, Sun H et al (2009) Diffusion-weighted imaging in predicting and monitoring the response of uterine cervical cancer to combined chemoradiation. Clin Radiol 64(11):1067–1074

Maldjian JA, Listerud J, Moonis G et al (2001) Computing diffusion rates in T2-dark hematomas and areas of low T2 signal. Am J Neuroradiol 22:112–118

Manfredi R, Gui B, Maresca G et al (2005) Endometrial cancer: magnetic resonance imaging. Abdom Imaging 30: 626–636

McCarthy S, Scott G, Majumdar S et al (1989) Uterine junctional zone: MR study of water content and relaxation properties. Radiology 171:241–243

McVeigh PZ, Syed AM, Milosevic M et al (2008) Diffusion-weighted MRI in cervical cancer. Eur Radiol 18:1058–1064

Moteki T, Ishizaka H (2000) Diffusion-weighted EPI of cystic ovarian lesions: evaluation of cystic contents using apparent diffusion coefficients. J Magn Reson Imaging 12:1014–1019

Naganawa S, Sato C, Kumada H et al (2005) Apparent diffusion coefficient in cervical cancer of the uterus: comparison with the normal uterine cervix. Eur Radiol 15:71–78

Nakayama T, Yoshimitsu K, Irie H et al (2005) Diffusion weighted echo-planar MR imaging and ADC mapping in the differential diagnosis of ovarian cystic masses: usefulness of detecting keratinoid substances in mature cystic teratomas. J Magn Reson Imaging 22:271–278

Namimoto T, Yamashita Y, Awai K et al (2009) Combined use of T2-weighted and diffusion-weighted 3-T MR imaging for differentiating uterine sarcomas from benign leiomyomas. Eur Radiol 19(11):2756–2764

Payne GS, Schmidt M, Morgan VA et al (2010) Evaluation of magnetic resonance diffusion and spectroscopy measurements as predictive biomarkers in stage 1 cervical cancer. Gynecol Oncol 116(2):246–252

Prat J (2004) Prognostic parameters of endometrial carcinoma. Hum Pathol 35:649–662

Sahdev A, Sohaib SA, Wenaden AE et al (2007) The performance of magnetic resonance imaging in early cervical carcinoma: a long-term experience. Int J Gynecol Cancer 17:629–636

Sala E, Priest AN, Kataoka M et al (2010) Apparent diffusion coefficient and vascular signal fraction measurements with magnetic resonance imaging: feasibility in metastatic ovarian cancer at 3 Tesla – technical development. Eur Radiol 20(2):491–496

Shen SH, Chiou YY, Wang JH et al (2008) Diffusion-weighted single-shot echo-planar imaging with parallel technique in assessment of endometrial cancer. Am J Roentgenol 190:481–488

Shimada K, Ohashi I, Kasahara I et al (2004) Differentiation between completely hyalinized uterine leiomyomas and ordinary leiomyomas: three-phase dynamic magnetic resonance imaging (MRI) vs. diffusion-weighted MRI with very small b-factors. J Magn Reson Imaging 20:97–104

Takeuchi M, Matsuzaki K, Nishitani H (2009) Diffusion-weighted magnetic resonance imaging of endometrial cancer: differentiation from benign endometrial lesions and preoperative assessment of myometrial invasion. Acta Radiol 50(8):947–953

Takeuchi M, Matsuzaki K, Nishitani H (2009) Hyperintense uterine myometrial masses on T2-weighted magnetic resonance imaging: differentiation with diffusion-weighted magnetic resonance imaging. J Comput Assist Tomogr 33(6):834–837

Takeuchi M, Matsuzaki K, Nishitani H (2010) Diffusion-weighted magnetic resonance imaging of ovarian tumors: differentiation of benign and malignant solid components of ovarian masses. J Comput Assist Tomogr 34(2): 173–176

Tamai K, Koyama T, Saga T et al (2007) Diffusion-weighted MR imaging of uterine endometrial cancer. J Magn Reson Imaging 26(3):682–687

Tamai K, Koyama T, Saga T, Morisawa N, Fujimoto K, Mikami Y et al (2008) The utility of diffusion-weighted MR imaging for differentiating uterine sarcomas from benign leiomyomas. Eur Radiol 18:723–730

Wang J, Yu T, Bai R et al (2010) The value of the apparent diffusion coefficient in differentiating stage IA endometrial carcinoma from normal endometrium and benign diseases of the endometrium: initial study at 3-T magnetic resonance scanner. J Comput Assist Tomogr 34(3):332–337

Whittaker CS, Coady A, Culver L et al (2009) Diffusion-weighted MR imaging of female pelvic tumors: a pictorial review. Radiographics 29(3):759–774

Xue HD, Li S, Sun F et al (2008) Clinical application of body diffusion weighted MR imaging in the diagnosis and preoperative N staging of cervical cancer. Chin Med Sci J 23(3):133–137

Yamashita Y, Harada M, Sawada T et al (1993) Normal uterus and FIGO stage I endometrial carcinoma: dynamic gadolinium-enhanced MR imaging. Radiology 186:495–501

Yu SP, He L, Liu B et al (2010) Differential diagnosis of metastasis from non-metastatic lymph nodes in cervical cancers: pilot study of diffusion weighted imaging with background suppression at 3 T magnetic resonance. Chin Med J Engl 123(20):2820–2824

DWI of the Breast

10

Joaquim Barceló, Joan C. Vilanova, and Antonio Luna

10.1 Introduction

Dynamic contrast-enhanced MRI (DCE-MRI) of the breast has a high sensitivity for breast cancer detection (89–100%) but lacks specificity for characterizing breast tumors. An overlap between the MRI findings of benign and malignant lesions still exists, resulting in variable specificity (37–86%). Hence, several studies have investigated the role of advanced MRI techniques, such as DWI, to improve the specificity of MRI in the evaluation of breast lesions and also improve the positive predictive value (PPV).

DWI is an unenhanced MRI sequence that measures the mobility of water molecules (Brownian motion) in vivo (in tissues) and provides different and potentially complementary information to DCE-MRI. The diffusivity of water molecules is restricted in environments of high cellularity, intracellular and extracellular edema, high viscosity, and fibrosis because these conditions become barriers to the movement of water molecules. DWI can be performed without a significant increase in examination time, especially if low *b* values are used. It is possible to calculate the ADC using a DWI sequence, a quantitative measure that is directly proportional to the water diffusion. DWI depicts the areas of restriction of water molecules' diffusivity in malignant tissue as regions with high signal intensity with low ADC values (Fig. 10.1).

10.2 Quantification in Breast DWI

A ROI (region of interest) is defined for each DCE-MRI detected lesion at the corresponding location in the combined DWI series. The ROI encompasses as much of the abnormality as possible in the DWI or color map ADC. Care must be taken to avoid regions of fibrosis and regions with high T2 value within a lesion, such as cyst, hematoma, or necrosis. When a lesion is not hyperintense on DWI, the ROI should be drawn on the DCE-MRI abnormality and then pasted at the corresponding location. Some authors have proposed alternative less simplistic methods of ADC measurements than mean or median ADC. The use of histograms better reflects tumor heterogeneity. Furthermore, Koh and colleagues have proposed the use of ADC thresholds to create ADC thresholds maps in the monitorization of sequential ADC changes with treatment.

Although several studies have shown no significant effect on ADC of breast tissue if the DWI sequence is performed after the administration of a gadolinium-based contrast agent, it may be preferable to acquire the DWI sequence before contrast injection to avoid any confounding effects.

As DWI forms part of clinical breast MRI protocols, it is usually performed in the second week of the menstrual cycle, as it is necessary for DCE-MRI. Besides, in that moment, ADC of breast tissue is slightly lower due to reduced water content in the breast. Reported ADC values of normal breast tissue ranged from 1.51 to 2.37×10^{-3} mm²/s. Anyhow, the

J. Barceló (✉) • J.C. Vilanova
Department of Radiology,
Clínica Girona-Hospital Sta. Caterina,
Girona, Spain
e-mail: jbarcelo@cetir.es; kvilanova@comg.cat

A. Luna
Chief of MRI, Health Time Group, Jaén, Spain
e-mail: aluna70@sercosa.com

A. Luna et al., *Diffusion MRI Outside the Brain*,
DOI 10.1007/978-3-642-21052-5_10, © Springer-Verlag Berlin Heidelberg 2012

normal fluctuation of ADC values in the normal fibroglandular tissue during the menstrual cycle has been shown to be small and nonsignificant, with a coefficient of variation during the cycle of about 5.5% in the case of the menstrual cycle, whereas in patients with postmenopausal replacement therapy, its suspension is recommended 6–8 weeks in advance to avoid any hormonal variability in breast structure.

10.3 Assessment of Breast Lesions

Promising findings from preliminary DWI studies of the breast have shown significantly lower ADC measures for breast carcinomas (Fig. 10.1) than for benign breast lesions or normal tissue. High cell proliferation in malignant tumors increases cellular density, creating more barriers to the extracellular water diffusion, reducing thus the ADC value. Furthermore, preliminary data have related DWI to the growth patterns of carcinomas, including cellular density and architectural features of the stroma. Besides, very recently, ADC quantification has been related to prognostic factors such as positive expression of estrogen receptors and negative expression of c-erbB-2 in patients with invasive ductal carcinoma. Therefore, DWI appears to be a useful tool for tumor detection and characterization, as well as for monitoring and predicting treatment response. Improved diagnostic accuracy for breast lesion characterization has been extensively reported when DWI information is added to DCE-MRI data.

After some years of clinical application of breast DWI, there is no consensus regarding the optimal *b* value in diagnosis of breast cancer. Recent studies from Pereira et al. have proven that the ADC values calculated from *b* value of 0 and 750 s/mm^2 are slightly better than others combination of *b* values at 1.5 T magnets, showing a sensitivity of 92% and a specificity of 96%, with a cutoff ADC value of 1.24×10^{-3} mm^2/s for the diagnosis of benign and malignant lesions. Bogner and colleagues reported optimum DWI quality and ADC determination using *b* values of 50 and 850 s/mm^2 at 3 T magnets. In this series, distinction of benign and malignant tumors was optimal with an ADC threshold of 1.25×10^{-3} mm^2/s with an accuracy of 95%.

Another recent study by Partridge et al. showed the added value of DWI to DCE-MRI for improving the PPV for lesions of various types and sizes. This series evaluated 70 women with 83 suspicious lesions on DCE-MRI, all of them posteriorly biopsied. The DWI acquisition included two *b* values of 0 and 600 s/mm^2. A 100% sensitivity was obtained using an ADC threshold of 1.8 x10^{-3} mm^2/s with a PPV of 47% versus 37% for DCE-MRI alone, which would have avoided biopsy for 33% of benign lesions without missing any cancer. In this study, DWI increased PPV similarly for masses and non-mass-like enhancement, preferentially improving PPV for lesions smaller than 1 cm. However, a considerable overlap in ADC of benign and malignant lesions was also found.

Two recent meta-analyses have shown the great variability in reported ADC measurements for malignant and benign tumors ranging from 0.87 to 1.61 and 1.00 to 2.01×10^{-3} mm^2/s, respectively, resulting in recommended threshold values of ADC ranging from 0.90 to 1.76×10^{-3} mm^2/s. Furthermore, if the meta-analysis by Chen and colleagues demonstrated a great variability even in the subgroup of studies using a maximum *b* value of 1000 s/mm^2, the minimum and maximum ADC threshold values were 1.10×10^{-3} mm^2/s and 1.38×10^{-3} mm^2/s. Therefore, lack of standardization diminishes reproducibility of DWI data at this moment. However, the performance of DWI in the distinction between benign and malignant lesions is high. In the meta-analysis by Chen et al., the pooled weighted sensitivity and specificity within one subgroup of studies using a maximum *b* value of 1000 s/mm^2 were 84% (range 80–87%) and 84% (range 79–88%), respectively. In the meta-analysis of Tsushima and colleagues, the results were similar with pooled sensitivity and specificity of 89% (range 85–91%) and 77% (range 88–92%) respectively. The purpose of the MRI examination may determine the chosen threshold ADC. Therefore, in cases of screening where it is important not to miss any cancer, a higher cutoff value is necessary. Conversely, in a clinical setting, it is more important to avoid false positive of DCE-MRI, which needs of a lower threshold.

Currently, there is some controversy about the role of ADC measurement in breast cancer grading, as several studies have not found significant differences in ADC values between the different subtypes of invasive carcinomas or between intraductal carcinoma and invasive carcinoma, whereas other reports have shown significant differences. Although further research is needed, there is a trend toward DCIS to show higher ADC values than invasive ductal carcinoma and lower ADC values than normal breast tissue.

Regarding pitfalls, false-negative results can be present in tumors with low cellularity and with higher

ADC values, such as the malignant phyllodes tumor (Fig. 10.5), pure mucinous carcinoma (rich in mucina) (Fig. 10.2), apocrine carcinoma, invasive micropapillary carcinoma, scirrhous carcinoma and the non-mass-like part of DCIS (Fig. 10.3). False-positive presenting low ADC values have been reported in cases of non malignant lesions, such as intraductal papiloma, ductal adenoma, fibroadenoma (Fig. 10.4), benign proliferative disease, radial scars, lymph node, and abscess. Fibrocystic disease might show a high cell density and inflammatory reactions. This phenomenon restricts proton diffusion, a possible reason for low ADC values. However, the disparity between the ADC values of fibrocystic disease and malignancy could be further distinguished with a higher *b* value. This is because the effect of perfusion is smaller at higher *b* values and the reduction in ADC values of malignant lesions is more prominent than of benign lesions due to angiogenesis of malignant tumor.

Another subject of debate is the role of DWI in the evaluation of non-mass-like enhancement (Fig. 10.6). Lesions such as noninvasive ductal carcinomas, lobular carcinoma in situ, atypical ductal hyperplasia, papillomas, hormonal-related enhancement, and fibrocystic disease have shown this pattern of enhancement These lesions usually show less cellular density due to their heterogeneous and non-compact structure, being often interspersed with normal parenchyma. Higher ADC may be expected for these lesions. Contradictory data have been published about the usefulness of ADC measurements in their characterization, but we can conclude that DWI has a weak area in the evaluation of non-mass-like enhancement, although the addition of ADC measurements to DCE-MRI and morphological data improves lesional characterization.

10.4 Technical Considerations of Breast DWI

DWI has some technical limitations and challenges:

(a) As previously commented, lack of standardization in the technical approach limits reproducibility. The most extended sequence is SS EPI because it has demonstrated better lesion visibility than HASTE approach. SS EPI DWI is prone to susceptibility artifacts and distortions and HASTE DWI to image blurring. Spectral fat saturation such as CHESS, SPIR, or SPAIR is preferred to STIR.

(b) Common artifacts secondary to SS EPI DWI are magnetic susceptibility and chemical shift, which are another potential source of spatial misregistration in breast DWI. Parallel imaging techniques have limited these problems and enable DWI to produce images clinically acceptable.

(c) DWI can fail to categorize breast lesions because of the limited capability of recognizing diffuse and small lesions on the DWI and ADC maps, especially lesions smaller than 1 cm. Generally, DWI has low SNR, partial volume averaging, and low special resolution. Compared to DCE-MRI, in several reports, DWI has shown a detection rate between 89% and 100% of lesions, although smaller and benign lesions are harder to detect. This may be an important limitation to apply ADC quantification as not visible lesions on DWI may not be quantified.

(d) Therefore, a door is open to research the role of DWI at 3 T magnets in breast lesion detection. The use of parallel imaging allows mitigating artifacts secondary to the increase in magnetic field. Moreover, recent published data have reported better lesion delineation at 3 T and similar diagnostic accuracy to series using 1.5 T magnets. Therefore, 3 T magnets probably will outperform 1.5 T in the evaluation of lesions smaller than 1 cm.

(e) ADC measures are influenced by the degree of diffusion sensitization (*b* value) applied during DWI acquisition; therefore the ADC range for benign and malignant lesions obtained with a *b* value of 700 s/mm^2 may not be the same for DWI obtained at higher or lower *b* values. However, a recent report by Peters and colleagues reflected that ADC of lesions varied according to the different *b* values used for calculation, although characterization of lesions was not significantly distinct using different combinations of *b* values, if the appropriate ADC threshold was chosen.

(f) Patient movement during the acquisition of the DWI sequences may lead to wrong ADC values, although this may be partially solved applying a coregistration software before ADC measurements are performed. In order to avoid motion artifacts, some authors advocate obtaining only two *b* values, which is the minimum requirement for ADC calculation, although the use of more *b* values increases the precision of ADC measurements.

(g) Microvessel density is higher in malignant than benign breast tumor. The microperfusion effect may potentially increase ADC values. To reduce this effect, some authors have advocated obtaining DWI after contrast media injection due to postulated suppression by the contrast of the microperfusion effect. Others have preferred to increase the higher *b* value up to 1500 s/mm^2 to reduce this effect. The use of perfusion-insensitive ADC value excluding *b* value lower than 50–100 s/mm^2 has been anecdotally tested for breast MRI, but it has been a common approach in other organs. More sophisticated analysis of diffusion signal decay, as the IVIM approach, is now being tested in the breast. In our experience, it completely avoids microperfusion effect on tumors, achieving a more accurate estimation of tumoral diffusion (Fig. 10.7). Recently a series by Tamura et al., suggest comparison of parameters derived from biexponential fitting demonstrated no significant difference between benign and malignant lesions, although the fast component fraction of DWI of noninvasive ductal carcinoma was statistically greater than that of invasive ductal carcinoma. Conversely, recent results by Sigmund et al. suggest the potential of IVIM vascular and cellular biomarkers for initial grading, progression monitoring, or treatment assessment of breast tumors. Therefore, further research is needed in this field.

(h) Water movement in the breast is isotropic, although in the more structured breast parenchyma, low-to-moderate anisotropic diffusion has been described. FA measurements have been higher in the outer posterior region of the breasts, indicating heterogeneous anisotropy between breast regions related to microstructural differences. Lower FA values have been reported for malignant tumors than for normal tissue, but not different from those of benign lesions. DTI has not still extensively been used for lesion characterization, which should be tested in the near future.

10.5 Breast Cancer: Monitorization and Prediction of Response to Treatment with DWI

As for other tumors, DWI is under evaluation for predicting and monitoring response to treatment, especially for neoadjuvant chemotherapy (NAC). Locally advanced cancers are usually treated with NAC to downstage the disease for potential posterior curative surgery. Several authors related response to NAC with patient survival. RECIST criteria for evaluation of breast cancer response are based on gross morphology. DCE-MRI and now DWI offer earlier and functional information of tumor response to NAC (Figs. 10.8 and 10.9). Responders to NAC will show higher cellular reduction than nonresponders which will be reflected in higher increase of ADC values after therapy. Moreover, several reports have shown than this ADC elevation occurs before changes in tumor volume. Furthermore, they may be detected as soon as 1 week after the start of therapy, related to cellular damage and lysis, loss of integrity of cellular membrane, and reduced cellularity. Series by Pickles, Sharma, and Fangberget have pointed out the role of DWI in the early discrimination of responders and nonresponders to treatment. Although these data have been obtained in reduced populations and should be considered with caution, according to them, ADC may be a useful tool for personalized treatment management.

ADC may be a useful imaging biomarker for assessing overall response to therapy in breast tumors. Furthermore, Woodhands and colleagues reported an accuracy of 96% for depicting residual tumor after NAC for DWI compared with an accuracy of 89% for DCE-MRI (Fig. 10.10). Therefore, according to this series, DWI could be considered at least as good as DCE-MRI in this task.

Another area of research is the prediction of response to treatment with DWI. Pretreatment low ADC values have been related to responding tumors, as lower ADC values will reflect the presence of less necrosis which potentially enables a majority of cells to be targeted by the chemotherapeutic agents. Although without significant results, in a series by Sharma et al. and Park and colleagues, a trend toward better response of breast cancer with low pretreatment ADC may be confirmed. Larger series correlating pretreatment ADC with partial and complete response are needed to confirm these data.

10.6 Breast Cancer: Screening and Staging with DWI

MRI screening using DCE-MRI in high-risk population for breast cancer is increasing. In this field, DWI is an attractive alternative as it is fast, allows for quantitative information, has high sensitivity, and avoids the use of contrast. DCE-MRI is currently superior in lesion detection as previously commented. Lack of enough data precludes at this moment its clinical implementation as either a screening tool or to avoid the use of contrast agents in breast MRI, although, for sure, further studies will define its role in this field. In this sense, Yabauichi et al. evaluated 42 patients with non-palpable breast cancer in asymptomatic women. DWI along with T2-weighted sequence showed higher observer performances for the detection of non-palpable breast cancer than mammograms alone but lower than those of DCE-MRI

DWI has also been proposed for locoregional staging of breast cancer. There is a progressive increase in ADC from the core of the tumor to peritumor tissues to normal tissues, with an area of about 5 mm surrounding the border of the known tumor. The possibility of locoregional stadiation, proposed by Yili et al., is a potential application of DWI to define the necessary volume of free breast tissue surrounding the cancer for conservative surgery. For staging purposes, whole-body DWI has been used in breast cancer with very promising results, especially in bone staging (Fig. 16.2). Another area which may be a field of research for DWI is the noninvasive evaluation of axillary lymph node metastases according to its recently described capability to accurately distinguish malignant and inflammatory lymph nodes in pelvic and mediastinal territories (see chapter 14).

Case 10.1: Invasive Ductal Carcinoma

A 42-year-old woman presented with a palpable mass on the left breast. Biopsy confirmed invasive ductal carcinoma grade II. A breast MRI was requested for preoperative staging.

Comments

Invasive ductal carcinoma is the most common type of breast cancer representing 60–75% of cases. Currently, the most common indication for breast MRI is locoregional staging of cancer in order to plan the most appropriate treatment.

MRI allows to knowing the real extension of the tumor and its distribution within the breast, which is critical to assess both conservative treatment and the surgical approach of the lesions. MRI offers the best correlation with histology concerning the size, especially in the case of focal lesions or tumors, as in non-focal lesions, MRI tends to overestimate the size. Moreover, MRI is able to exclude multifocal, multicentric, or bilateral tumors, to detect the presence of a possible intraductal component and to evaluate the axillary lymph nodes or even the ones in internal mammary chain.

According to the literature, MRI is able to modify the treatment strategy in 20–40% of cases.

According to recent reports, DWI sequence might be able to distinguish malignant from benign lesions according to different ADC values. The mean ADC values for malignant lesions have been shown to be significantly lower than for benign lesions. Although comparative results for DWI have suggested different ADC thresholds according to the different *b* values used for ADC calculation. For breast DWI, a higher *b* value of 600–700 s/mm^2 in 1.5 T magnets is recommended, as it improves both sensitivity an specificity.

The restriction of water diffusion in malignant tumors is mainly due to increased cell density that creates barriers to the diffusion of extracellular water reducing the ADC. On DWI, false-positive results might be possible for intraductal papilloma, ductal adenoma, fibroadenoma, benign proliferative disease (mastopathy), radial scar, and lymph node abscess.

Imaging Findings

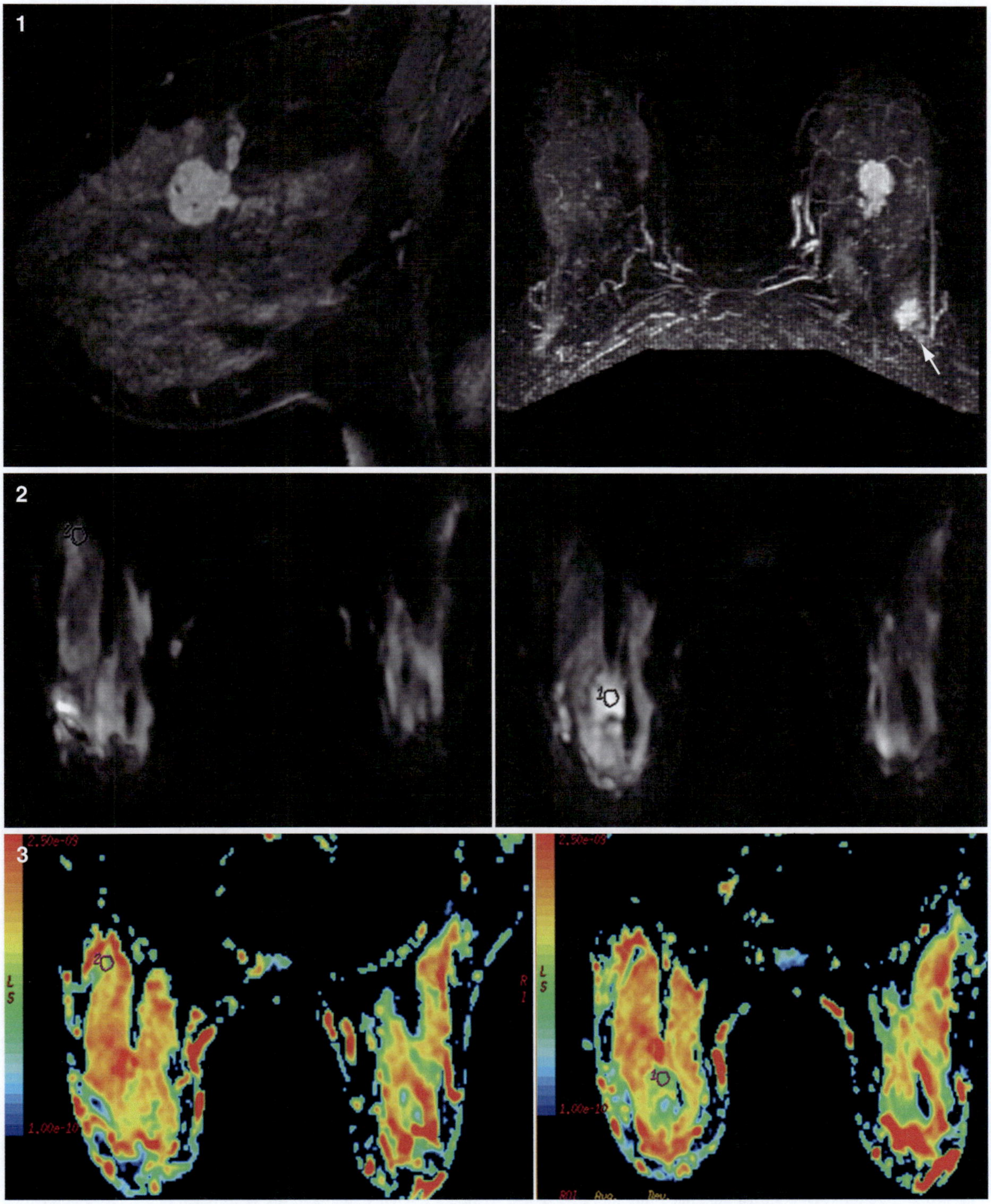

Fig. 10.1 Sagittal 3D contrast-enhanced fat-suppressed dynamic GE T1-weighted sequence and axial reconstruction from the same series shows an anterior irregular mass due to invasive carcinoma, and a posterior, previously unknown, area of focal enhancement (*arrow*) (**10.1.1**). This area was posteriorly biopsied with the result of mastopathy. Axial isotropic DWI (*b*: 700 s/mm^2) image (**10.1.2**) shows high signal intensity in the anterior mass (ROI number 1) and isointensity in the posterior focal area (ROI number 2). Axial ADC color map (**10.1.3**) shows restriction of diffusion of the anterior invasive ductal carcinoma mass with an ADC value of 1.16×10^{-3} mm^2/s (ROI number 1) and absence of restriction of diffusion in the posterior area of mastopathy with an ADC value of 1.53×10^{-3} mm^2/s (ROI number 2)

Case 10.2: Pure Mucinous Carcinoma

A 77-year-old woman was referred for a mass in the left breast. The biopsy yielded pure mucinous carcinoma.

Comments

Mucinous carcinoma of the breast is a relatively rare tumor that accounts for 1–7% of all cases of breast cancer.

There are two types of mucinous carcinoma. In the pure type, all tumoral cells are completely surrounded by mucin, and the tumor does not have any invasive ductal components. In the mixed type, invasive ductal carcinoma is present but not embedded in extracellular mucin.

ADC value and DWI signal intensity of mucinous carcinoma of the breast vary depending on amount of mucina, cellularity, and fibrous stroma.

Mucinous carcinoma of the breast has a much higher ADC, than other malignant breast tumors. The low cellularity and high ratio of mucin within the tumor might be responsible for this effect of high ADC value.

The mean ADC of mucinous carcinoma is higher than that of benign lesions and other malignant tumors. The mean ADC value of pure type mucinous carcinoma is higher than that of mixed type mucinous carcinoma. The homogeneity of signal intensity on diffusion-weighted images correlates with homogeneity of histologic structures of mucinous carcinoma. On diffusion-weighted images, the low signal intensity reflects the presence of mucin and low cellularity, but if there is high signal intensity, it might reflect the presence of fibrovascular bundles and increased cell density.

Imaging Findings

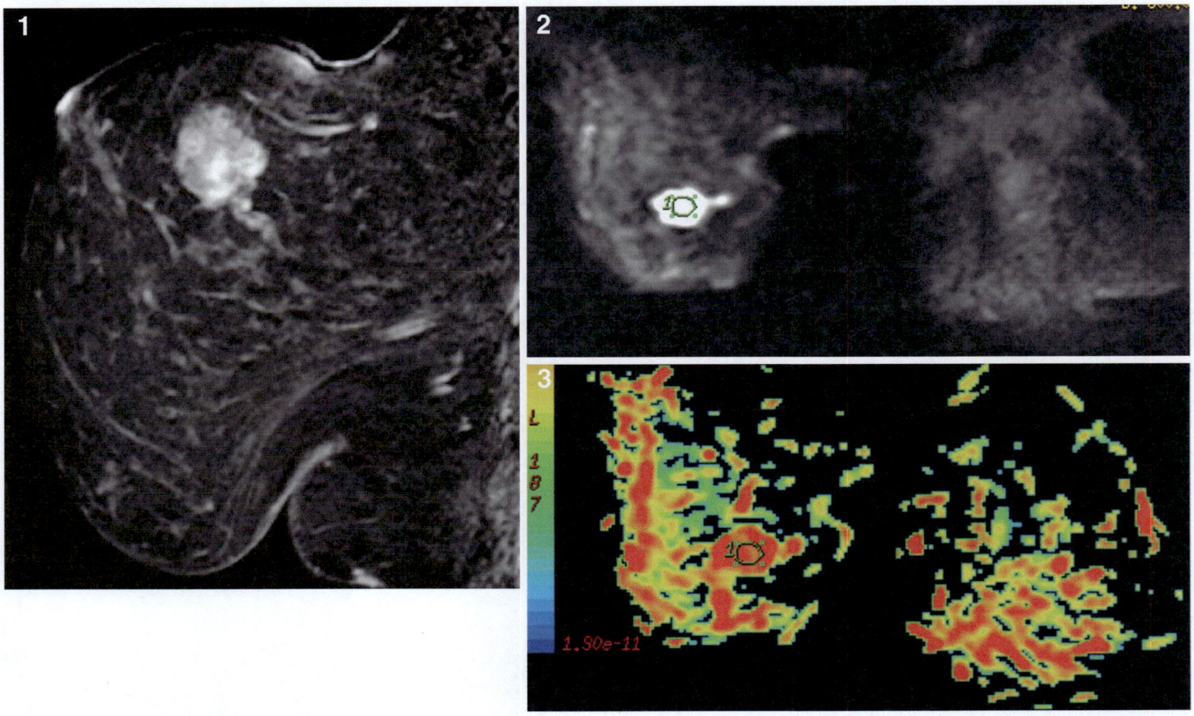

Fig. 10.2 Sagittal 3D contrast-enhanced fat-suppressed GE T1-weighted image (**10.2.1**) shows a lobulated 3-cm tumor in the left breast with a heterogeneous signal enhancement. Axial isotropic DWI (*b*: 700 s/mm^2) image (**10.2.2**) shows a high signal intensity tumor in the left breast. Axial ADC color map image (**10.2.3**) demonstrates the tumor with an ADC value of 2.2×10^{-3} mm^2/s

Case 10.3: Ductal Carcinoma In Situ

A 45-year-old asymptomatic woman presented at our Radiology Department in which a breast MRI examination was performed after an ultrasound study detected a mass in the right breast.

Comments

Ductal carcinoma in situ (DCIS) is a noninvasive malignancy characterized by clonal proliferation of malignant epithelial cells originating in the terminal ductal lobular unit, with no histologic evidence of invasion of the basement membrane. It is most often asymptomatic and may involve multiple sites separated by normal tissue in the same ductal system or in different ductal systems.

DCIS accounts for 20–30% of breast cancers detected at screening mammography and approximately 14–75% of cases may progress to invasive carcinoma.

When DCIS is treated with surgery achieving negative margins and no radiation therapy, the recurrence rate is 22%. Whole-breast radiation therapy reduces the recurrence rate by 52%, and treatment of estrogen receptor–positive cases with tamoxifen reduces this risk by another 50%. The sensitivity of MRI for detection of DCIS is lower than that of invasive carcinoma ranging from 77% to 96%, perhaps because of differences in tumor size, degree of angiogenesis, and histology.

On contrast-enhanced dynamic MRI, DCIS can manifest in a range of appearances. It more frequently presents as a clumped non-mass-like enhancement, in a ductal or segmental distribution, and most commonly showing rapid initial contrast uptake with plateau, persistent enhancement or washout kinetics in the delayed phase. Less common distributions can be seen in DCIS such as regional and focal area of enhancement.

In some studies, the ADC value of DCIS has been shown to be higher than invasive carcinoma, reflecting the endoductal cellular distribution with lower cellular density. In other reports, no significant differences in ADC values have been found between DCIS and invasive carcinoma.

The ADC value of pure DCIS tends to be lower than that of benign masses, although this difference has been shown not to be statistically significant in other studies.

Comedo-type DCIS tumor shows necrosis, hemorrhage, and calcification. The high degree of oxidation, as a consequence of necrosis, affects the high ADC value. Specifically, the strong effect of magnetic susceptibility is one of the reasons for high ADC values in DCIS due to the presence of bleeding.

The scattering, small foci and sparse distribution of DCIS limits the spatial resolution of DWI, which makes it difficult to represent the ADC values, thus reducing the sensitivity of the sequence.

Imaging Findings

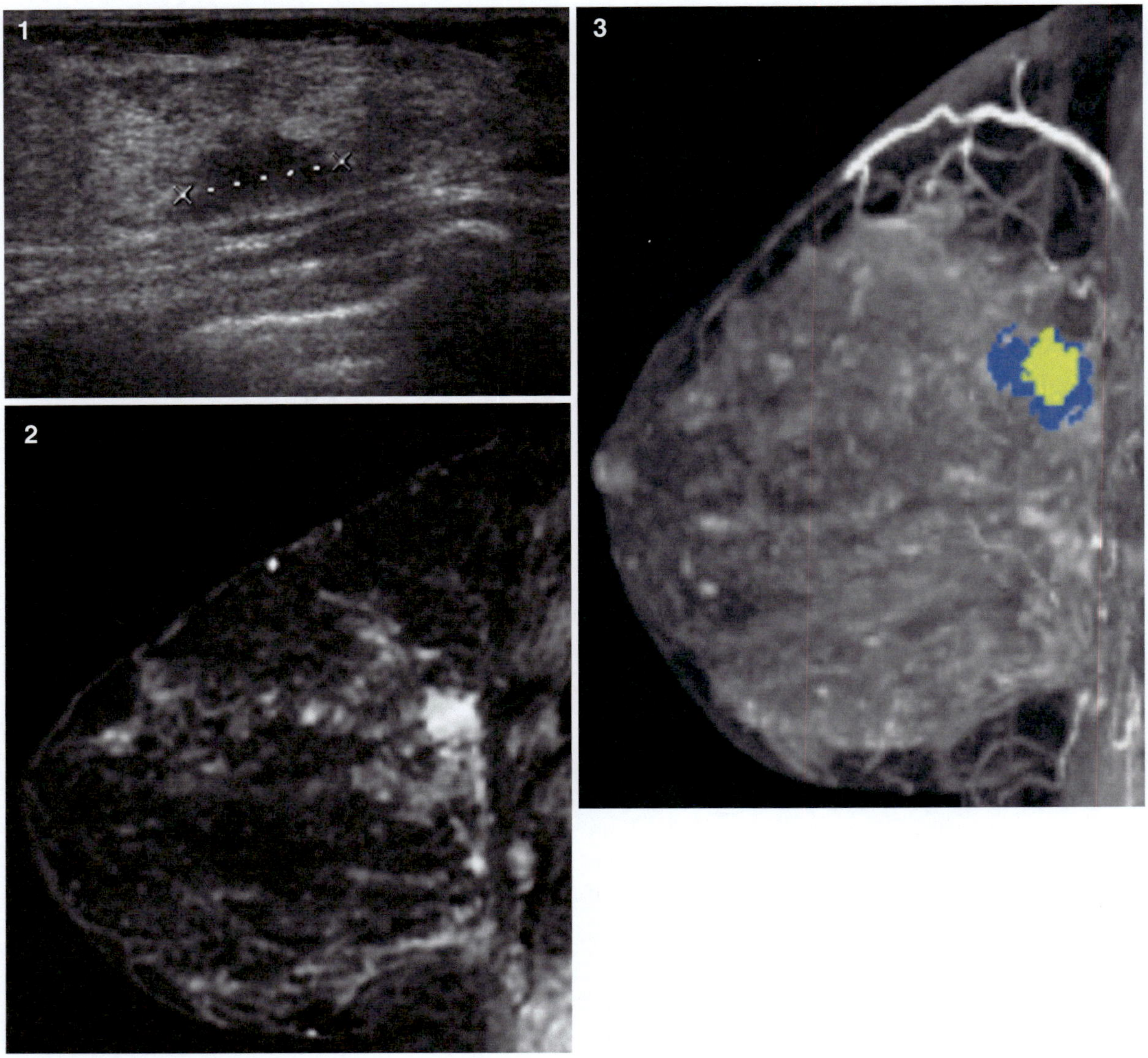

Fig. 10.3 Ultrasound examination shows a solid spiculated mass posteriorly (**10.3.1**) in the right breast, corresponding to a biopsy-proven DCIS grade III. Sagittal 3D contrast-enhanced fat-suppressed GE T1-weighted image (**10.3.2**) demonstrates the prepectoral enhanced spiculated mass in the right breast. Overlay of color parametric map of enhancement kinetics on sagittal MIP of post-contrast phase of dynamic series (**10.3.3**) shows the tumor with kinetic type II in the center (*yellow color*) and type I in the periphery (*blue color*). Axial isotropic DWI (*b*: 700 s/mm^2) image (**10.3.4**) shows high signal intensity within the mass. Axial ADC color map image (**10.3.5**) confirms the restriction of diffusion of the mass with an ADC value of 1.21×10^{-3} mm^2/s (ROI number 1)

Fig. 10.3 (continued)

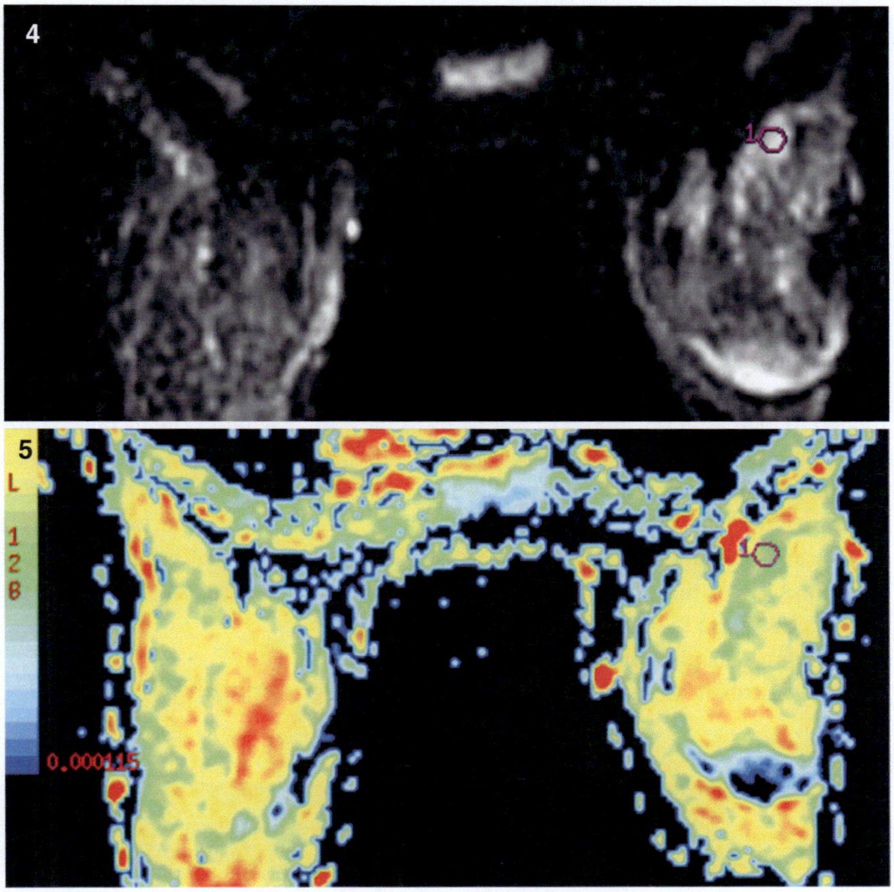

Case 10.4: Fibroadenoma

A 31-year-old woman presented at our department with a palpable tumor in the left breast.

Comments

Fibroadenoma (FA) is the most common benign tumor of the breast. It occurs in 10–15% of all women, with increased incidence in black race. It is most common before the third decade and its cause appears to be related to increased sensitivity to estrogens as they are more common in premenopausal women, pregnant and menopausal women receiving hormone replacement therapy.

FA can occur alone, in groups or as a complex mass. The presence of multiple or complex fibroadenomas may slightly raise the risk of breast cancer.

FA represents proliferation of both fibrous and epithelial elements in varying proportions, demonstrating marked histopathologic variability. The resultant variability in MR appearance limits the ability to distinguish between benign and malignant masses on the bases of signal intensity and enhancement alone. FA frequently has high T2 signal with enhancement, but also can show low T2 signal without enhancement in cases associated with more sclerotic stroma and older patient age. After the administration of contrast, only 22% of FA might show a suspicious signal intensity-time course.

FA often has lobular, oval, or round shape (83%), well-defined margins (87%), and internal septations without enhancement (30–60%), which appears to correlate with collagenous bands.

The mean ADC value of benign lesions, such as fibroadenoma, is frequently higher ($1.6 \pm 0.5 \times 10^{-3}$ mm²/s) than malignant ones, but not all FA will show high ADC values, as it depends on their internal structure.

Imaging Findings

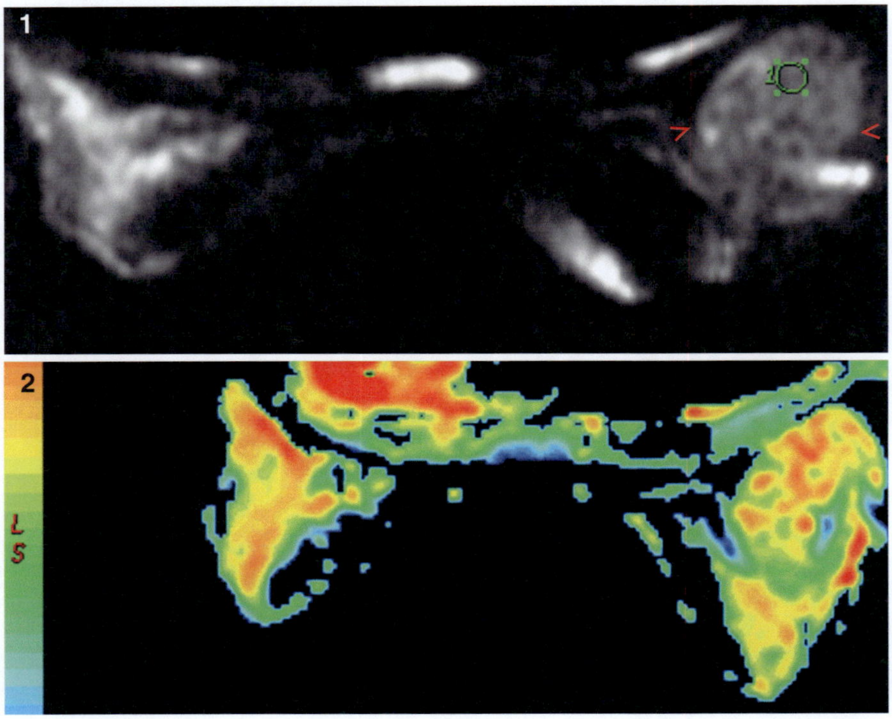

Fig. 10.4 Axial isotropic DWI (*b*: 700 s/mm²) image (**10.4.1**) shows a round and well-circumscribed mass in the right breast, with isointensity and heterogeneous signal (*arrowheads*, ROI number 1). Axial ADC color scale map image (**10.4.2**) demonstrates the tumor without significant diffusion restriction and an ADC value of 1.91×10^{-3} mm²/s. These findings are typical of a benign tumor (in this case a fibroadenoma)

Case 10.5: Borderline Phyllodes Tumor

A 43-year-old woman presented with a large palpable tumor in the left breast, which has grown on a fast rate during last month.

Comments

Phyllodes tumors (PT) are fibroepithelial neoplasms composed of an epithelial and a cellular stromal component. They may be considered benign, borderline, or malignant depending on histologic features. Approximately 20–50% of PT are reported to be malignant.

They account for less than 1% of all breast neoplasms, and they are found predominantly in adult women (age range of 40 to 50 years) prior to the menopause. These tumors are usually very fast growing.

Treatment of both benign and malignant PT requires a complete surgical excision with wide margins owing to the high recurrence rate in patients with resection margins of less than 1 cm around the primary tumor.

Some studies have shown findings suggestive of histopathologically malignant PT of the breast such as tumor signal intensity higher than normal breast tissue, high signal intensity on T1-weighted images (corresponding to hemorrhage), cystic changes with irregular walls (corresponding to necrotic changes), tumor signal intensity lower than or equal to normal breast tissue signal intensity on T2-weighted images, and/or low ADC on diffusion-weighted images.

The ADC value for benign PT has been shown higher than borderline ones; and malignant PT has even demonstrated the lowest ACD values between all subtypes of PT. These low ADC values in malignant PT have been attributed to stromal hypercellularity.

Tumor size, cystic changes with smooth wall, and time-signal intensity curve pattern have not correlated significantly with histologic grade of PT.

Imaging Findings

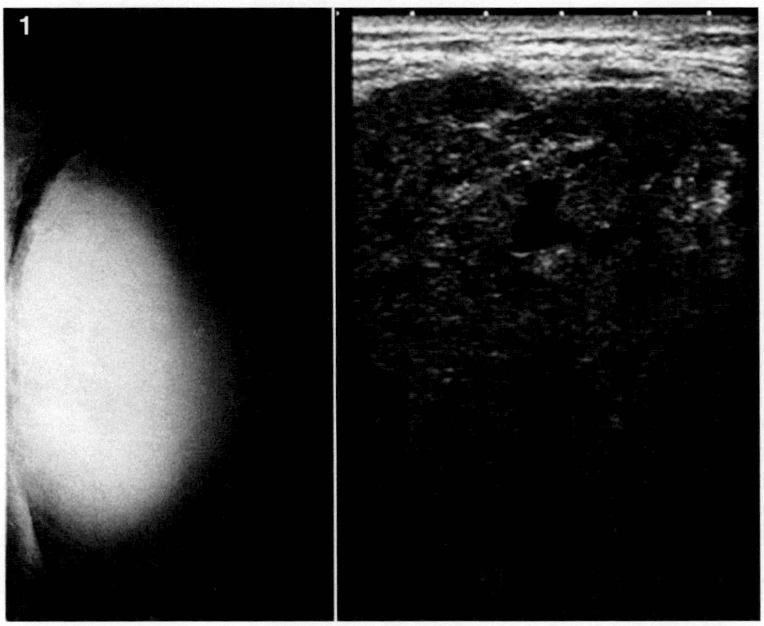

Fig. 10.5 Plain oblique mammography and ultrasound (**10.5.1**) show a large well-defined round lesion in the left breast with irregular walls (corresponding to necrotic changes). Axial FSE T1-weighted and fat-suppressed FSE T2-weighted images (**10.5.2**, top and bottom, respectively) show a lobulated, well-defined mass with septa. Sagittal 3D contrast-enhanced fat-suppressed GE T1-weighted image acquired 2 minutes after contrast injection image (**10.5.3**) shows an enhancing lesion with enhancement kinetics type II–III. The septa do not show enhancement. Axial isotropic DWI (*b*: 700 s/mm^2) image (**10.5.4**) demonstrates predominantly high signal intensity within the large tumor. Axial ADC color scale map image (**10.5.5**) shows an ADC value of 1.8×10^{-3} mm^2/s. This was a false-negative result according to DCE and DWI findings

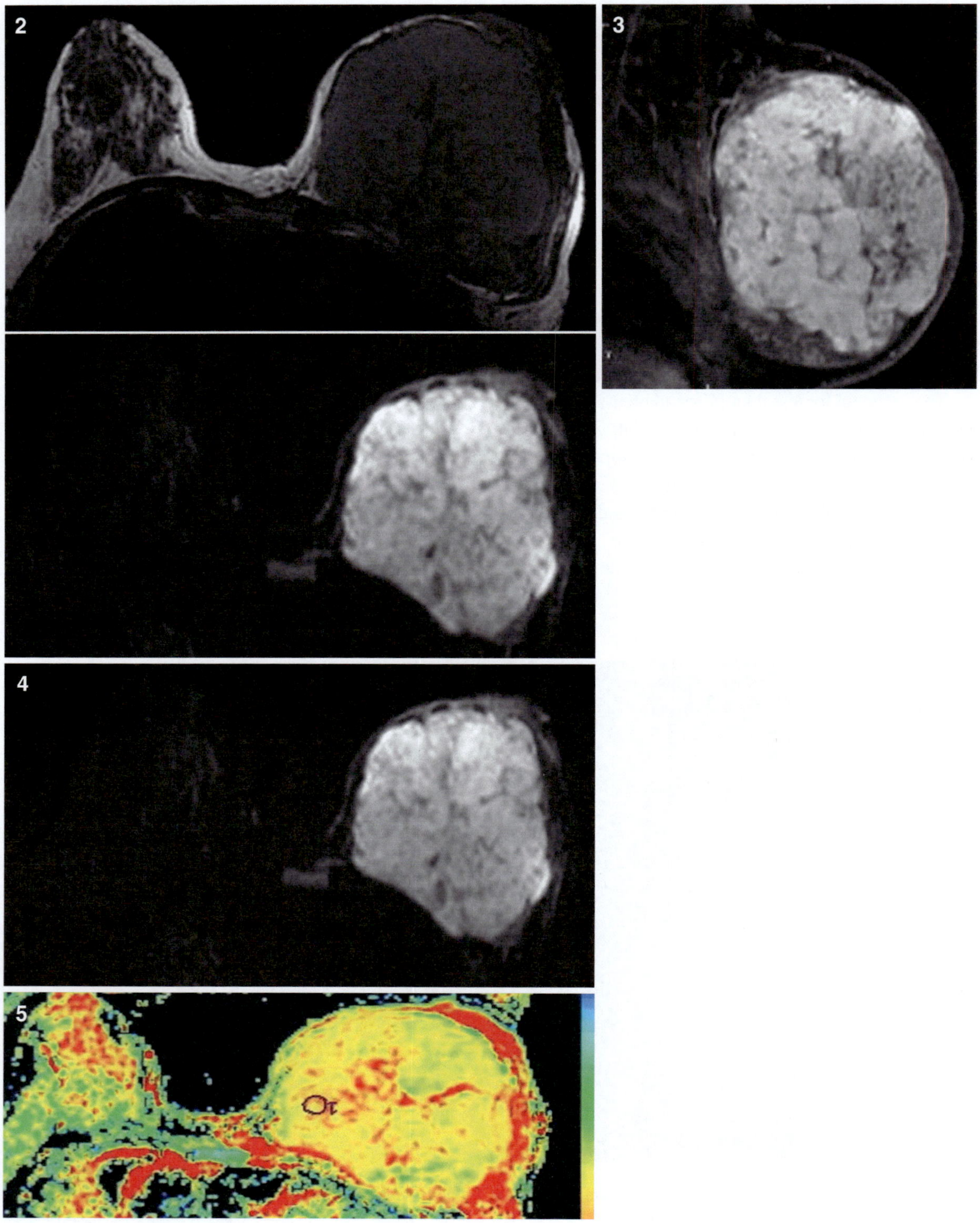

Fig. 10.5 (continued)

Case 10.6: Infiltrating Lobulillar Carcinoma

A 73-year-old female presented in a mammography a intermediate concern cluster of micro calcifications in upper outer quadrant of right breast, which were unchanged in comparison with previous mammogram performed 1 year before. The patient was sent to our center to perform a functional breast MRI in a 3 T magnet for further characterization as she was reluctant to undergo a biopsy.

Comments

In this example, an invasive lobulillar carcinoma showed a mild restriction of free water movement, in the range of benign lesions, when using a monoexponential signal decay approach. However, DCE-MRI clearly suggested malignancy. This finding reinforces the concept of tumor heterogeneity, as sometimes different functional techniques will yield distinct results indicating the complex structure and nature of cancer. Therefore, the concept of multiparametric imaging is necessary to integrate information from different functional imaging or MRI techniques.

Besides, some controversy exists about the role of ADC measurement in breast cancer grading, as several studies have not found significant differences in ADC values between intraductal and invasive carcinomas, whereas other reports have shown significant differences.

Fig. 10.6 A new appearing cluster of suspicious microcalcifications was identified in routine screening mammography in right upper outer quadrant (**10.6.1**, right cranio-caudal mammography). Dynamic contrast-enhanced MRI confirmed a regional enhancement with maximum diameter of 5 cm (**10.6.2**), whose enhancement pattern was consistent with malignancy (**10.6.3**) Axial MIP of the first dynamic postcontrast series (**10.6.4**) better depicted the tumoral extension, the absence of additional foci, and the presence of enlarged right axillary lymph nodes (*arrows*). Axial DWI with *b* value of 1000 s/mm^2 (**10.6.5**) at the same level as that of Fig. **10.6.2** showed a moderately high signal intensity of the lesion, which also demosntrated a moderate restriction on ADC map, with a mean ADC value of 1.48×10^{-3} mm^2/s (**10.6.6**). A core biopsy confirmed infiltrating lobulillar carcinoma of right breast with right axillary nodal metastases

Imaging Findings

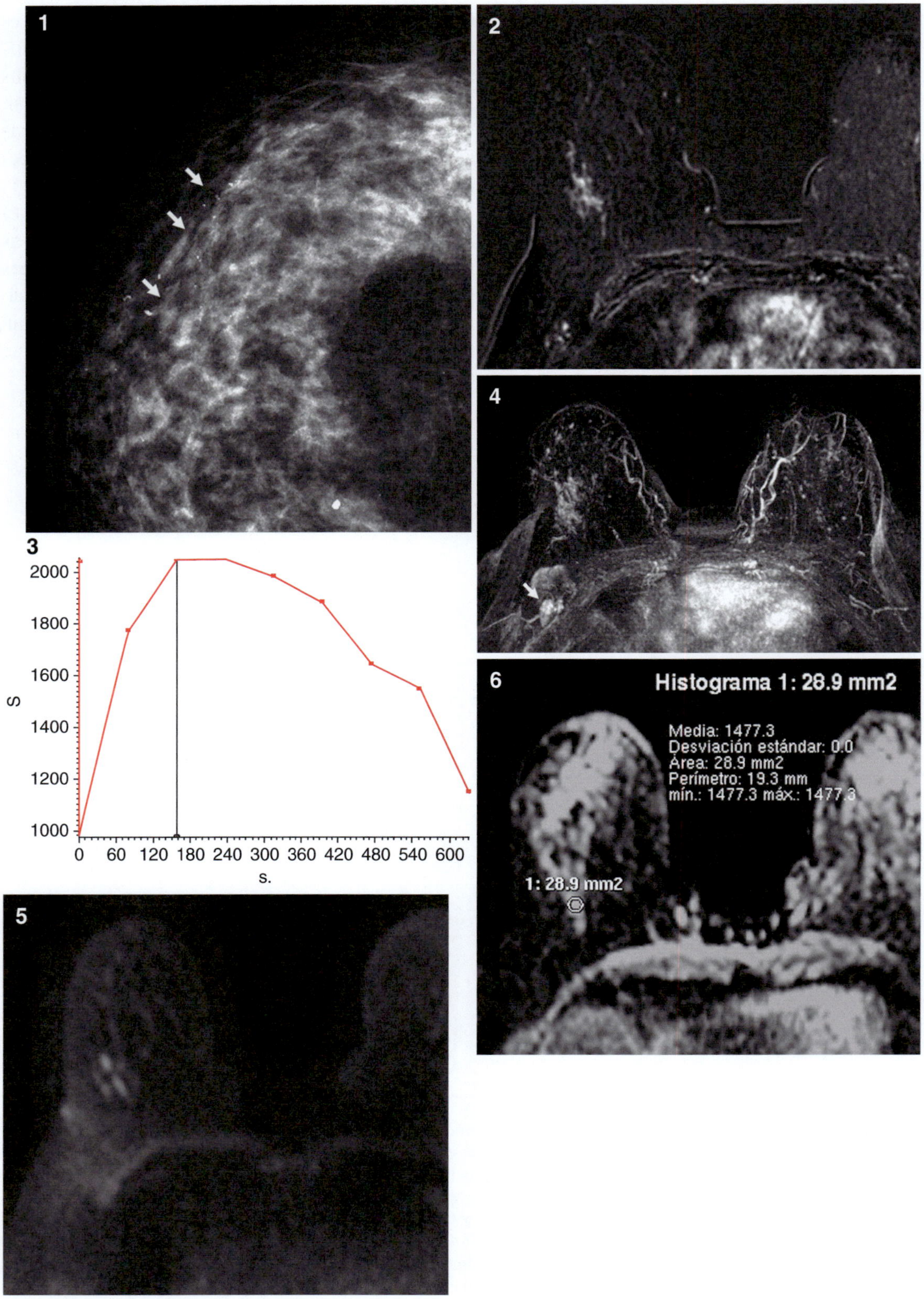

Case 10.7: Invasive Lobulillar Carcinoma – IVIM Approach

Same case as Fig. 10.6. Additional information for breast lesion characterization was obtained by means of the IVIM analysis of DWI and spectroscopy.

Comments

Biexponential analysis of diffusion signal decay in the breast has been little studied. The IVIM approach allows us to separate the perfusion and diffusion of the tissues, avoiding the microperfusion effect in the quantification of tumor diffusion. Therefore, true diffusion (*D*) is potentially a more accurate parameter than ADC, and perfusion fraction may reflect the microvascularization of cancer (microvascular density). In this example, a difference exists between *D* and ADC values, being *D* value lower than ADC, and in the range of malignant lesions.

Tamura et al. described in a recent report that the signal decay of normal mammary glands, most cysts, and some fibroadenomas fitted to a monoexponential model of DWI signal decay, but intraductal papilloma and malignant tumors were better fitted by a biexponential function. However, the authors found no significant difference between benign and malignant lesions derived from the biexponential fitting, although the fast component fraction of DWI of noninvasive ductal carcinoma was statistically greater than that of invasive ductal carcinoma. Similarly, recent results by Sigmund et al. found that normal tissue was better fitted to a monoexponential approach and lesions to a biexponential one. Their data indicated significant differences between normal fibroglandular tissue and malignant lesions in mean ADC and *D*. They found differences in f values for invasive ductal carcinoma versus other malignant lesions. In their series, correlation of IVIM-derived biomarkers with DCE-MRI ones was only moderate. Therefore, further research is needed in this field, as the IVIM approach may increase the applications of DWI for breast diseases.

Fig. 10.7 (**10.7.1**) Axial DWI with a *b* value of 25 s/mm^2 at the same level as that of Fig. **10.6.5** was part of our breast IVIM DWI sequence that included 7 *b* values (0, 25, 50, 100, 250, 500, 1,000 s/mm^2). (**10.7.2**) Graph of the biexponential signal decay of the tumor showed a first fast decay related to tumoral perfusion with *b* values under 100 s/mm^2 and a more flattened slope of signal decay with *b* values over 100 s/mm^2 related to true diffusion. (**10.7.3**, **10.7.4**) *D* (true diffusion) and *f* (perfusion fraction) parametric maps of the tumor, respectively. Notice the correlation with the relative enhancement map derived from a monocompartmental analysis of the dynamic postcontrast series (**10.7.5**). Tumoral perfusion fraction measured with the IVIM approach was that of 12%. Tumoral *D* value of 1.34×10^{-3} mm^2/s was lower than ADC obtained from monocompartmental analysis of diffusion signal decay, and more suspicious for malignancy. Single-voxel spectroscopy demonstrated the presence of elevated choline, consistent with malignancy (**10.7.6**). As spectroscopy was performed before the dynamic series, DWI was used to correctly place the voxel (**10.7.7**). A core biopsy confirmed infiltrating lobulillar carcinoma of right breast with right axillary nodal metastases

Imaging Findings

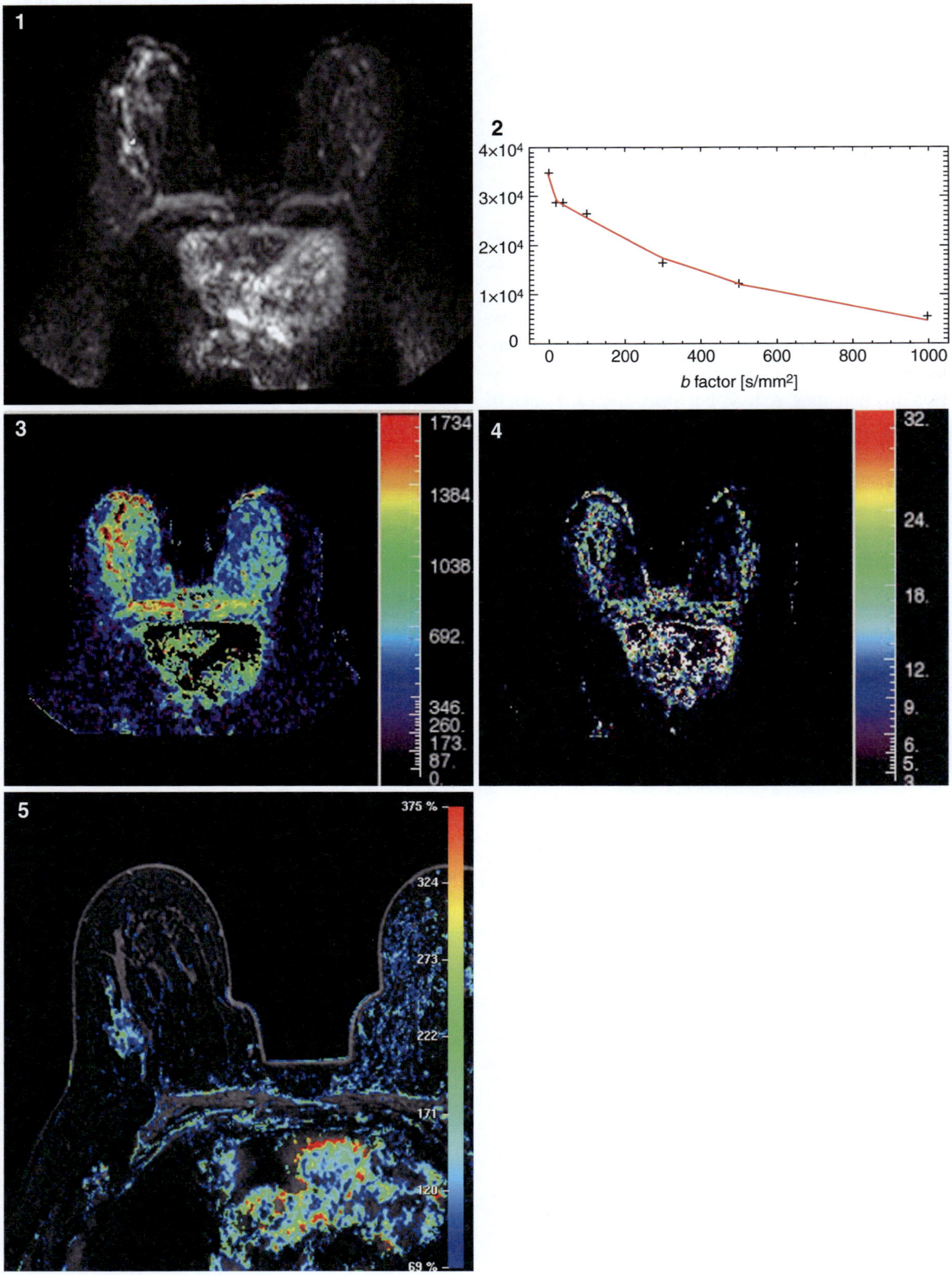

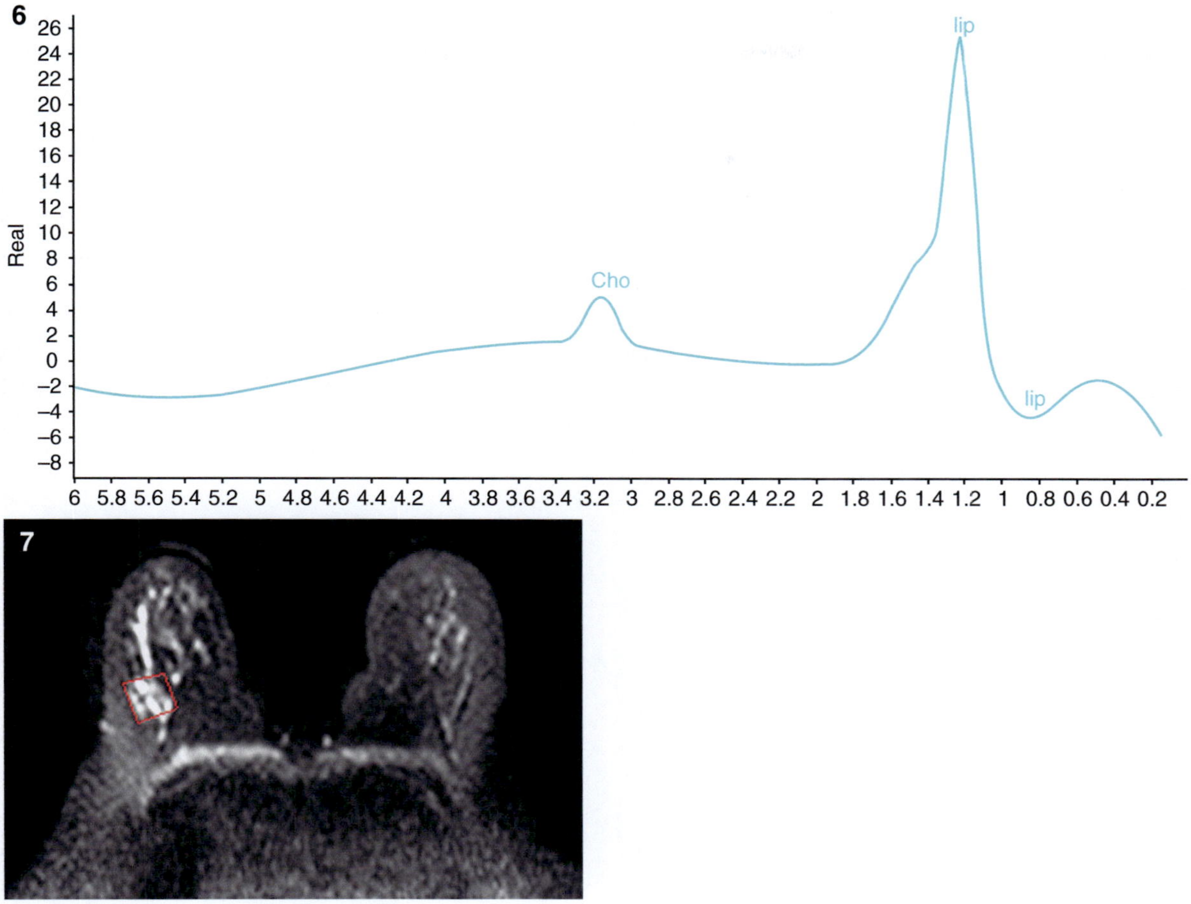

Fig. 10.7 (continued)

Case 10.8: Post-treatment Monitorization of Lobulillar Carcinoma

A 53-year-old female with confirmed lobulillar carcinoma of left breast is sent to our center to exclude additional areas of malignancy.

Comments

Functional information derived for DWI is under evaluation for monitoring response to NAC. Responders will show a significant elevation of ADC before changes in volume and size occur. These changes have been described as soon as 48 h after the start of therapy. Therefore, DWI may be used as an early biomarker of tumor response or to assess overall response. Recently, Woodhams and colleagues evaluated 72 patients with 73 breast cancers treated with chemotherapy, they could accurately depict residual tumor with DWI. Reported accuracy was 96% for DWI, compared with an accuracy of 89% for DCE-MRI. According to this data, DWI may be considered a valid alternative to DCE-MRI in this task. In the example presented, there is a nice correlation in both pre- and posttreatment MRI studies between DWI and DCE-MRI.

Imaging Findings

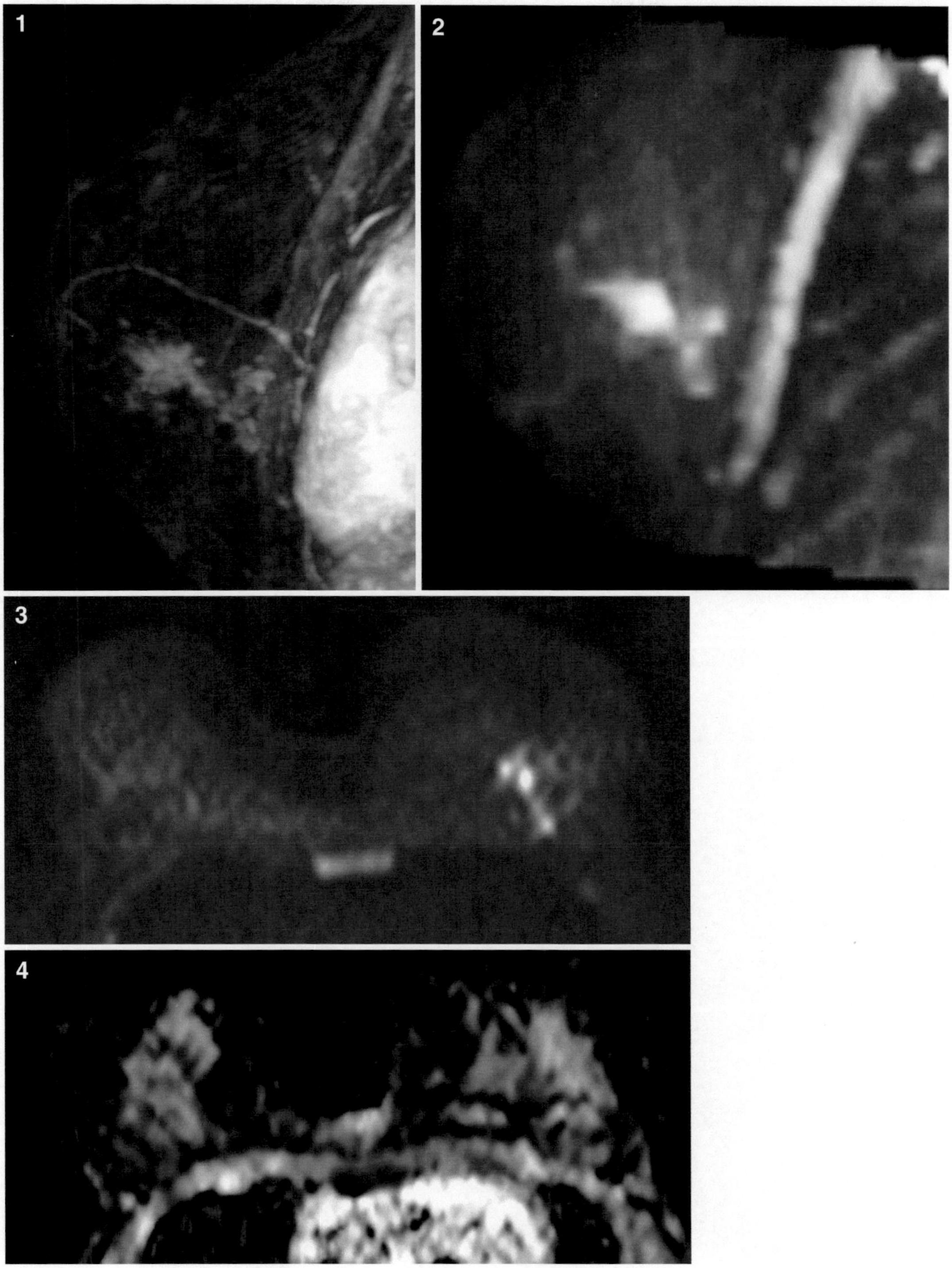

Fig. 10.8 (**10.8.1–10.8.4**) Pretreatment MRI. Sagittal MIP of the first postcontrast dynamic series demonstrated a spiculated mass of 57 × 29 mm in the lower quadrants of left breast (**10.8.1**). Similar findings may be found in a sagittal MIP from DWI with a *b* value of 1000 s/mm^2 (**10.8.2**). Axial DWI with a *b* value of 1000 s/mm^2 (**10.8.3**) confirmed the mass as a high-intensity lesion related to impeded free water motion, as confirmed in the ADC map (**10.8.4**). Mean ADC value was 0.9×10^{-3} mm^2/s. (**10.8.5–10.8.8**) Posttreatment MRI after 6 months of chemotherapy. Corresponding images to first MRI demonstrated a moderate reduction in size of the mass, which presented maximum diameters of 23 × 21 mm, and reduction of restriction of diffusion, with an ADC value of 1.1×10^{-3} mm^2/s. All these findings suggested only partial response according to RECIST criteria

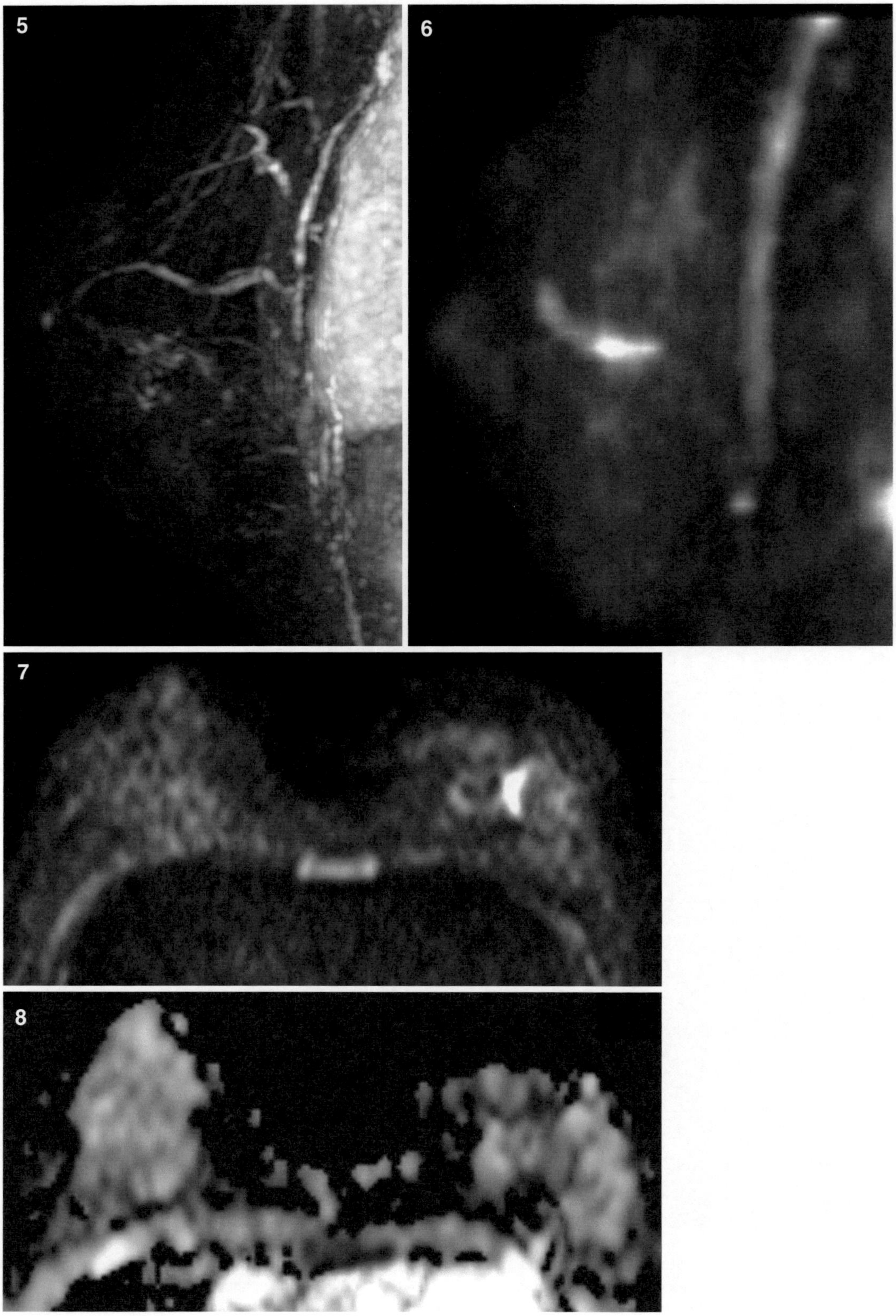

Fig. 10.8 (continued)

Case 10.9: Post-treatment Monitorization of Multifocal Infiltrating Ductal Carcinoma

A 78-year-old female is sent to our department for staging of infiltrating ductal carcinoma.

Comments

In this case, the reduction of tumor volume and lesions is consistent with only partial response, although the marked elevation of ADC suggests a better prognosis than in cases in which this elevation does not occur. As previously commented, DWI is a useful biomarker in monitoring response to chemotherapy.

Another area of research is the prediction of response to treatment with DWI. Pretreatment low ADC values have been related to responding tumors, as lower ADC values indicate viable tissue with high cellularity. Conversely, high ADC values indicate necrotic tissue with low cellularity. Therefore, lower pretreatment ADC values enable a major number of cells to be targeted by the chemotherapeutic agents. In the series by Park and colleagues, pretreatment mean ADC of responders was significantly lower than that of nonresponders and mean percentage ADC increase of responders was higher than that of nonresponders. In this series, the best pretreatment ADC cutoff to differentiate between responders and nonresponders was 1.17×10^{-3} mm²/s, which yielded a sensitivity of 94% and a specificity of 71%, using a DWI sequence with a maximum *b* value of 750 s/mm² in a 1.5 T magnet.

Imaging Findings

1

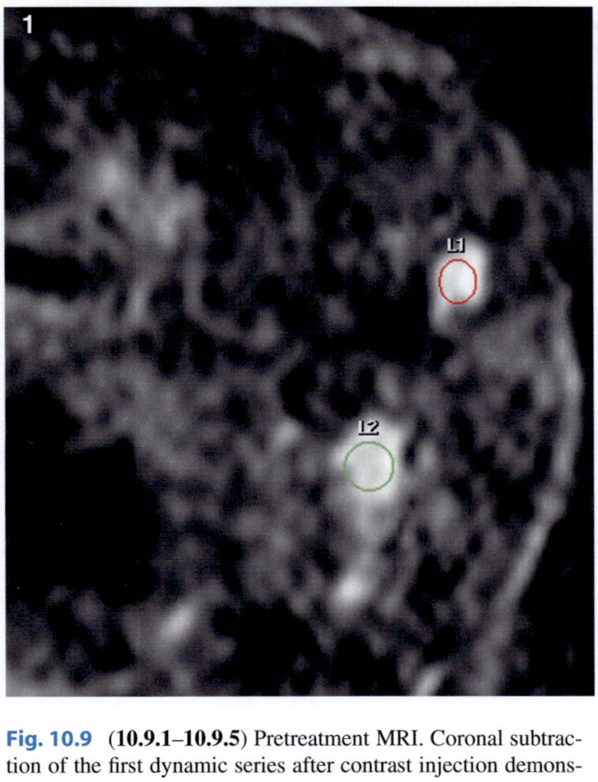

2

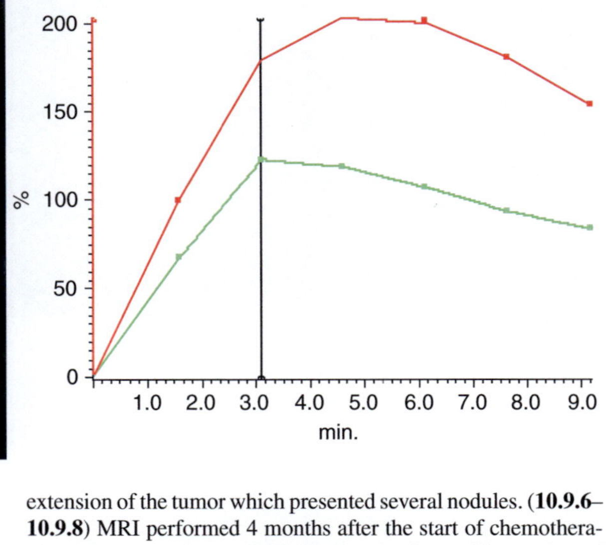

Fig. 10.9 (**10.9.1–10.9.5**) Pretreatment MRI. Coronal subtraction of the first dynamic series after contrast injection demonstrated two enhancing lesions (**10.9.1**), whose enhancement (signal intensity/time) curves are consistent with malignancy (**10.9.2**). Axial DWI with a *b* value of 1000 s/mm² and corresponding ADC map (**10.9.3** and **10.9.4** respectively) showed marked restriction of free water diffusion consistent with malignancy (ADC value: 1×10^{-3} mm²/s) (*arrows*). Sagittal MIP from DWI with a *b* value of 1000 s/mm² (**10.9.5**) demonstrated the extension of the tumor which presented several nodules. (**10.9.6–10.9.8**) MRI performed 4 months after the start of chemotheraphy demonstrated a marked reduction in size and in number of the nodules identified in the pretreatment MRI, as confirmed in sagittal MIP from DWI with a *b* value of 1000 s/mm² (**10.9.6**). ADC increased up to 1.9×10^{-3} mm²/s, as shown in axial DWI with a *b* value of 1000 s/mm² and corresponding ADC map (**10.9.7** and **10.9.8**, respectively), located at a similar level than Figs. **10.9.3** and **10.9.4**, respectively

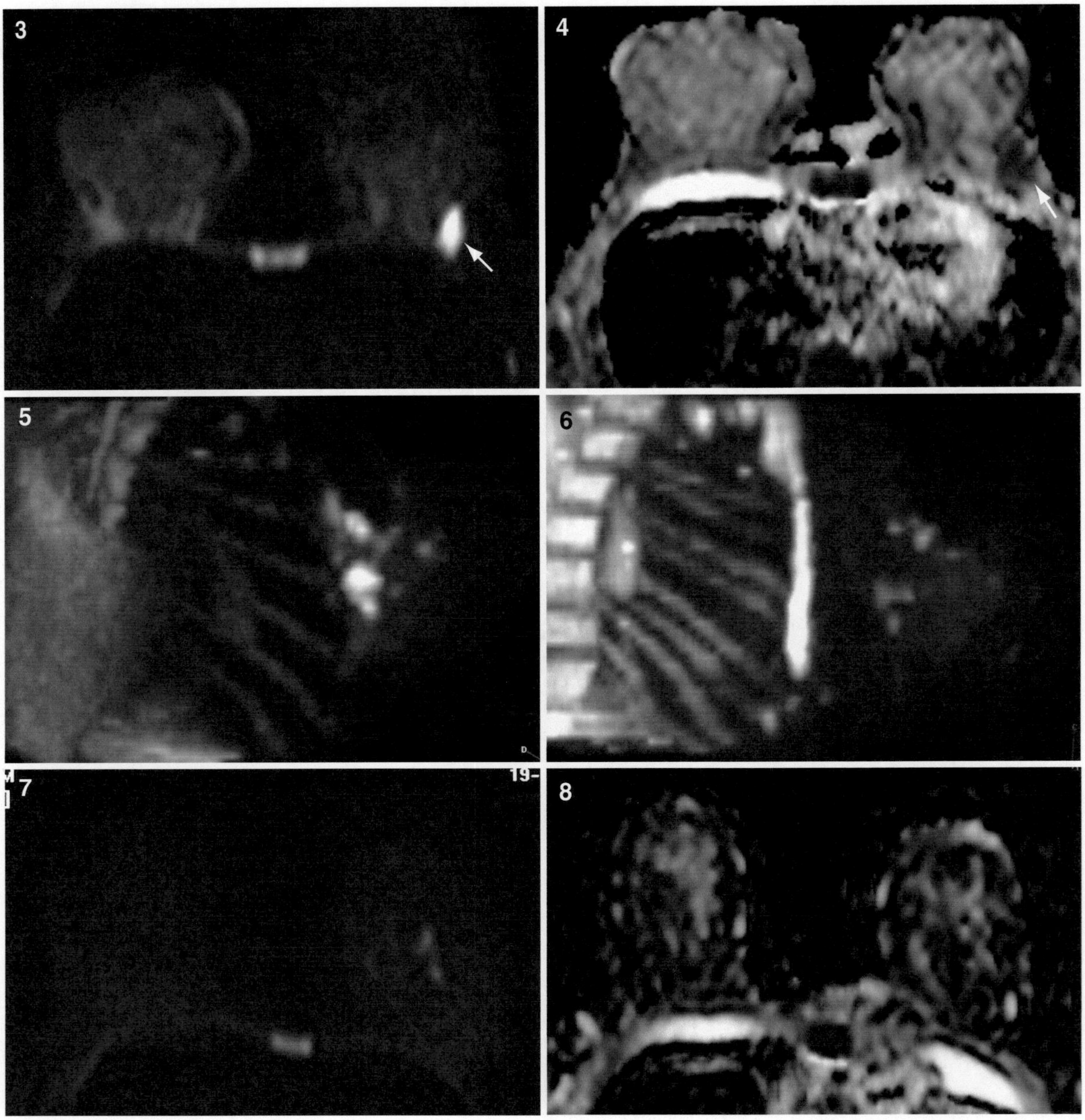

Fig. 10.9 (continued)

Case 10.10: Recurrent Invasive Ductal Carcinoma

A 71-year-old female with antecedent of left mastectomy 4 years ago for an invasive ductal carcinoma was submitted to our department to perform a breast MRI, after a nodule was suspected in physical examination of the scar.

Comments

Rinaldi and colleagues demonstrated than that ADC value of recurrences was statistically lower than that of scarring, in patients operated with breast cancer. DWI may be an adjunct tool to DCE-MRI in the evaluation of recurrent tumors as these are usually more hypercellular than fibrous tissue. This example shows the potential role of DWI for assessment of recurrence after breast cancer therapy.

Imaging Findings

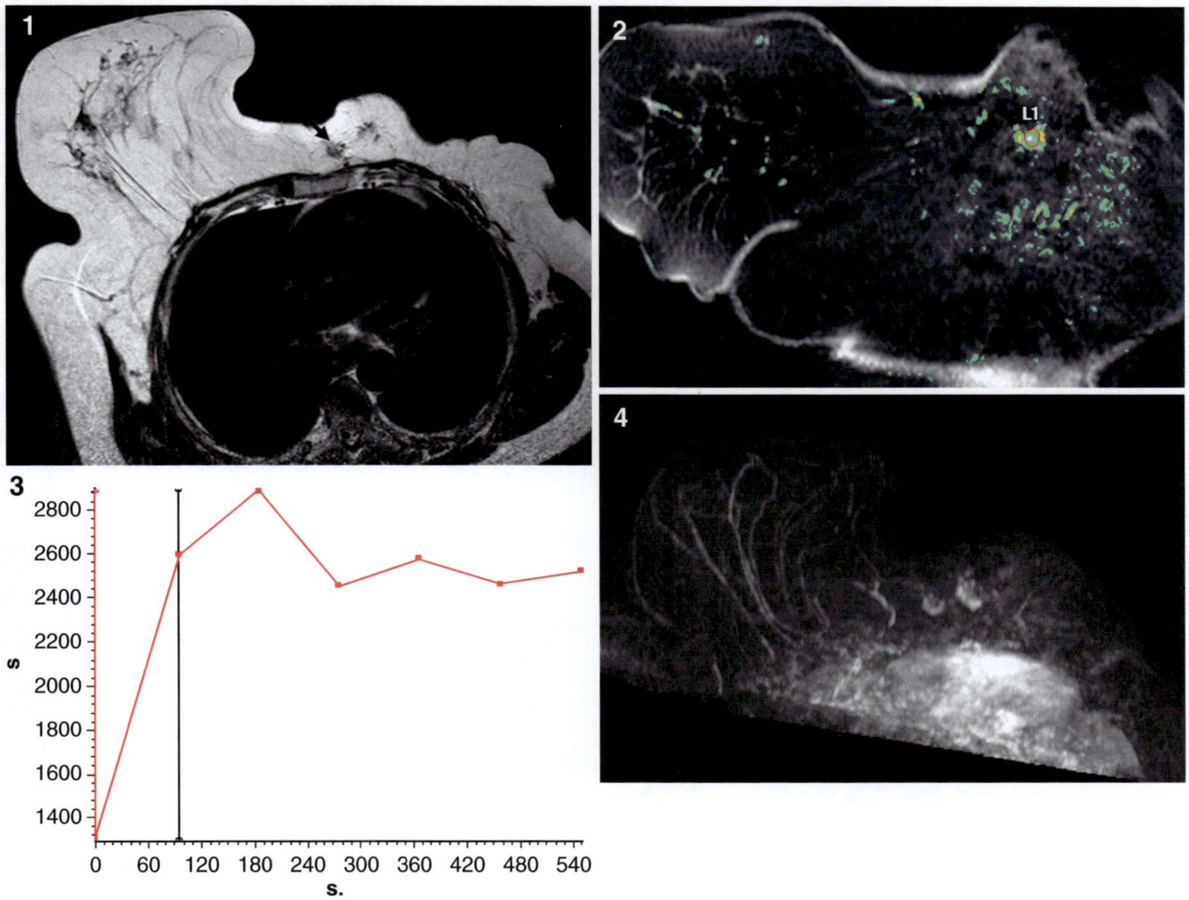

Fig. 10.10 Axial TSE T2-weighted image showed a nodule within the inferior aspect of the scar (**10.10.1**). In the postcontrast dynamic series, fast enhancement with posterior wash-out is seen suggesting malignancy (**10.10.2** and **10.10.3**). Axial MIP of the first postcontrast dynamic series demonstrated two hypervascular nodules adjacent to the scar area (**10.10.4**). Notice the nice correlation with the axial MIP obtained from DWI with a *b* value of 1000 s/mm^2 (**10.10.5**). Low ADC value of the largest nodule (ADC value: 0.8×10^{-3} mm^2/s) is consistent with malignancy, as it was confirmed on biopsy (**10.10.6**)

Fig. 10.10 (continued)

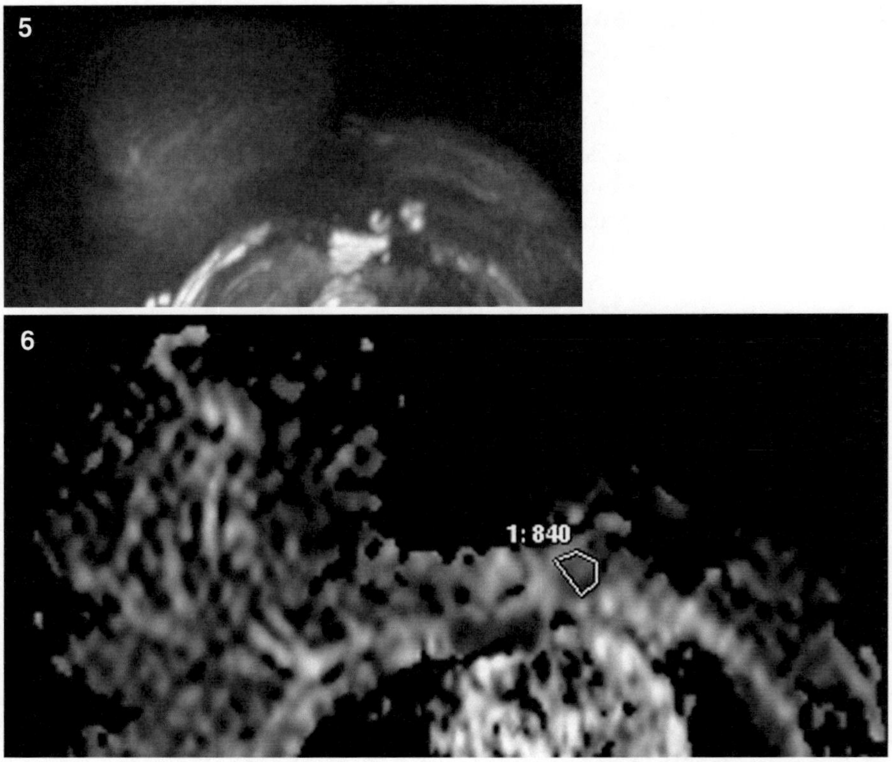

Further Reading

Arantes F, Martins G, Figueiredo E et al (2009) Assessment of breast lesions with diffusion-weighted MRI: comparing the use of different b values. Am J Roentgenol 193: 1030–1035

Baltzer PA, Benndorf M, Dietzel M et al (2010) Sensitivity and specificity of unenhanced MR mammography (DWI combined with T2-weighted TSE imaging, ueMRM) for the differentiation of mass lesions. Eur Radiol 20(5):1101–1110

Barceló J, Vilanova JC, Albanell J et al (2009) Breast MRI: the usefulness of diffusion-weighted sequences for differentiating between benign and malignant lesions. Radiología 51(5):469–476

Baron P, Dorrius MD, Kappert P et al (2010) Diffusion-weighted imaging of normal fibroglandular breast tissue: influence of microperfusion and fat suppression technique on the apparent diffusion coefficient. NMR Biomed 23(4):399–405

Bogner W, Gruber S, Pinker K et al (2009) Diffusion-weighted MR for differentiation of breast lesions at 3.0 T: how does selection of diffusion protocols affect diagnosis? Radiology 253(2):341–351

Chen X, Li WL, Zhang YL et al (2010) Meta-analysis of quantitative diffusion-weighted MR imaging in the differential diagnosis of breast lesions. BMC Cancer 29(10):693–704

Costantini M, Belli P, Rinaldi P et al (2010) Diffusion-weighted imaging in breast cancer: relationship between apparent diffusion coefficient and tumour aggressiveness. Clin Radiol 65(12):1005–1012

Ei Khouli RH, Jacobs MA, Mezban SD et al (2010) Diffusion-weighted imaging improves the diagnostic accuracy of conventional 3.0-T breast MR imaging. Radiology 256(1):64–73

Fangberget A, Nilsen LB, Hole KH et al (2011) Neoadjuvant chemotherapy in breast cancer-response evaluation and prediction of response to treatment using dynamic contrast-enhanced and diffusion-weighted MR imaging. Eur Radiol 21(6):1188–1199

Guo Y, Cai YQ, Cai ZL et al (2002) Differentiation of clinically benign and malignant breast lesions using diffusion-weighted imaging. J Magn Reson Imaging 16:172–178

Heusner TA, Kuemmel S, Hamami ME et al (2010) Diagnostic value of DWI MRI compared to FDG PET/CT for whole body breast cancer staging. Eur J Nucl Med Mol Imaging 37(6):1077–1086

Huang W, Fisher PR, Dulaimy K et al (2004) Detection of breast malignancy: diagnostic MR protocol for improved specificity. Radiology 232:585–591

Iacconi C (2010) Diffusion and perfusion of the breast. Eur J Radiol 76(3):386–390

Imamura T, Isomoto I, Sueyoshi E et al (2010) Diagnostic performance of ADC for non-mass-like breast lesions on MR imaging. Magn Reson Med Sci 9(4):217–225

Jacobs MA, Barker PB, Bluemke DA et al (2003) Benign and malignant breast lesions diagnosis with multiparametric MR imaging. Radiology 229:225–232

Jeh SK, Kim SH, Kim HS et al (2011) Correlation of the apparent diffusion coefficient value and dynamic magnetic resonance imaging findings with prognostic factors in invasive ductal carcinoma. J Magn Reson Imaging 33(1):102–109. doi:10.1002/jmri.22400

Kim SH, Cha ES, Kim HS et al (2009) Diffusion-weighted imaging of breast cancer: correlation of the apparent diffusion coefficient value with prognostic factors. J Magn Reson Imaging 30(3):615–620

Kinoshita T, Yashiro N, Ihara N et al (2002) Diffusion-weighted half-fourier single-shot turbo spin echo imaging in breast tumors: differentiation of invasive ductal carcinoma from fibroadenoma. J Comput Assist Tomogr 26:1042–1046

Kul S, Cansu A, Alhan E et al (2011) Contribution of diffusion-weighted imaging to dynamic contrast-enhanced MRI in the characterization of breast tumors. Am J Roentgenol 196(1): 210–217

Kuroki Y, Nasu K, Kuroki S et al (2004) Diffusion-weighted imaging of breast cancer with the sensitivity encoding technique: analysis of the apparent diffusion coefficient value. Magn Reson Med Sci 3:79–85

Marini C, Iacconi C, Giannelli M et al (2007) Quantitative diffusion-weighted MR imaging in the differential diagnosis of breast lesion. Eur Radiol 17:2646–2655

Matsubayashi RN, Fujii T, Yasumori K et al (2010) Apparent diffusion coefficient in invasive ductal breast carcinoma: correlation with detailed histologic features and the enhancement ratio on dynamic contrast-enhanced MR images. J Oncol 2010:pii: 821048, Epub Sep 2, 2010

Nunes LW, Schanall MD, Orel SG (2001) Update of breast MR imaging architectural interpretation model. Radiology 219: 484–494

Park SH, Moon WK, Cho N et al (2010) Diffusion-weighted MR imaging: pretreatment prediction of response to neoadjuvant chemotherapy in patients with breast cancer. Radiology 257(1):56–63

Partridge S, De Martini W, Kurland B et al (2009) Quantitative diffusion-weighted imaging as an adjunct to conventional breast MRI for improved positive predictive value. Am J Roentgenol 193:1716–1722

Partridge SC, Demartini WB, Kurland BF et al (2010) Differential diagnosis of mammographically and clinically occult breast lesions on diffusion-weighted MRI. J Magn Reson Imaging 31(3):562–570

Partridge SC, Mullins CD, Kurland BF et al (2010) Apparent diffusion coefficient values for discriminating benign and malignant breast MRI lesions: effects of lesion type and size. Am J Roentgenol 194(6):1664–1673

Partridge SC, Ziadloo A, Murthy R et al (2010) Diffusion tensor MRI: preliminary anisotropy measures and mapping of breast tumors. J Magn Reson Imaging 31(2):339–347

Partridge SC, Rahbar H, Murthy R et al (2011) Improved diagnostic accuracy of breast MRI through combined apparent diffusion coefficients and dynamic contrast-enhanced kinetics. Magn Reson Med. doi:10.1002/mrm.22762, Epub ahead of print

Pediconi F, Catalano C, Occhiato R et al (2005) Breast lesion detection and characterization at contrast-enhanced MR mammography: gadobenate dimeglumine versus gadopentetate dimeglumine. Radiology 237:45–56

Pereira FP, Martins G, Figueiredo E et al (2009) Assessment of breast lesions with diffusion-weighted MRI: comparing the use of different b values. Am J Roentgenol 193(4): 1030–1035

Pereira FP, Martins G, Carvalhaes de Oliveira Rde V (2011) Diffusion magnetic resonance imaging of the breast. Magn Reson Imaging Clin N Am 19(1):95–110

Peters NH, Vincken KL, van den Bosch MA et al (2010) Quantitative diffusion weighted imaging for differentiation of benign and malignant breast lesions: the influence of the choice of b-values. J Magn Reson Imaging 31(5): 1100–1105

Pickles MD, Gibbs P, Lowry M et al (2006) Diffusion changes precede size reduction in neoadjuvant treatment of breast cancer. Magn Reson Imaging 24(7):843–847

Rinaldi P, Giuliani M, Belli P et al (2010) DWI in breast MRI: role of ADC value to determine diagnosis between recurrent tumor and surgical scar in operated patients. Eur J Radiol 75(2):e114–e123

Rubesova E, Grell AS, De Maertelaer V et al (2006) Quantitative diffusion imaging in breast cancer: a clinical prospective study. J Magn Reson Imaging 24:319–324

Satake H, Nishio A, Ikeda M et al (2011) Predictive value for malignancy of suspicious breast masses of BI-RADS categories 4 and 5 using ultrasound elastography and MR diffusion-weighted imaging. Am J Roentgenol 196(1):202–209

Sharma U, Danishad KK, Seenu V et al (2009) Longitudinal study of the assessment by MRI and diffusion-weighted imaging of tumor response in patients with locally advanced breast cancer undergoing neoadjuvant chemotherapy. NMR Biomed 22(1):104–113

Sigmund EE, Cho GY, Kim S et al (2011) Intravoxel incoherent motion imaging of tumor microenvironment in locally advanced breast cancer. Magn Reson Med. doi:doi: 10.1002/mrm.22740, Epub ahead of print

Sinha S, Lucas-Quesada FA, Sinha U et al (2002) In vivo diffusion-weighted MRI of the breast: potential for lesion characterization. J Magn Reson Imaging 15:693–704

Tamura T, Usui S, Murakami S et al (2010) Biexponential signal attenuation analysis of diffusion-weighted imaging of breast. Magn Reson Med Sci 9(4):195–207

Thoeny HC, Ross BD (2010) Predicting and monitoring cancer treatment response with diffusion-weighted MRI. J Magn Reson Imaging 32(1):2–16

Tozaki M, Fukuma E (2009) ^{1}H MR Spectroscopy and difusión-weighted imaging of the breast: are they useful tools for characterizing breast lesions before biopsy? Am J Roentgenol 193:840–849

Tsushima Y, Takahashi-Taketomi A, Endo K (2009) Magnetic resonance (MR) differential diagnosis of breast tumors using apparent diffusion coefficient (ADC) on 1.5-T. J Magn Reson Imaging 30(2):249–255

Vilanova JC, Barcelo J (2008) Diffusion-weighted whole-body MR screening. Eur J Radiol 67:440–447

Woodhams R, Matsunaga K, Iwabuchi K et al (2005) Diffusion-weighted imaging of malignant breast tumors: the usefulness of apparent diffusion coefficient (ADC) value and ADC map for the detection of malignant breast tumors and evaluation of cancer extension. J Comput Assist Tomogr 29:644–649

Woodhams R, Matsunaga K, Kan S et al (2005) ADC mapping of benign and malignant breast tumors. Magn Reson Med Sci 4:35–42

Woodhams R, Kakita S, Hata H et al (2009) Diffusion-weighted imaging of mucinous carcinoma of the breast: evaluation of apparent diffusion coefficient and signal intensity in correlation with histologic findings. Am J Roentgenol 193:260–266

Woodhams R, Kakita S, Hata H et al (2010) Identification of residual breast carcinoma following neoadjuvant chemotherapy: diffusion-weighted imaging – comparison with contrast-enhanced MR imaging and pathologic findings. Radiology 254(2):357–366

Yabuuchi H, Matsuo Y, Sunami S et al (2011) Detection of non-palpable breast cancer in asymptomatic women by using unenhanced diffusion-weighted and T2-weighted MR imaging: comparison with mammography and dynamic contrast-enhanced MR imaging. Eur Radiol 21(1):11–17

Yili Z, Xiaoyan H, Hongwen D et al (2009) The value of diffusion-weighted imaging in assessing the ADC changes of tissues adjacent to breast carcinoma. BMC Cancer 14:9–18

11 Diffusion-Weighted Imaging of the Gastrointestinal Tract and Peritoneum

German A. Castrillon, Stephan Anderson, Jorge A. Soto, and Antonio Luna

The application of MRI to specifically evaluate the nonsolid abdominal organs such as the stomach, bowel, and colon has lagged behind the multiple uses that are now routine for evaluating the solid viscera. Consequently, the true clinical advantages offered by MRI are less understood. Successful imaging of the gastrointestinal tract organs has presented numerous challenges due to the usually long acquisitions times and the normal physiologic motion from breathing and, especially, from bowel peristalsis. The often subtle disease of the gastrointestinal tract can be very difficult to depict. Continued advances in MRI equipment hardware and software have overcome some of these initial limitations. Faster pulse sequences have made breath-hold acquisitions a routine component of imaging protocols, significantly decreasing or eliminating artifacts from physiologic motion. High-performance gradient systems have made high-resolution imaging feasible and can produce images with excellent detail and soft tissue contrast. All of this, with the added advantage of lack of ionizing radiation, has helped propel the use of MRI and made it the imaging modality of choice in certain specific situations where the suspected pathology involves primarily the gastrointestinal tract, such as in pregnant patients with acute abdominal pain and suspected acute appendicitis.

The use of diffusion-weighted imaging (DWI) of the abdomen provides additional information to evaluate abdominal pathology. The majority of the accepted applications of DWI studied so far and published in the literature focus on the evaluation of the solid abdominal and pelvic organs, including the liver, kidneys, adrenals, pancreas, prostate, uterus, and ovaries. These topics are the focus of other chapters in this book. The use of DWI to evaluate the gastrointestinal tract has been studied less extensively and, consequently, there is less evidence to support the use of DWI in such cases. Recently, DWI has been also used to evaluate peritoneal metastasis due to its higher sensitivity to detect small deposits against a suppressed background.

In order to describe the several uses of MRI and, specifically, DWI in the evaluation of the gastrointestinal tract, we will divide the gastrointestinal diseases into malignant and inflammatory diseases.

11.1 Malignant Lesions of GI Tract on DWI

Most malignant tumor tissues demonstrate restricted diffusion because of their high cellularity and the increased content of cell membranes per unit of volume. This results in a restriction of the movement of water molecules and, therefore, in a high signal intensity on DWI and low signal intensity on the corresponding ADC maps. Radiological imaging and endoscopic methods are commonly used to diagnose

G.A. Castrillon
Radiology Department, University of Antioquia, Medellin, Colombia

S. Anderson • J.A. Soto (✉)
Radiology Department, Boston University School of Medicine, Boston, MA, USA

A. Luna
Chief of MRI section, Health Time Group, Jaén, Spain
e-mail: aluna70@sercosa.com

A. Luna et al., *Diffusion MRI Outside the Brain*,
DOI 10.1007/978-3-642-21052-5_11,

gastrointestinal tract malignancies. Imaging findings provide additional information used for staging the tumor, which establishes the type of treatment that the patient will receive. The MRI findings can also help characterize the wall of the gastrointestinal tract and differentiate between tumoral and inflammatory thickening.

11.1.1 Colorectal Carcinoma

MRI has become increasingly important for evaluation of colorectal diseases, particularly in the anorectal region. MRI of this region is commonly used during the evaluation of rectal carcinoma, especially during preoperative staging and postoperative follow-up for detection of recurrence. Several factors contribute to a successful MRI examination of the rectum, including the fixed position of the rectum, lack of peristalsis, and the minimal effect of respiratory motion. In addition, pulse sequence and software developments in fast imaging techniques such as echo-planar imaging and parallel imaging methods have helped to overcome the difficulties and restrictions of abdominal MRI. DWI continues to grow as a diagnostic tool in neoplastic and inflammatory abdominal pathology. Because primary and recurrent malignancies and inflammatory diseases of the bowel wall both increase the wall thickness, DWI is a useful tool to differentiate between the two entities, with distinct advantages over conventional MR images. Furthermore, colon carcinomas show lower ADC values than active or fibrotic inflammatory bowel disease. Other articles have demonstrated the utility of DWI imaging with the combination of low and high *b* values as a potentially useful screening tool, with a high sensitivity near 100% in the detection of colon carcinoma (Fig. 11.1). Although the experience is still limited, the only reported false-negatives have corresponded to low-grade adenocarcinomas.

Several studies have also reported that DWI is a successful method to predict response to and evaluate the efficacy of treatment of colorectal carcinoma. For example, Dziik-Jurasz et al. reported that DWI could provide clinically important data that were useful in determining the patients' response to treatment. Their study revealed that the rate of treatment success increased when the pretreatment ADC values were high, indicating a high water content. They also found a decrease in the mean ADC value after several cycles of chemotherapy and radiation, likely secondary to cytotoxic edema and fibrosis. A more detailed explanation of this topic may be found in the chapter of DWI of the rectum (chapter 12).

11.1.2 Stomach

Carcinoma is the most important and common tumor of the stomach. The most common gastric carcinoma is adenocarcinoma. Predisposing conditions include atrophic gastritis, pernicious anemia, adenomatous polyps, dietary nitrates, and Japanese heritage. These tumors have a predilection for the lesser curvature of the antropyloric region. The goals of MRI in patients with gastric cancer are to demonstrate the primary tumor, to assess the depth of invasion, and to detect extra-gastric disease.

Adequate distention is necessary in order to evaluate the gastric wall. On T1-weighted sequences, gastric adenocarcinoma is isointense to normal stomach wall and may be apparent only as an area of focal wall thickening. On T2-weighted images, tumors usually are slightly higher in signal intensity than adjacent normal wall except for diffusely infiltrative carcinoma (linitis plastica), which tends to be lower in signal intensity than normal adjacent wall because of its desmoplastic nature. Tumors demonstrate a heterogeneous enhancement that may be decreased or increased relative to the gastric wall on early and/or on delayed images. Linitis plastica carcinoma enhances only modestly after intravenous contrast. Dynamic gadolinium-enhanced fat-suppressed gradient-echo images help in the identification of transmural spread, including peritoneal disease, tumor involvement of lymph nodes, and metastases. As it may be expected, gastric adenocarcinoma shows restriction of the free water diffusion (Fig. 11.2). In the only published series of gastric adenocarcinoma evaluated with DWI in comparison to CT, both techniques perform equivalently in detection and staging of 15 patients with gastric cancer.

The stomach is the site of the gastrointestinal tract most commonly involved with non-Hodgkin's lymphoma, accounting for approximately 50% of such cases. Gastric lymphoma is classified as infiltrative, ulcerative, polypoid, or nodular. The infiltrative form of gastric lymphoma is depicted on MRI as marked concentric mural and rugal thickening. The appearance can be similar to Menetrier's disease or severe gastritis. Gastric lymphoma may also be seen on MRI as a polypoid or ulcerated gastric mass that is indistinguishable from gastric adenocarcinoma. Our experience with diffusion-weighted MR pulse sequences has shown that there is high signal intensity with *b* factors of 400 and 800 s/mm^2 and low signal intensity on the ADC maps, indicating restriction of diffusion in both gastric adenocarcinoma and lymphoma (Fig. 11.3).

11.1.3 Small Bowel Tumors

Bowel distension is the main requisite for any imaging method of the small intestine, as revealed by years from experience with X-ray barium studies. In fact, a collapsed bowel loop can hide lesions or simulate pathological wall thickening. The presence of a lesion generating small bowel obstruction creates a natural distension of the lumen and affords the possibility of examining the patient without the need for a specific preparation. In contrast, the relative collapse of normal caliber bowel loops has motivated researchers to look for methods to achieve appropriate luminal distension and uncover non-obstructive lesions. Currently, there are two approaches to achieve this necessary distention: using oral administration of contrast material or introducing the oral contrast through a naso-enteric tube. Both methods have advantages and disadvantages. The specific approach preferred may be radiologist dependent or determined by the main suspected pathology in each patient. In the majority of cases, we prefer the administration of an adequate amount of a contrast agent orally, usually polyethylene glycol (PEG). PEG has similar MRI signal properties as water, but it is not absorbed through the intestinal wall due to the large size of the molecule; thus, better distension of distal ileum is achieved. The patient intakes about 1,500–1,800 mL of water mixed with PEG, divided into 3 or 4 doses, to be ingested every 15–20 min starting approximately 1 h before the examination. A final cup of contrast agent should be administered immediately before entering the scanner room to improve proximal jejunal distention. Concomitant administration of an intravenous or intramuscular spasmolytic agent (such as glucagon or Buscopan) at the beginning of the examination, to reduce motion artifacts from peristalsis, is optional.

With regards to the specific MRI technique, we prefer using fast sequences, which are able to acquire T1- and T2-weighted images within a single breath-hold. Dynamic contrast-enhanced sequences are also routinely acquired as part of the imaging sequence. Finally, we acquire the DWI with *b* factors of 100, 400, and 800 s/mm^2, along with the corresponding ADC maps. Large-gradient body coils are necessary for adequate resolution and a sufficiently large field of view. An initial thick-slab T2-weighted MRI cholangiopancreatography-type sequence helps confirm passage of contrast material into the right colon. Coronal and axial balanced gradient-echo (true FISP) images are then obtained, providing a rapid overview of the entire abdomen and assessment of luminal distention. At this stage, if there is inadequate distention of the ileum, the patient can return to the waiting room to drink more oral contrast material. Subsequently, T2-weighted HASTE sequences are acquired in the coronal and axial planes. Fat-saturated HASTE sequences may be added to allow detection of wall and mesenteric edema, as well as differentiation of focal wall fatty infiltration from edema. A baseline coronal 3D fast low-angle shot fat-saturated T1-weighted sequence (VIBE) is then performed. Coronal VIBE sequences are performed 30 and 70 s after gadolinium-based contrast material injection, followed by axial imaging beginning 90 s after injection and covering the entire abdomen. This allows assessment of bowel and nodal enhancement, and it often aids in the demonstration of fistulas.

Malignant tumors of the small intestine are uncommon, occurring in fewer than 2 in 100,000 persons in the United States each year. Adenocarcinoma is the most common cell type, accounting for approximately one-half of small bowel cancers. Other histological types include carcinoid tumors, leiomyosarcoma, lymphoma, metastases, and malignant gastrointestinal stromal tumors. The clinical presentation of patients with small bowel tumors is often nonspecific, resulting in a delay in diagnosis. Small bowel tumors are usually isointense to small bowel on T1-weighted images and demonstrate a heterogeneous enhancement, greater than adjacent normal bowel on gadolinium-enhanced spoiled gradient-echo imaging. In our experience, most tumors show a high signal intensity on diffusion-weighted images and low signal intensity on the ADC maps.

The GI tract is the most common primary extranodal site of involvement by lymphoma. Primary GI lymphoma comprises a group of distinct clinical and pathological entities that may be either B-cell or T-cell type. The most common lymphomas involving bowel are non-Hodgkin's lymphomas that arise from lymphoid tissue associated with the GI tract or that secondarily affect the bowel in patients with widespread abdominal and pelvic lymphoma. The lymphoid tissue associated with the GI tract is found in the epithelium, lamina propria, submucosa, and mesenteric lymph nodes. This lymphoid tissue is collectively known as MALT tissue.

The MRI appearance of GI tract lymphomas depends on the specific location and the morphological appearance of the tumor. After the stomach, the small intestine is the next most commonly involved site, especially the distal ileum which is the segment containing a larger volume of lymphoid tissue. Lymphoma of the small bowel can present as disseminated disease, as a solitary mass (Fig. 11.4) or as multiple independent small bowel masses. Primary small bowel lymphoma begins in the wall of the small intestine. On MRI, there is focal small bowel mural thickening, or multifocal mural masses. The tumor may extend beyond the bowel serosa to involve the adjacent mesentery and lymph nodes. The caliber of the intestine may be narrowed; however, bowel obstruction is not frequent due to the fact that the wall of the small bowel remains pliable. Alternatively, the intestinal lumen may appear focally dilated in patients with GI lymphoma. This dilatation is thought to be due to the destruction of the autonomic nerves within the bowel wall and the tumor replacement of the normal muscularis layer of the intestinal wall. Small bowel lymphoma may also result in a huge cavitary mass that communicates with the intestinal lumen ("aneurysmal dilatation"). Extensive extraintestinal lymphoma may secondarily involve the GI tract. Large mesenteric nodal masses may extend to the mesenteric border of the bowel and then directly invade the small intestine.

On MRI, bowel lymphoma may be depicted as multiple large mesenteric nodal masses that distort the adjacent bowel loops. Associated mural thickening is direct evidence of intestinal tumor invasion and spread. On DWI, lymphoma shows a high signal intensity with multiple *b* factors of 400 and 800 s/mm^2, and low signal intensity on the ADC maps (Fig. 11.4).

11.1.4 Esophagus

Incidence of esophageal cancer has increased in recent decades. Cancer of the esophagus is three times more common in men than in women and three times more common in blacks than whites. The distal esophagus is the most common site of involvement by tumor. Nowadays, adenocarcinomas are more common than squamous cell carcinoma in the United States and Europe. Esophageal adenocarcinoma is associated with Barret's esophagus and symptomatic gastroesophageal reflux. Preoperative imaging of patients with esophageal carcinoma must include the thorax and abdomen. Oral water is administered to distend the stomach and optimally delineate the gastroesophageal junction. MRI examinations of the distal esophagus and stomach can be obtained with thin section images in multiple planes, combined with routine T1-weighted and T2-weighted images with fat suppression and contrast-enhanced sequences. MRI is useful to evaluate more extensive tumors with mediastinal invasion or distant metastases. Invasion of the pericardium, aorta, and tracheobronchial tree can be depicted with MRI with moderate accuracy. However, detection of disease in normal size lymph nodes remains problematic.

There is little experience of DWI with esophageal cancer (Fig. 11.5 and 14.4). In our experience, the use of respiratory and cardiac trigger is necessary to obtain adequate DWI images, mainly in retrocardiac lesions. Sakurada and colleagues demonstrated a poor detection rate of esophageal cancer of 49.4% using DWIBS, the depiction of early tumors being especially problematic. Moreover, average patient-based sensitivity and specificity for the detection of node metastasis were 77.8% and 55.6%, respectively. ADC values of node metastases of esophageal cancer unexpectedly were significantly higher than that of nonmetastatic lymph nodes, although there was an overlap in the ADCs of both groups. The higher ADC values of node metastases may be related to areas of microscopic necrosis. More recently, DWIBS has also shown similar potential than 18F-FDG-PET for detecting postoperative recurrent squamous cell esophageal cancer and nodal metastases. Both recurrent tumors and nodal metastases showed low ADC values.

11.2 Inflammatory Diseases

Until recently, MR imaging of the small bowel had been a relatively unexplored field of application for this imaging modality. Multiple reasons accounted for this limited use in small bowel disease, as has already been delineated in the Introduction to this Chapter. There is also a limited intrinsic contrast between normal and diseased bowel wall on conventional MRI pulse sequences. However, the use of MRI for evaluating bowel pathology has grown exponentially in recent years. Developments in hardware (gradients, multichannel coils) and software (fast and ultrafast sequences) described previously helped circumvent some of the limitations, but the introduction of new pulse sequences with higher contrast resolution (such as DWI) and the ability to obtain some functional information were just as important. In addition, the increased awareness of the need to limit the amount of radiation delivered to patients with diseases that require frequent surveillance or follow-up with imaging has also shifted the emphasis away from CT to MRI in specific clinical circumstances. Common everyday uses of MRI in gastrointestinal diseases include pregnant patients with acute abdominal pain and suspected acute appendicitis and patients with Crohn disease in remission who require periodic surveillance with imaging or who present with acute flares and possible complications.

Successful MRI imaging of the small bowel demands a rigorous approach in technique to obtain images with diagnostic image quality. Maximum bowel loop distention is required, together with a focused scanning protocol including the most appropriate fast (single breath-hold) T1- and T2-weighted sequences combined with dynamic contrast-enhanced sequences. As DWI sequences have been incorporated into the routine protocol of most abdominal MRI examinations, there is also a growing experience on how these sequences may be applied to the evaluation of stomach and small bowel diseases. However, more studies will be necessary in order to ascertain the exact role and the meaning of findings seen only on diffusion images.

11.2.1 Acute Appendicitis

Acute appendicitis is the most common acute gastrointestinal disease that requires surgery in pregnant and nonpregnant patients. The usual clinical manifestations of appendicitis, such as leukocytosis, fever, and right lower quadrant pain, are nonspecific during pregnancy. Furthermore, in pregnant patients, the appendix is not located in its usual position, as it is displaced by the gravid uterus. This makes the evaluation of the appendix as the source of pain more difficult, both clinically and sonographically. For this reason, MRI has become the accepted second choice as an imaging modality in this setting and provides diagnostic information that is not available with ultrasonography. However, since the potential untoward effects of exposing the fetus to the high magnetic field and radiofrequency waves of MRI are not completely known, ultrasonography remains as the first-line test requested, followed rapidly by MRI if sonographic findings are negative or nonspecific.

A typical MRI protocol for appendicitis includes (a) breath-hold single-shot T2-weighted fast SE sequences in the axial, coronal, and sagittal planes with and without fat suppression and (b) breath-hold axial T1-weighted in-phase and out-of-phase gradient-echo sequences. Additional sequences may be acquired as deemed necessary. No gadolinium-based intravenous contrast should be administered in pregnant patients. Administration of an oral contrast agent (a combination of barium sulfate and iron oxide) is strongly recommended. Inci and colleagues have recently communicated their experience with the use of DWI, obtaining very promising results. They were able to detect all, except 1, of 79 patients with acute appendicitis treated with surgery. The characteristic findings on DWI were hyperintensity on high *b* value acquisitions (up to *b* 1,000 s/mm^2) and significantly lower ADC values ($1.28+0.18\times10^{-3}$ mm^2/s) than in normal appendix in the diagnosis of acute appendicitis. Therefore, many institutions (including ours) have been acquiring DWI as an integral part of the protocol for abdominal MRI. We acquire DWI with *b* factors of 0, 50, 400, and 600–800 s/mm^2, with the corresponding ADC maps. MRI has high reported sensitivity (97–100%) and specificity (92–93%) for the diagnosis of acute appendicitis, which may potentially be increased with the addition on DWI. The imaging criteria of non-perforated acute appendicitis are similar to those found with other cross-sectional modalities and include appendiceal diameter and wall thickness greater than 7 and 2 mm, respectively, and inflammatory changes in the periappendiceal fat. The T2-weighted images with fat saturation show the edema and inflammation which appear as areas of high signal intensity within the wall or in the adjacent fat. DWI demonstrates the inflamed appendix and surrounding fat as bright, secondary to a restriction in water diffusion (Fig. 11.6). Periappendiceal abscesses, which can complicate a perforated appendix, also exhibit high T2 signal and restricted diffusion. A similar appearance may show hepatic abscesses, which may occur secondarily to complicated appendicitis

(Fig. 5.6). An important limitation of MRI (compared to CT) that should be kept in mind in the sicker patients is the difficulty in detecting extraluminal gas collections and even significant free pneumoperitoneum, although DWI is probably one of the most sensitive sequence for detection of free air due to the susceptibility artifact it produces (Fig. 12.8).

11.2.2 Acute Diverticulitis

Acute diverticulitis is a common inflammatory condition that usually affects the left colon but can involve the right colon as well, mimicking appendicitis. Imaging is often necessary to confirm the diagnosis and assess for complications. CT is the imaging test of choice to diagnose acute diverticulitis. However, MRI is also able to demonstrate the findings of acute diverticulitis. Acute diverticulitis may be found with MR in pregnant patients with nonspecific abdominal pain or with suspected acute appendicitis or in patients with underlying inflammatory bowel disease who also happen to have colonic diverticula. The typical imaging protocol consisting of HASTE sequences in multiple planes and pre- and post-gadolinium-enhanced T1-weighted fat-suppressed GE sequences allows the diagnosis of acute diverticulitis and its complications, including abscess formation and venous thrombosis (Figs. 11.7 and 12.9). At our institutions, oral and intravenous (in nonpregnant patients) contrast agents are used routinely. Free perforation into the peritoneal cavity may be more difficult to detect than with CT. By characterizing the pattern and degree of colonic wall thickening, the DWI and ADC maps can help establish the diagnosis of diverticulitis firmly and differentiate it from colon carcinoma. Additional definitive findings in this differential diagnosis include the presence of peritoneal and hepatic metastases. Ultimately, though, colonoscopy with biopsy proof remains as the gold standard for the diagnosis of colorectal carcinoma and inflammatory bowel disease.

MRI findings of acute diverticulitis include increased signal on T2-weighted and DWI, representing the fluid and edema in the adjacent inflamed mesenteric fat surrounding the affected diverticulum. Gadolinium-enhanced T1-weighted fat-suppressed gradient-echo images demonstrate the inflamed diverticulum as a low signal intensity outpouching of the colon and surrounding inflammation. The inflammatory involvement of the adjacent fascial planes results in a thickened and hyperenhancing mesocolon on gadolinium-enhanced sequences. Diverticular abscesses appear as low signal intensity fluid with rim-enhancement on T1-weighted sequences and increased signal on T2-weighted and DWI sequences (Fig. 11.7).

11.2.3 Colitis and Enteritis

Bowel wall thickening is a nonspecific finding that can be seen in a variety of infectious, inflammatory, ischemic, and neoplastic diseases of bowel. Mural stratification (target sign) can be seen on axial images of CT and MRI and is highly suggestive of an inflammatory process. Mural thickening is well illustrated on T2- and T1-weighted sequences and can help assess the presence of activity of inflammatory disease, especially in Crohn disease. Furthermore, the presence of mural enhancement and increased mesenteric vascularity are good indicators of inflammatory activity. Kiryu and colleagues have recently reported sensitivity, specificity, and accuracy over 80% for active disease detection upon a visual assessment of a breath-hold DWI. Ono et al. confirmed and improved these results. Therefore, DWI and ADC maps are useful tools to help demonstrate the inflammatory activity as well. In acute flares of Crohn disease and in patients with proven active disease, there is restricted diffusion. Thus, the hyperintensity on DWI and hypointensity on the ADC map are associated with inflammatory activity (Fig. 11.8), whereas the presence of hypointensity in both is more characteristic of the fibrostenotic stage. Both mentioned series detected lower ADC values in segments with active inflammation compared to fibrotic or normal ones (Fig. 11.9). The restriction of free water diffusion in active inflammatory segments has been related to infiltration by inflammatory cells, presence of aphtoid ulcers with lymphoid aggregates, dilated lymphatic channels, hypertrophied neuronal tissue, and the development of granulomas.

11.2.4 Epiploic Appendagitis and Omental Infarction

Epiploic appendagitis is an acute inflammatory process that affects the epiploic appendages secondary to torsion and infarction. The clinical manifestations are almost identical to acute appendicitis and diverticulitis depending on the location of the torsed appendage. Treatment is conservative. On MRI, T2-weighted images demonstrate the enlarged appendage with a central high signal focus and a low signal rim. On T1-weighted images, epiploic appendagitis appears as an oval shaped lesion with a high signal intensity center and low signal intensity rim. After administration of intravenous gadolinium chelates, the rim is seen to enhance, while the central area shows low signal intensity.

Omental infarction is an uncommon cause of acute abdominal pain. It occurs more frequently in young males and is usually located in the right lower quadrant, clinically mimicking acute appendicitis. The treatment is conservative. The MRI findings include a fat-containing omental mass generally located anteromedial to the ascending colon with increased signal on T2-weighted sequences and mild enhancement on contrast-enhanced sequences. Although there are no publications with a large number of patients confirming a role for DWI in the diagnosis of epiploic appendagitis or omental infarction, it is expected that, as with other inflammatory/ischemic conditions, findings would include high signal intensity and restricted diffusion.

11.3 Evaluation of the Peritoneum

Imaging has an essential role in the presurgical evaluation of peritoneal metastases. CT is the most extended technique, although MRI is able to detect smaller peritoneal metastases, mainly with the use of 5 min post-contrast fat-suppressed 3D isotropic GE T1-weighted sequences. DWI has demonstrated to be highly sensitive to peritoneal metastasis, with advantages over morphological MRI sequences to detect small deposits in challenging anatomical sites as a right subdiaphragmatic space, omentum, root of the mesentery, and serosal surface of the small bowel (Fig. 11.10). Furthermore, two series has shown higher sensitivity, specificity, and accuracy for the detection of peritoneal metastasis with the addition of DWI with high *b* value to standard MRI protocols, being specially useful for less experienced radiologists.

Case 11.1: Colon Carcinoma

A 74-year-old-male patient with several months of evolution of weight loss and abdominal pain. Colonoscopy showed an irregular and ulcerated mass in the transverse colon and the pathological diagnoses was a colon adenocarcinoma. A MRI examination was performed for staging the tumor.

Comments

The incidence of colorectal cancer (CRC) in the United States amounts to 130,000 per year with 50,000 cases of death. CRC is the second most common cancer in both genders in the Western world. Up to 90% of CRC cases originate from preexisting benign adenomas. Hence, the incidence of CRC could be considerably reduced by more than 80% if polyps are detected and removed before their malignant transformation.

Despite the availability of several screening options, CRC remains a considerable cause of morbidity and mortality. The main use of MR images in colon carcinoma is as preoperative imaging for staging. Early reports of the accuracy of CT scanning and MRI in preoperative staging of colon carcinoma showed an overall staging accuracy of 70% with only approximately 45% sensitivity for identifying nodal metastases. However, many refinements in MRI of colorectal cancer have since occurred, taking advantage of high-performance gradients, faster pulse sequences, and higher resolution images. Technical improvements include MRI using endorectal coil, the addition of various types of intravenous contrast agents, the use of oral and rectal contrast agents to improve bowel distention, and, more recently, the introduction of DWI, which improve detection of nodal metastases and hepatic metastases. The combined use of intraluminal agents with intravenous contrast material facilitates depiction of the wall of the colon and rectum and allows an estimation of the depth of tumor involvement of the bowel wall. A combination of thin section T2-weighted images and contrast-enhanced sequences can be used to evaluate colon and rectal cancers. A partial thickness involvement of the bowel indicates a stage T1 tumor. A tumor with full thickness involvement correlates with a stage T2 tumor. A tumor with full thickness involvement and nodular tumor extension into the adjacent pericolonic or perirectal fat suggests a T3 tumor. A T4 tumor is indicated by gross extracolonic tumor extension with invasion into adjacent organs.

The depiction of nodal metastases is still limited by the difficulty to detect tumor in normal sized lymph nodes. Furthermore, enlarged lymph nodes could be inflammatory. The prediction of nodal involvement on MRI is improved by using the border contour and signal intensity characteristics of lymph nodes involved, instead of size criteria alone. However, depicting tumor in normal sized lymph node may require the use of additional contrast agents directed at imaging nodal metastatic disease or the use of DWI sequences, which has recently shown promising results in this task.

Imaging Findings

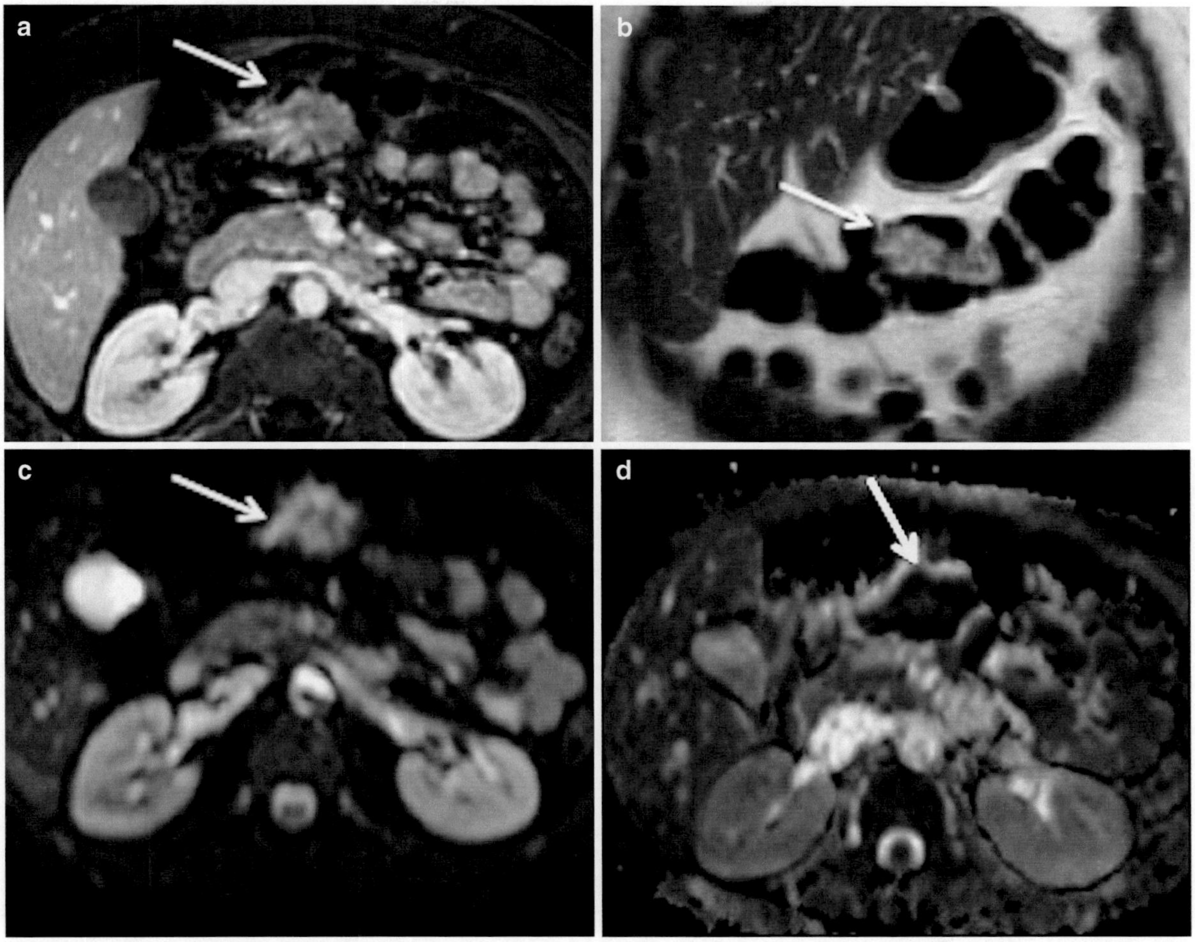

Fig. 11.1 (**a**) Axial contrast-enhanced GE T1-weighted gradient-echo image with fat suppression shows a heterogeneous mass with an intraluminal polypoid component arising from the transverse colon (*arrow*). (**b**) Coronal T2-weighted image shows the mass with high signal intensity in the transverse colon (*arrow*). (**c**) DWI with *b* factor of 1,000 s/mm^2 and (**d**) ADC map images show the corresponding high signal intensity in the DWI and low signal intensity in the ADC map in the mass, indicating restricted diffusion by colon adenocarcinoma (*arrows*)

Case 11.2: Gastric Carcinoma

A 70-year-old-female patient who complained of progressive weight loss and abdominal pain. A gastric mass was found on endoscopy. Pathological diagnosis was gastric adenocarcinoma. A CT and MRI were performed for staging the tumor.

Comments

The use of DWI of the abdomen and pelvis provides a new contrast mechanism to evaluate patients with abdominal malignancy. However, description of the application of DWI to assess the hollow abdominal viscera, including the gastrointestinal tract and peritoneum, is less extensive. Most tumors, including tumors from the gastrointestinal tract, show restricted diffusion because of the higher cellularity and their increase in cell membranes per volume unit, resulting in restriction of water movement and corresponding high signal intensity on DWI and low signal intensity in the corresponding ADC map. DWI has shown excellent results in the detection and staging of gastric carcinoma with the limited available data. There is lack of information about the role of DWI in the distinction of the different types of gastric carcinoma and assessment and prediction of treatment response.

Imaging Findings

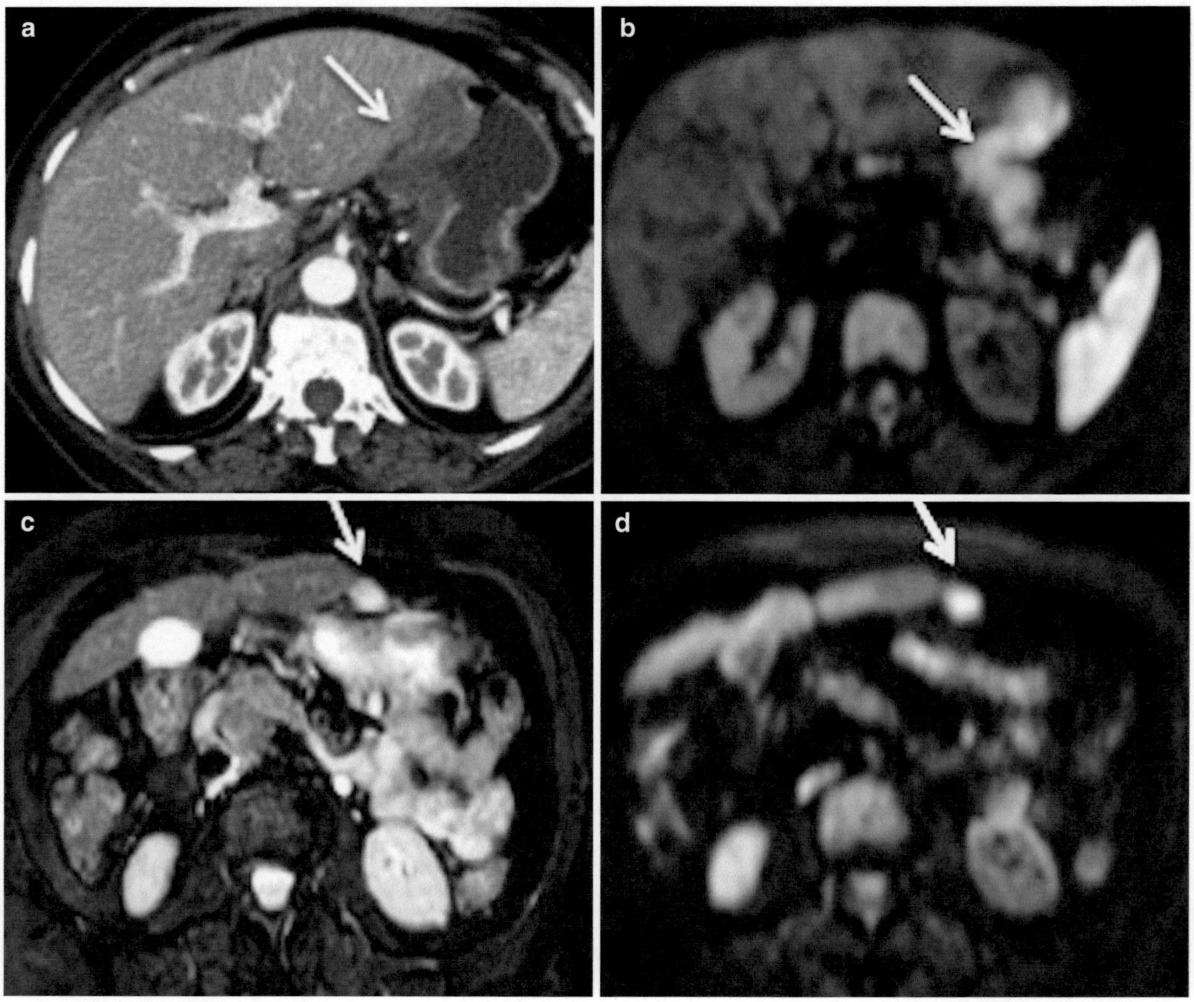

Fig. 11.2 (**a**) Contrast-enhanced CT image shows focal thickening of the gastric wall, suspicious for gastric cancer (*arrow*). (**b**) DWI acquired with a *b* factor of 1,000 s/mm^2 shows high signal intensity in the thickened gastric wall indicating restricted diffusion by gastric carcinoma (*arrow*). (**c**) Axial fat-suppressed T2 weighted image and (**d**) corresponding DWI with a *b* factor of 1,000 s/mm^2 show perigastric adenopathy with restricted diffusion, indicating involvement with tumor (*arrows*)

Case 11.3: Gastric Lymphoma

A 45-year-old-male with HIV infection and several weeks of fever, weight loss, and abdominal pain. Physical examination disclosed a palpable abdominal mass. The MRI examination was performed for localization and staging of the tumor. Pathological findings yielded the diagnosis of non-Hodgkin's lymphoma.

Comments

The stomach is the site of the gastrointestinal tract most commonly involved with non-Hodgkin's lymphoma, accounting for approximately 50% of the cases. The GI tract is also the most common primary extranodal site of involvement by lymphoma. Primary GI lymphoma comprises a group of distinct clinical and pathologic entities that may be either B-cell or T-cell type. The most common lymphoma involving bowel is non-Hodgkin's lymphoma that arises from lymphoid tissue associated with the GI tract or that secondarily affects the bowel in patients with widespread abdominal and pelvic lymphoma. Lymphoid tissue associated with the GI tract is found in the epithelium, lamina propria, submucosa, and mesenteric lymph nodes. This lymphoid tissue is collectively known as MALT tissue. Immunodeficiency-related GI lymphoma can occur as a complication of acquired immune deficiency syndrome (AIDS). Non-Hodgkin's lymphoma is the second most common neoplasm in patients with AIDS.

Imaging may depict gastric involvement indicated by concentric mural thickening or multiple mural tumors. The findings on MRI include irregularly thickened mucosal folds, irregular submucosal infiltration, annular constricting lesion, exophytic tumor growth, mesenteric masses, and mesenteric/retroperitoneal lymphadenopathy. The tumors usually show homogeneous or intermediate signal intensity on T1-weighted images. On T2-weighted images, the tumors usually exhibit heterogeneous increased signal intensity. Mild-to-moderate enhancement after intravenous administration of gadolinium chelates is usually present. In our experience, DWI demonstrates restriction of tissue diffusion with high signal intensity on the DWI and low signal on the corresponding ADC map.

Imaging Findings

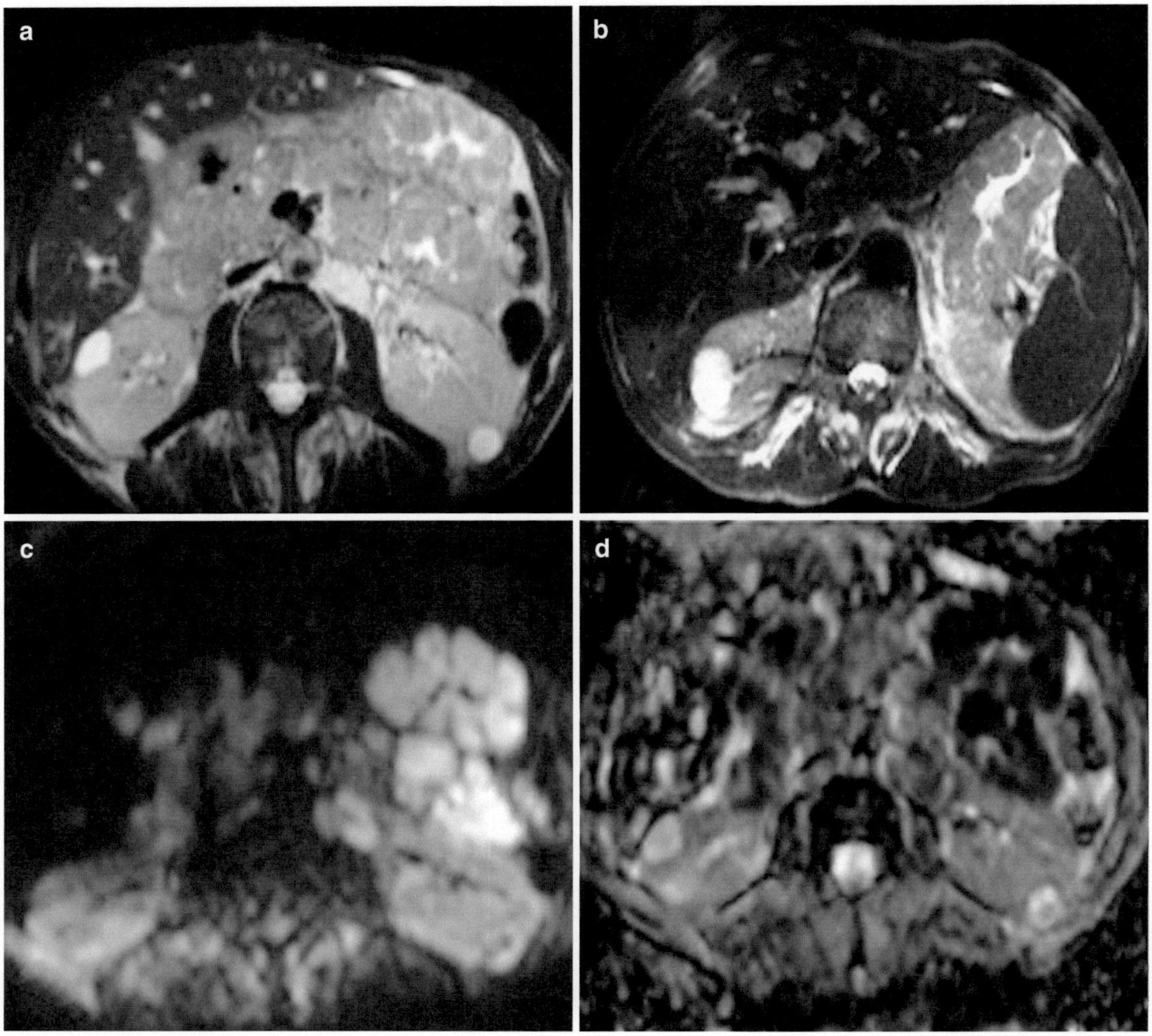

Fig. 11.3 (**a**, **b**) Axial T2-weighted images with fat saturation at two different levels show marked nodular thickening of the gastric wall along with multiple enlarged retroperitoneal lymph nodes. (**c**) DWI acquired with a *b* factor of 1,000 s/mm^2 and (**d**) ADC map image show high signal intensity on the DWI and low signal intensity on the ADC map in the thickened gastric wall and the enlarged nodes, indicating restricted diffusion and involvement by lymphoma

Case 11.4: Duodenal Non-Hodgkin Lymphoma

A 54-year-old-male with wasting syndrome and dyspepsia. A duodenal mass was found on upper endoscopy with pathological diagnosis of high-grade non-Hodgkin lymphoma. MRI was performed for staging.

Comments

Non-Hodgkin B-cell lymphoma is the most common subtype in the small bowel, arising from mucosa-associated lymphoid tissue (MALT). T-cell lymphoma of the small bowel is unusual, and it is associated to previous celiac disease. MR enterography has recently showed its role in the evaluation of small bowel pathology, and it has also been used to analyze small bowel lymphoma, as it allows concurrent evaluation of luminal integrity, mural deformity, and distant extraluminal disease extent. With regard to histological differentiation, a correlation between small bowel luminal stricturing and the presence of low-grade disease has been reported, and also mesenteric fat infiltration in the absence of discrete lymphadenopathy in relation to the presence of high-grade NHL.

WB-DWI has shown excellent results in nodal and bone marrow staging of lymphoma and leukemia and it is a perfect tool for surveillance evaluation. Although to our knowledge there is no available data in the literature regarding the role of DWI for small bowel lymphoma, it may be speculated that DWI has the potential to easily detect it, due to high cellular packing and content. Furthermore, it may have a role in posttreatment monitorization, staging, and histologic grading.

Imaging Findings

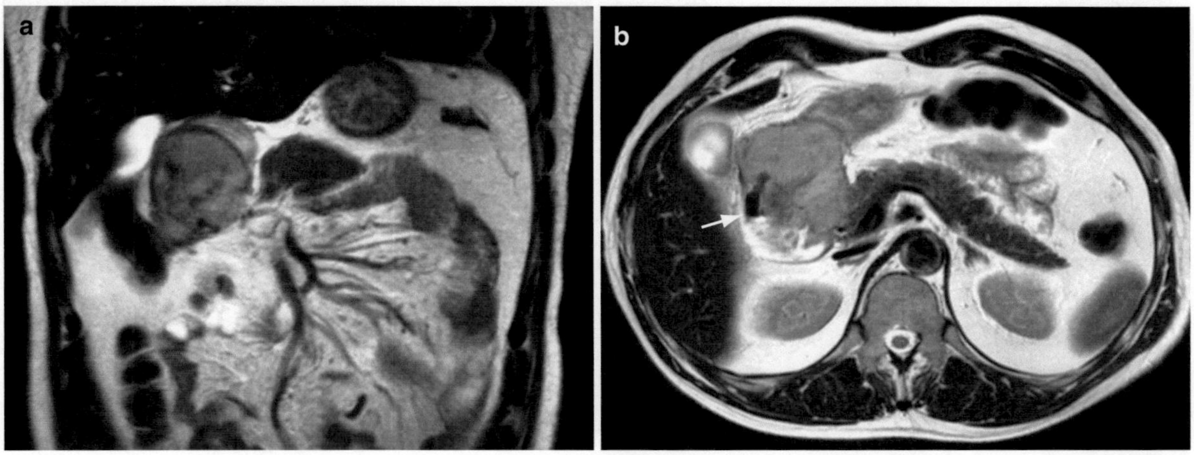

Fig. 11.4 Coronal HASTE (**a**) and axial TSE T2-weighted (**b**) sequences show a diffuse and eccentric mural thickening on the medial aspect of the 2nd duodenal portion, which causes moderate luminal narrowing and fatty stranding. The mass is of intermediate signal with a central area of lower intensity (*arrow*). (**c**, **d**) Axial pre- and postcontrast THRIVE sequences demonstrate intense enhancement of the mass, except the central area of lower intensity on T2-weighted sequences (*arrows*), which is clearly hypovascular and moderately hyperintense on precontrast image. (**e**, **f**) DWI with *b* values of 0 and 1,000 s/mm² better depict the borders of the tumor, confirming the infiltration of the pancreatic head. Notice the absence of hyperintensity on both images of the central hypovascular area (*arrows*). (**g**) ADC map demonstrates hypercellularity of the whole mass (*ADC* value: 1.2×10^{-3} mm²/s). Notice decreased signal on ADC of the central area (*arrow*) above mentioned (*ADC* value: 0.8×10^{-3} mm²/s), corresponding to the site of previous biopsy (T2-dark-through effect)

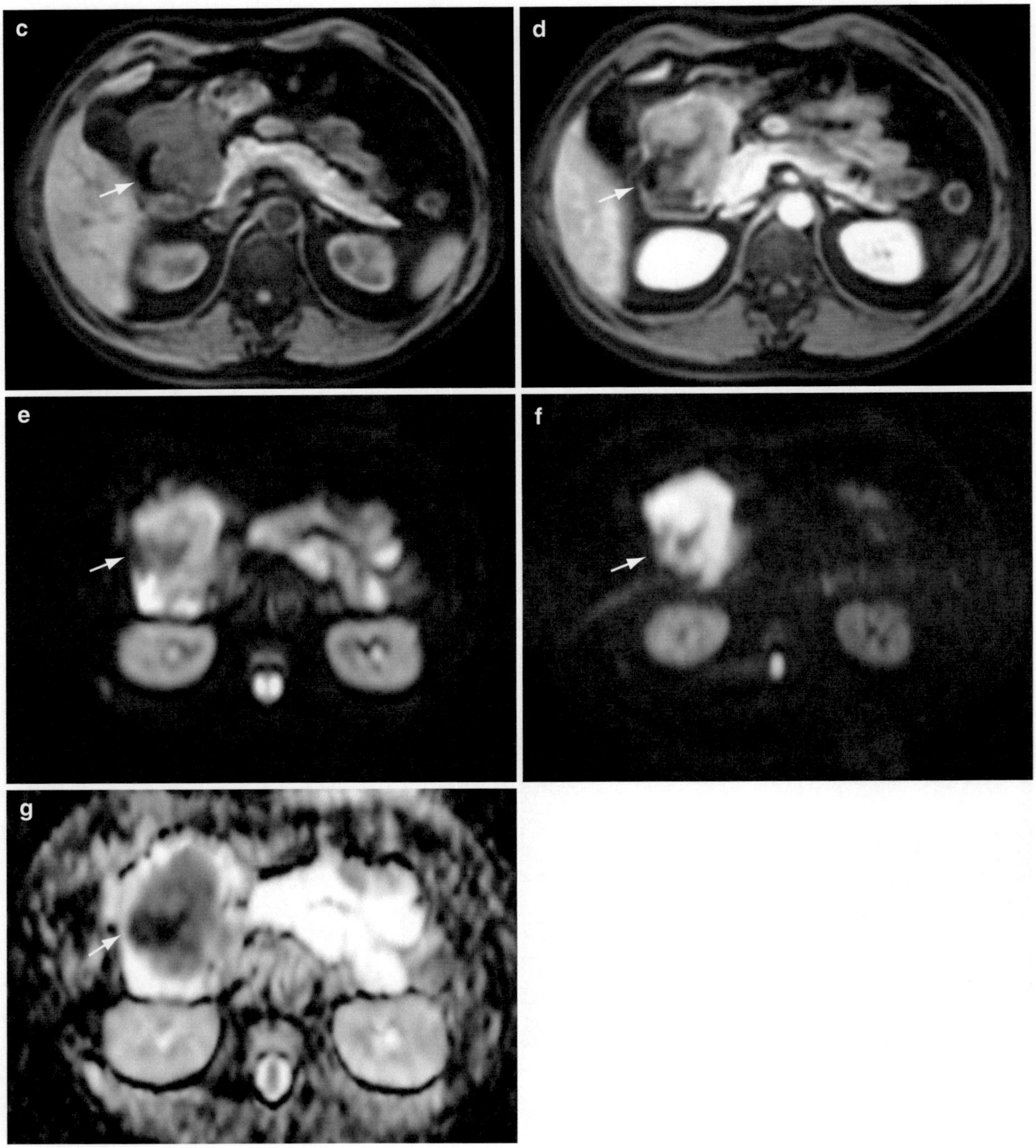

Fig. 11.4 (continued)

Fig. 11.5 (**a**) Axial contrast-enhanced T1-weighted gradient-echo image with fat suppression shows the thickened distal esophageal wall (*arrow*). (**b**) Axial FSE T2-weighted image shows a periportal lymph node, which is only minimally enlarged (*arrow*). (**c**, **d**) DWI acquired with a *b* factor of 800 s/mm^2 show a high signal intensity in the distal esophageal wall and the periportal node (*arrows*). Surgical exploration subsequently proved involvement with adenocarcinoma at both sites

Case 11.5: Esophageal Carcinoma

A 74-year-old-male patient with progressive weight loss and dysphagia, and an esophageal mass found on upper endoscopy. Pathological diagnosis was esophageal adenocarcinoma.

Comments

The incidence of esophageal cancer has increased in recent decades. Cancer of the esophagus is three times more common in men than in women and three times more common in blacks than whites. The distal esophagus is the most common site of involvement with tumor. Adenocarcinoma is now more common than squamous cell carcinoma in Western countries. Esophageal adenocarcinoma is associated with Barrett's esophagus and symptomatic gastroesophageal reflux. Preoperative imaging of patients with esophageal carcinoma must include the thorax and abdomen. Water is administered orally to distend the stomach and optimally delineate the gastroesophageal junction. MR examinations of the distal esophagus and stomach can be obtained with thin section images in multiple planes, with routine T1-weighted and T2-weighted images with fat suppression and contrast-enhanced sequences. MRI is useful to evaluate extensive tumors with mediastinal invasion or distant metastases. Direct invasion of the pericardium, aorta, and tracheobronchial tree can be depicted with MRI with moderate accuracy. However, detection of tumor involvement in normal size lymph nodes remains problematic. DWI can help establish the presence of tumor in normal size lymph nodes, by showing evidence of restricted diffusion.

Imaging Findings

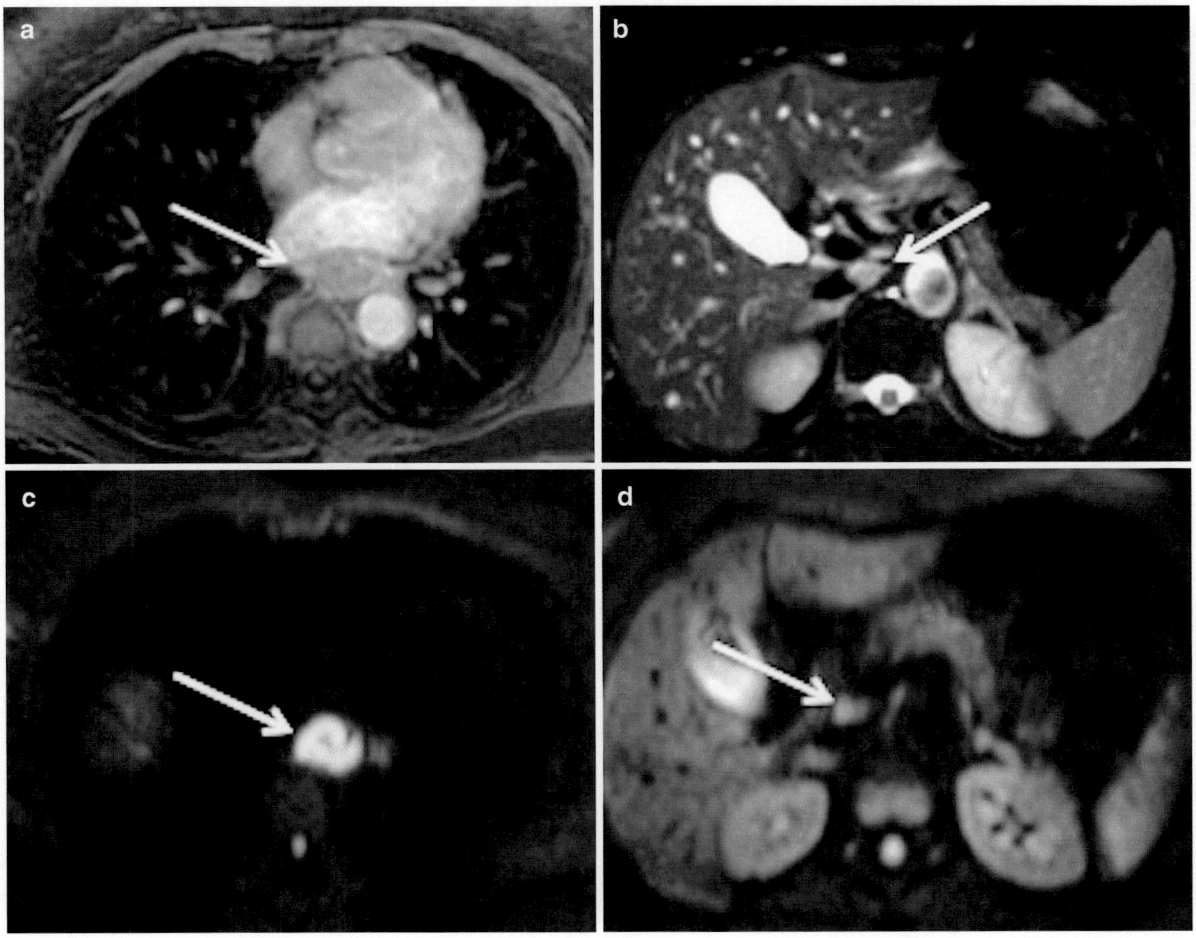

Case 11.6: Acute Appendicitis

A 45-year-old-female pregnant patient with right lower quadrant pain and fever. US was non-confirmatory. The MRI was performed in order to establish the cause of the abdominal pain cause.

Comments

Acute appendicitis is the most common acute gastrointestinal disease that requires surgery in pregnant and nonpregnant patients. The usual clinical manifestations of appendicitis are leukocytosis, fever, and right lower quadrant pain. With the available data, MRI may be recommended as a second imaging test for patients with suspected appendicitis and a negative ultrasound. It has also demonstrated to be valid in pregnant women. Although, sometimes it is enough with the acquisition of HASTE sequences to perform the diagnosis of appendicitis. Additional sequences may be acquired as deemed necessary. Since no gadolinium-based intravenous contrast should be administered to pregnant patients, DWI is especially important in this group of patients due to its reported high sensitivity and specificity. In our experience, DWI demonstrates the inflamed appendix and surrounding fat as bright, secondary to a restriction in water diffusion, and it may also rule out accurately complications as abscess.

Radiological Findings

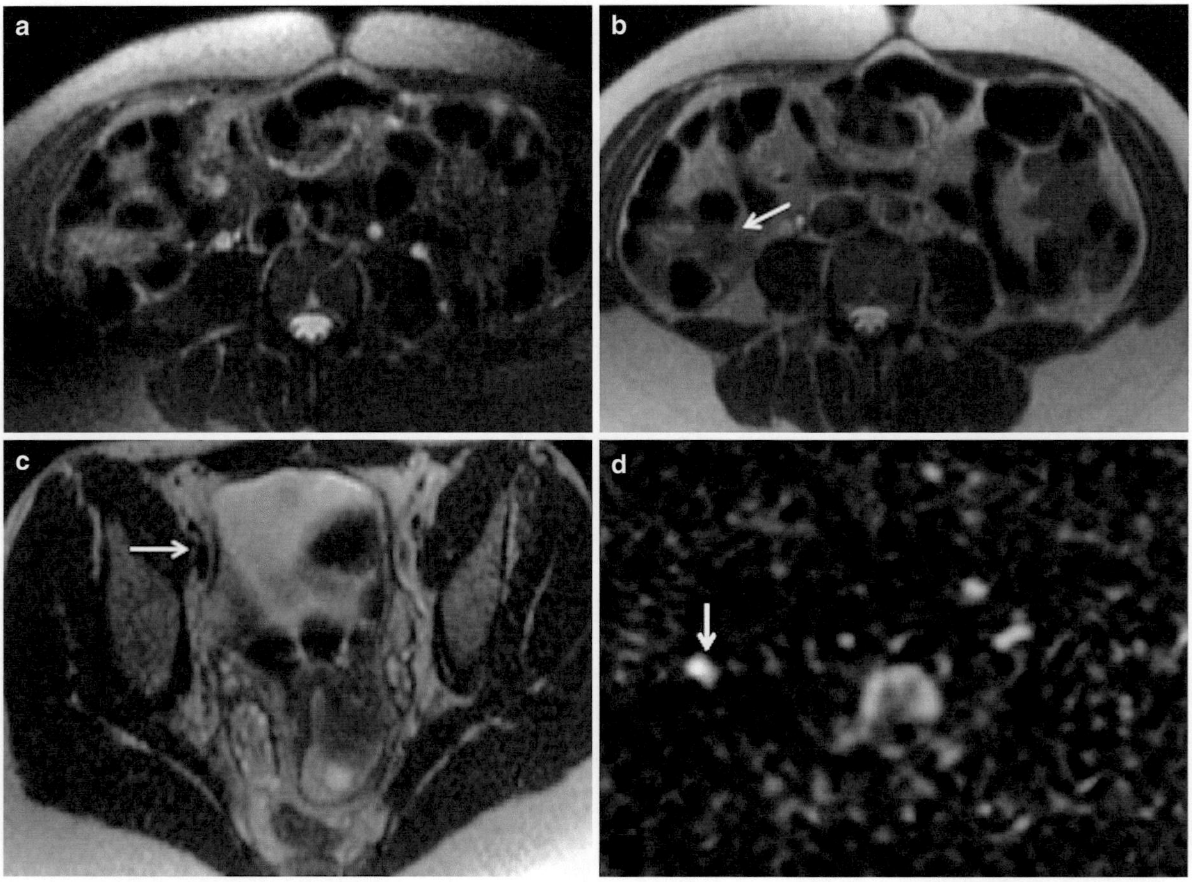

Fig. 11.6 (**a**) Axial FSE T2-weighted image shows stranding of the periappendiceal fat with mild periappendiceal increased T2-weighted signal caused by inflammatory changes. (**b**, **c**) Axial and oblique coronal FSE T2-weighted images demonstrate a mildly thickened wall and dilated appendiceal lumen (*arrows*). (**d**) DWI acquired with a *b* factor of 1,000 s/mm^2 shows high signal intensity in the fluid-filled appendiceal lumen, indicating inflammatory changes and restricted diffusion

Case 11.7: Acute Diverticulitis with Abscess Formation

A 68-year-old female patient with acute left lower quadrant pain and fever. The MRI was done as the initial examination due to chronic renal failure and contraindications to intravenous contrast.

Comments

Acute diverticulitis is a common inflammatory condition that usually affects the left colon but can involve the right colon as well, mimicking appendicitis. Imaging is often necessary to confirm the diagnosis and assess for complications. CT is the imaging test of choice to diagnose acute diverticulitis. However, MRI is also able to demonstrate the characteristic imaging findings and its complications, including abscess formation and venous thrombosis. However, free perforation into the peritoneal cavity may be more difficult to detect. The addition of DWI to the MRI protocol may increase its accuracy. In this sense, a recent series evaluating rectosigmoid inflammatory and neoplastic involvement with DWI and quantification of ADC values demonstrate the accurate differentiation between active inflammatory bowel disease and malignant tumors based on ADC quantification. Active inflammatory lesions presented a higher ADC value than carcinomas, with an ADC of 1.21 (0.08) × 10^{-3} mm^2/s and 0.97 (0.14) × 10^{-3} mm^2/s, respectively.

Abscesses in different locations have been reported to present restricted diffusion, mainly in the periphery. This is due to its viscous content. This characteristic has made DWI an adequate tool to differentiate cysts and abscesses in the liver and brain. Therefore, abscesses are also a potential pitfall for malignancy on DWI. As with maturation, the central part of abscess may liquefy, the restriction of the central part of the abscess gradually decreases as ADC increases, which may be used to evaluate response to antibiotic treatment.

Imaging Findings

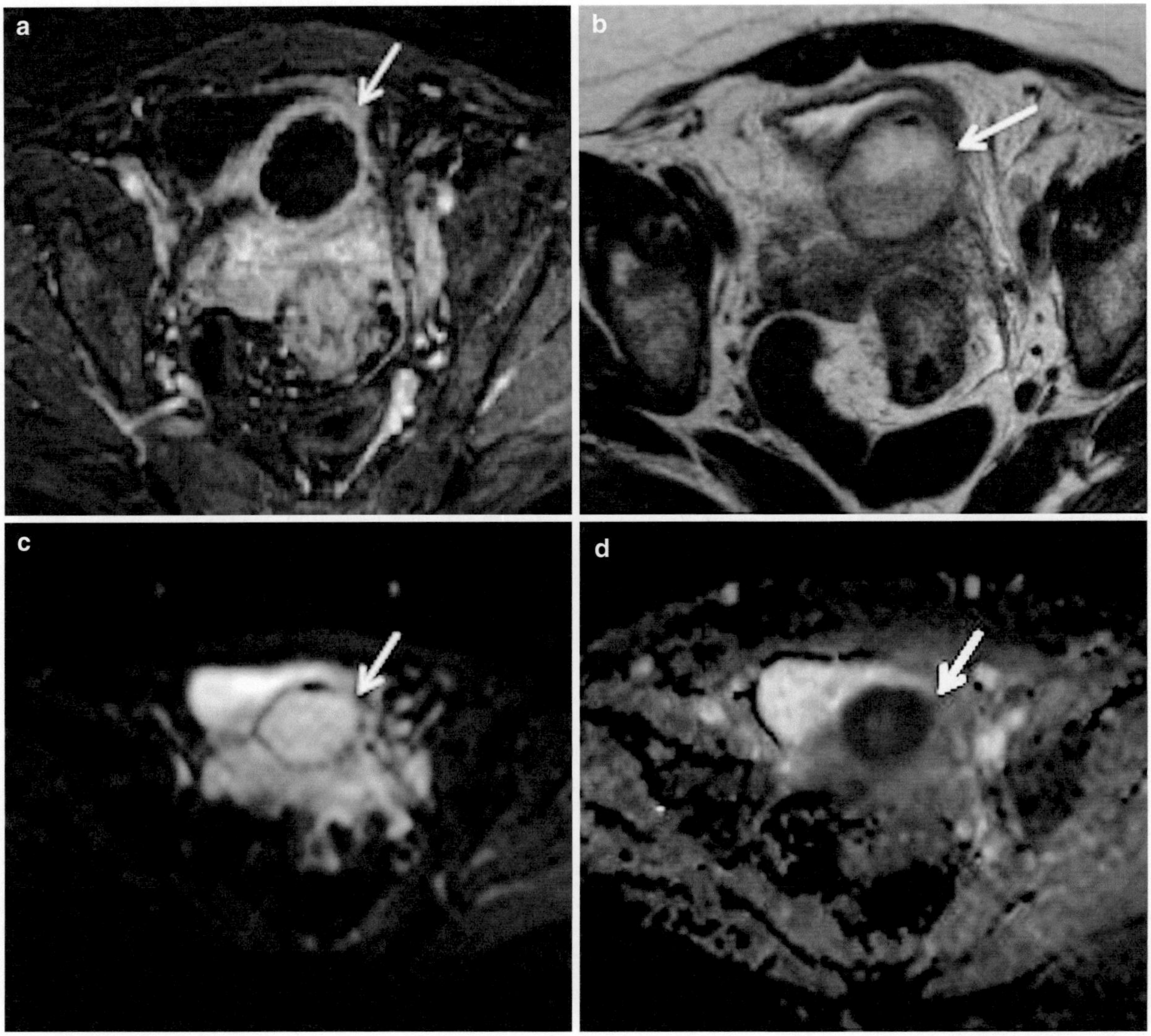

Fig. 11.7 (**a**) Axial T1 GE image with fat suppression shows a round, ring-enhancing fluid collection consistent with abscess (*arrow*). (**b**) Axial FSE T2-weighted image demonstrates the fluid collection (*arrow*) as predominantly hyperintense with a hypointense capsule and surrounding fat stranding. Notice the presence of a small air-fluid level, indicating intralesional air suggesting communication with the GI tract. (**c**, **d**) DWI acquired with a *b* factor of 1,000 s/mm^2 and corresponding ADC map demonstrates the fluid collection and inflammatory changes in the adjacent fat which show high signal intensity on DWI and low signal intensity on the ADC map indicating restricted diffusion in the abscess secondary to acute diverticulitis (*arrows*)

Fig. 11.8 (**a**, **b**) Axial postcontrast GE T1-weighted and FSE T2-weighted images, both with fat suppression show the thickened distal ileum wall which enhances avidly with gadolinium, consistent with inflammatory process (*arrows*). (**c**) DWI acquired with *b* factor of 800 s/mm^2 shows the intestinal wall with high signal intensity (*arrow*). (**d**) The ADC map image demonstrates low signal intensity in the abnormal bowel wall, indicating restricted diffusion caused by active inflammatory stage of Crohn's disease (*arrow*)

Case 11.8: Crohn's Disease – Active Inflammation

Thirty-eight-year-old woman complaining of weight loss, abdominal pain, and diarrhea. The MRI examination was performed for evaluating the cause of these symptoms.

Comments

Crohn's disease can affect any segment of the small bowel, with a predilection for the terminal ileum. The main advantage of MRI over other techniques for detection of small bowel abnormalities is the ability to evaluate the complete small bowel and extramural disease manifestations without the use of ionizing radiation. The imaging protocol enables both the diagnosis and the extent of the disease. Functional information can be used to differentiate between collapsed but normal bowel wall, active disease, inactive disease, and bowel wall stenosis. The contrast-enhanced series contribute to the differentiation between active and chronic disease. Specific characteristics for Crohn's disease – that is, creeping fat (increased mesenteric fat), skip lesions, and fistulas – are also readily identified. Findings of active inflammation are bowel wall edema, ulcerations, increased mesenteric vascularization, increased enhancement of the bowel wall, and mesenteric lymph nodes. In acute inflammation, the bowel wall can have a layered pattern. A double-halo sign is related to submucosal edema. Although DWI has not been routinely used in Crohn's disease, the reported experience has demonstrated that active inflammation may be demonstrated as areas of restricted diffusion within the bowel wall, as illustrated in this case. Furthermore, ADC measurements allow to differentiate active from fibrotic segments, which opens a door for posttreatment monitorization. Another potential advantage of DWI is the chance to obviate contrast administration.

Imaging Findings

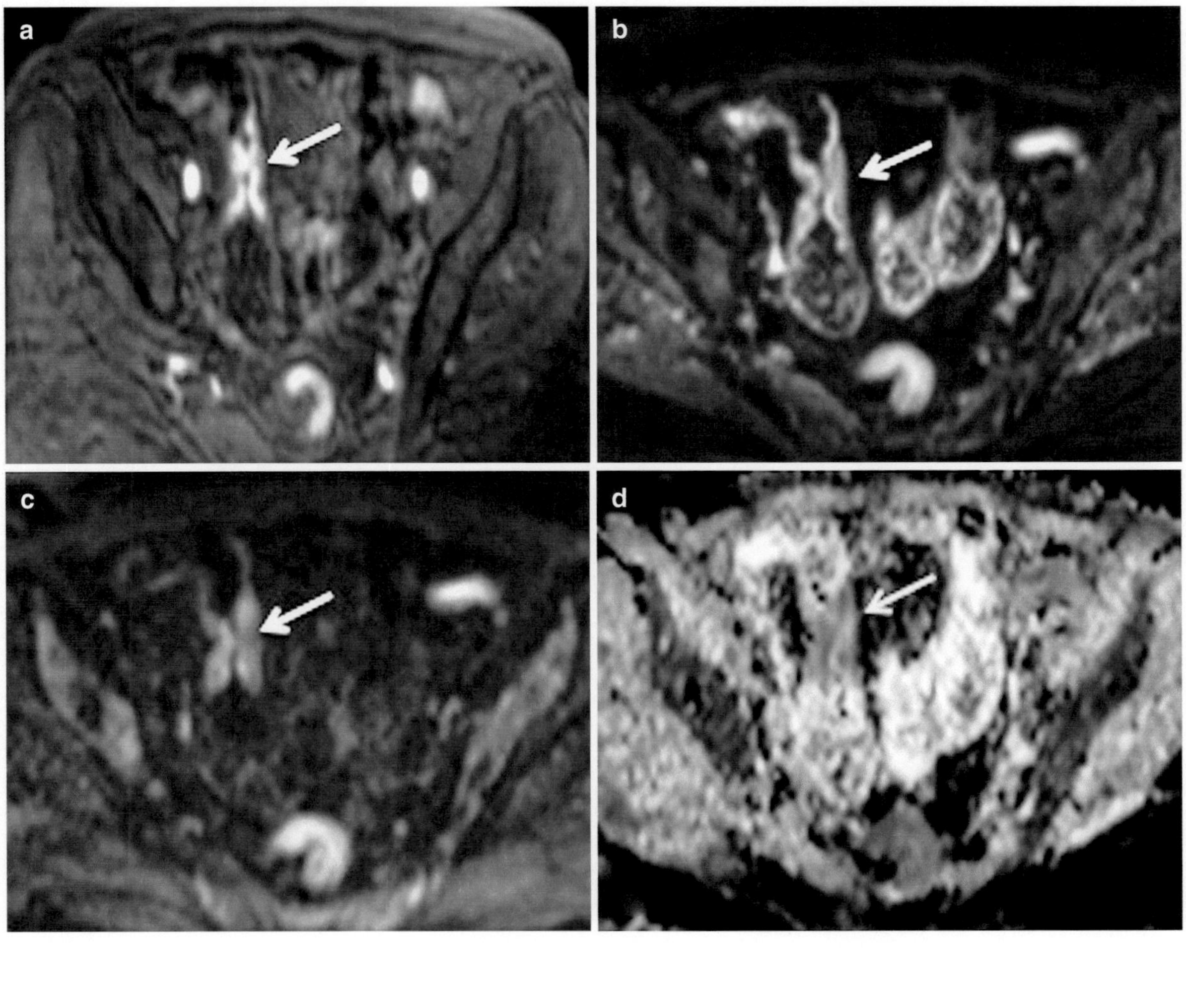

Case 11.9: Crohn's Disease: Fibrostenotic Stage

A 31-year-old man with Crohn's disease. Main current complaint was recurrent episodes of abdominal pain and distention. MR enterography was requested to evaluate possible bowel stenosis and mechanical obstruction.

Comments

Crohn's disease can be localized in every segment of the small bowel, with a predilection for the terminal ileum. MR enterography is helpful to detect evidence of active disease and to diagnose complications. Fat accumulation in the submucosa can be found in the subacute or chronic stage. The contrast-enhanced MR series also contribute to the differentiation between active and chronic disease. Inactive disease is characterized by absence of abnormalities (i.e., optimal distention of bowel loops, healthy peristalsis, and no stenosis) or bowel wall thickening with relatively low signal intensity representing fibrosis with limited, homogeneous contrast enhancement. MRI can show infiltration of mesenteric fat that may evolve into a fistula. Intraluminal fluid and the use of an IV contrast medium can improve the ability to detect fistulas. Abscesses are more readily identified on the sequences performed after the injection of IV contrast medium as well. MRI also allows the evaluation of other complications associated with Crohn's disease, including intussusception, stricture formation, and carcinoma. DWI can be helpful for characterizing Crohn's disease and for detecting complications. Furthermore, it has been recently reported that DWI can help differentiate between the active and inactive phases of the disease, which is important to determine the adequate course of treatment.

Imaging Findings

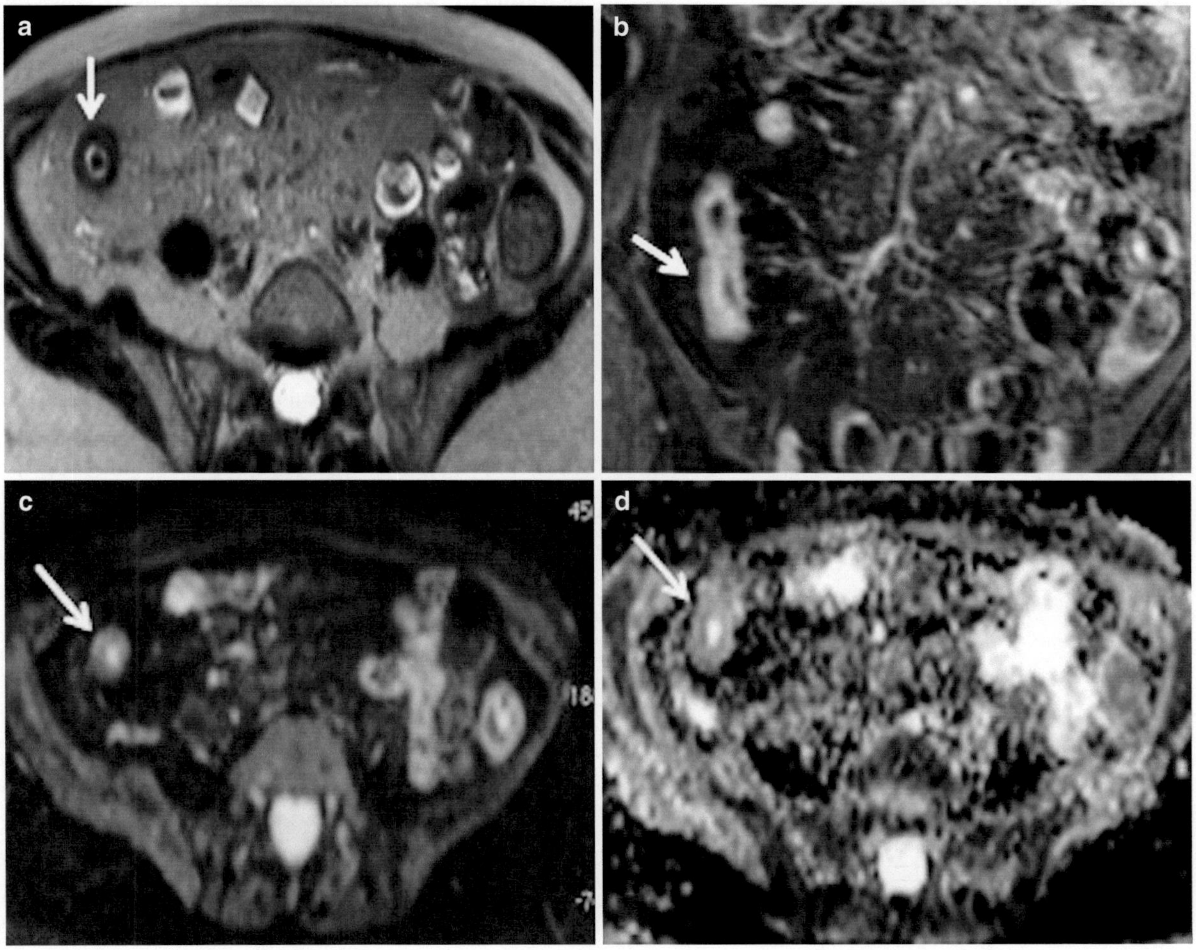

Fig. 11.9 (**a**) Axial FSE (*arrow*) T2-weighted image shows the thickened distal ileum wall with low signal intensity. (**b**) Coronal contrast-enhanced GE T1-weighted gradient-echo image with fat suppression demonstrates enhancement of the bowel wall and preservation of mural stratification (target sign), consistent with inflammatory process (*arrow*). (**c**) DWI acquired with *b* factor of 800 s/mm^2 shows the thickened bowel wall with low signal intensity (*arrow*). (**d**) The ADC map image demonstrates intermediate signal intensity indicating lack of significant restriction in the affected segment of bowel (*arrow*). This is an example of the fibrostenotic stage of Crohn's disease

Case 11.10: Peritoneal Metastases of Ovarian Carcinoma

A 53-year-old female, with surgically removed ovarian carcinoma 2 years before and in clinical complete remission, is submitted to our imaging department to perform a follow-up MRI.

Comments

Primary tumors of the peritoneum are rare, whereas metastatic disease is the most commonly encountered neoplastic process involving the peritoneum. MRI, using 5-min postcontrast fat-suppressed VIBE sequences, is the preferred imaging technique for evaluation of the metastatic peritoneum. Addition of DWI with high *b* value to conventional MRI increases the detection of peritoneal deposits, being specially useful in specific challenging regions and increasing the conspicuous city of lesions smaller than 4 mm. Reported data has used a highest *b* value between 500 and 800 s/mm^2, although in our experience, the use of higher *b* values up to 1,400 s/mm^2 enables better differentiation of lesions against the suppressed background, including structures that normally show restricted diffusion with smaller *b* values, as small bowel mucosa, endometrium, or ovaries. Although DWI with very high *b* values show lower SNR and is more prone to artifacts, it is feasible to use the maximum higher strength, parallel imaging, and spectral fat suppression. The use of fusion software also allows better anatomical localization of the small peritoneal deposits, as shown in this case.

Imaging Findings

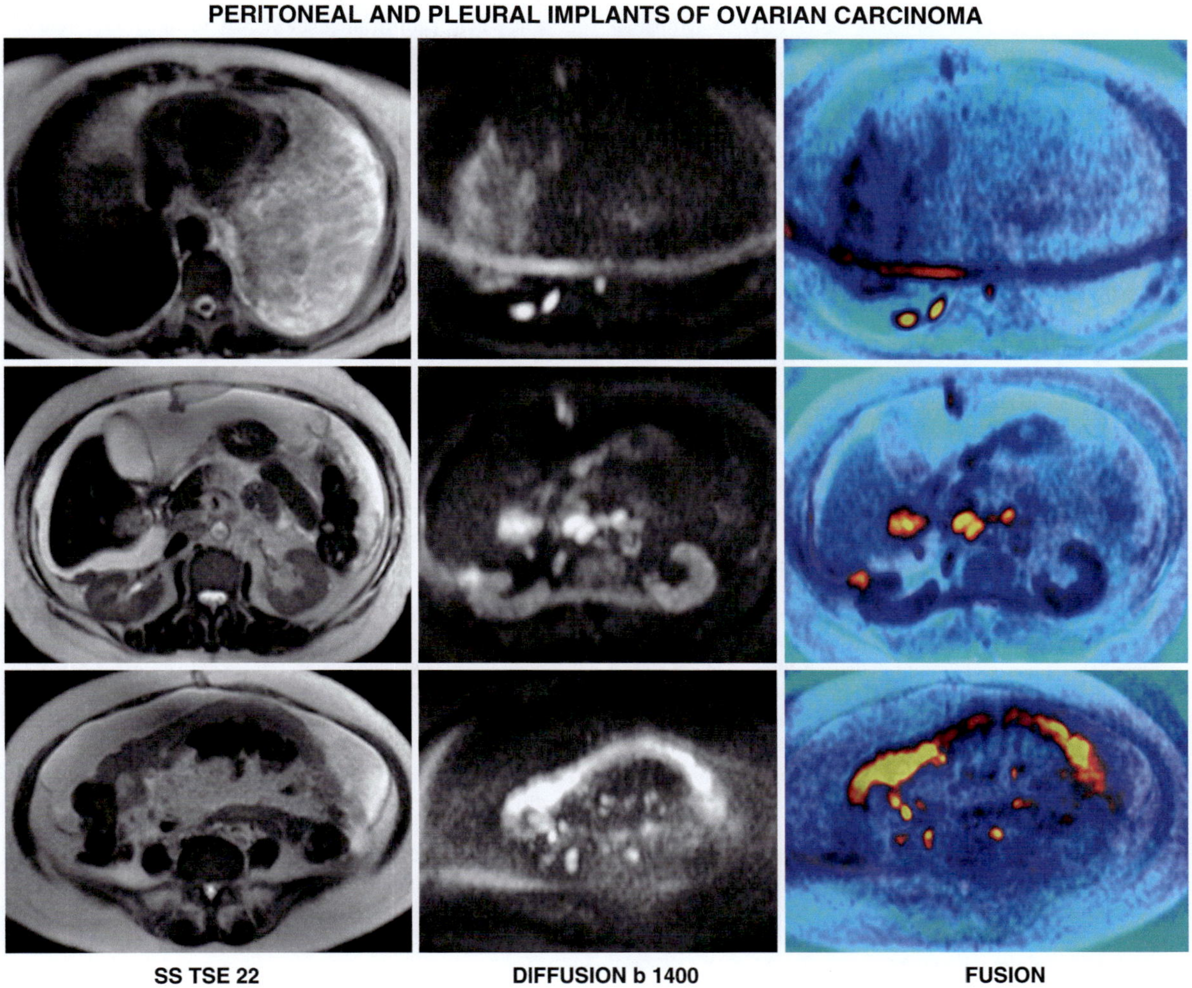

Fig. 11.10 HASTE (*left column*), free-breathing DWI with spectral fat suppression and *b* value of 1,400 s/mm^2 (*central column*) and fusion of both sequences (*right column*) at three different levels demonstrate diffuse peritoneal carcinomatosis, omental cake and right basal pleural metastasis. Notice how DWI and the fusion images better depict the small metastatic foci even in challenging regions such as the root of the mesentery, pleura, and hepatic subcapsular space

Further Reading

Blumenfeld YJ, Wong AE, Jafari A et al (2011) MR imaging in cases of antenatal suspected appendicitis – a meta-analysis. J Matern Fetal Neonatal Med 24:485–488

Bozkurt M, Doganay S, Kantarci M et al (2010) Comparison of peritoneal tumor imaging using conventional MR imaging and diffusion-weighted MR imaging with different b values. Eur J Radiol Jul 1, 2010 [Epub ahead of print]

Bruegel M, Holzapfel K, Gaa J et al (2008) Characterization of focal liver lesions by ADC measurements using a respiratory-triggered diffusion weighted single-shot echo-planar MR imaging technique. Eur Radiol 18:477–485

Dzik-Jurasz A, Domenig C, George M et al (2002) Diffusion MRI for prediction of response of rectal cancer to chemoradiation. Lancet 360(9329):307–308

Feuerlein S, Pauls S, Juchems MS et al (2009) Pitfalls in abdominal diffusion-weighted imaging: how predictive is restricted water diffusion for malignancy. Am J Roentgenol 193(4):1070–1076

Fidler JL, Guimaraes L, Einstein DM (2009) MR imaging of the small bowel. Radiographics 29(6):1811–1825

Hammond NA, Miller FH, Yaghmai V et al (2008) MR imaging of acute bowel pathology: a pictorial review. Emerg Radiol 15(2):99–104

Ichikawa T, Erturk SM, Motosugi U et al (2006) High-B-value diffusion-weighted MRI in colorectal cancer. Am J Roentgenol 187:181–184

Inci E, Kilickesmez O, Hocaoglu E et al (2011) Utility of diffusion-weighted imaging in the diagnosis of acute appendicitis. Eur Radiol 21:768–775

Kilickesmez O, Atilla S, Soylu A et al (2009a) Diffusion-weighted imaging of the rectosigmoid colon: preliminary findings. J Comput Assist Tomogr 33(6):863–866

Kilickesmez O, Atilla S, Soylu A et al (2009b) Diffusion-weighted imaging of the recto sigmoid colon: preliminary findings. J Comput Assist Tomogr 33(6):863–866

Kiryu S, Dodanuki K, Takao H et al (2009) Free-breathing diffusion-weighted imaging for the assessment of inflammatory activity in Crohn's disease. J Magn Reson Imaging 29(4):880–886

Koh DM, Collins DJ (2007) Diffusion-weighted MRI in the body: applications and challenges in oncology. Am J Roentgenol 188:1622–1635

Kyriazi S, Collins DJ, Morgan VA et al (2010) Diffusion-weighted imaging of peritoneal disease for noninvasive staging of advanced ovarian cancer. Radiographics 30(5):1269–1285

Lohan DG, Alhajeri AN et al (2008) MR enterography of small-bowel lymphoma: potential for suggestion of histologic subtype and the presence of underlying celiac disease. Am J Roentgenol 190(2):287–293

Low RN (2007) MR imaging of the peritoneal spread of malignancy. Abdom Imaging 32:267–283

Low RN, Gurney J (2007) Diffusion-weighted MRI (DWI) in the oncology patient: value of breath hold DWI compared to unenhanced and gadolinium-enhanced MRI. J Magn Reson Imaging 25:848–858

Low RN, Barone RM, Gurney JM et al (2008) Mucinous appendiceal neoplasms: preoperative MR staging and classification compared with surgical and histopathologic findings. Am J Roentgenol 190:656–665

Low RN, Sebrechts CP, Barone RM et al (2009) Diffusion-weighted MRI of peritoneal tumors: comparison with conventional MRI and surgical and histopathologic findings, a feasibility study. Am J Roentgenol 193(2):461–470

Malagò R, Manfredi R, Benini L et al (2009) Assessment of the extension and the inflammatory activity in Crohn's disease: comparison of ultrasound and MRI. Abdom Imaging 34(2):141–148

Masselli G, Brunelli R, Casciani E et al (2010) Acute abdominal and pelvic pain in pregnancy: MR imaging as a valuable adjunct to ultrasound? Abdom Imaging Oct 30, 2010 [Epub ahead of print]

Oto A, Zhu F, Kulkarni K et al (2009) Evaluation of diffusion-weighted MR imaging for detection of bowel inflammation in patients with Crohn's disease. Acad Radiol 16(5):597–603

Padhani AR, Liu G, Koh DM et al (2009) Diffusion-weighted magnetic resonance imaging as a cancer biomarker: consensus and recommendations. Neoplasia 11(2):102–125

Sakurada A, Takahaara T, Kwee TC et al (2009) Diagnostic performance of diffusion-weighted MRI in esophageal cancer. Eur Radiol 19:1461–1469

Shinya S, Sasaki T, Nakagawa Y et al (2007) The usefulness of diffusion-weighted imaging (DWI) for the detection of gastric cancer. Hepatogastroenterology 54(77):1378–1381

Shinya S, Sasaki T, Nakagawa Y et al (2009) The efficacy of diffusion-weighted imaging for the detection of colorectal cancer. Hepatogastroenterology 56(89):128–132

Shuto K, Saito H, Ohira G et al (2009) Diffusion-weighted MR imaging for postoperative nodal recurrence of esophageal squamous cell cancer in comparison with FDG-PET. Gan To Kagaku Ryoho 36(12):2468–2470

Sugita R, Yamazaki T, Furuta A et al (2009) High b-value diffusion-weighted MRI for detecting gallbladder carcinoma: preliminary study and results. Eur Radiol 19:1794–1798

Sugita R, Ito K, Fujita N et al (2010) Diffusion-weighted MRI in abdominal oncology: clinical applications. World J Gastroenterol 16(7):832–836

Thoeny HC, De Keyzer F (2007) Extracranial applications of diffusion-weighted magnetic resonance imaging. Eur Radiol 17:1385–1393

Van Weyenberg SJ, Meijerink MR, Jacobs MA et al (2010) MR enteroclysis in the diagnosis of small-bowel neoplasm's. Radiology 254(3):765–773

Diffusion-Weighted Imaging of Anorectal Region

12

Lidia Alcalá, Teodoro Martín, and Antonio Luna

12.1 Technical Considerations

DWI is a functional sequence which has shown to be able to indirectly determine the degree of cellularity of a lesion as more cellular lesions constrain diffusion of free water in the interstitial space. Even more, the diffusion within a tissue may be quantified by measuring the ADC.

In the anorectal region, we perform a SS-DWI sequence with SPIR. We use a free-breathe approach as there are no artifacts from either respiratory movement or vascular pulsation. As in other pelvic organs, the use of the shortest TE available and parallel imaging is desirable. The use of a phase-array coil is important in order to improve the signal to noise ratio (SNR).

Although the optimum *b* value in this anatomic area is not well established, a maximum *b* value of 1,000 s/mm^2 is generally accepted since lower values are less specific for lesion detection due to the intrinsic high signal intensity of the rectal mucosa on DWI. Using high *b* values, we can diminish the normal hypersignal of the rectal mucosa. Our DWI sequence includes five different *b* values (*b* 0 s/mm^2, *b* 250 s/mm^2, *b* 500 s/mm^2, *b* 750 s/mm^2 and *b* 1,000 s/mm^2) in order to improve the image quality of ADC maps. We always co-register the acquisitions obtained with different *b* values before calculating the ADC maps.

As DWI is extending its role in rectal cancer imaging, it is essential to standardize imaging protocols and data analysis methods. This includes the way to draw ROIs for ADC measurements and the selection of the areas of analysis. There is general consensus in avoiding areas of necrosis and susceptibility artifacts in ADC measurements. The use of the mean ADC of the whole tumor seems to be a simplistic approach that will probably be substituted by histogram or voxel-wise analyses which are able to evaluate tumor heterogeneity

The use of antiperistaltic agents may improve imaging quality although in our experience, it is not essential. It is important to avoid susceptibility artifacts derived from the presence of air within the rectum. In this sense, the use of cleansing enemas before the test or to fill-in the rectum with ultrasound gel can help.

12.2 Clinical Applications

12.2.1 Rectal Cancer Detection

One of the most common clinical applications of DWI in the rectum is rectal cancer detection. DWI has shown to increase the detection of rectal cancer in combination with T2-weighted images as compared to the use only of T2-weighted images. There are several series of detection of rectal cancer using only DWI with high *b* values, all of them showed a sensitivity near 100%, using only a qualitative approach. The specificity ranged between 65% and 94%. According to the same reports, ADC calculation allows to reduce the number

Lidia Alcalá (✉)
Body Section, Clínica Las Nieves, SERCOSA,
Jaén, Spain
l.alcala.o@htime.org

T. Martín
MRI section, Clínica Las Nieves, SERCOSA,
Jaén, Spain

A. Luna
Chief of MRI, Health Time Group,
Jaén, Spain
aluna70@sercosa.com

A. Luna et al., *Diffusion MRI Outside the Brain*,
DOI 10.1007/978-3-642-21052-5_12, © Springer-Verlag Berlin Heidelberg 2012

of false positives as rectal cancer usually shows lower ADC values. The cutoff ADC value in several series is around 1.2×10^{-3} mm²/s. The most common cause of false negatives was the presence of a circumference (ring-shaped) area of high signal in the lower rectum in high *b* values. One of the reasons of the increase in sensitivity of DWI compared to morphological MRI sequences is the presence of small polyps, which are sometimes impossible to detect with morphological MRI sequences. These polyps usually demonstrate marked restriction of diffusion (Fig. 12.1). Even more, in rectal cancer staging, DWI may be used as a scout sequence to locate the tumor and plan the axial high-resolution T2-weighted sequences, which will allow an accurate locoregional staging.

12.2.2 Rectal Cancer Staging

DWI is also useful for delineating the cancer extension in the initial staging of rectal carcinomas, since some of them show fibrous and inflammatory changes that hinder the correct staging which is very important to decide the therapeutic approach. The TNM classification is the most commonly used. On the one hand, if either the tumor extends beyond the muscularis mucosa (T3 and T4 stages) or if there are more than three nodes in the mesorectal fat (N2 stage), the appropriate treatment will be chemoradiation. On the other hand, if the rectal cancer is confined to the rectal muscular wall (T2 stage) or less than three metastatic nodes in the mesorectal fat are present (N0 or N1 stages), a total mesorectal excision should be performed. In cases of tumors located within the rectal mucosa and/or submucosa (T1 stage), a limited endorectal resection will be the appropriate surgical approach. Therefore, it is crucial to differentiate between T2 and T3 stage carcinomas. In our experience, DWI may be useful in this task in some cases, mainly when desmoplastic changes are presented, since these usually show a lesser degree of restriction than rectal cancer, allowing a better depiction of tumor borders.

DWI also allows the detection of a greater number of lymph nodes, even those smaller than 3 mm, compared to morphological MRI sequences (Fig. 12.2). Small lymph nodes can be easily missed, mainly if they are adjacent to vessels or bowel loops, in the presence of ascites or when there is scarce pelvic fat. The use of fusion software improves lymph node location, which may be sometimes challenging with high *b* values DWI images due to poor SNR and background suppression.

One of the major problems in the MRI staging of rectal carcinoma is to differentiate between metastatic and reactive or inflammatory lymph nodes. Morphological criteria such as a size superior to 3–5 mm, ill-defined edges, and a heterogeneous signal intensity on T2-weighted sequences similar to or lower than the primary tumor have been demonstrated to be insufficient and limited, as they are observer dependent. Until the definitive advent of ultrasmall iron-based particles (USPIO), contrast materials that will hopefully bring real improvement in lymph node characterization, MRI, as all other imaging methods, is clearly limited in this area. Several studies have proposed DWI and ADC quantifications as helpful imaging tools in the discrimination between benign and malignant lymph nodes in head and neck and gynecological cancer staging. Normal lymph nodes are hypercellular appearing as high signal spots on DWI with high *b* values. Therefore, ADC quantification is necessary to characterize lymph nodes. At this moment, there is only a report evaluating the differentiation between metastatic and benign lymph nodes in the primary staging of rectal carcinoma. In this series, metastatic lymph nodes were significantly larger and showed a lower ADC value than benign ones, allowing for preoperative characterization. The most accurate parameter to identify metastatic lymph nodes was ratio of lymph node ADC value to the primary tumor ADC value. Larger series are necessary to confirm these preliminary results.

12.2.3 Prediction of Rectal Cancer Outcome and Early Detection of Tumor Response

Perhaps, the most revolutionary application that has emerged from DWI in rectal cancer evaluation is the ability to predict whether a patient with rectal cancer will respond to neoadjuvant chemotherapy and radiotherapy, so that, nonresponding patients will not be exposed to such an aggressive and expensive treatment. This is possible by quantifying both the cellularity of the lesions and the integrity of the cell membrane with DWI. Therefore, in several series rectal cancers with a lower ADC values showed a good response to neoadjuvant treatment (Fig. 12.3), while those with higher ADC values demonstrated a poorer outcome (Fig. 12.4). It must be taken into consideration that the presence of necrosis, a factor that indicates a high tumor aggressiveness, increases the ADC value and that tumoral necrosis is related to hypoxia-related radioresistance. In these series, the criteria for responding tumors were a tumoral volume reduction of 50% or a T-downstaging after chemoradiation. Contrarily, other reports have shown the absence of relationship between pretreatment ADC value of rectal cancer and treatment outcome when the pathological complete response was the reference standard. Therefore, we can conclude with the available data that rectal cancers with lower ADC values will show at least a partial response to treatment, although a complete response cannot be assured. Further research is needed to evaluate the real role of DWI in the prediction of rectal cancer to chemoradiation.

In the early stages of treatment, as soon as 2 weeks after treatment, DWI is able to depict relatively small effects of the treatment such as modified permeability of cell membranes, cell swelling, and early cell lysis and apoptosis-induced cell death. This allows the early monitorization of the response to chemotherapy of rectal cancer with DWI, as rectal cancer with good response will show a gradual increase in the ADC values at first, which will not significantly vary in nonresponders. After a certain time, a reequilibrium in ADC values may happen with a decrease at the end of the treatment, due to the development of postradiation fibrosis. Inflammatory and edematous areas may also arise around the treated tumor. These areas of inflammation are a common cause of false-positive results in PET. Responding tumors may also show areas of mucinous differentiation which will increase the ADC value at the end of treatment. The early assessment of chemoradiation provided by DWI prevents from overstaging of morphological MRI and may allow the development of individualized therapies in the near future.

12.2.4 Posttreatment Restaging and Detection of Recurrence

DWI is a useful tool in the restaging of rectal cancer after neoadjuvant therapy. It is difficult to distinguish posttreatment fibrosis from residual tumor with conventional morphological sequences, including postcontrast acquisitions, as early fibrosis may enhance with gadolinium in a similar manner to recurrent cancer. Postchemoradiation ADC values of rectal cancer can reliably differentiate responders from nonresponders according to recent data. An ADC cutoff value between 1.2 and 1.3×10^{-3} mm^2/s has been proposed, with negative predictive values near 100%. However, a poor predictive positive value around 50–60% has been achieved in the same series, probably related to the limitations of DWI in the differentiation between complete response from near-complete response and in the discrimination between residual tumor from inactive mucin areas.

In the late posttreatment assessment, DWI may also distinguish between old fibrosis and recurrent tumor, as fibrosis tends to demonstrate less restriction of diffusion than recurrent viable tumor. Therefore, DWI is also useful in detecting tumor recurrence, which will commonly show similar ADC values than the non-treated primary tumor (Fig. 12.5).

An accurate nodal restaging after chemoradiation is important in order to ensure that the true node-negative patients are accurately selected. In patients with complete response, new more conservative therapeutic strategies are in debate, such as a local excision or a wait-and-see policy, with the aim of reducing treatment-related morbidity and mortality. Morphological criteria for nodal restaging after chemoradiation work better than in primary staging, because only nodes that remain large are likely to be malignant. In a recent series by Lambregts, 30 patients with locally advanced distal cancer, treated with chemoradiation and resection, were submitted to postchemoradiation MRI, including T2-weighted and DWI sequences with ADC measurements, for assessment of nodal staging with direct histological comparison. DWI improved nodal detection compared to TSE T2-weighted sequences alone, although visual assessment of DWI did not help in nodal characterization. ADC values of nodal metastasis were significantly higher than nonmetastatic ones, although there was a considerable overlap in values and ADC was impossible to calculate in a important number of nodes due to the presence of artifacts or the small size of the nodes. However, the addition of DWI to T2-weighted sequences did not improve the diagnostic accuracy and T2 weighted-MRI alone was considered sufficiently accurate.

12.2.5 Applications of DWI in Other Rectal Tumors

DWI is also useful for further characterization of rectal lesions other than rectal adenocarcinoma or perirectal lesions. In this sense, benign lesions such as enteric cyst or retrorectal cystic hamartomas show higher ADC values than malignant ones, indicating both their cystic nature and absence of hypercellularity (Fig. 12.6). In occasions, lesions with a mucin rich content may show false restriction (Fig. 4.9).

Anorectal location of gastrointestinal stromal tumors (GIST) occurs approximately between 5% and 10% of the times. They are more commonly mural lesions of well-defined borders, with internal areas of hemorrhage and lack of perirectal lymphadenopathies. Besides rectal adenocarcinoma, other uncommon rectal lesions such as lymphoma, malignant melanoma, carcinoid, leiomyoma, and leiomyosarcoma must be considered in the differential diagnosis of these tumors. These tumors are treated with drugs such as imitanib that causes destruction of the cell membrane, producing areas of necrosis within the tumors, which will usually increase in size early after treatment. This feature may lead to misinterpretation as disease progression if only morphological imaging is used. Because of this, RECIST criteria should be applied with caution in GIST, as tumor size is not an early predictor of tumor response, while structural and perfusion modifications are readily observed. Functional techniques such as DWI are being tested in order to distinguish GIST imitanib responders from nonresponders (Fig. 12.7).

12.2.6 Inflammatory Conditions

DWI has been proposed as a promising imaging tool to detect inflammatory conditions in an acute clinical setting. Areas of active inflammation and abscesses usually show restricted diffusion and low ADC values, being a potential mimicker of malignant processes (Fig. 12.8). Therefore, information provided by DWI may be helpful in distinguishing necrotic tumors from abscesses and in the detection of complications from diverticulitis and inflammatory bowel disease (Fig. 12.9).

DWI is being used in the evaluation of inflammatory bowel disease to identify areas of activity and to distinguish acute and chronic areas of inflammation. Even more, in the rectosigmoid colon, DWI has demonstrated its capability to accurately differentiate between inflammatory bowel disease and neoplastic involvement.

12.2.7 Evaluation of Fistula-In-Ano

The inflammatory pathology is the most prevalent disease in anus, being fistula-in-ano, the most frequent by far. Nowadays, endoanal examination under anesthesia, endoanal ultrasound, and contrast-enhanced anorectal MRI are considered the three diagnostic pillars to detect anal fistula, although it has been demonstrated that MRI is the most sensitive of them and that it also allows assessing the activity of the fistula (Fig. 12.10).

DWI, in combination with T2-weighted sequences, has recently shown to be superior in the detection of anal fistula compared to only T2-weighted sequences and to perform similarly to postcontrast sequences and T2-weighted sequences together. DWI may also differentiate between inactive fibrous fistula and active inflammatory ones, as active fistulas will show lower ADC values. Therefore, DWI may be considered as an alternative to contrast agent administration in patients with renal insufficiency in this clinical setting.

12.3 Conclusions

DWI is a functional MRI sequence, which provides additional information to the basal sequences in the anorectal region. DWI is capable of increasing the sensitivity of tumoral and inflammatory disease detection. It may help in the staging of rectal carcinoma, with a great potential in the prediction of response to treatment, posttreatment monitorization, and detection of posttreatment recurrence.

Case 12.1: T1-Stage Concurrent Carcinomatous Rectal Polyps

A 76-year-old male with constipation for months. A polypoid mass in the lower third of the rectum was demonstrated in rigid rectoscopy. Biopsy demonstrated a rectal adenocarcinoma. MRI was performed for tumor staging.

Comments

Rectal carcinoma is one of the most common tumors in developed countries and the most common between all gastrointestinal tract carcinomas. Up to 98% of rectal carcinomas are adenocarcinomas. It is very important to determine tumor extension according to TNM staging in order to establish the therapeutic approach:

- T1-stage: The tumor affects only the mucosa and submucosa. The preferred treatment is endoscopic transanal resection.
- T2-stage: The tumor invades muscularis mucosa but does not affect the mesorectal fat. The treatment would be total excision of the mesorectum without previous neoadjuvant treatment.
- T3-stage: Tumor invades mesorectal fat without infiltrating neighboring organs. The treatment would be receiving neoadjuvant treatment with radiation therapy and subsequent total mesorectum excision.
- T4-stage: Tumor invades adjacent organs or the sphincter complex. The patient receives chemotherapy and radiotherapy, with subsequent restaging for surgical evaluation.

N-stage is defined by the number of metastatic lymph nodes in mesorectal fat and its location respect to the mesorectal fascia. If more than three lymph nodes in mesorectal fat are involved, this is N2 stage and the patient will receive neoadjuvant chemotherapy independently of the T-stage.

Currently, the imaging method of choice for the staging of rectal carcinoma is MRI, as it offers very high spatial resolution for locoregional staging and it also allows the assessment of lymph nodes in mesorectal fat. MRI morphological sequences have demonstrated some limitations with regard to the assessment of small lymph nodes in the mesorectal fat, as they may have less than 3 mm in diameter and in the detection of small fibrous polypoid cancers. T2-weighted sequences may also confound focal areas of wall thickening secondary to peristaltic contractions with tumors. Some of these issues may be partially solved by means of DWI, which can detect very small hypercellular lesions, such as small carcinogenic rectal focus and also increases the detection of lymphadenopathies.

Imaging Findings

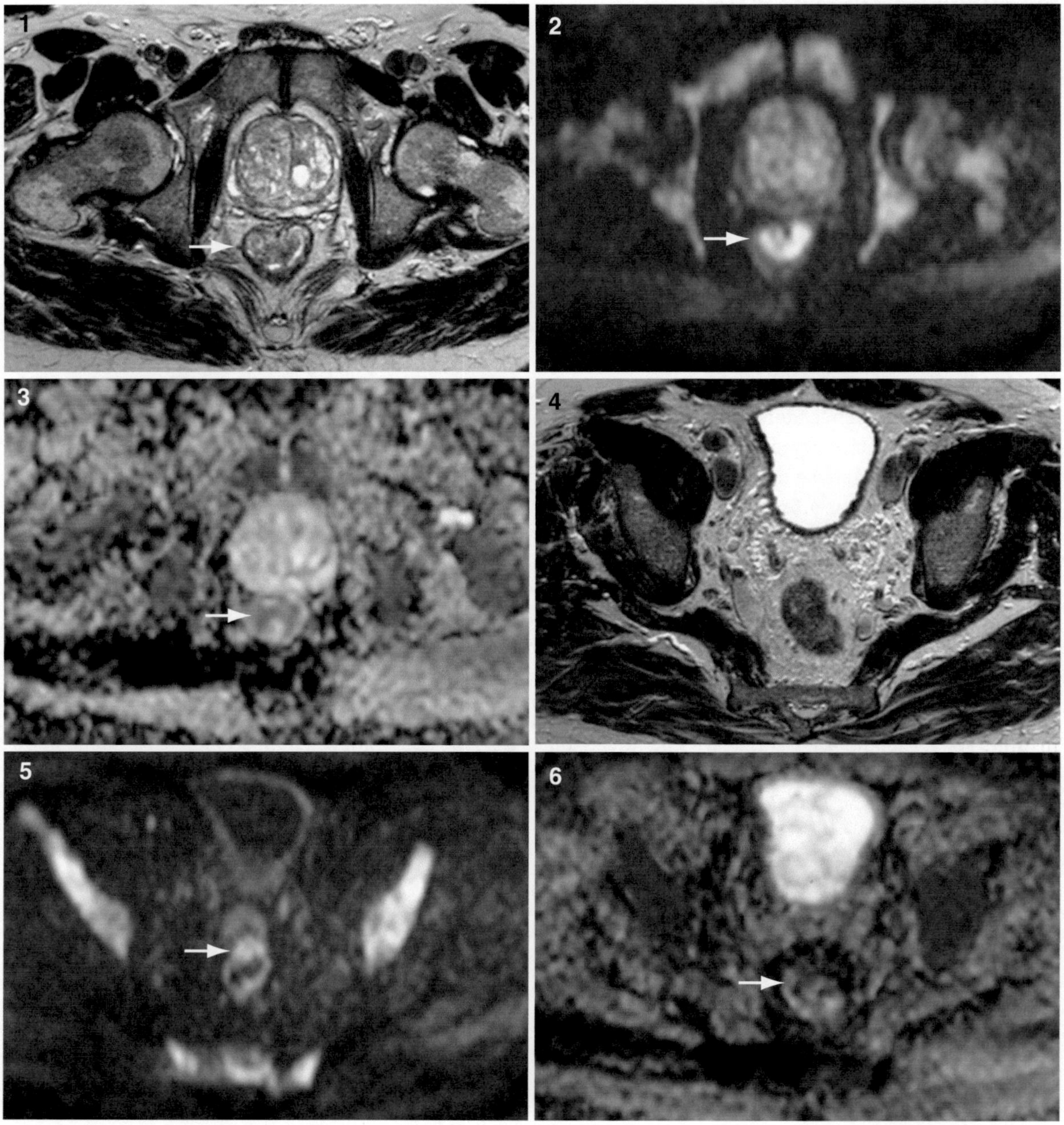

Fig. 12.1 The presence of a polypoid mass located in the lower third of the rectum was confirmed on TSE T2-weighted and more clearly on the DWI series with a *b* value of 1,000 m^2/s (*arrows*) (**12.1.1** and **12.1.2**). It was confined to the mucosa and submucosa and demonstrated a marked restriction of diffusion, with an ADC value of 0.7 ×10^{-3} mm^2/s (*arrow*) (**12.1.3**). Additionally, a second lesion was located in the upper third of the rectum. It was not visualized on T2-weighted sequence (**12.1.4**) and it was more clearly depicted on the DWI series (**12.1.5**) as an area of restricted diffusion with an ADC value of 1×10^{-3} mm^2/s (*arrow*) (**12.1.6**). Both lesions presented a local T1-stage

Case 12.2: Detection of Mesorectal Lymphadenopathies Using DWI

A 69-year-old male who was diagnosed of a stenosing rectal carcinoma was sent to our department for initial tumor staging.

Comments

Accurate N-staging of rectal cancer is crucial in order to determine patient management. If three or less metastatic lymph nodes are found in the mesorectal fat, N1-stage, the patient will not receive neoadjuvant chemotherapy, but if four or more metastatic lymph nodes are detected, N2-stage, neoadjuvant chemotherapy should be applied.

MRI detection of lymph nodes improves with the use of DWI, mainly in the assessment of small nodes adjacent to vessels or bowel loops. The biggest drawback of presurgical staging of rectal cancer with MRI is the difficulty to distinguish between metastatic and inflammatory nodes. Morphological criteria such as a size larger than 3 mm, ill-defined borders, and signal intensity similar or lower than the rectal tumor on T2-weighted sequences have demonstrated to be insufficient for local N-staging, although these criteria work better in a restaging setting than on primary nodal staging. In gynecological malignancies, DWI has shown to increase the number of detected lymph nodes and there were differences in the ADC values between benign and malignant lymph nodes. Depending on the report, malignant lymph nodes showed higher or lower ADC values than benign ones. Different sequences, *b* values, and magnets were used, making it difficult to compare results. With regard to rectal cancer, there is a report evaluating the role of ADC quantification for nodal staging after chemoradiation. In the series by Lambregts et al., ADC measurements showed potential for nodal characterization, although the addition of DWI to T2-weighted sequences did not improve the accuracy of nodal staging compared with T2-weighted sequences. Besides, ADC of malignant nodes was significantly higher than that of benign nodes, although an important overlap was described. Analyzing all the literature regarding lymph nodes characterization in different anatomical locations, higher ADCs in metastatic nodes are found after radiation due mainly to necrotic changes. Before treatment, in all the series, the ADC of metastatic lymph nodes was lower than that of benign ones. In a similar manner, in the only published series evaluating the role of DWI in the primary nodal staging of rectal cancer, metastatic lymph nodes showed a significant lower ADC value than reactive ones.

Imaging Findings

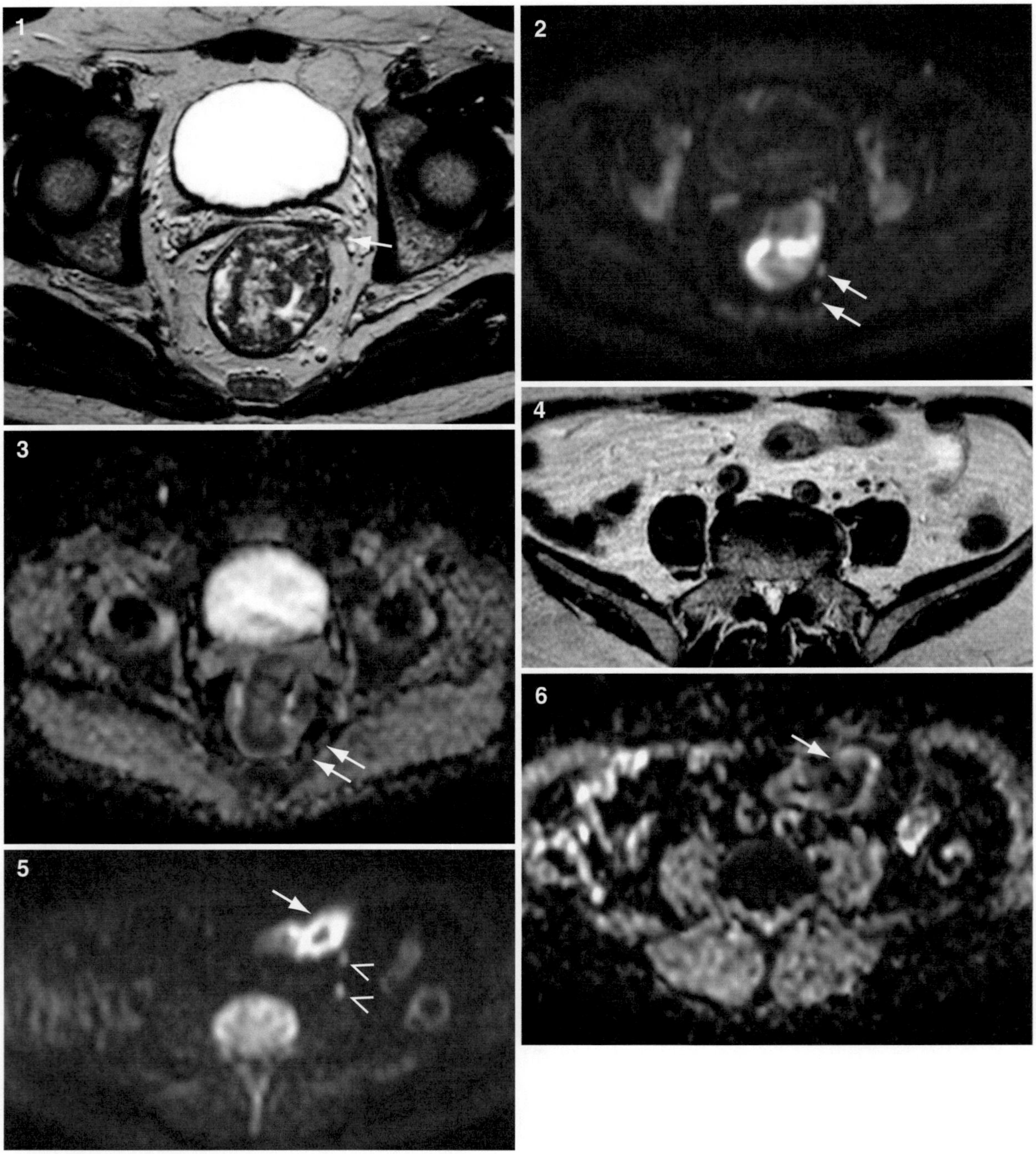

Fig. 12.2 A large concentric tumor causing almost complete stenosis was detected on T2-weighted and DWI images (**12.2.1**, **12.2.2**) in the middle third of the rectum. This tumor infiltrated all layers of the rectal wall, invaded the mesorectal fat, and contacted with the anterior aspect of the mesorectal fascia (*arrow* on **12.2.1**). The tumor showed restriction of diffusion with an ADC value of 0.8×10^{-3} mm^2/s (**12.2.3**). Its locoregional MRI staging was T3b. Eight lymph nodes larger than 3 mm in the mesorectal fat were detected on the DWI sequence, five of them not visualized on T2 weighted sequences (*arrows* on **12.2.2**). Their ADC values did not exceed 0.8×10^{-3} mm^2/s, favoring a metastatic origin (*arrows* on **12.2.3**). We considered a N2 nodal staging. In the same MR examination, a second lesion was identified in the sigmoid colon (**12.2.4**, **12.2.5**). The lesion was better depicted on DWI (*arrow* on **12.2.5**) than on T2-weighted sequences (**12.2.4**). It showed restriction of diffusion, with an ADC value of 0.9×10^{-3} mm^2/s (**12.2.6**). It was suggestive of a synchronous carcinoma in a patient who had undergone an incomplete colonoscopy due to the stenosing rectal tumor. This second lesion was also concentric, but only affected the inner layers of the sigma, without exceeding the serosa. Four lymph nodes were identified on DWI (*arrowheads*), not visualized on T2-weighted images. Their ADC values were all between 1.2 and 1.6×10^{-3} mm^2/s, favoring a reactive origin. A IIA-stage of Dukes' classification was confirmed in the posterior resection

Case 12.3: Prediction of Response to Neoadjuvant Treatment

A 78 year-old male submitted to our department for MRI staging of middle third rectal carcinoma after 3 months of neoadjuvant treatment.

Comments

One of the most important applications of DWI in rectal cancer evaluation is the prediction of outcome and evaluation of response to neoadjuvant treatment.

On the one hand, DWI has been proposed as a tool to predict which rectal carcinomas are candidates to response to neoadjuvant and which ones not. Tumors that will respond to radiotherapy and chemotherapy have ADC values much lower than nonresponders, this is because tumors with high ADC values usually present a highly necrotic component, indicating high aggressiveness and poor response to treatment. Anyway, there are contradictory results in this regard in the literature.

On the other hand, DWI is able to differentiate between residual tumor and desmoplastic changes within the same mass. This differentiation is difficult to assess early after treatment with morphological MRI sequences, even using dynamic contrast MRI, as fibrosis in early stages enhances after gadolinium administration in a similar manner than residual tumors. Conversely, on DWI, fibrosis, even in an early stage usually shows ADC values higher than the tumoral remnants.

Imaging Findings

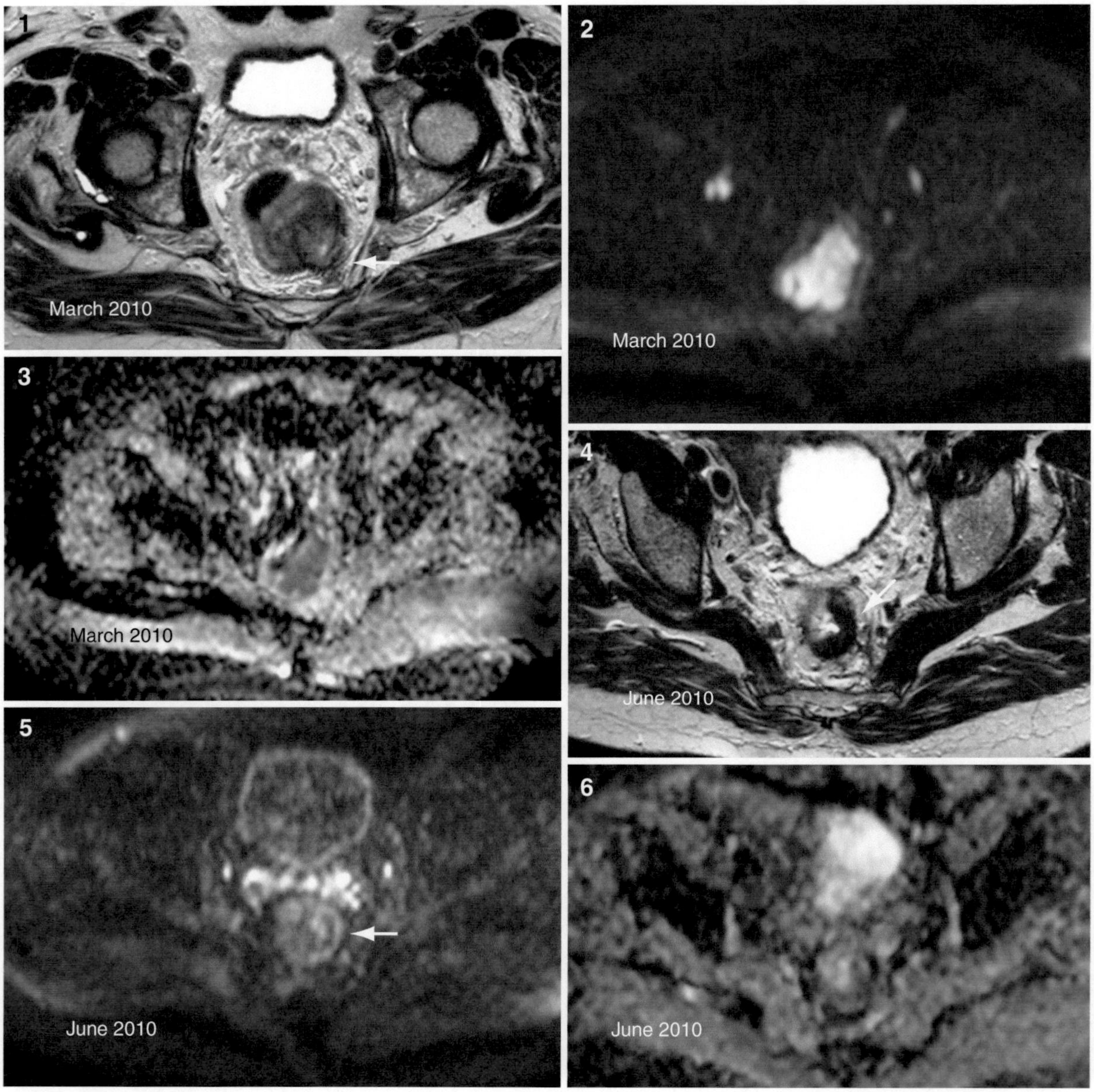

Fig. 12.3 At primary staging MRI (**12.3.1–12.3.3**), the tumor involved all layers of the rectal wall and invaded the mesorectal fat to contact with the mesorectal fascia in its posterior aspect, without exceeding it (*arrow* on **12.3.1**). Thus, local staging was that of T3b. The tumor showed a marked restriction of diffusion with a low ADC value of 0.6×10^{-3} mm^2/s. This low ADC value favors good outcome after neoadjuvant therapy. At the restaging MRI after neoadjuvant treatment (**12.3.4–12.3.6**), there was a significant reduction in size of the tumor which displayed a horseshoe shape and a markedly hypointense signal on T2-weighted sequences (*arrow*) (**12.3.4**). On DWI, there was only a minimal internal area of restriction (*arrow*) (**12.3.5**). The mass showed an increased ADC value of 1.5×10^{-3} mm^2/s (**12.3.6**), which indicates good response to treatment, with a T1-stage, since the mass affects only the mucosa

Case 12.4: Mucinous Adenocarcinoma of the Rectum with Poor Response to Treatment

A 73 -year-old male was referred to our department for staging and assessment of response to treatment of rectal carcinoma with inflammatory characteristics.

Comments

Mucinous colorectal adenocarcinomas are rare, constituting 0.09% of colorectal carcinomas; their most common location is the rectum followed by the descending colon. They typically affect the rectal wall concentrically, not affecting the mucosa, which is usually intact, with invasion of the muscularis mucosa and the mesorectal fat at the initial diagnosis. Because of the lack of involvement of the innermost layer, they tipically present with an insidious clinical picture of diarrhea, alternating with subacute bowel occlusion without bleeding.

These tumors show little restriction of diffusion and higher ADC values than ordinary adenocarcinomas, since most of its volume corresponds to mucin. These type of rectal tumors only show small foci of restricted diffusion in solid areas, and also in lymph nodes and tumoral implants that often exist in the mesorectal fat. These tumors are poor responders to neoadjuvant treatment. Therefore, after treatment, there are little changes either in their morphology or free water diffusion. Even more, they may increase cellularity, increasing the restriction of diffusion during treatment.

Imaging Findings

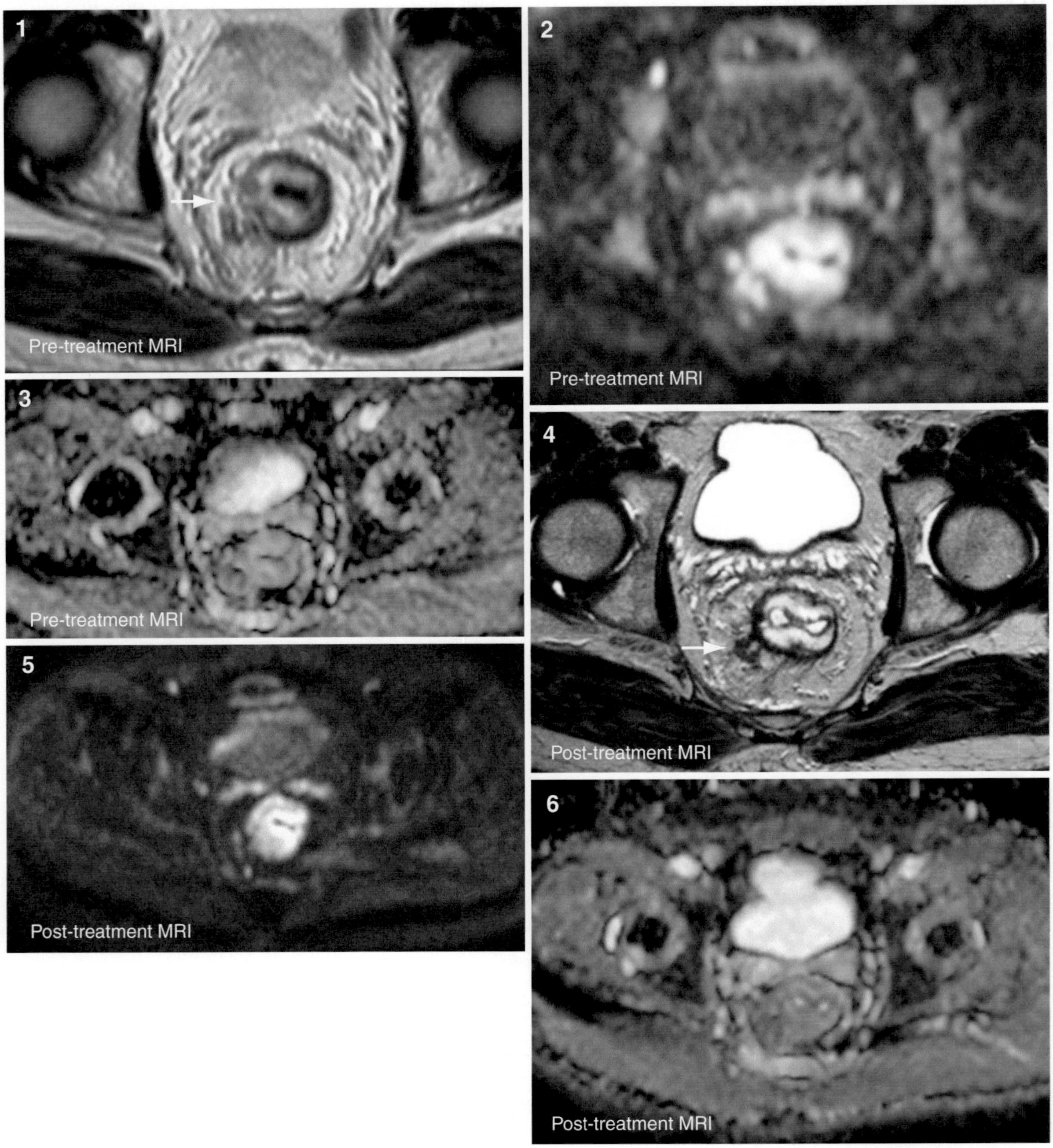

Fig. 12.4 A concentric tumor located in the distal third of the rectum was confirmed at pretreatment MRI. This mass demonstrated high signal intensity on T2-weighted sequences with infiltration of all layers of the rectal wall and a 15 mm in-depth invasion of the mesorectal fat in its right lateral aspect (*arrow*) (**12.4.1**). The tumor showed only a moderate restriction of diffusion (**12.4.2**), with an ADC value of 1.6×10^{-3} mm^2/s (**12.4.3**). These characteristics favour a mucinous adenocarcinoma, which usually shows poor response to neoadjuvant treatment. Six-week posttreatment MRI study confirms the stability of the tumor in size (**12.4.4**), perirectal fat invasion depth (*arrow*), restriction of diffusion (**12.4.5**), and unchanged ADC value (1.6×10^{-3} mm^2/s) (**12.4.6**)

Case 12.5: Diagnosis and Monitoring of Presacral Recurrence of Rectal Carcinoma

A 76-year-old male, treated with an abdominoperitoneal amputation for adenocarcinoma of the rectum, with perianal pain but without discharge or fever.

Comments

DWI helps to differentiate between posttreatment fibrosis and tumor recurrence early and late after treatment. In an early phase, the tumor size does not predict early response to chemoradiation, as an increase in size may occur in an early period, due to apoptosis and cell necrosis. The use of DWI may help in the differentiation between responders from nonresponders. Thus, tumors with a good response to treatment would present an increase in ADC and nonresponding tumors will show an unchanged or lower ADC value. Additionally, DWI may be an adjunct tool to PET-CT in the evaluation of presacral scar, as this technique has shown excellent sensitivity although limited specificity in this task.

Imaging Findings

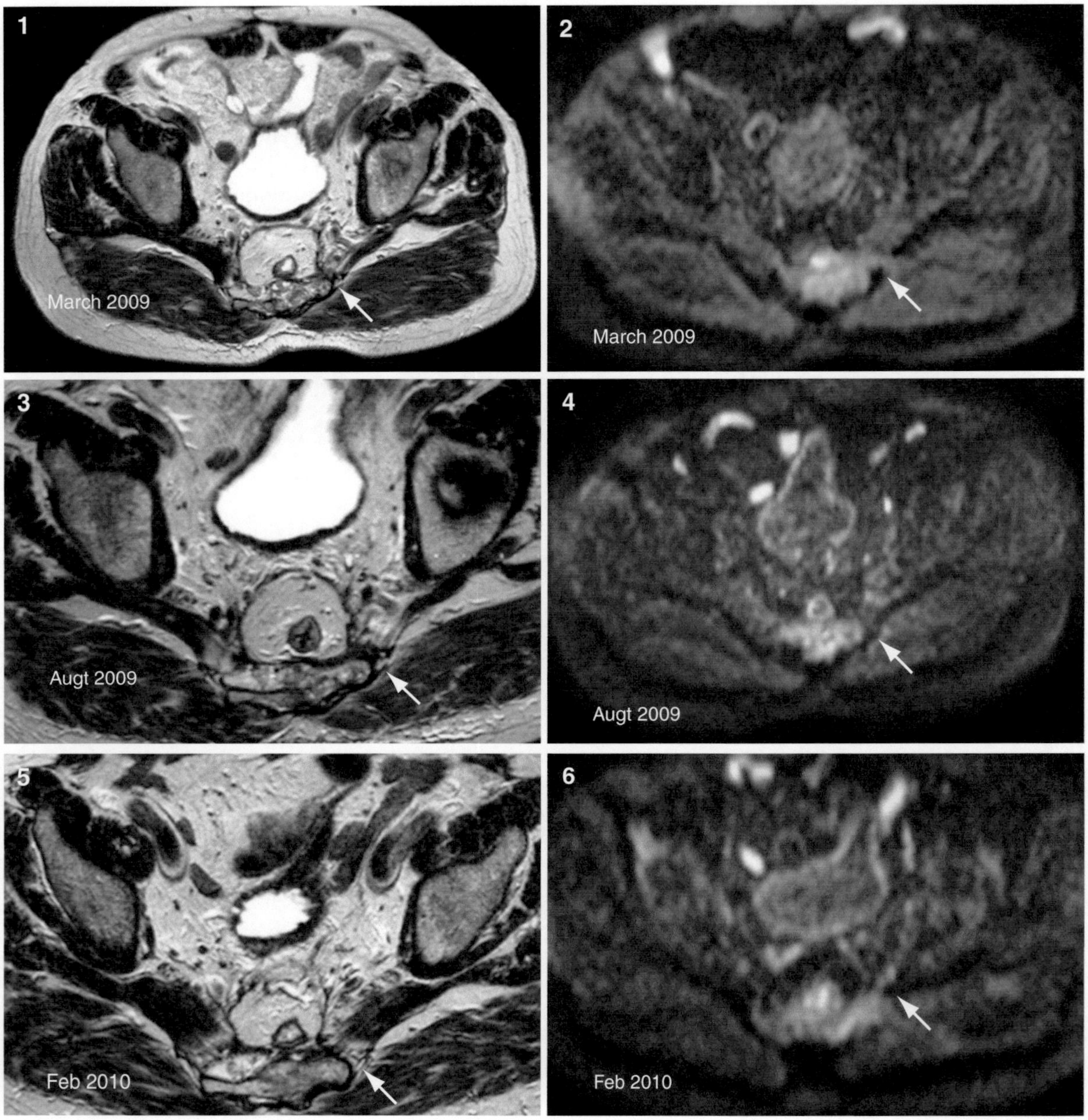

Fig. 12.5 In the first MRI performed in March of 2009, a presacral mass invading the 3rd sacral vertebra was evident with a size of 5.8 × 2.4 × 4.1 cm (*arrow* on **12.5.1**) and demonstrating restricted diffusion (*arrow*) (ADC value: 1.3 $\times 10^{-3}$ mm^2/s) (**12.5.2**). In the following study after chemoradiation in August of 2009, the lesion volume remains unchanged (*arrow* on **12.5.3**), although the DWI signal has slightly disminished (*arrow*) and the ADC value had increased up to 1.6 $\times 10^{-3}$ mm^2/s (**12.5.4**), suggesting a partial response to treatment. In the latest study performed in February of 2010, the tumor has decreased in size (4.4 × 3.4 × 1.4 cm) (*arrow*) (**12.5.5**) and does not present significant restriction of diffusion (*arrow*) (ADC value: 2 $\times 10^{-3}$ mm^2/s) (**12.5.6**)

Case 12.6: Cystic Retrorectal Hamartoma or Tailgut Cyst

A 49-year-old male was referred for anorectal MRI due to pain and mass sensation in the anal canal.

Comments

The tailgut cysts are a rare congenital tumor, included in the group of the enteric cysts, which originates from embryonic tissue located in the presacral space. They are more common in middle-aged women. These tumors usually are multicystic in appearance, demonstrating well-defined borders. It may show mucinous content, which demonstrates high signal intensity on T1-weighted and T2-weighted sequences. The presence of mucinous material is a key feature for its characterization. The presence of tiny calcifications is rare. Peripheral wall enhancement after gadolinium administration may be found.

The most common complications are infection and malignant degeneration. Tailgut cysts may degenerate into adenocarcinomas, developing solid components and with infiltration of the rectal wall or adjacent structures.

To our knowledge, the characteristics on DWI of tailgut cyst have not been reported. In this case, the tumor showed absence of restriction, with high ADC values, in both the purely cystic and mucinous areas. DWI may help in the characterization of its cystic nature and in excluding complications.

Imaging Findings

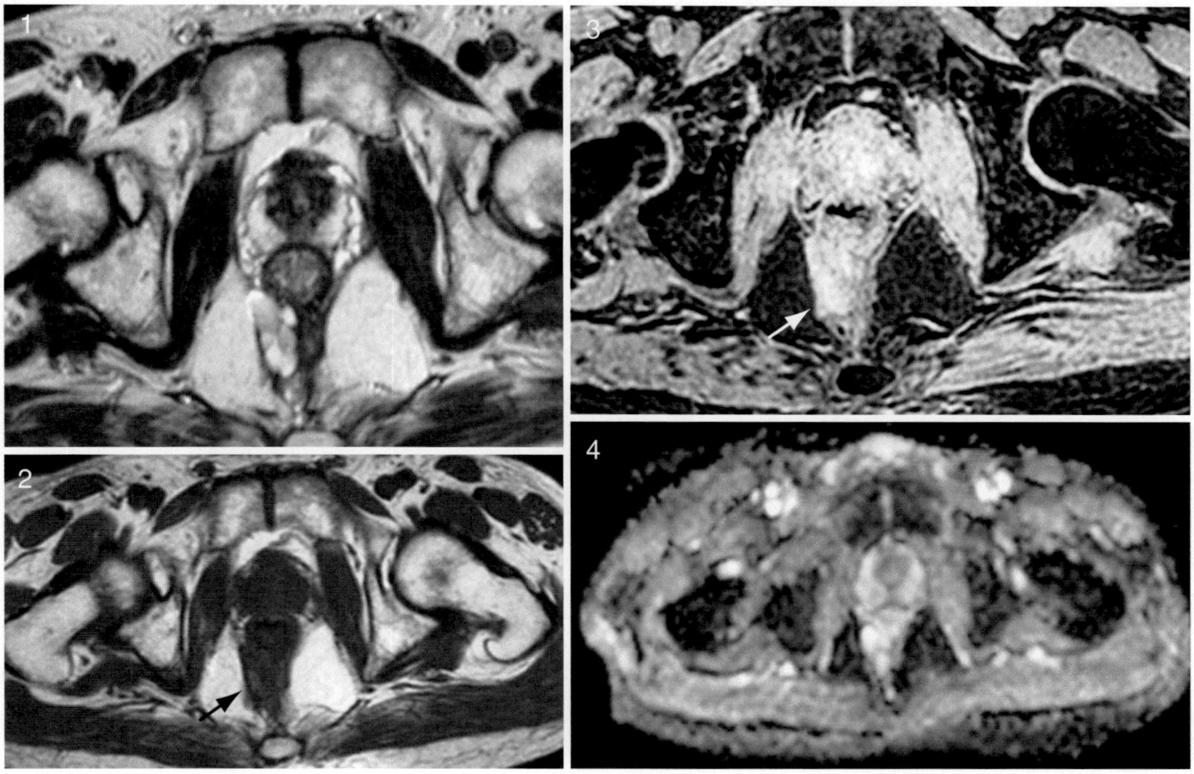

Fig. 12.6 A complex cystic lesion located in right ischiorectal fossa which showed typical appearance of cystic lesions: hyperintensity on T2-weighted sequence (**12.6.1**), hypointensity on pre- (**12.6.2**) and postcontrast (**12.6.3**) T1-weighted sequences. Areas of high signal intensity on T1-weighted image corresponded to mucinous content (*arrows*). ADC map shows absence of free water restriction of the lesion (**12.6.4**)

Case 12.7: Monitorization of Response to Treatment with Imatinib of a Rectal GIST

A 78-year-old patient who has a rectal GIST, treated with Imatinib, was submitted to consecutive MRI exams for monitoring response to treatment during 2 years.

Comments

GIST are the most common mesenchymal tumor, although in our environment, they are a very rare entity (12.4 patients per million). They lack the traditional features of smooth muscle or Schwann cells, and now are thought to derive from a precursor of the interstitial cells of Cajal. They are a distinct entity than leiomyomas or leiomyosarcomas. Their histologic presentation ranges from a predominance of either spindle or epitheloid cells or a mixture of both. Most of the time, the final diagnosis is made by identifying *KIT* (CD117), a tyrosine kinase receptor in the interstitial cells of Cajal. They show different biological behavior, from completely benign to highly aggressive. A specific diagnosis is necessary, because a new KIT-tyrosine kinase inhibitor (Imatinib [Gleevec]; Novartis, Basel, Switzerland) has been shown to be of clinical utility in treating patients with GISTs.

Although they may appear in any area of the gastrointestinal tract, peritoneum, and retroperitoneum, their most common location is the stomach (37%). The rectal presentation is the fifth in frequency with an incidence of approximately a 5–10%. Patients with neurofibromatosis type 1 (NF1) have an increased prevalence of GISTs. In the rectum, they are most commonly mural lesions with frequent external spread. They usually are focal well-circumscribed lesions with areas of necrosis and hemorrhage and heterogeneous enhancement.

GIST response to Imitanib is different from that of other tumors, because the decrease in size typically occurs months after the beginning of therapy. Because of this, GIST response is difficult to include in Response Evaluation Criteria in the Solid Tumor (RECIST). Early after treatment, cell destruction occurs, which can lead to an increase in tumor size due to internal bleeding and myxoid degeneration. CT is the most common imaging tool used in the posttreatment monitorization of these tumors. Soon after therapy, a positive response is detected in contrast-enhanced CT as a change in the enhancement pattern from a heterogeneous hyperattenuating pattern to a homogeneous hypoattenuating one. This change occurs in the interval of 1 week to 1 month after therapy. The quantification of changes in tumor density has been proposed as a valid tool in treatment monitorization. A decrease in the maximum standardized uptake value (SUV) has been also demonstrated in PET when the response is positive.

The role of MRI in the posttreatment monitorization of GIST tumors is also under evaluation, especially with functional techniques as DWI. In the example shown, an increase in ADC helps to predict good response to treatment before increase in size occurs.

Fig. 12.7 An anterior excrescent mass attached to the anterior wall of the lower rectum was confirmed in several consecutive MRI exams performed before therapy in October 2008 (**12.7.1–12.7.3**) and at 3 months (**12.7.4–12.7.6**), 9 months (**12.7.7–12.7.9**), and 18 months (**12.7.10**, **12.7.11**) after the start of therapy with Imanitib. In the pretreatment MRI, the mass showed intermediate signal intensity on T2-weighted sequence (*arrow*) (**12.7.1**), severe restriction of diffusion with *b* value of 1,000 s^2/mm (**12.7.2**), and an ADC value of 0.8 10^{-3} mm^2/s (**12.7.3**). In the first follow-up study, an increase in size is visualized (*arrow*) (**12.7.4**), although there is a decrease in the restriction of diffusion (**12.7.5**) and elevation of ADC value (1.1×10^{-3} mm^2/s) (**12.7.6**), suggesting a good response to treatment. In the two following examinations, a decrease in tumor size (*arrows*) (**12.7.7**, **12.7.10**), a decrease in diffusion restriction (**12.7.8, 12.7.11**), and a progressive increase in ADC values (1.3 and 1.5×10^{-3} mm^2/s respectively) (**12.7.9**) confirm the positive outcome

Imaging Findings

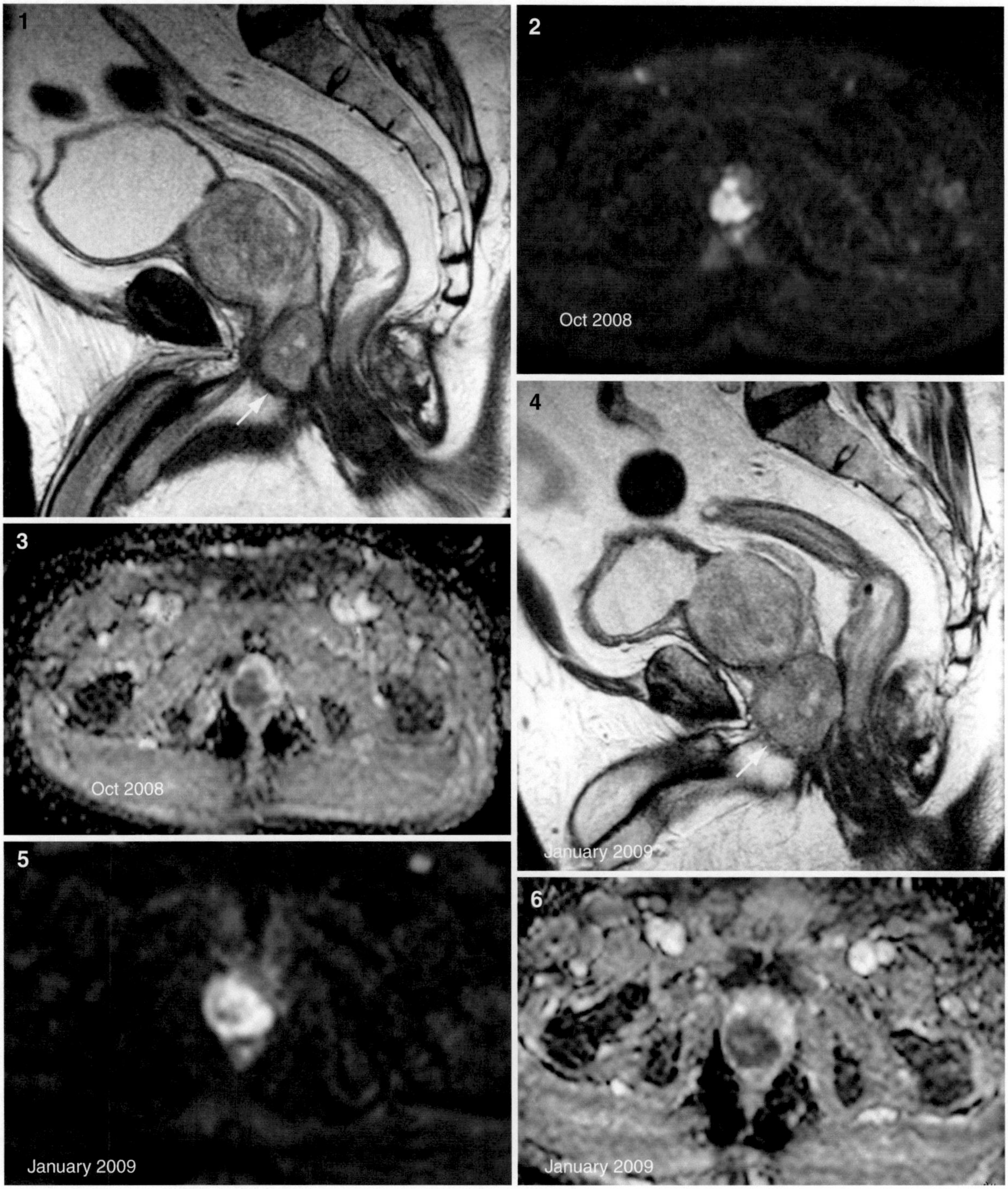

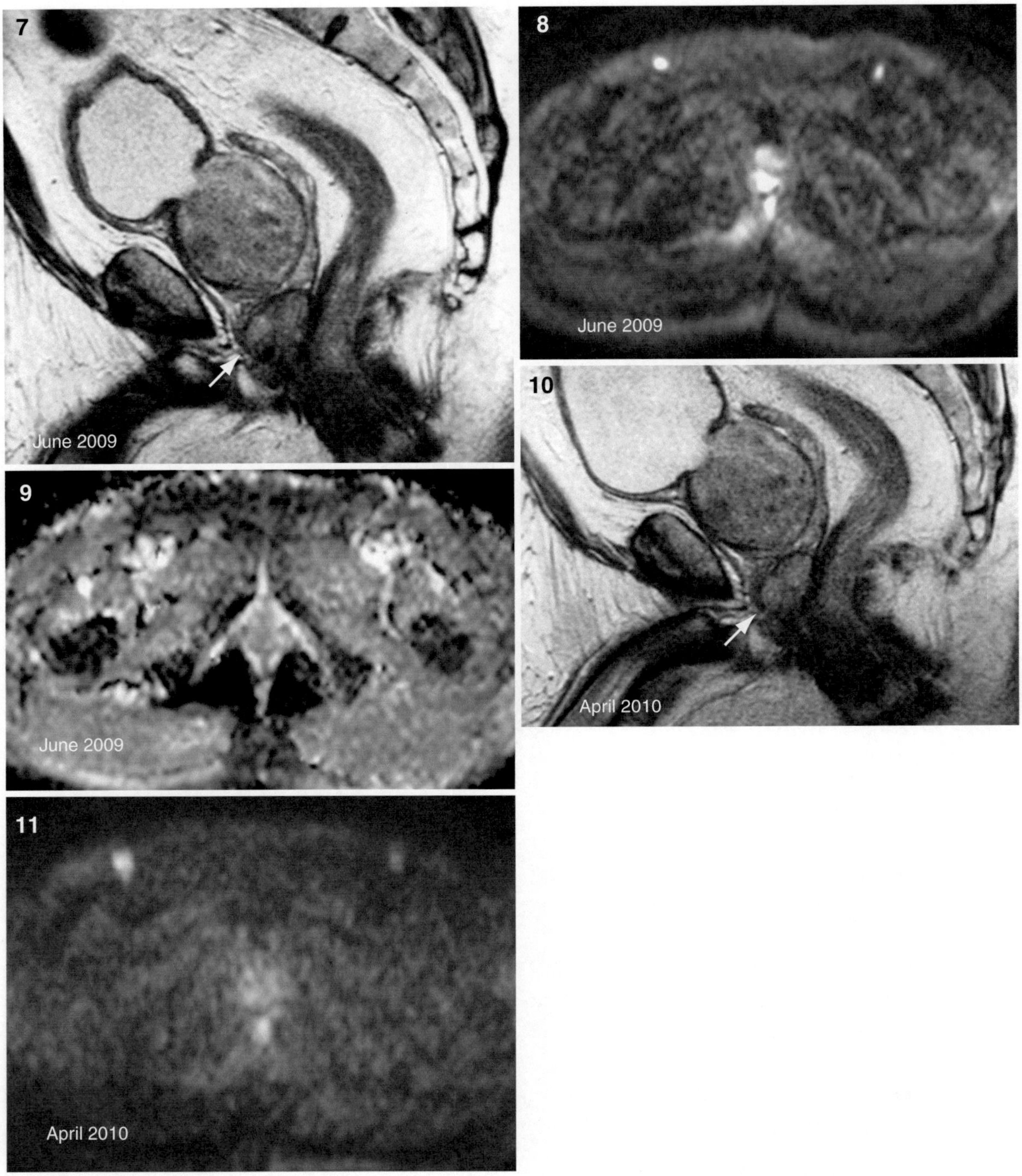

Fig. 12.7 (continued)

Case 12.8: Perirectal Abscess Secondary to Postsurgical Dehiscence of Sutures

A 63-year-old male who had undergone low anterior resection for rectal carcinoma 1 month before, presented fever and pain in right gluteal region during a week. Clinically an abscess was suspected. MRI is performed for further assessment.

Comments

DWI has demonstrated its potential to detect abscesses in the abdomen and pelvis with a similar accuracy to postcontrast images. Acute pyogenic abscesses usually show marked restriction of diffusion, appearing very bright with high *b* values against a suppressed background. This is due to the high viscosity and cellularity within their content. Later on, as liquefaction occurs, the restriction of diffusion should diminish in a similar manner.

On morphological MRI sequences, both cystic and necrotic tumors demonstrate a central area of hyperintense signal on T2-weighted sequences, in a similar manner to inflammatory collections. DWI helps in this differential diagnosis as areas of cystic degeneration or necrosis will show little restriction of diffusion and high ADC values, and abscess content will appear brighter on diffusion with high *b* values and low ADC values.

Imaging Findings

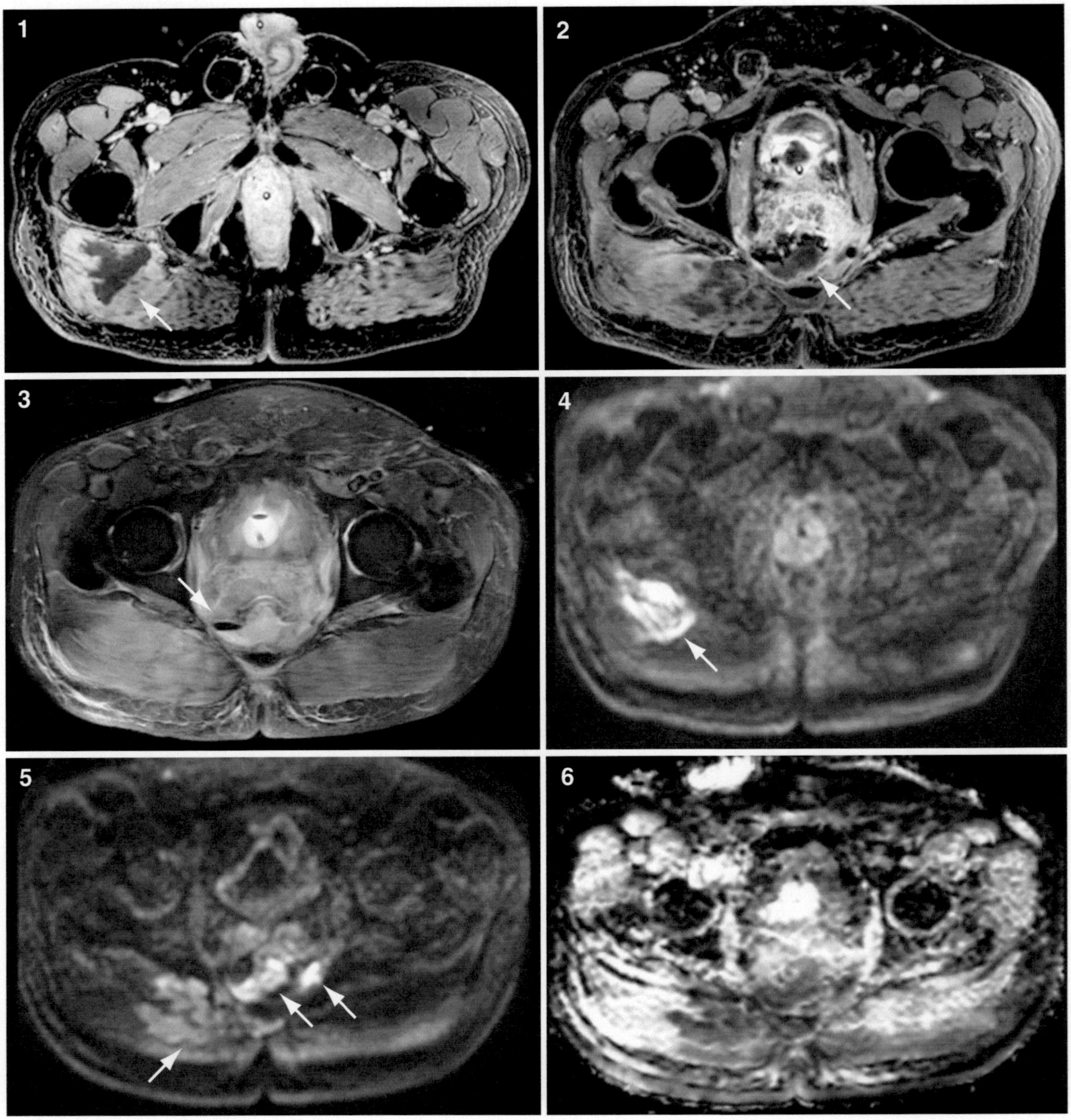

Fig. 12.8 Axial postcontrast THRIVE sequence at two different levels shows a large collection in the right gluteus maximus muscle (**12.8.1**) that communicates with another complex collection in the presacral space (**12.8.2**) (*arrows*). On STIR, a sinus tract (*arrow*) that communicates this collection with the posterior aspect of the rectum is detected (**12.8.3**). The perirectal collection shows several internal fluid-air levels. These collections have an intense peripheral uptake after administration of gadolinium. DWI with a *b* value of 800 s^2/mm helps to better define the limits of both gluteal and perirectal collections (*arrows*) (**12.8.4** and **12.8.5**). Both lesions demonstrate a significant restriction, mainly in the central area of the collection, with very low ADC values (between 0.6 and 0.7 $\times 10^{-3}$ mm^2/s) (**12.8.6**), suggesting the diagnosis of abscesses caused by a dehiscence of sutures at the level of sigmoid colon-terminal rectum anastomosis

Case 12.9: Complicated Acute Diverticulitis

A 84-year-old female, with constitutional symptoms and long-standing fever, but normal abdominal physical examination. CT showed a mass in the sigmoid colon, being unable to differentiate between sigmoid diverticulitis and carcinoma. A pelvic MRI with and without gadolinium was performed for further characterization.

Comments

Diverticulosis affects 10% of individuals over 45 years and 80% of individuals over 85 years. Among this percentage of the population, between 10% and 25% of individuals have diverticular inflammation, causing acute diverticulitis. The most common complications of diverticulitis include the presence of abscess, intestinal perforation, and fistula formation to adjacent structures (bladder, vagina, or small bowel). In our case, the symptoms were not very suggestive of acute diverticulitis since pain was not present.

The classic radiographic signs that can differentiate between diverticulosis and diverticulitis are: the extent of the disease, which is usually larger in the inflammatory processes; and the presence of abscesses and fistulas which are more common in complicated diverticulitis, although there are some infiltrating colonic adenocarcinomas that may show a similar presentation, making it almost impossible to differentiate between the two diseases.

Both acute inflammatory processes and malignant tumors show restriction of free water movement. DWI with high *b* values may help to define the borders of the pathological process. In a recent series, DWI with quantification of ADC values allowed to accurately differentiate active inflammatory bowel disease from malignant tumors in the rectum, based on ADC quantification. Active inflammatory lesions presented a higher ADC value than carcinomas, with an ADC of 1.21 (0.08) $\times 10^{-3}$ mm^2/s and 0.97 (0.14) $\times 10^{-3}$ mm^2/s, respectively.

Imaging Findings

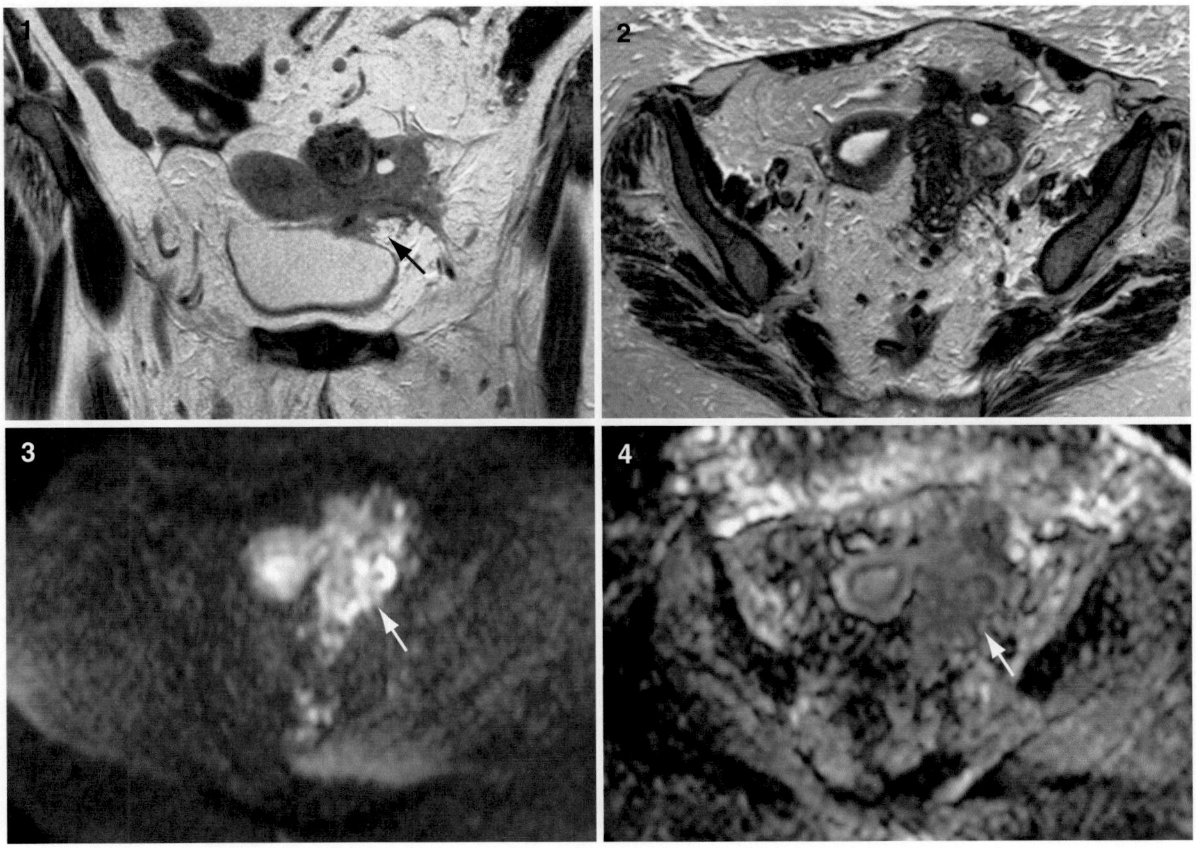

Fig. 12.9 Coronal and axial T2-weighted sequences (**12.9.1**, **12.9.2**) show a segmentary concentric thickening of the sigmoid colon with extension to adjacent fat, left ovary, and left Fallopian tube. A sinus tract from the area of divetticulitis to the superior aspect of the bladder is detected on coronal acquisition (*arrow*). DWI with a *b* value of 1,000 s^2/mm helps to define the borders (*arrow*) of the lesion (**12.9.3**), which shows an ADC of 1.2×10^{-3} mm^2/s (*arrow*) (**12.9.4**). These findings favor a perforated acute diverticulitis

Case 12.10: Crohn's Disease and Perianal Fistulas

A 28-year-old male with Crohn's disease, featuring anal discharge and perineal pain for months.

Comments

The incidence of perianal disease in patients with active Crohn's disease is between 14% and 38%, causing a significant increase in morbidity. A recent report has demonstrated that the detection rate of fistulas is similar using T2-weighted sequence and DWI than using T2-weighted sequence and postcontrast-enhanced sequences, suggesting that it would not be necessary to administer intravenous contrast for the detection of perianal fistulas, thus reducing side effects and costs of examination.

The way to differentiate between active and nonactive fistulas with DWI is by measuring its ADC value, being lower in active disease (ADC value: $1.52 \pm 0.43 \times 10^{-3}$ mm^2/s) than in chronic inactive fistulas (ADC value: $2.31 \pm 0.59 \times 10^{-3}$ mm^2/s). In that series, they use 2 *b* values of 0 and 800 s^2/mm for ADC calculation.

Besides, DWI has recently shown in several reports to accurately identify active areas of inflammation in the small bowel, colon, and rectum in a similar fashion to dynamic contrast-enhanced MRI.

Imaging Findings

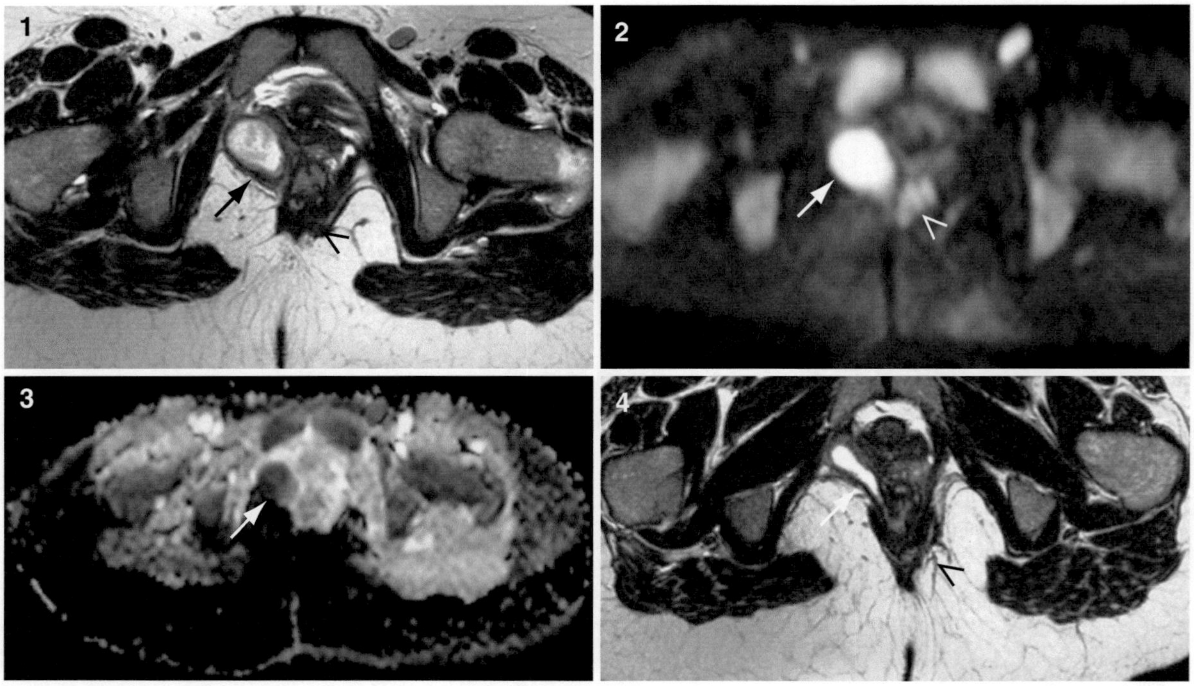

Fig. 12.10 On T2-weighted sequence (**12.10.1**), an anterior right perianal collection is visualized (*arrow*). It originates from a transphincteric fistula-in-ano with origin at 8 o'clock position. On DWI (**12.10.2**), this collection is clearly visualized (*arrow*) along with the fistulous tract. A second fistula-in-ano with a horseshoe shape and originating at 5 o'clock position is better visualized on DWI than on T2-weighted sequence (*arrowheads*). Both the collection (*arrow*) and the fistulas show low ADC values, between 0.5 and 0.9×10^{-3} mm^2/s (**12.10.3**), indicating active disease in a patient who refused contrast administration in this examination. A second MRI was repeated after a month of conservative treatment with antibiotics (**12.10.4–12.10.6**) where we keep on identifying the perianal collection (*arrows*) and both fistulae that show a decrease in size, less hypersignal on DWI, and increase of ADC values, indicating partial response to treatment

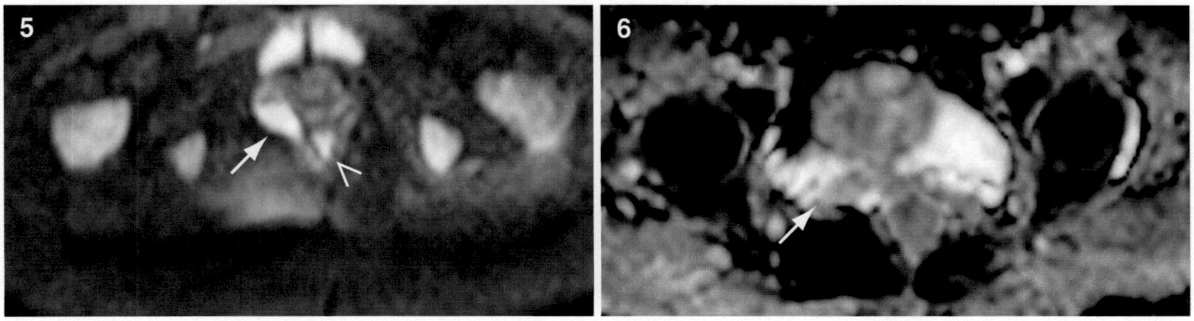

Fig. 12.10 (continued)

Further Reading

Barbaro B, Vitale R, Leccisotti L et al (2010) Restaging locally advanced rectal cancer after chemoradiation therapy with MR imaging. Radiographics 30(3):699–716

Dahan H, Arrivé L, Wendum D et al (2001) Retrorectal developmental cysts in adults: clinical and radiologic-histopathologic review, differential diagnosis, and treatment. Radiographics 21(3):575–584

DeVries AF, Kremser C, Hein PA et al (2003) Tumor microcirculation and diffusion predict therapy outcome for primary rectal carcinoma. Int J Radiat Oncol Biol Phys 56(4):958–965

Dzik-Jurasz A, Domenig C, George M et al (2002) Diffusion MRI for prediction of response of rectal cancer to chemoradiation. Lancet 360(9329):307–308

Hein PA, Kremser C, Judmaier W et al (2003) Diffusion-weighted magnetic resonance imaging for monitoring diffusion changes in rectal carcinoma during combined, preoperative chemoradiation: preliminary results of a prospective study. Eur J Radiol 45(3):214–222

Heverhagen JT, Klose KJ (2009) MR imaging for acute lower abdominal and pelvic pain. Radiographics 29(6): 1781–1796

Hori M, Oto A, Orrin S et al (2009) Diffusion-weighted MRI: a new tool for the diagnosis of fistula in ano. J Magn Reson Imaging 30(5):1021–1026

Hosonuma T, Tozaki M, Ichiba N et al (2006) Clinical usefulness of diffusion-weighted imaging using low and high b-values to detect rectal cancer. Magn Reson Med Sci 5(4):173–177

Ichikawa T, Ertuk SM, Motosugi U et al (2006) High-b-value diffusion weighted MRI in colorectal cancer. Am J Roentgenol 187:181–184

Kilickesmez O, Atilla S, Soylu A et al (2009) Diffusion-weighted imaging of the rectosigmoid colon: preliminary findings. J Comput Assist Tomogr 33(6):863–866

Kim DJ, Kim JH, Lim JS et al (2010) Restaging of rectal cancer with MR imaging after concurrent chemotherapy and radiation therapy. Radiographics 30(2):503–516

Kim JK, Kim KA, Park BW et al (2008) Feasibility of diffusion-weighted imaging in the differentiation of metastatic from nonmetastatic lymph nodes: early experience. J Magn Reson Imaging 28:714–719

Kim SH, Lee JM, Hong SH et al (2009) Locally advanced rectal cancer: added value of diffusion-weighted MR imaging in the evaluation of tumor response to neoadjuvant chemo- and radiation therapy. Radiology 253(1):116–125

Kim SH, Lee JY, Lee JM et al (2011) Apparent diffusion coefficient for evaluating tumour response to neoadjuvant chemoradiation therapy for locally advanced rectal cancer. Eur Radiol 21(5):987–995

Koh DM, Chau I, Tait D et al (2008) Evaluating mesorectal lymph nodes in rectal cancer before and after neoadjuvant chemoradiation using thin-section T2-weighted magnetic resonance imaging. Int J Radiat Oncol Biol Phys 71:456–461

Lambrecht M, Deroose C, Roels S et al (2010) The use of FDG-PET/CT and diffusion-weighted magnetic resonance imaging for response prediction before, during and after preoperative chemoradiotherapy for rectal cancer. Acta Oncol 49(7):956–963

Lambregts DM, Maas M, Riedl RG et al (2011) Value of ADC measurements for nodal staging after chemoradiation in locally advanced rectal cancer-a per lesion validation study. Eur Radiol 21(2):265–273

Levy AD, Remotti HE, Thompson WM et al (2003) Gastrointestinal stromal tumors: radiologic features with pathologic correlation. Radiographics 23(2):283–304

Lin G, Ho KC, Wang JJ et al (2008) Detection of lymph node metastasis in cervical and uterine cancers by diffusion-weighted magnetic resonance imaging at 3T. J Magn Reson Imaging 28:128–135

Menu Y (2007) Evaluation of tumour response to treatment with targeted therapies: standard or targeted criteria? Bull Cancer 94(7 Suppl):F231–F239

MERCURY Study Group (2007) Extramural depth of tumor invasion at thin-section MR in patients with rectal cancer: results of the MERCURY study. Radiology 243(1): 132–139

Nasu K, Kuroki Y, Kuroki S et al (2004) Diffusion-weighted single shot echo planar imaging of colorectal cancer using a sensitivity-encoding technique. Jpn J Clin Oncol 34: 620–626

Ono K, Ochiai R, Yoshida T et al (2009) Comparison of diffusion-weighted MRI and 2-[fluorine-18]-fluoro-2-deoxy-D-glucose positron emission tomography (FDG-PET) for detecting primary colorectal cancer and regional lymph node metastases. J Magn Reson Imaging 29: 336–340

Oussalah A, Laurent V, Bruot O et al (2010) Diffusion-weighted magnetic resonance without bowel preparation for detecting colonic inflammation in inflammatory bowel disease. Gut 59(8):1056–1065

Padhani AR, Liu G, Koh DM et al (2009) Diffusion-weighted magnetic resonance imaging as a cancer biomarker: consensus and recommendations. Neoplasia 11(2):102–125

Rao SX, Zeng MS, Chen CZ et al (2008) The value of diffusion-weighted imaging in combination with T2-weighted imaging for rectal cancer detection. Eur J Radiol 65(2): 299–303

Shankar S, Dundamadappa SK, Karam AR et al (2009) Imaging of gastrointestinal stromal tumors before and after imatinib mesylate therapy. Acta Radiol 50(8):837–844

Soyer P, Lagadec M, Sirol M et al (2010) Free-breathing diffusion-weighted single-shot echo-planar MR imaging using parallel imaging (GRAPPA 2) and high b value for the detection of primary rectal adenocarcinoma. Cancer Imaging 10(1):32–39

Sun YS, Zhang XP, Tang L et al (2010) Locally advanced rectal carcinoma treated with preoperative chemotherapy and radiation therapy: preliminary analysis of diffusion-weighted MR imaging for early detection of tumor histopathologic downstaging. Radiology 254(1):170–178

Yasui O, Sato M, Kamada A (2009) Diffusion-weighted imaging in the detection of lymph node metastasis in colorectal cancer. Tohoku J Exp Med 218(3):177–183

Diffusion-Weighted Imaging in the Evaluation of Lung, Mediastinum, Heart, and Chest Wall

13

Antonio Luna, Teodoro Martín, and Javier Sánchez González

13.1 Introduction

The fields of applications of DWI have increased considerably in the last few years due to recent technological improvements such as more powerful gradients and phased-array coils, development of fast imaging techniques such as echo-planar sequences (EPI) and parallel imaging. In spite of these developments, DWI of the chest is technically challenging and not always feasible due to obvious shortcomings such as motion artifacts related to breathing and heart and vascular pulsation and susceptibility artifacts associated to air–tissue interfaces. In spite of all these limitations, the clinical applications of DWI in the chest are increasing.

13.2 Technical Considerations

Different pulse sequences have been employed for DWI of the chest. Although, EPI suffers from gross geometrical distortion in the presence of B0 inhomogeneities, these sequences are commonly used. Different strategies have been proposed to diminish EPI-related artifacts, such as the segmentation of the echo train length of the EPI acquisition in different shots, the application of motion correction techniques like navigation echoes, the use of the Periodically Rotated Overlapping Parallel Lines with Enhanced Reconstruction acquisition (PROPELLER) which is less sensible to motion artifacts and the use of parallel imaging. Furthermore, improvements in gradient systems with reduced eddy-current effects have allowed faster EPI readout which can decrease geometric distortions.

The use of fat suppression is mandatory in DWI of the chest because fat signal usually overlaps on the studied anatomy. DWI with STIR has been most commonly used in the chest, in sequences such as diffusion-weighted image with background suppression (DWIBS). In order to overcome the limited SNR of these sequences, spectral fat suppression techniques, such as Spectral Presaturation Inversion Recovery (SPIR) and Spectral Selection Attenuated Inversion Recovery (SPAIR), have been included in DWI sequences.

Although most of the reported applications of DWI of the chest have been performed in 1.5 T magnets, the use of higher field magnets, such as 3 T, has been advocated due to the associated signal improvement. The acquisition problems inherent to DWI increase in 3 T magnets, due to higher magnetic field variation and susceptibility artifacts, which can be overcome using appropriately the higher strength of the gradient systems in combination with parallel imaging and advanced fat suppression sequences. Gill and colleagues reported recently the first clinical series of DWI performed on a 3 T magnet, and also in our experience, with an adequate technical tuning, DWI of the chest is feasible at 3 T magnets.

A. Luna (✉)
Chief of MRI, Health Time Group, Jaén, Spain
aluna70@sercosa.com

T. Martin
Neuroradiology Section, Clínica Las Nieves, SERCOSA, Health Time Group, Jaén, Spain
t.martin.f@htime.org

J.S. González
Clinical Scientist, Philips Medical Systems, Madrid, Spain
javier.sanchez.gonzalez@philips.com

A. Luna et al., *Diffusion MRI Outside the Brain*,
DOI 10.1007/978-3-642-21052-5_13,

Disclosures Javier Sánchez is an employee of Philips Medical Systems as an MR clinical scientist in Spain.

Synchronization is a critical factor when performing chest DWI (Fig. 13.1). The use of respiratory trigger improves the quality of DWI sequences compared to those using breath-holding. The use of cardiac trigger is also useful to avoid pulsation artifacts, but it is not always necessary except in the case of lesions located immediately around the heart or in dedicated cardiac acquisitions, as it is time consuming.

Our sequence design, when possible, is:

- Single-shot spin-echo EPI
- Phased-array surface coil
- *b* values: several values between 0 and 100 s/mm^2 until 1,000 s/mm^2
- FOV: 320–400
- Parallel imaging acceleration factor of 2
- Pixel resolution 2.5 × 2.5 × 7 mm^3
- Spectral fat suppression
- Number of slices 24
- TR: 5,000 ms
- TE: 53 ms (shortest)
- Respiratory triggered
- Three orthogonal motion-probing gradients

In the evaluation of pulmonary or mediastinal lesions, ADC quantification is needed. The use of coregistration software limits motion and susceptibility artifacts (Fig. 3.8). Very recently, Luna et al. have proposed the use of a bicompartmental model for the analysis of pulmonary lesion, with potential improvement in lesional characterization by using the parameter *D* (diffusion coefficient) instead of the ADC calculation, which is usually higher than *D* due to perfusion effect (Fig. 13.2). The use of an IVIM DWI sequence with several *b* values allows us to separate the two components of the diffusion signal decay, the one due to perfusion at low *b* values and the true diffusion one that occurs with *b* values over 100 s/mm^2.

13.3 Clinical Applications

13.3.1 Detection of Pulmonary Nodules

Scarce data exist about the capabilities of DWI for detection of pulmonary nodules. DWIBS has demonstrated similar accuracy and sensitivity to PET and PET-CT in the depiction of pulmonary metastases with similar rates of false-positive lesions. Noninvasive adenocarcinomas, bronchioloalveolar carcinomas (BAC), and metastasis smaller than 1 cm may produce false-negative results in both PET and DWI. Besides, STIR sequence is usually preferable to DWI for pulmonary lesional detection according to the available series.

13.3.2 Pulmonary Nodule Characterization

DWI has been applied to pulmonary nodule characterization, achieving good results in the differentiation between benign and malignant nodules. In malignant lesions, the increased cellularity, higher tissue disorganization, and increased extracellular space tortuosity limit the diffusion of interstitial water compared to benign ones (Figs. 13.2 and 13.3). Therefore, malignant nodules tend to show higher signal on high *b* value DWI acquisitions and lower ADC values than benign lesions. Comparison of results of different series is limited due to the different types of performed sequence, *b* values selection, and approach of assessment, using either visual or semiquantitative or even quantitative analysis.

Liu and colleagues proposed a threshold ADC value of 1.4 × 10^{-3} mm^2/s, which allowed the distinction between benign and malignant lesions with a sensitivity of 83% and a specificity of 74%. Mori and colleagues used a cutoff ADC value of 1.1 × 10^{-3} mm^2/s in the distinction of benign from malignant pulmonary nodules, obtaining a sensitivity of 70% and specificity of 97%, compared to 72% and 79%, obtained by PET. Besides, DWI allowed reducing the rate of false-positive lesions compared to PET.

Limitations of the technique are the presence of a significant number of false-positives related mainly to benign inflammatory lesions and potential false-negatives are low-grade adenocarcinomas and metastasis (Fig. 13.2). In general, DWI performs equivalently to PET in pulmonary lesion characterization, with similar limitations, although DWI tends to have less false-positive lesions.

13.3.3 Lung Cancer Evaluation

DWI has also been proposed to evaluate histological grading of lung cancer. For example, Matoba and colleagues demonstrated an adequate correlation between the ADC values of lung cancer with tumor cellularity. In this report, well-differentiated adenocarcinomas showed higher ADC values than those of more aggressive adenocarcinomas and epidermoid carcinomas in a significant manner (Fig. 13.4). In the investigation of 66 pulmonary nodules by Liu and colleagues, small cell lung cancer (SCLC) demonstrated statistically significant lower ADC values than non-small cell lung cancer (NSCLC). Furthermore, very recently, Razek and colleagues have proposed the potential role of ADC measurements as a new prognostic parameter for lung cancer. In their series, they evaluated 31 patients with lung cancer, with a DWI sequence with a maximum *b* value of 600 s/mm^2. Significant differences were found in the mean ADC value of SCLC from NSCLC and between poorly and well-differentiated compared to moderately differentiated lung cancer, and between patients with N0 and N3 stages. Therefore, the lowest the ADC value of lung cancer, the highest the tumor grade and metastatic mediastinal node stage. Furthermore, Kanauchi and colleagues studied, with DWI using a visual qualitative analysis, 41 patients with clinical stage IA NSCLC who had undergone curative resection. DWI was found to be an independent predictive factor to detect patients with invasive cancer with a sensitivity of 90%, a specificity of 81%, a positive predictive value of 60%, and a negative predictive value of 96%.

Contradictory data have been reported in the evaluation of adenocarcinomas with DWI. On the one hand, Tanaka and colleagues studied 46 peripheral adenocarcinomas smaller than 3 cm, with DWI with a higher *b* value of 1,000 s/mm^2. They were able to significantly differentiate invasive adenocarcinomas from BAC, as invasive adenocarcinomas usually showed higher signal intensity (Fig. 13.4). On the other hand, Koyama and colleagues evaluated 33 adenocarcinomas with DWI and a higher *b* value of 1,000 s/mm^2, demonstrating lack of usefulness of ADC values in the differentiation of the subtypes of adenocarcinoma.

A correct depiction of tumoral borders is critical for radiotherapy planning. In this task, DWI is able to distinguish central lung cancer from postobstructive consolidation, with more accurate results than either T2-weighted sequences or enhanced CT (Fig. 13.5). DWI is also a powerful tool to study lesions located in pulmonary apices, such as Pancoast tumors or infection. DWI in lung cancer may also have a role in the posttreatment monitorization and detection of recurrent active tumor after treatment. Pretreatment prediction and early evaluation of response to treatment with DWI has still to be fully explored in lung cancer. Very recently, Zhou and colleges reported their preliminary experience of the role of DWI in treatment follow-up in 19 patients with lung cancer. DWI was performed 1 week before and 1 month after the beginning of chemotherapy. They found a positive correlation between the percentage of changes in ADC values of the tumors and the percentage of changes of the maximum, minimum, and the mean diameter, respectively. Therefore, these data opens a door for future research of the role of ADC in early postchemotherapy monitorization. In the same direction, Okuma and colleagues evaluated prospectively 17 patients with 20 malignant lung lesions which underwent CT-guided radiofrequency ablation. DWI with ADC calculation was performed immediately before and 3 days after treatment. The posttreatment ADC of the lesions without local progression was significantly higher than that of the lesions with local progression.

13.3.4 Staging of NSCLC with DWI

Local staging (T-staging) of NSCLC has not been extensively studied with DWI. Conversely, DWI has shown promising results in the N-staging (Fig. 13.6). A distinction has to be made in the results between series using a dedicated chest DWI sequence with respiratory trigger and spectral fat suppression and those using a free-breath DWIBS sequence, commonly included in whole-body protocols. With the first type of sequence, Nomori and colleagues demonstrated that DWI was significantly more accurate than PET in the N-staging of NSLC due to less overstaging and fewer false-positive lesions in the former. They used a threshold ADC value of 1.6×10^{-3} mm^2/s, and they were able to detect node metastases with a minimum size of 4 mm. Other series confirmed the potential of DWI in the characterization of mediastinal node involvement of NSCLC using either visual assessment or ADC measurements.

In contrast to these results, the results of DWIBS in the N-staging of lung cancer have achieved less accuracy than PET-CT. Lichy and colleagues included in their series 3 patients with lung cancer and 11 metastatic thoracic lymph nodes detected on PET-CT, of which DWIBS could only detected one. More recently, Chen and colleagues obtained a significant difference in the accuracy of lymph node metastases detection, favoring PET-CT compared to DWIBS in 56 patients with NSCLC. In contrast, similar results in the M-staging of NSCLC for whole-body DWIBS and PET-CT were found in the same report, although better detection rates were achieved with the last technique. In a previous series, Ohno et al. demonstrated that whole-body DWIBS is useful for M-stage of NSCLC patients with accuracy as good as that of PET-CT, although most of the false-positive and false-negative lesions with both techniques corresponded to brain and pulmonary lesions. They stated that whole-body DWIBS should be used along with morphological whole-body sequences in order to improve the diagnostic accuracy of this technique. Chen and colleagues did not used conventional MRI sequences in their series, which may justify the differences in results compared to Ohno's report.

13.3.5 Mediastinum

Several reports have demonstrated a potential role for DWI in the characterization of mediastinal lymph nodes, as previously reported for the head and neck region. Kosucu et al. demonstrated that DWI and ADC measurements allowed distinguishing between benign and metastatic lymph nodes of SCLC and NSCLC. More recently, Razek and colleagues studied with DWI 35 patients with mediastinal lymphadenopathy. The differentiation between benign and malignant lymph nodes was optimal using an ADC threshold of 1.85×10^{-3} mm²/s, obtaining an accuracy of 83.9%, a sensitivity of 96.4%, a specificity of 71.4%, a negative predictive value of 95.2%, a positive predictive value of 77.1%, and an area under the curve of 0.98. There were not significant differences between metastatic and lymphomatous lymph nodes in this report. Mean ADC value of malignant lymph nodes was $1.06 \pm 0.3 \times 10^{-3}$ mm²/s and that of benign lymphadenopathy corresponds to $2.39 \pm 0.7 \times 10^{-3}$ mm²/s. In contrast, Sakurada and colleagues demonstrated that ADC value of metastatic lymph nodes of esophageal cancer were higher than that of non-metastatic lymph nodes, although there was an overlap in the ADCs of both groups.

The characterization of mediastinal masses with DWI has also been investigated by different researchers with promising results. For example, Razek et al. obtained an accuracy of 95%, sensitivity of 96%, specificity of 94%, positive predictive value of 94%, negative predictive value of 96%, and area under the curve of 0.938 in the differentiation between benign and malignant tumors using a cutoff ADC value of 1.56×10^{-3} mm²/s in 45 patients with mediastinal tumors excluding the purely cystic ones. These results have been confirmed in other series using a DWIBS sequence.

13.3.6 Pleural Disease

Some researchers have advocated DWI as an adjunct tool for noninvasive characterization of pleural effusions. In the limited series available, exudative pleural effusions have shown significantly lower ADC values than transudative ones (Fig. 13.7).

Following a prognostic classification, malignant pleural mesothelioma (MPM) may be divided into epithelioid and nonepithelioid (biphasic and sarcomatoid) subtypes. Gill et al. demonstrated in a group of 57 patients with MPM using a 3 T magnet that the sarcomatoid subtype showed significantly lower ADC values than the epithelial one. The ADC values of biphasic MPM had a wide range of overlap with the ADC values of other subtypes.

13.3.7 Hyperpolarized Gases DWI

Gases, such as ^{129}Xe and more frequently ^{3}He, may be hyperpolarized to be administered into the lungs and imaged with MRI. Although their use is still limited to research centers, DWI of inhaled hyperpolarized gases gives information of quantitative MRI-derived ventilation and microstructural pulmonary changes in various diseases, such as asthma or chronic obstructive pulmonary disease (COPD), through measurements of their ADC. This information is obtained by measuring the degree of restriction that suffers the inhaled hyperpolarized gas by the walls of the airways. Increases in ADC have been related with the enlargement of the airspaces in both emphysema and COPD, and in healthy smokers, such as an early marker of alveolar breakdown.

13.3.8 Chest Wall

DWI has shown in other locations the potential to detect and help in the characterization of soft tissue and bone tumors. In a similar manner, DWI may be applied to the study of lesions of the chest wall. Kwee et al. have also advocated the use of DWI in cases of traumatic injury of the chest wall to detect occult rib fractures or areas of contusion (Fig. 13.8).

13.3.9 Cardiac DWI and DTI

Recent technological advances have made it possible to get diffusion information from the heart. When using cardiac synchronization with the diastolic part of the heart cycle, fine-tuning is necessary to reduce the TE to the minimum, to apply the maximum gradient strength during the DWI acquisition, and to use breath-holding or respiratory trigger. We usually perform a modified conventional spin-echo Stejskal–Tanner sequence, with a maximum b value of 300 s/mm^2. In our experience, it is possible to detect myocardial edema as areas of increased signal due to restricted diffusion, showing ADC values in the edematous area lower than in normal myocardium in cases of infarction and acute myocarditis. There is limited data available in the literature of the role of DWI in cardiac applications, although as reported by Laissy and colleagues, DWI may help to differentiate necrotic from viable myocardium, and it has the potential to further characterize cardiac and paracardiac tumors (Fig. 13.9).

Another area of research in cardiac imaging is the application of DTI to analyze the different layers and 3D structure of the myocardium (Fig. 13.10). Most of the reports have used ex vivo acquisitions, although nowadays, cardiac DTI is feasible in vivo for animals and humans but far from being ready for the clinical arena. DTI is under investigation to monitor the sequential changes of postinfarction remodeling.

13.4 Conclusions

Clinical applications of DWI of the chest have been limited by susceptibility and motion artifacts. Improvements in gradient strength, parallel imaging, and synchronization have recently allowed its use in lung nodule characterization, lung cancer evaluation, and investigation of mediastinum, pleura, and chest wall. In the near future, cardiac DWI and DTI and lung DWI after administration of hyperpolarized gases may expand the applications of MRI in the thorax.

Case 13.1: Synchronization on Chest DWI

Five different approaches under different strategies of motion compensation of the same DWI sequence are shown, using the same *b* value (300 s/mm^2) at a 3 T magnet, in a patient with SCLC.

Comments

Synchronization is critical in chest DWI, as the macroscopic movement produced by the respiratory motion and heartbeat destroys the microscopic information of the diffusion signal. Different strategies have been proposed and carefully studied in the liver, with a short experience in the chest. ADC values of normal liver and focal lesions acquired with respiratory-triggered and breath-hold strategies were similar and in good agreement in the series by Kandpal and colleagues. Respiratory-triggered DWI acquisitions were longer but showed higher SNR in normal liver and higher CNR between normal liver and focal lesion than with breath-hold sequences. In contrast, Kwee et al. found equivalent ADC values when using breath-hold and free-breathing sequences, while respiratory-triggered acquisitions systematically showed an overestimation in the ADC values. Finally, in another report by Kwee and colleagues, they studied the effect of the heart motion on DWI of the liver, showing a strong degradation of those images acquired during the heart systole due to the effect of the heart movement, which should affect the ADC measurements. These results may be also valid for chest DWI. Therefore, breath-holding DWI may be an option due to faster acquisitions, although the use of respiratory trigger usually improves the quality of DWI sequences. The use of cardiac trigger is necessary in cases of lesions located immediately around the heart or in dedicated cardiac acquisitions, as it is time consuming.

Fig. 13.1 (**13.1.1**) Free-breathing DWI, (**13.1.2**) breath-hold DWI, (**13.1.3**) breath-hold DWI with cardiac trigger, (**13.1.4**) respiratory trigger DWI, and (**13.1.5**) DWI with respiratory and cardiac trigger. Higher signal of the mediastinal mass is shown in acquisitions with cardiac and respiratory control (**13.1.3** and **13.1.5**), due to reduction of the signal loss on DWI related to respiratory and cardiac movement. On the contrary, in acquisitions without cardiac synchronization (**13.1.1**, **13.1.2** and **13.1.4**), a loss of signal within the tumor is evident due to the cardiac movement effect over the DWI signal

Imaging Findings

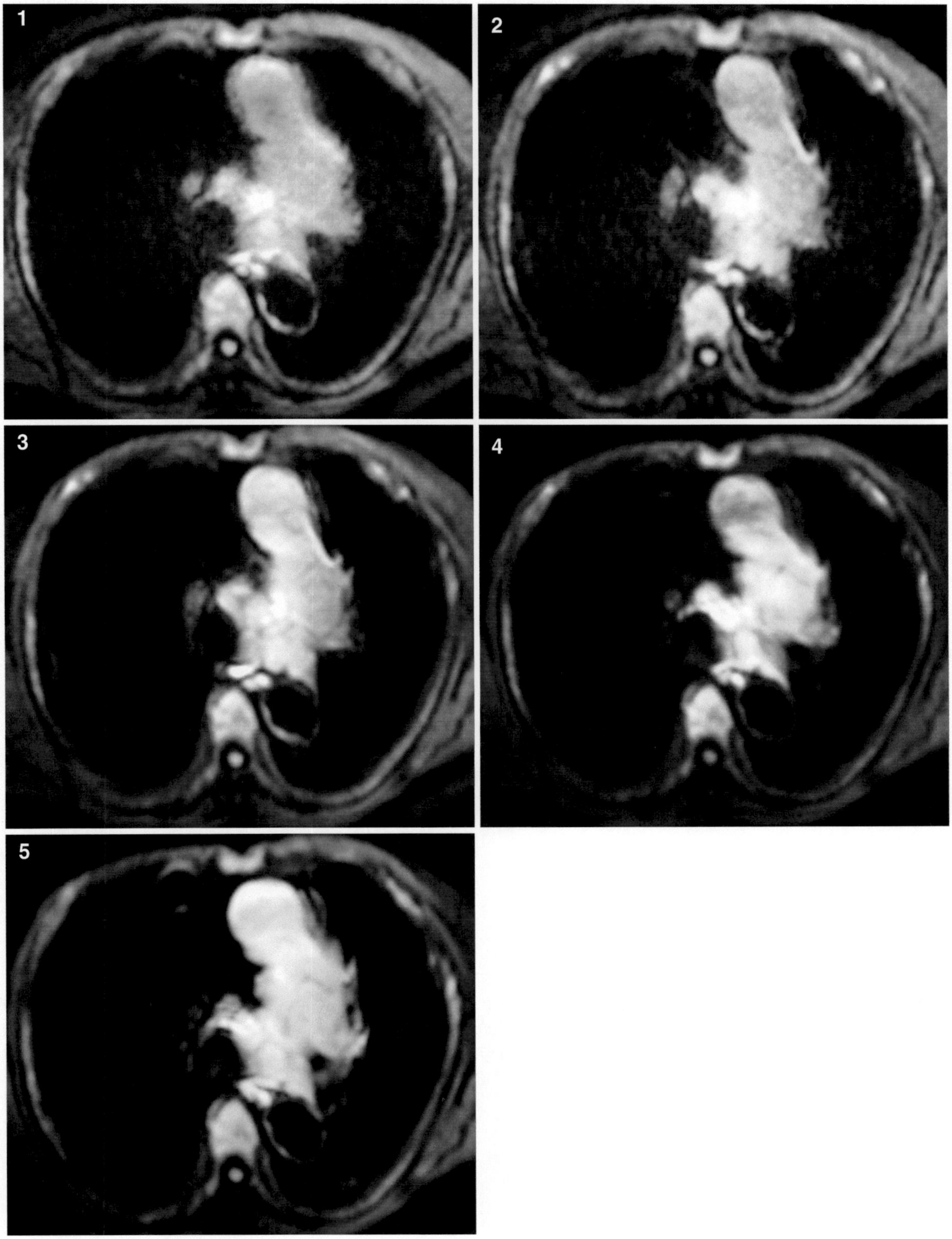

Case 13.2: Pulmonary Metastasis of Renal Cell Carcinoma

A 56-year-old male with renal cell carcinoma. On staging CT, a solitary pulmonary nodule of 2 cm was found in left lower lobe. MRI was performed for further characterization.

Comments

Tissue perfusion has demonstrated to affect ADC calculation in several organs. In the same sense, Uto and colleagues correctly stated that ADC calculations of pulmonary lesions were significantly affected by perfusion phenomena. They proposed to increase the higher *b* value over 1,000 s/mm^2 to prevent perfusion effects, as DWI sequences obtained with higher *b* values are more sensitive to diffusion. Another approach in order to avoid perfusion contamination, it is to avoid *b* values under 100 in the ADC quantification minimizing perfusion effects.

A more sophisticated and accurate option to avoid the effect of perfusion over DWI quantifications is to use the IVIM model. This approach has demonstrated that microvascular perfusion is detected at low *b* values (under 100 s/mm^2), allowing to calculate the perfusion free diffusion parameter (*D*) in several organs such as brain, abdominal organs, or muscle. ADC values are usually significantly higher than *D* values, as demonstrated in abdominal organs. The IVIM model is feasible in the thorax, although it is time consuming. Luna et al. suggested than the *D* value may be more exact than ADC measurements for lung nodule characterization, as in this case, although this theory still has to be validated.

Fig. 13.2 A nodule in the left lower lobe is identified on axial black blood TSE T2-weighted image (**13.2.1**). DWI using an IVIM approach was performed (not shown). Parametric maps obtained from a bicompartimental model of analysis of the signal decay of diffusion allowed to obtain the perfusion fraction (*f*) and true diffusion (*D*) parametric maps (**13.2.2** and **13.2.3**, respectively). The perfusion fraction of the nodule was high corresponding to that of 31%. The perfusion effect over diffusion is the cause of the difference between the ADC value (ADC = 1,6 × 10^{-3} mm^2/sg) and the *D* value (*D* = 1.3 × 10^{-3} mm^2/sg) as shown in the graph of the signal decay of diffusion (**13.2.4**) according to a monocompartmental (*gray line*) and bicompartmental model (*black line*), respectively. The ADC value was in the limit between benign and malignant lesions in this case. However, the *D* value suggested a malignant lesion, as posteriorly confirmed by percutaneous biopsy, corresponding to a renal cell carcinoma metastasis

Imaging Findings

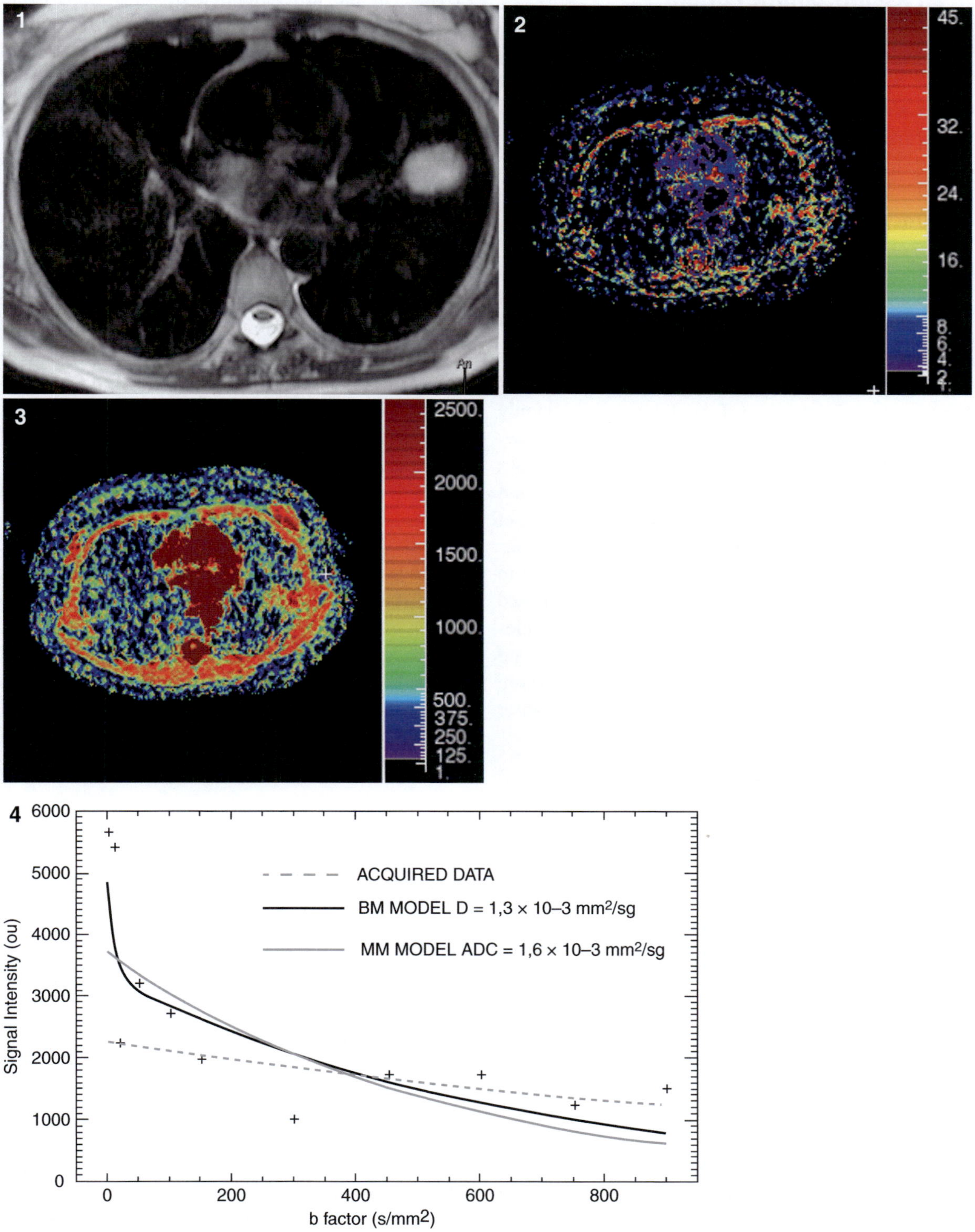

Case 13.3: Solitary Benign Lung Nodule in an Asymptomatic Patient

A 75-year-old male that presents incidentally a lung nodule in right lower lobe in a plain chest film without any clinical symptoms. Thorax MRI was performed for further assessment.

Comments

The noninvasive characterization of pulmonary nodules is still a common clinical problem. As the probability of malignancy increases with the nodule's size, it is critical to accurately characterize nodule as small as possible. In this purpose, different imaging modalities have been investigated. CT is the most commonly used, but still is based on morphologic criteria, showing obvious limitations. Dynamic enhanced CT shows an excellent sensitivity but a limited specificity, and PET has demonstrated to be also useful in this task, but it is also limited in the detection of adenocarcinomas and shows an important false-positive rate due to inflammation. Conventional MRI has been proposed for the evaluation of solitary pulmonary nodules according to their relaxation times with significant overlap between benign and malignant tumors. More recently, dynamic enhanced MRI has shown better specificity and accuracy than MDCT and coregistered PET/CT in the differentiation between benign and malignant nodules, although an overlap is still present in the patterns of enhancement between malignant and inflammatory lesions.

Characterization of pulmonary nodules has been also investigated using DWI, based on the concept that malignant lesions demonstrate increased cellularity, higher tissue disorganization, and increased extracellular space tortuosity compared to benign ones; diffusion of interstitial water should be restricted in cases of lung cancer. Visual assessment is a valid option, although small metastasis and some nonsolid adenocarcinomas were predominantly hypointense on DWI with high *b* value and granulomas, active inflammatory and fibrous nodules showed occasionally high signal intensity in a similar fashion to malignant lesions. Semiquantitative and quantitative approaches have demonstrated similar results. Different ADC cutoff values, between 1.1 and 1.4 × 10^{-3} mm^2/s, have been used with excellent results in this task. In the series by Mori and colleagues, better results in the distinction of benign from malignant pulmonary nodules were achieved with DWI with a *b* value of 1,000 s/mm^2 compared to PET. Therefore, DWI may be considered an adjunct tool for pulmonary nodule characterization, although further research is needed in this field.

Fig. 13.3 (**13.3.1**, **13.3 2**) Coronal TSE T2-weighted and axial black blood STIR images showed a well-defined hyperintense nodule in a peripheral location in the right posterobasal segment. Note the presence of a small fluid-fluid level inside the nodule (*arrow*). SS EPI DWI with *b* values of 0, 500, and 800 s/mm^2 (**13.3.3–13.3.5**, respectively) show disappearance of the lesion with higher *b* values, consistent with absence of restriction of diffusion as confirmed in the ADC map (**13.3.6**). The lesional mean ADC value was 2.3 × 10^{-3} mm^2/s. Those findings suggest a benign inflammatory origin which was proved by biopsy

Imaging Findings

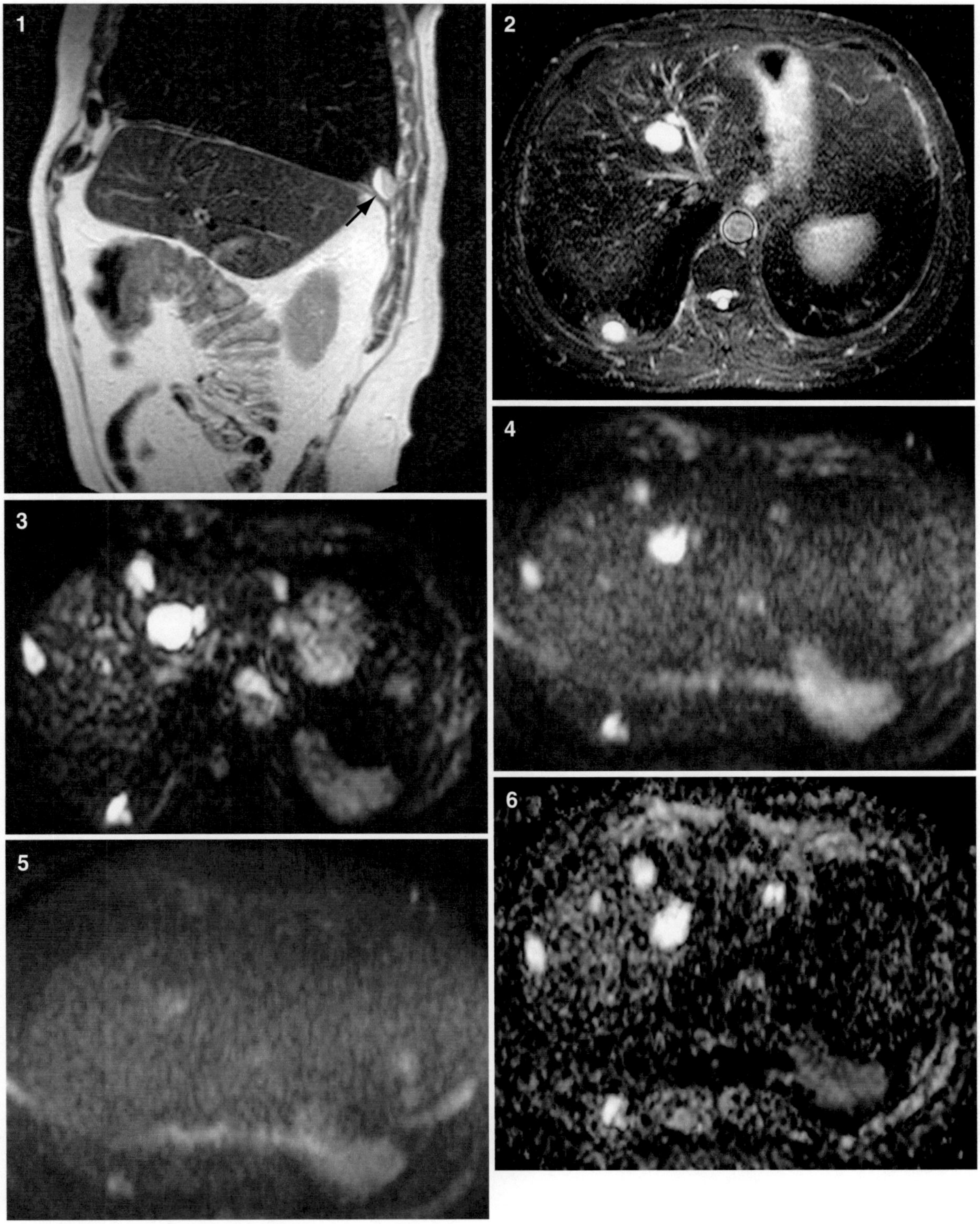

Case 13.4: Histological Grading and Prediction of Response and Posttreatment Monitorization of Lung Adenocarcinoma

A 62-year-old smoker male with partial atelectasis of left superior lobe on chest X-ray. In chest CT, a central mass was suspected although it was difficult to depict. A bronchoscopy with biopsy confirmed a low-grade adenocarcinoma. Chest MRI was performed for staging purposes, as it was complicated to define the extent of the central lesion.

Comments

DWI has been defined as an in vivo biomarker of tumoral grade and differentiation in oncologic lesions in other organs, as more aggressive lesions are more hypercellular than well-differentiated ones. This has also been investigated for lung cancer, especially for adenocarcinoma. Matoba and colleagues studied with DWI 30 patients with lung carcinoma, demonstrating an adequate correlation between the ADC values of lung cancer with tumor cellularity. Although, there was an overlap between the ADC values of the different types of lung carcinoma, they demonstrated that well-differentiated adenocarcinomas showed higher ADC values than those of more aggressive adenocarcinomas and epidermoid carcinomas in a significant manner, as well-differentiated adenocarcinomas showed lesser tumor cellularity and cellular differentiation than the other types of pulmonary carcinoma. In another series, Tanaka and colleagues studied 46 peripheral adenocarcinomas lesser than 3 cm, with DWI with a higher *b* value of 1,000 s/mm^2. They made a visual assessment of the signal intensity on DWI of the nodules compared to spinal cord. They were able to significantly differentiate invasive adenocarcinomas from BAC, as invasive adenocarcinomas usually showed higher signal intensity. Besides, Koyama and colleagues evaluated 33 adenocarcinomas with DWI and a higher *b* value of 1,000 s/mm^2. The ADC values were not useful to differentiate the subtypes of adenocarcinoma.

DWII can also be used for predictive purposes in different types of tumors as rectal and breast cancer or hepatic metastasis of colorectal carcinoma. The prediction of response to treatment with DWI can lead to a change in the management of lung cancer. The relationship between pretreatment ADC value and response to treatment is complex, and it is related to organ of interest, histological subtype, and type of treatment. In lung cancer, the role of DWI in the prediction of response to treatment has still to be investigated, although potentially tumors with higher ADC values, indicating a less aggressive biological nature, should respond better to chemotherapy as in this case. Besides, DWI has also been advocated a biological marker to assess response to chemotherapy of lung cancer, with the potential to evaluate its response as early as 1 month after the start of treatment

Imaging Findings

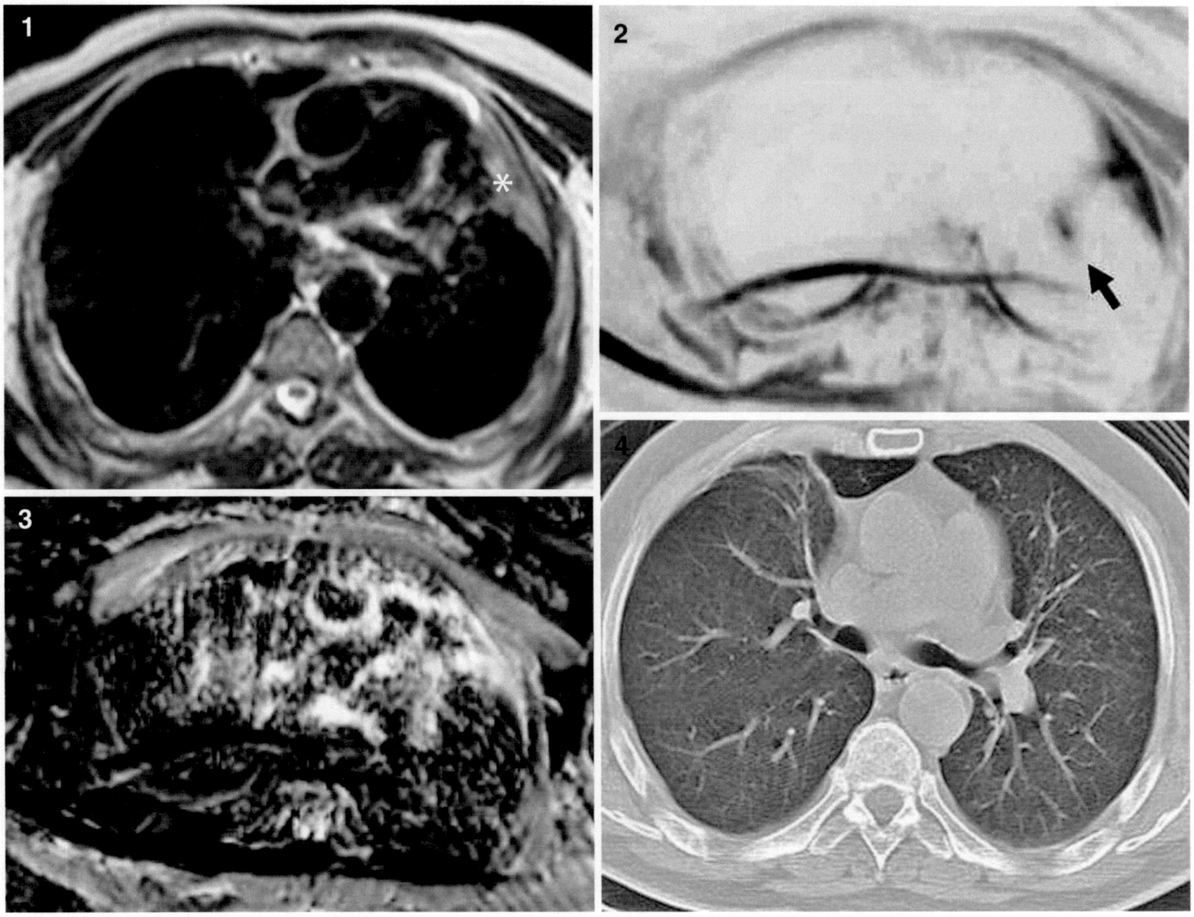

Fig. 13.4 (**13.4.1**) Axial TSE T2-weighted image shows the collapse of the apical segment of the left superior lobe (*asterisk*), although the mass is difficult to identify. However, a low intensity hilar lesion (*arrow*) is identified on DWI image with a *b* value of 1,000 s/mm^2 and inverted gray-scale (**13.4.2**). A mean ADC value of 1.9 × 10^{-3} mm^2/s (**13.4.3**) is consistent with tumor histology of low-grade adenocarcinoma. On the CT performed 3 months after chemotherapy (**13.4.4**), a complete remission of the disease is demonstrated

Case 13.5: Distinction of Central Bronchogenic Carcinoma and Peripheral Obstructive Atelectasis

A 54-year-old smoker male with confirmed central epidermoid carcinoma and complete atelectasis of left lung. MRI was requested to distinguish between central tumor and associated postobstructive pneumonitis, which was unclear on enhanced CT (not shown).

Comments

Up to one half of cases of central bronchial carcinomas are usually associated with peripheral lung collapse or obstructive pneumonia, due to compression or invasion of proximal bronchi. The imaging technique of choice to study pulmonary oncological lesions is still CT, but CT may not clearly distinguish the primary tumor from pulmonary atelectasis due to limited soft tissue contrast. This differentiation is of great importance with diagnostic, therapeutic, and prognostic implications. Furthermore, T-staging of lung cancer may be misinterpreted due to an erroneous depiction of the extent of collapse obstruction. Besides, proper delimitation of the primary tumor is critical in planning radiation therapy to adjust both the dose and the radiation field and to minimize the adverse side effects, especially with the newer high-dose, high-precision radiotherapeutic techniques. Last but not least, it is critical to assess the therapeutic effect of radiotherapy.

Classical T2-weighted sequences have been used to differentiate between central cancer and postobstructive collapse according to their signal intensity. Several series have demonstrated that T2-weighted sequences may achieve this difference in approximately 70–80% of the cases. Since the advent of chest DWI, it has been proposed to discriminate the cancer limits from the obstructive atelectasis, according to differences in signal intensity in DWI acquisitions with high *b* values. It was supposed that central bronchogenic carcinomas will show higher signal intensity and lower ADC values than benign obstructive atelectasis, according to differences in cellularity and grade of occupancy of the interstitium. Qui et al. compared the accuracy of CT, T2-weighted sequences and DWI in this task. They studied 33 patients with central lung cancer and obstructive atelectasis with a breath-hold DWI sequence with a maximum *b* value of 500 s/mm^2. Enhanced CT was able to achieve this difference in 14 patients, T2-weighted sequences in 21 cases, and DWI in 26 cases. The best result was performed using a combination of T2-weighted and DWI with an accuracy of 88% (29/33 patients). They concluded that in doubtful cases for CT, MRI using DWI and T2-weighted sequences would increase the ability to define properly the postobstructive collapse. Furthermore, in our experience, the use of fusion software to integrate information from T2-weighted and DWI software increases the accuracy of MRI. In another series, Baysal and colleagues studied 27 patients with central lung cancer and obstructive atelectasis with a DWI sequence with a maximum *b* value of 1,000 s/mm^2. They obtained a significant difference between both entities, as mean ADC value of central lung carcinomas was that of $1.83 \pm 0.75 \times 10^{-3}$ mm^2/s and the one of obstructive consolidation corresponded to $2.50 \pm 0.76 \times 10^{-3}$ mm^2/s.

Imaging Findings

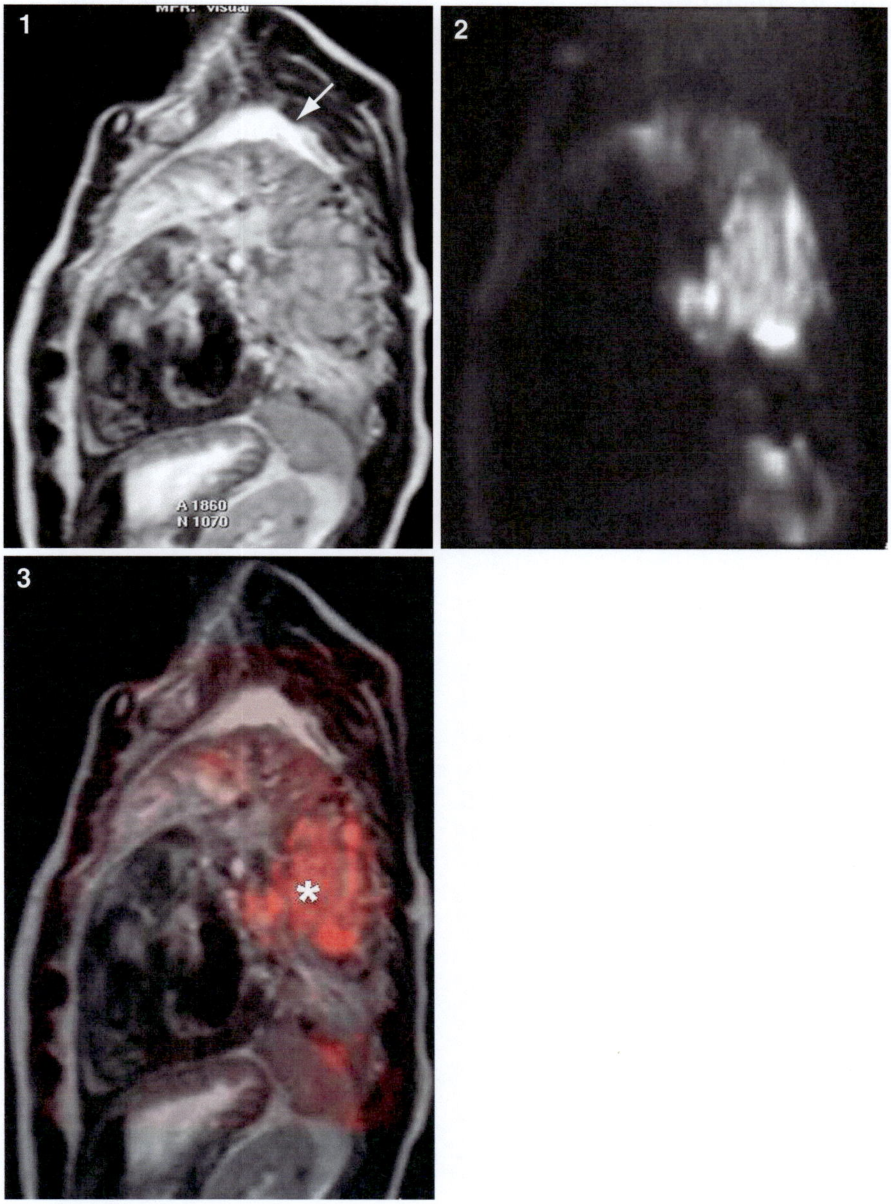

Fig. 13.5 (**13.5.1**) Sagittal TSE T2-weighted image shows extensive collapse of left lung without clear definition of central bronchogenic carcinoma borders. Note the presence of apical loculated pleural effusion (*arrow*). (**13.5.2**) Sagittal MPR of a SS EPI DWI using a *b* value of 1,000 s/mm^2 at the same level as that of Fig. **13.5.1** shows a central area of restricted diffusion corresponding to an epidermoid carcinoma. (**13.5.3**) Fusion imaging of T2-weighted and DWI allows better differentiation of the tumor borders (*asterisk*) from postobstructive pneumonitis

Case 13.6: Staging and Posttreatment Monitorization of Small Cell Lung Carcinoma

A 59-year-old male was referred for abdominal MRI in the work-up of hepatomegaly and altered liver function. Multiple liver metastases and an incidental thoracic mass were found. In the same session, thoracic MRI was performed under the suspicion of lung cancer, which was confirmed (SCLC).

Comments

Lung cancer remains a challenge for medicine, because despite advances indiagnostic techniques and therapeutic resources, the treatment results are not fully satisfactory, as evidenced by the few cures in relation to the number of patients cared for. CT still remains as the first diagnostic tool in many centers for the detection and characterization of lung cancer. But, MRI due to its high ability for tissue characterization is being used for staging especial cases, as those where it is necessary to exclude invasion of neighboring structures, such as chest wall or mediastinal great vessels. The routine inclusion of DWI sequences in the MRI protocol for lung cancer could probably increase its accuracy in TNM-staging.

Although, DWI may help in local T-staging, its role in this task has not been fully investigated. DWI may increase the accuracy in the measurement of the distance of the tumor to the carina and tumor size. This sequence also facilitates the distinction of tumor borders from adjacent structures in order to exclude great vessels, pleural, pericardial, or chest wall invasion, and it also allows accurate differentiation between obstructive atelectasis and central tumor. In the case of NSCLC, DWI has demonstrated a role in the N- and M-staging with similar results to PET/CT.

However, TNM-staging is not usually performed for SCLC as the therapeutic management is independent of the stage. DWI has also been proposed for histological grading of lung cancer. In several series such as the one by Liu and colleagues or the recent report by Razek and colleagues, SCLC demonstrated statistically significant lower ADC values than non-small cell lung cancer NSCLC, indicating its more aggressive biological behavior. Although there is still little data in the evaluation of posttreatment monitorization of lung cancer for DWI, recent data opens the door to its use in the early and standard evaluation of response to treatment. As extensively demonstrated in other organs, functional information provided by DWI will change before tumoral volume, suggesting the necessity or not for a change in drug treatment.

Fig. 13.6 (**13.6.1**) Axial balanced TFE shows a large right mediastinal mass (*asterisk*) with hiliar and prevascular lymph nodes (*arrows*). (**13.6.2, 13.6.3**) SS EPI DWI with a *b* value of 800 s/mm^2 and ADC map show severe restriction of diffusion within the mass (*asterisk*). Note the hyperintensity on DWI of thoracic vertebral body, ribs, and scapula in relation to bone metastasis (*arrows*). (**13.6.4**) Fusion image of Figs. **13.6.1** and **13.6.2** allows a better depiction and localization of hypercellular areas as red and dark blue areas. Note the absence of restricted diffusion in the right upper lobe subsegmental atelectasis (*arrow*). (**13.6.5, 13.6.6**) DWI with *b* values of 0 and 800 s/mm^2 respectively demonstrate the infiltration of the main right pulmonary artery by the mass. (**13.6.7**) DWI with a *b* value of 800 s/mm^2 demonstrates several focal liver lesions with restricted diffusion corresponding to metastasis. MR-staging was that of stage IV (T4 N3 M1b). (**13.6.8, 13.6.9**) Follow-up MRI 4 months after chemotherapy. DWI with *b* values of 0 and 800 s/mm^2 respectively, at approximately the same level as that of Figs. **13.6.5** and **13.6.6**, show reduction of hilar tumor volume and disminished restriction of diffusion. ADC of the tumor markedly increased (not shown) consistent with adequate response to treatment. (**13.6.10**) Posttreatment liver DWI with a *b* value of 800 s/mm^2 at approximately the same level as that of Fig. **13.6.7** confirmed the drastic reduction in number and volume of focal liver lesions

Imaging Findings

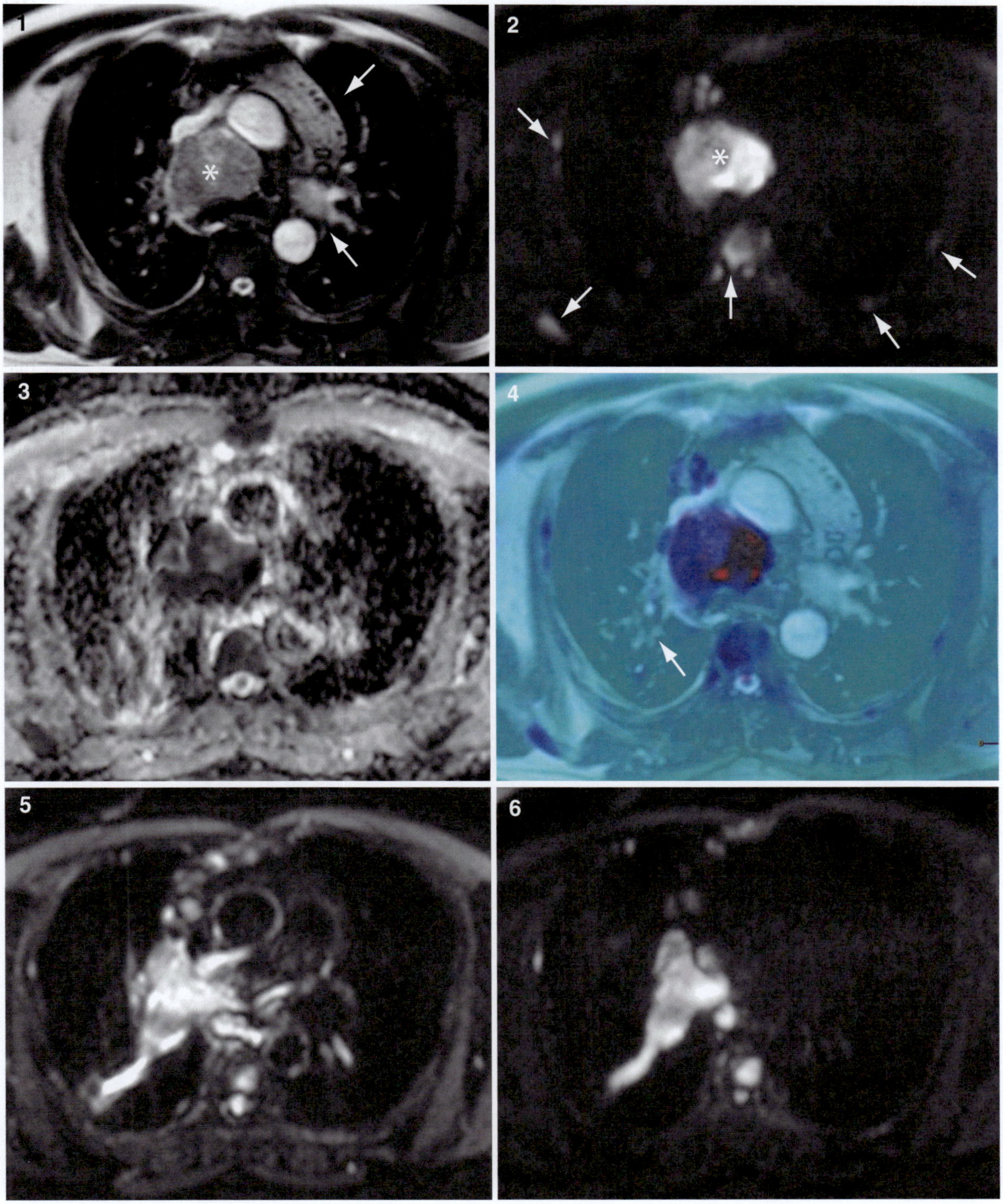

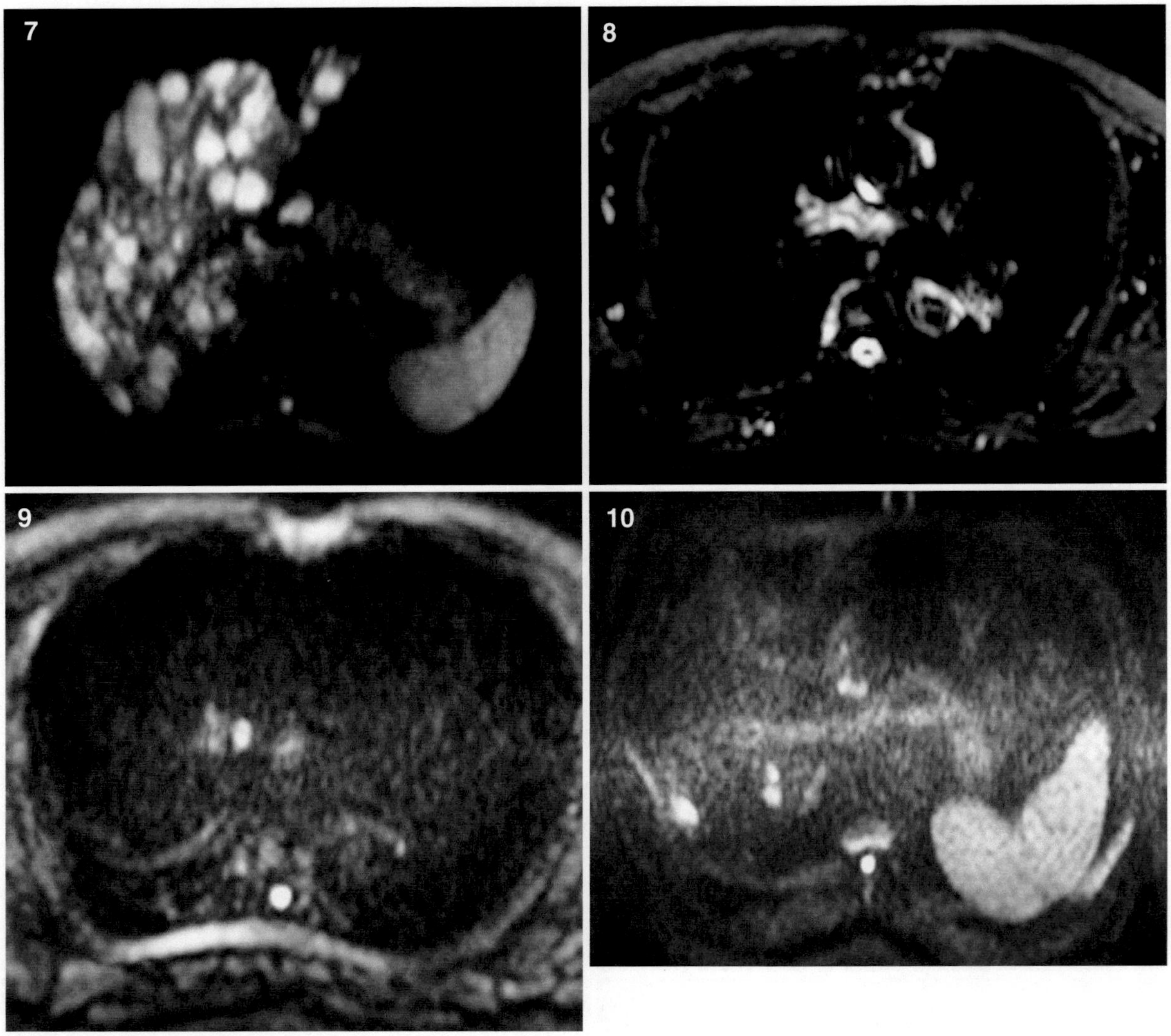

Fig. 13.6 (continued)

Case 13.7: Exudative Pleural Effusion

A 62-year-old female with extensive right pleural effusion. CT identified an anterior mediastinal mass with involvement of the chest wall. MRI was performed for further assessment.

Comments

The differentiation between transudative and exudative pleural effusion has been a classical challenge for clinicians. The importance of this issue lies on making diagnostic and therapeutic decisions based on the nature of pleural fluid. Nowadays, the gold standard technique for fluid characterization is pleurocentesis and further biochemical analysis is based on Light's criteria (mainly LDH/protein ratio). Although minimal, this procedure is linked to a few complications such as pneumothorax, bleeding, or infection, especially in patients with comorbidities.

These are the reasons why noninvasive tests have been investigated in an attempt to characterize pleural effusion. First, chest MRI with gadolinium chelates injection was used for this purpose. Several authors suggested that exudative effusion would enhance instead transudative fluid with no definitive results. DWI was also tested for this purpose in the series by Baysal and colleagues, and more recently by Inan and colleagues. According to their results, a cutoff ADC value between 3.38×10^{-3} mm^2/s and 3.6×10^{-3} mm^2/s could accurately differentiate exudative from transudative pleural effusion. ADC values of exudative fluid were lower than the ones of transudative effusions in both reports. In visual assessment, transudative effusions showed similar signal intensity to paraspinal muscle with high *b* value. However, exudative effusion demonstrated higher signal intensity than paraspinal muscle. These studies conclude that the use of DWI would allow a high sensitivity and specificity for differentiating probably benign (transudative) effusions from probably malignant (exudative) ones.

Imaging Findings

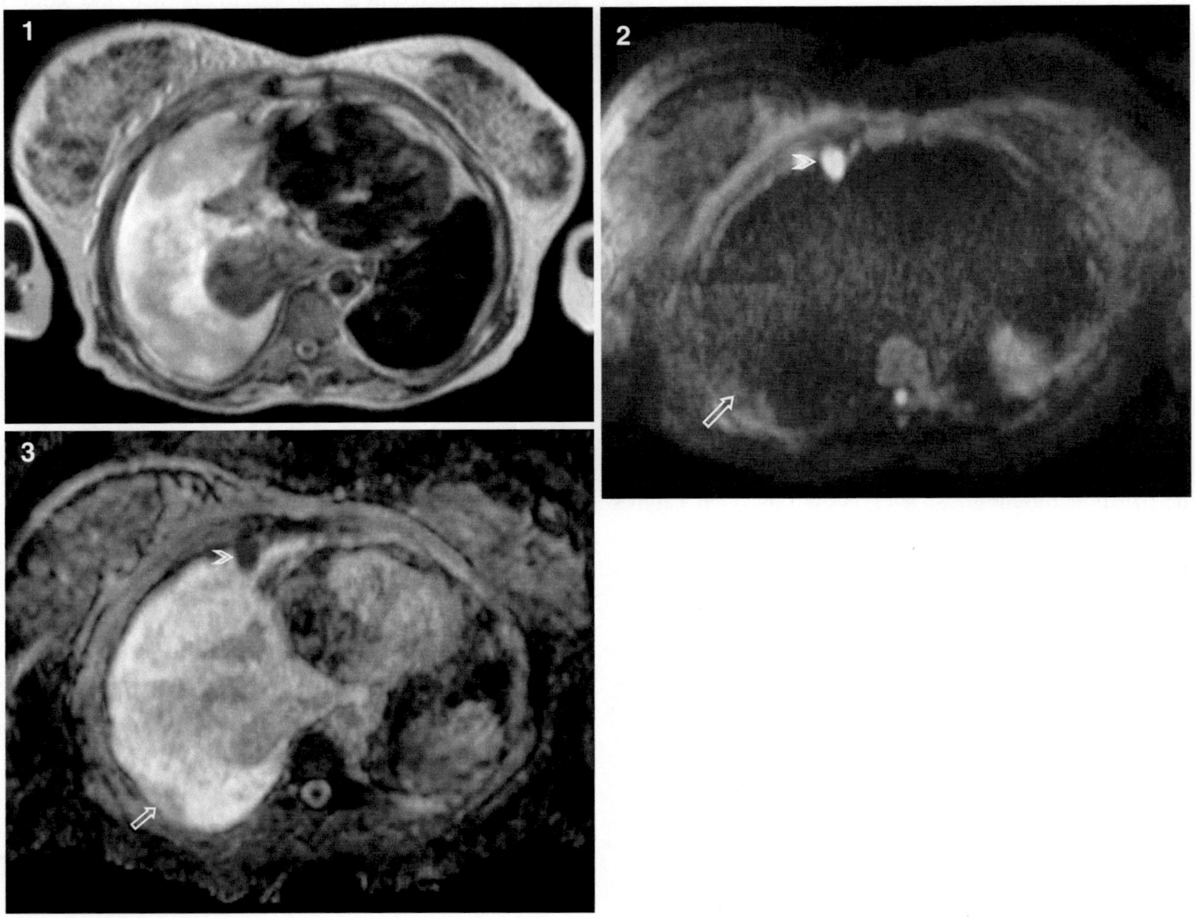

Fig. 13.7 (**13.7.1**) Transverse black blood TSE T2-weighted image shows a large right pleural effusion with secondary lung collapse. (**13.7.2**) DWI with a *b* value of 800 s/mm^2 shows how most of the pleural effusion is not visible, except a hyperintense area in the posterior aspect of right hemithorax (*open arrow*) and a hyperintense nodule in the anterior right pleura (*arrowhead*), which corresponds to a pleural metastasis. (**13.7.3**) Areas of restricted diffusion (*open arrow*) are identified within the effusion with ADC values between 2.9×10^{-3} mm^2/s and 3.1×10^{-3} mm^2/s, which suggest malignant effusion. Thoracentesis and cytology proved adenocarcinoma cells. Posterior work-up demonstrated a primary breast adenocarcinoma

Case 13.8: Chronic and Occult Acute Rib Fractures

A 61-year-old woman with right flank pain during the last 2 months. She had no recent history of trauma. Chest plain film showed multiple rib lesions. Clinicians requested an MRI to investigate the differential diagnosis between benign fractures, metastases, or multiple myeloma.

Comments

DWI may be used not only to assess oncological diseases. New applications are arising to help in the diagnosis of traumatic and orthopedic questions. Chest trauma is one of the most common clinical reasons for consultation at ER department. Classical chest plain film or CT is used to rule out rib injuries and underlying lung complications. However, occasionally, chest X-ray or even CT may not adequately depict rib fractures or contusion. In addition, once a rib fracture is detected, it is necessary to define if it is acute or chronic. This issue is more important in certain types of patients, such as in cases of suspicion of elder or children abuse, athletes, etc. There are classical radiological criteria to answer that question, but in many cases, the level of activity of the fracture, its date, or the phase of the consolidation process cannot be elucidated. Furthermore, it is sometimes difficult to detect small fissures or fractures in inaccessible locations such as costovertebral or chondrosternal regions.

In the last decade, the MRI study of rib injuries has begun based primarily on T1-weighted sequences due to its high sensitivity for the detection of bone edema. Otherwise, fat-suppressed T2-weighted sequences are used for the assessment of both bone and adjacent tissue edema. However, these sequences have the limitation of significant background noise, with poor image contrast. The introduction of DWI, especially DWIBS, has increased the capacity of MRI for detection of ribs fractures. The chance to perform multiplanar reconstructions allows us to verify the distribution and number of them. The biological basis for explaining the detection of rib fractures and bruises by DWI is not entirely clear. In fact, according to some experiments in animal models, it is thought that the detection is based more on prolonged T2 relaxation time (due to edema or associated with the fracture hematoma) than on a true restriction of diffusion. Following this theory, chronic fractures may not show signal changes in DWIBS unlike acute ones.

Finally, returning to the broadcast oncology applications, another problem of daily practice is the differential diagnosis of rib fracture and metastasis. To our knowledge, there are currently studies only for differentition between collapsed vertebrae from pathologic fractures based on DWI signal intensity and ADC values. With DWIBS, we obtain a PET-like image that allows us to assess the distribution of rib injuries and, together with clinical data, to approximate the diagnosis of fractures (classical arrangement following consecutive lines of strength) or metastasis (random distribution). Additional data such as the presence of a soft tissue mass or involvement of adjacent tissues may help in this differential.

Imaging Findings

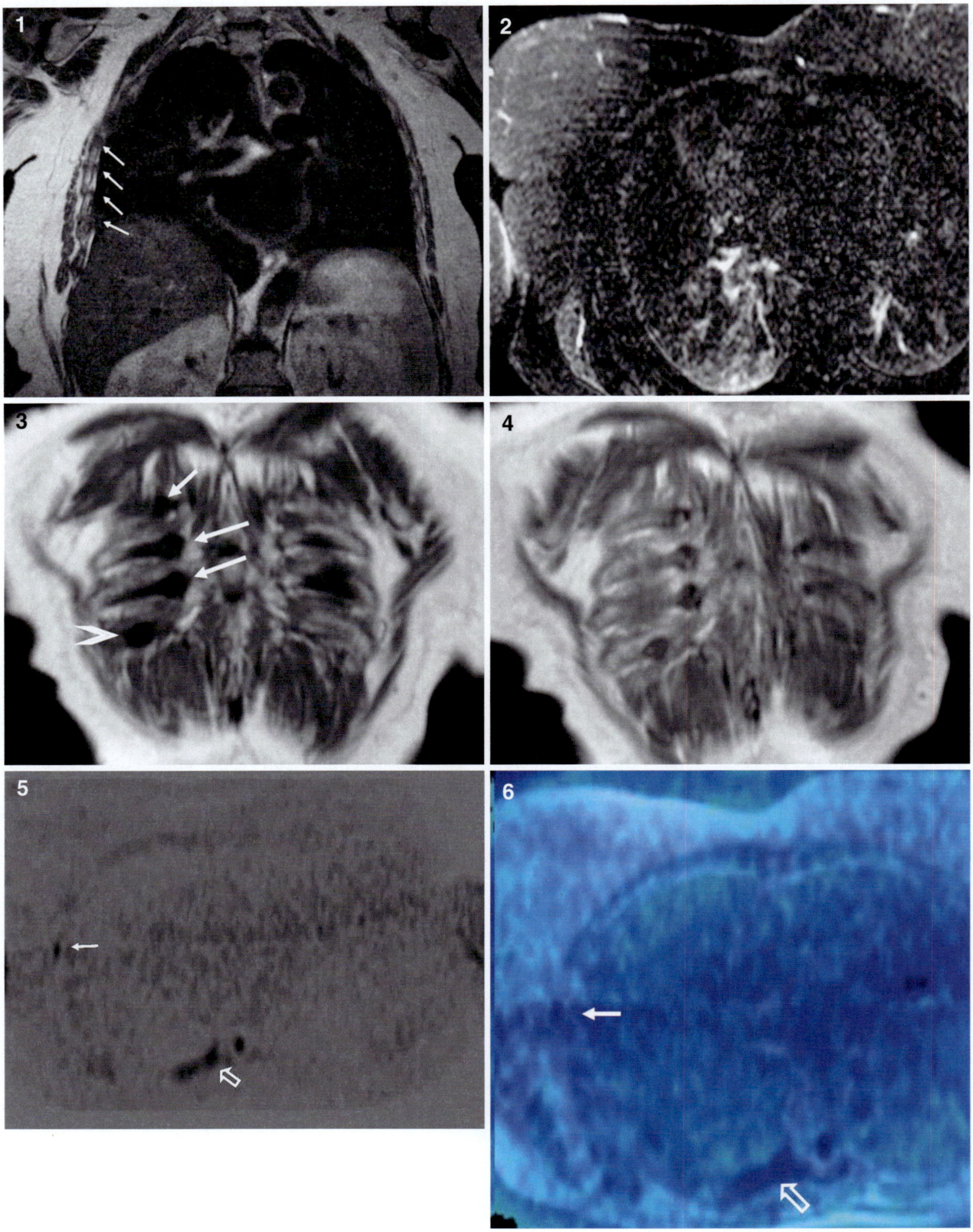

Case 13.9: Pericardial Neuroblastoma

A 49-year-old male referred to our MRI unit with suspicion of dilated right atrial appendage in chest CT examination. A cardiac MRI study was performed.

Comments

Neuroblastoma is a frequent malignant tumor in children, being the most common extracranial neoplasm at this group of age, but it is very rare in adults. It originates in neural crest cells of the sympathetic nervous system. Nearly two-thirds of neuroblastomas are located in the abdomen, and use to locate next to the vertebrae. These tumors have a particular histological composition mainly based on small cells with little cytoplasm.

Some authors have studied the MRI characteristics of abdominal neuroblastomas on DWI. They have tried to characterize and differentiate them from other tumors of similar histological origin, although with a more benign behavior such as ganglioneuroma or ganglioneuroblastoma. In those studies, an ADC threshold value of 1.13×10^{-3} mm^2/s was able to significantly discriminate between both groups of tumors. The average ADC value of neuroblastoma was 0.8×10^{-3} mm^2/s and for ganglioneuroma or ganglioneuroblastoma, it corresponded to 1.1×10^{-3} mm^2/s. DWI may help in their differentiation, and to distinguish areas of viable and nonviable tumor. Furthermore, whole-body DWI has been used for the staging of abdominal neuroblastomas. To our knowledge, no pericardial neuroblastoma has been reported.

Fig. 13.8 (**13.8.1**) Coronal TSE T2-weighted image shows multiple consolidated rib fractures (*arrows*) without apparent signs of inflammation. (**13.8.2**) Axial STIR shows no areas of edema, suggesting old healed fractures. (**13.8.3**, **13.8.4**) *Pre- and post-contrast* coronal TSE T1-weighted image show bone edema at costovertebral junctions (*arrows*) and a posterior rib acute fracture (*arrowhead*) with minimal enhancement after contrast injection. There was no associated soft tissue mass. (**13.8.5**) SS EPI DWI with a *b* value of 800 s/mm^2 at the same level as that of STIR image (**13.8.2**) shows high signal at the costovertebral junction (*open arrow*) and in the right lateral rib arch (*arrow*) consistent with acute or instable fracture. (**13.8.6**) Fusion image of T2-weighted and DWI improves the depiction and localization of these fractures. Notice that among the multiple consolidated fractures of right lateral ribs demonstrated in Fig. **13.8.1**, there was an acute one that showed restricted diffusion (*arrow*)

Imaging Findings

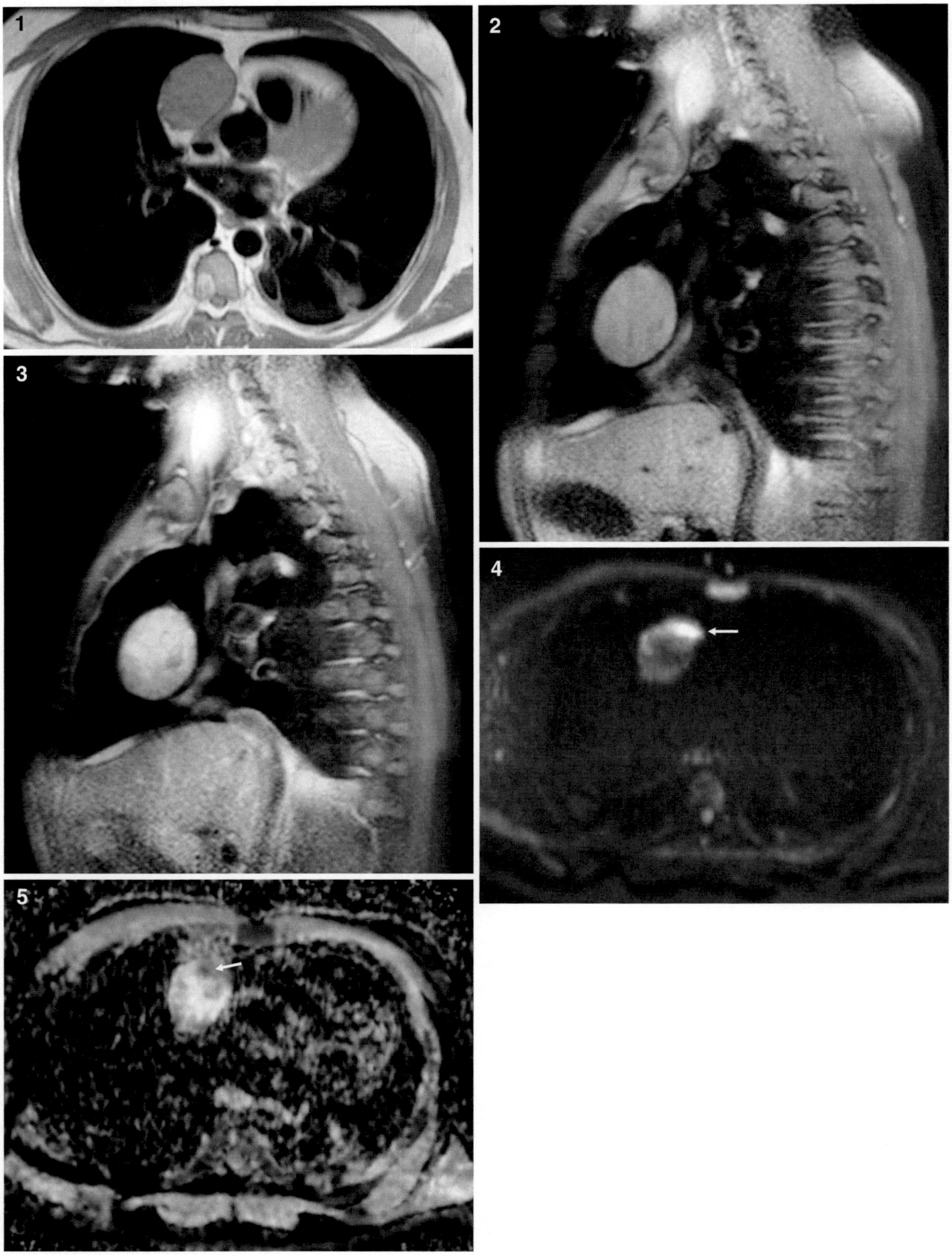

Case 13.10: Ex Vivo DTI of a Pig Heart

A conventional SE DWI sequence with a *b* value of 800 s/mm^2 was performed in a 3 T magnet to study the fiber structure of the pig heart.

Comments

Cardiac DTI is a growing area of research. Ex vivo and recently in vivo acquisitions allow knowing the 3D organization of myocardial fibers which is determinant of cardiac torsion, strain, and stress. In order to acquire this information, it is necessary to perform DWI in at least six different diffusion directions that permit to build the tensor information. Clinical applications of cardiac DTI are still very limited, although areas of altered cardiac structure after subacute myocardial infarction revealed changes in mean diffusivity and fractional anisotropy. Furthermore, DTI has been useful in the monitorization of postischemic injury remodeling, with an association between sequential zonal improvement of tissue integrity and fiber architecture remodeling with sequential recovery of zonal wall thickening of the infarcted area. Therefore, the clinical role of cardiac DTI needs further research.

Fig. 13.9 (**13.9.1–13.9.3**). Black blood TSE T1-weighted and pre- and postcontrast sagittal SPIR black blood TSE T1-weighted images shows a large paracardiac mass, located between both pericardial leaves, which is isointense to myocardium and enhances strongly and heterogeneously after contrast administration. No signs of cardiac or mediastinal invasion were showed. (**13.9.4**) DWI with a *b* value of 800 s/mm^2 shows heterogeneous signal intensity of the mass. (**13.9.5**) ADC map. ADC ranged between 0.9×10^{-3} mm^2/s in the hypointense regions (*arrow*), corresponding to viable tumor, to 1.9×10^{-3} mm^2/s in the necrotic hyperintense areas on the ADC map. This patient underwent cardiac surgery with pathologic diagnosis of pericardial neuroblastoma

Imaging Findings

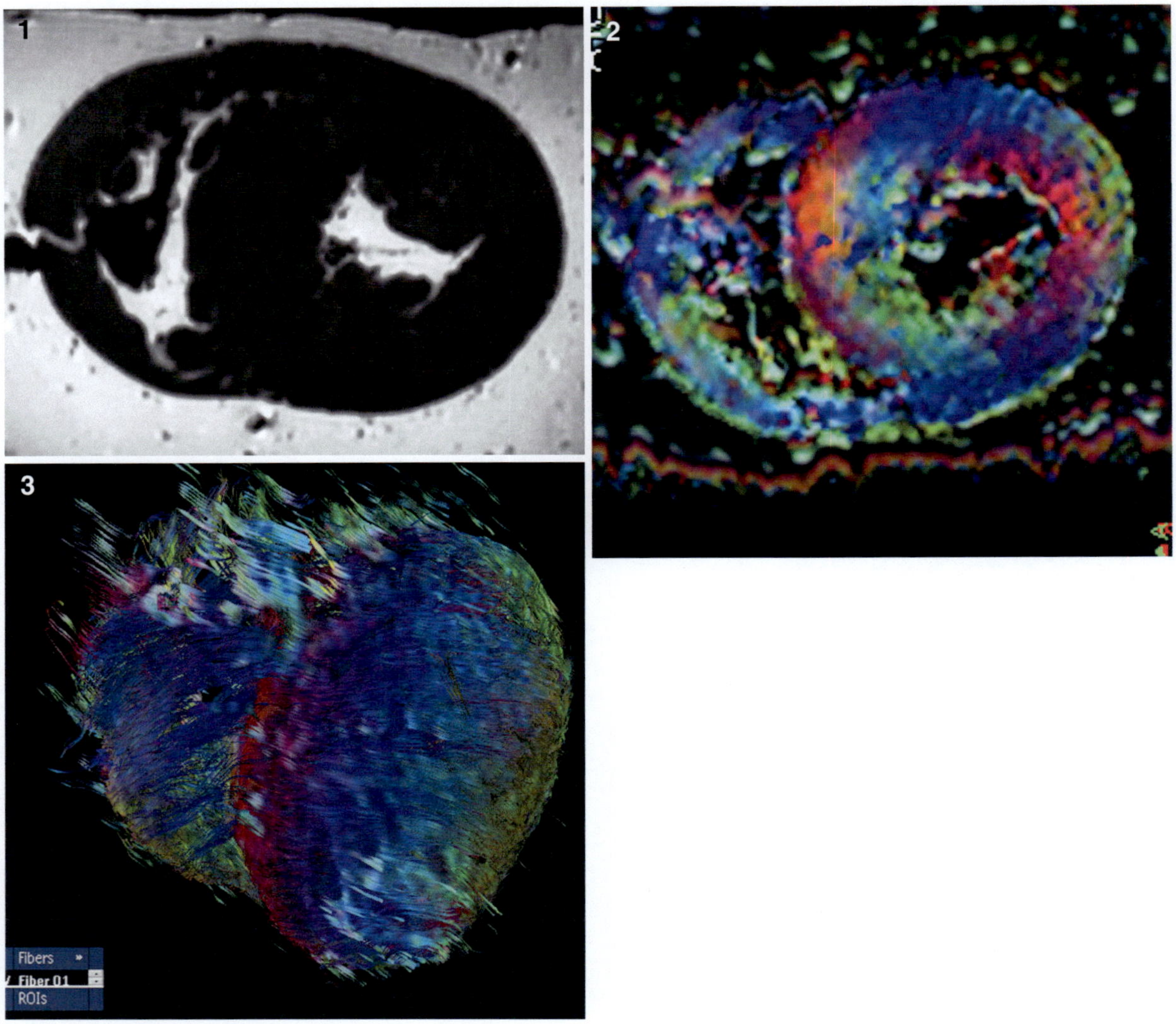

Fig. 13.10 (**13.10.1**) Short-axis black blood TSE T2-weighted image. (**13.10.2**) Short-axis source fractional anisotropy image of the heart. (**13.10.3**) A 3D DTI reconstruction reveals the organization and pathways of the heart fibers

Further Reading

Baysal T, Bulut T, Gökirmak M et al (2004) Diffusion-weighted MR imaging of pleural fluid: differentiation of transudative vs exudative pleural effusions. Eur Radiol 14(5):890–896

Baysal T, Mutlu DY, Yologlu S (2009) Diffusion-weighted magnetic resonance imaging in differentiation of postobstructive consolidation from central lung carcinoma. Magn Reson Imaging 27(10):1447–1454

Bruegel M, Gaa J, Woertler K et al (2007) MRI of the lung: value of different turbo spin-echo, single-shot turbo spin-echo, and 3D gradient-echo pulse sequences for the detection of pulmonary metastases. J Magn Reson Imaging 25(1):73–81

Chen W, Jian W, Li H et al (2010) Whole-body diffusion-weighted imaging vs. FDG-PET for the detection of non-small-cell lung cancer. How do they measure up? Magn Reson Imaging 28:613–620

Deng J, Miller FH, Salem R et al (2006) Multishot diffusion-weighted PROPELLER magnetic resonance imaging of the abdomen. Invest Radiol 41(10):769–775

Dietrich O, Reiser MF, Schoenberg SO (2008) Artifacts in 3-T MRI: physical background and reduction strategies. Eur J Radiol 65:29–35

Fain SB, Panth SR, Evans MD et al (2006) Early emphysematous changes in asymptomatic smokers: detection with 3He MR imaging. Radiology 239(3):875–883

Frericks BB, Meyer BC, Martus P et al (2008) MRI of the thorax during whole-body MRI: evaluation of different MR sequences and comparison to thoracic multidetector computed tomography (MDCT). J Magn Reson Imaging 27(3):538–545

Gahr N, Darge K, Hahn G et al (2011) Diffusion-weighted MRI for differentiation of neuroblastoma and ganglioneuroblastoma/ganglioneuroma. Eur J Radiol 79(3):443–446

Gill RR, Umeoka S, Mamata H et al (2010) Diffusion-weighted MRI of malignant pleural mesothelioma: preliminary assessment of apparent diffusion coefficient in histologic subtypes. Am J Roentgenol 195(2):W125–W130

Goo HW (2010) Whole-body MRI of neuroblastoma. Eur J Radiol 75(3):306–314

Hasegawa I, Boiselle PM, Kuwabara K et al (2008) Mediastinal lymph nodes in patients with non-small cell lung cancer: preliminary experience with diffusion-weighted MR imaging. J Thorac Imaging 23(3):157–161

Henzler T, Schmid-Bindert G, Schoenberg SO et al (2010) Diffusion and perfusion MRI of the lung and mediastinum. Eur J Radiol 76(3):329–336

Inan N, Arslan A, Akansel G et al (2009) Diffusion-weighted MRI in the characterization of pleural effusions. Diagn Interv Radiol 15(1):13–18

Jeong YJ, Lee KS, Jeong SY et al (2005) Solitary pulmonary nodule: characterization with combined wash-in and wash-out features at dynamic multi-detector row CT. Radiology 237(2):675–683

Kanauchi N, Oizumi H, Honma T et al (2009) Role of diffusion-weighted magnetic resonance imaging for predicting of tumor invasiveness for clinical stage IA non-small cell lung cancer. Eur J Cardiothorac Surg 35(4):706–710; discussion 10-1

Kandpal H, Sharma R, Madhusudhan KS et al (2009) Respiratory-triggered versus breath-hold diffusion-weighted MRI of liver lesions: comparison of image quality and apparent diffusion coefficient values. Am J Roentgenol 192:915–922

King AD, Ahuja AT, Yeung DK et al (2007) Malignant cervical lymphadenopathy: diagnostic accuracy of diffusion-weighted MR imaging. Radiology 245(3):806–813

Komori T, Narabayashi I, Matsumura K et al (2007) 2-[Fluorine-18]-fluoro-2-deoxy-D-glucose positron emission tomography/computed tomography versus whole-body diffusion-weighted MRI for detection of malignant lesions: initial experience. Ann Nucl Med 21(4):209–215

Koşucu P, Tekinbaş C, Erol M et al (2009) Mediastinal lymph nodes: assessment with diffusion-weighted MR imaging. J Magn Reson Imaging 30(2):292–297

Koyama H, Ohno Y, Kono A et al (2008) Quantitative and qualitative assessment of non-contrast-enhanced pulmonary MR imaging for management of pulmonary nodules in 161 subjects. Eur Radiol 18(10):2120–2131

Koyama H, Ohno Y, Aoyama N et al (2010) Comparison of STIR turbo SE imaging and diffusion-weighted imaging of the lung: capability for detection and subtype classification of pulmonary adenocarcinomas. Eur Radiol 20(4):790–800

Kwee TC, Takahara T, Koh DM et al (2008) Comparison and reproducibility of ADC measurements in breath hold, respiratory triggered, and free-breathing diffusion-weighted MR imaging of the liver. J Magn Reson Imaging 28(5):1141–1148

Kwee TC, Takahara T, Niwa T et al (2009) Influence of cardiac motion on diffusion-weighted magnetic resonance imaging of the liver. Magn Reson Mater Phy 22:319–325

Kwee TC, Takahara T, Niwa T (2010) Diffusion-weighted whole-body imaging with background body signal suppression facilitates detection and evaluation of an anterior rib contusion. Clin Imaging 34(4):298–301

Laissy JP, Serfaty JM, Messika-Zeitoun D et al (2009) Cardiac diffusion MRI of recent and chronic myocardial infarction: preliminary results. J Radiol 90(4):481–484

Li S, Xue HD, Li J et al (2008) Application of whole body diffusion-weighted MR imaging for diagnosis and staging of malignant lymphoma. Chin Med Sci J 23:138–144

Lichy MP, Aschoff P, Plathow C et al (2007) Tumor detection by diffusion-weighted MRI and ADC-mapping – initial clinical experiences in comparison to PET-CT. Invest Radiol 42:605–613

Liu H, Liu Y, Yu T et al (2010) Usefulness of diffusion-weighted MR imaging in the evaluation of pulmonary lesions. Eur Radiol 20(4):807–815

Luna A, Sánchez-Gonzalez J, Caro P (2011) Diffusion-weighted imaging of the chest. Magn Reson Imaging Clin N Am 19(1):69–94

Mathew L, Kirby M, Etemad-Rezai R, et al (2011) Hyperpolarized 3He magnetic resonance imaging: preliminary evaluation of phenotyping potential in chronic obstructive pulmonary disease. Eur J Radiol 79(1):140–146

Matoba M, Tonami H, Kondou T et al (2007) Lung carcinoma: diffusion-weighted MR imaging – preliminary evaluation with apparent diffusion coefficient. Radiology 243(2):570–577

Mori T, Nomori H, Ikeda K et al (2008) Diffusion-weighted magnetic resonance imaging for diagnosing malignant pulmonary nodules/masses: comparison with positron emission tomography. J Thorac Oncol 3(4):358–364

Nakayama J, Miyasaka K, Omatsu T et al (2010) Metastases in mediastinal and hilar lymph nodes in patients with non-small cell lung cancer: quantitative assessment with diffusion-weighted magnetic resonance imaging and apparent diffusion coefficient. J Comput Assist Tomogr 34(1):1–8

Nomori H, Mori T, Ikeda K et al (2008) Diffusion-weighted magnetic resonance imaging can be used in place of positron emission tomography for N staging of non-small cell lung cancer with fewer false-positive results. J Thorac Cardiovasc Surg 135(4):816–822

Ohba Y, Nomori H, Mori T et al (2009) Is diffusion-weighted magnetic resonance imaging superior to positron emission tomography with fludeoxyglucose F 18 in imaging non-small cell lung cancer? J Thorac Cardiovasc Surg 138(2):439–445

Ohno Y, Hatabu H, Takenaka D et al (2004) Metastases in mediastinal and hilar lymph nodes in patients with non-small cell lung cancer: quantitative and qualitative assessment with STIR turbo spin-echo MR imaging. Radiology 231(3): 872–879

Ohno Y, Koyama H, Onishi Y et al (2008) Non-small cell lung cancer: whole-body MR examination for M-stage assessment-utility for whole-body diffusion-weighted imaging compared with integrated FDG PET/CT. Radiology 248(2): 643–654

Ohno Y, Koyama H, Takenaka D et al (2008) Dynamic MRI, dynamic multidetector-row computed tomography (MDCT), and coregistered 2-[fluorine-18]-fluoro-2-deoxy-D-glucose-positron emission tomography (FDG-PET)/CT: comparative study of capability for management of pulmonary nodules. J Magn Reson Imaging 27(6):1284–1295

Okayama S, Uemura S, Saito Y (2009) Detection of infarct-related myocardial edema using cardiac diffusion-weighted magnetic resonance imaging. Int J Cardiol 133(1):20–21

Okuma T, Matsuoka T, Yamamoto A et al (2009) Assessment of early treatment response after CT-guided radiofrequency ablation of unresectable lung tumours by diffusion-weighted MRI: a pilot study. Br J Radiol 82(984):989–994

Qi LP, Zhang XP, Tang L et al (2009) Using diffusion-weighted MR imaging for tumor detection in the collapsed lung: a preliminary study. Eur Radiol 19(2):333–341

Razek AA, Elmorsy A, Elshafey M et al (2009) Assessment of mediastinal tumors with diffusion-weighted single-shot echo-planar MRIJ. Magn Reson Imaging 30:535–540

Razek AA, Elkammary S, Elmorsy AS et al (2011) Characterization of mediastinal lymphadenopathy with diffusion-weighted imaging. Magn Reson Imaging 29(2): 167–172

Razek AA, Fathy A, Gawad TA (2011) Correlation of apparent diffusion coefficient value with prognostic parameters of lung cancer. J Comput Assist Tomogr 35(2):248–252

Reese TG, Weisskoff RM, Smith RN et al (1995) Imaging myocardial fiber architecture in vivo with magnetic resonance. Magn Reson Med 34:786–791

Sakurada A, Takahaara T, Kwee TC et al (2009) Diagnostic performance of diffusion-weighted MRI in esophageal cancer. Eur Radiol 19:1461–1469

Satoh S, Kitazume Y, Ohdama S et al (2008) Can malignant and benign pulmonary nodules be differentiated with diffusion-weighted MRI? Am J Roentgenol 191(2):464–470

Sosnovik DE, Wang R, Dai G et al (2009) Diffusion MR tractography of the heart. J Cardiovasc Magn Reson 11:47–61

Takano A, Oriuchi N, Tsushima Y et al (2008) Detection of metastatic lesions from malignant pheochromocytoma and paraganglioma with diffusion-weighted magnetic resonance imaging: comparison with 18 F-FDG positron emission tomography and 123I-MIBG scintigraphy. Ann Nucl Med 22(5):395–401

Tanaka R, Horikoshi H, Nakazato Y et al (2009) Magnetic resonance imaging in peripheral lung adenocarcinoma: correlation with histopathologic features. J Thorac Imaging 24(1):4–9

Turner R, Le Bihan D, Maier J et al (1990) Echo-planar imaging of intravoxel incoherent motion. Radiology 177(2):407–414

Uto T, Takehara Y, Nakamura Y et al (2009) Higher sensitivity and specificity for diffusion-weighted imaging of malignant lung lesions without apparent diffusion coefficient quantification. Radiology 252(1):247–254

Van Beek EJ, Wild JM, Kauczor HU et al (2004) Functional MRI of the lung using hyperpolarized 3-helium gas. J Magn Reson Imaging 20:540–554

Wahidi MM, Govert JA, Goudar RK et al (2007) Evidence for the treatment of patients with pulmonary nodules: when is it lung cancer?: ACCP evidence-based clinical practice guidelines (2nd edition). Chest 132(3 Suppl):94S–107S

Wang C, Altes TA, Mugler JP et al (2008) Assessment of the lung microstructure in patients with asthma using hyperpolarized 3He diffusion MRI at two time scales: comparison with healthy subjects and patients with COPD. J Magn Reson Imaging 28(1):80–88

Wu MT, Tseng WY, Su MY et al (2006) Diffusion tensor magnetic resonance imaging mapping the fiber architecture remodeling in human myocardium after infarction: correlation with viability and wall motion. Circulation 114(10): 1036–1045

Wu MT, Su MY, Huang YL et al (2009) Sequential changes of myocardial microstructure in patients postmyocardial infarction by diffusion-tensor cardiac MR: correlation with left ventricular structure and function. Circ Cardiovasc Imaging 2(1):32–40

Zhou R, Yu T, Feng C et al (2011) Diffusion-weighted imaging for assessment of lung cancer response to chemotherapy. Zhongguo Fei Ai Za Zhi 14(3):256–260

14 Role of DWI in the Evaluation of Tumors of the Head and Neck and in the Assessment of Lymph Nodes

Inmaculada Rodriguez, Teodoro Martín, and Antonio Luna

14.1 DWI in Head and Neck Regions

14.1.1 Technical Aspects and Field-Strength

Since the advent of the EPI sequences for evaluating the rate of microscopic water diffusion in tissues, DWI has been used to evaluate many different processes in brain. Its most known application has been the early diagnosis and management of cerebral ischemia, but its utility in white matter disorders or others brain diseases, especially the differentiation of the brain tumors according to their rate of cellularity, has also been extensively reported. Brain tumors have shown a clear inverse relationship between ADC values and cellular density. Therefore, it is suggested that a greater presence of cells within tumors is associated with a more restricted diffusivity. Therefore, ADCs are expected to vary according to the microstructures of tissues or pathologic states.

Ultimately, DWI and ADC measurements are being considered as potentially useful in the evaluation and characterization of head and neck extracranial lesions (Fig. 14.1). Although initial technical difficulties to warrant good quality DWI images of the head and neck regions have limited its clinical application, recent technical improvements allow to surpass the susceptibility artifacts in this area, which are prone to occur during EPI-DWI acquisitions, particularly in the neck. The presence of dental fillings with metallic materials, the air-bone-soft tissue interfaces, involuntary or deglutition motions and physiologic vascular pulsation cause susceptibility-related image distortions and difficulties with these techniques. According to some investigators, up to one third of all the cases showed susceptibility artifacts using EPI-DWI. The use of SS-EPI sequences with parallel imaging or navigator-eco may improve these results. Nyquist's artifact is also frequent in EPI-DWI in the head and neck regions. In this artifact, image ghosts appear in half the FOV in the phase-encoding directions, which can be reduced by using a pre-scan calibration with the phase-encoding gradient turned off.

Other approaches, such as line-scan DWI, have shown very good results as they are insensitive to susceptibility artifacts. Other DWI techniques insensitive to artifacts, such as split acquisition of fast spin-echo signals (SPLICE) and fast asymmetric SE (FASE), have been explored, although with scarce clinical experience. DWIBS may also be used in the head and neck regions, although it suffers from important anteroposterior distortion and the ADC values obtained with this technique are lower than with conventional EPI-DWI. In order to reduce motion artifact, it is interesting to reduce acquisition time as much as possible, with a maximum scan time of 5 mins as a good reference. The DWI-PROPELLER acquisition reduces motion-related artifact, as it benefits from a modified radial acquisition scheme with rotating parallel lines, which inherently oversamples the k-space center and can be used to

I. Rodriguez (✉) and T. Martín
Neuroradiology Section, Clínica Las Nieves, SERCOSA, Health Time Group, Jaén, Spain
e-mail: i.rodriguez.o@htime.org; t.martin.f@htime.org

A. Luna
Chief of MRI, Health Time Group, Jaén, Spain
e-mail: aluna70@sercosa.com

A. Luna et al., *Diffusion MRI Outside the Brain*,
DOI 10.1007/978-3-642-21052-5_14, © Springer-Verlag Berlin Heidelberg 2012

correct in-plane motion. This approach is also insensitive to susceptibility artifacts and hemorrhage and offers better conspicuity for lesions located at the air–tissue interface, although it has limited SNR and requires longer acquisition times. The acquisition of the DWI in sagittal orientation has been proposed to diminish the vascular pulsation artifact of large vessels.

These shortcomings are even more pronounced at 3T, as distortion and field inhomogeneity at tissue boundaries increases compared to 1.5T. Conversely, the increase in field-strength allows for a better SNR (Fig. 14.2). It is also necessary to take into account that ADC values could vary at 3 T compared to 1.5 T, although the association between increased cellularity, malignancy with low ADC is similar for both types of magnets. However, more DWI studies comparing the ADC values at different field strengths from the head and neck regions are necessary.

In general, the acquisition of several *b* values is recommended to improve image quality, minimize the noise, and diminish movement artifacts. A high *b* value between 800 and1,000 s/mm^2 has been the most used in scientific literature. We usually perform a SS EPI sequence with SPIR with 5 *b* values between 0 and 1,000 s/mm^2. The differentiation between true diffusion from perfusion may be accomplished in the head and neck regions using an IVIM sequence, and analyzing the bicompartmental scheme of the diffusion (Fig. 14.2). There is scarce clinical experience exploring the potential advantages of this approach, which has shown advantages in other regions, such as the liver.

14.1.2 Characterization of Benign and Malignant Tumors

As conventional MRI is often nonspecific for the distinction between most tumors in the head and neck, the application of DWI in this task is promising. DWI has shown to be a reliable tool to distinguish malignant from benign lesions and normal tissues, using either at 1.5T or 3T magnets, with proposed threshold ADC values of 1.22 and 1.30×10^{-3} mm^2/s, respectively (Figs. 14.2–14.7). It has also been well documented the usefulness of the ADC value in the differentiation of squamous cell carcinoma (SCC), the most common tumor of the head and neck (Fig. 14.2), from lymphoma, as it is also frequent in this region (Fig. 16.8). Mean ADC of malignant lymphomas is also significantly lower than that of SCC. Differentiation between the different subtypes of SCC is possible using ADC measurements, as highly or moderately differentiated SCCs tend to show higher ADC values than those of poorly differentiated SCCs. This difference has been related to a more abundant macromolecular protein content along with hypercellularity and a higher nuclear: cytoplasmic ratio associated with poorly differentiated SCC and the presence of a high degree of small foci of liquefactive necrosis in well-differentiated SCC. Histologically, lymphomas tend to have more cellularity, larger nuclei with more abundant macromolecular proteins, and less extracellular space than well or moderately differentiated SCC. The distinction between lymphomas and very poorly differentiated carcinomas on the basis of ADC value is more challenging, with contradictory results in the literature. Non-Hodgkin lymphoma shows lower ADC values than Hodgkin subtype, which may show overlap with SCC. Besides, DWI has been able to differentiate using ADC measurements lymphoma from carcinoma in the cavernous sinus.

In a similar manner to contrast enhanced-perfusion MRI, DWI is able to distinguish between the viable and necrotic portions of head and neck tumors (Fig. 14.5). Razek et al. reported that the mean ADC value of viable tumors was significantly lower than that of necrotic portions. This could be useful to choose the biopsy site in the more cellular areas of a tumor. There is controversy about if the presence of micronecrosis within a tumor may vary its ADC value, as it seems to be difficult for DWI and ADC maps to be able to detect areas of microscopic necrosis which are smaller than the used voxel size. The application of the bicompartmental model of the diffusion gives the chance to estimate the tumoral perfusion without using contrast (Fig. 14.2).

As in the brain, abscesses in the head and neck regions usually show restricted diffusion due to their viscous content (Fig. 14.6). However, abscesses and necrotic lymphadenitis are commonly hyperintense on DWI with high *b* values and tumoral necrosis or metastatic nodal necrosis are usually hypointense with higher ADC values. Therefore, DWI helps in their differentiation.

DWI is especially indicated for characterizing lesions in children avoiding the use of contrast. During childhood, there is a high incidence of congenital lesions and cysts which should be distinguished from malignant tumors that are often very aggressive at these ages. Epidermal cysts typically associate restricted diffusion and low ADC values due to their keratinous content. These lesions are frequently found in head and neck regions during the first decade of life. Fewer differences in ADC values among cystic lesions are caused by protein component variations in the fluid and the changes in the viscosity of the contents.

14.1.3 Salivary Gland Tumors

Although salivary gland tumors are uncommon, their accurate presurgical assessment is crucial as there are different therapeutic options which differ even in cases of benign tumors. These differences are more evident for the more frequent parotid gland tumors. Besides, controversy remains in the value of pretreatment CT, MRI and fine needle aspiration cytology. Although there is limited experience with DWI of tumors of the major salivary glands, the results are contradictory, and the presurgical characterization of different histological subtypes or the differentiation between benign and malignant lesions is not possible according to the reported data. There is a clear trend for pleomorphic adenomas to show high ADC values and for Warthin tumor to show low ADC values. This is probably due to their different histologic origin, as pleomorphic adenomas show a heterogeneous composition of epithelial, myoepithelial, and stromal cells with areas of fluid within the epithelial glandular areas, and Warthin tumors have a lymphoid origin. Furthermore, acinic cell carcinoma of the parotid gland shows intermediate ADC values between pleomorphic adenomas and Warthin tumors, because they are hypercellular lesions but commonly less than Warthin tumors (Fig. 14.7). Lymphoma of major salivary glands usually demonstrates very low ADC value. Yabuuchi et al. recently demonstrated the usefulness of the addition of ADC value to dynamic contrast-enhanced MRI in the characterization of parotid tumors. For example, in several series, the mean ADC values varied as follows: pleomorphic adenoma between 1.5 and 2×10^{-3} mm^2/s; Warthin tumor between 0.7 and 1.1×10^{-3} mm^2/s; carcinoma between 1 and 1.4×10^{-3} mm^2/s; and malignant lymphoma $0.7–0.9 \times 10^{-3}$ mm^2/s. Adenoid cystic carcinoma tends to show the higher ADC values among all the malignant carcinomas of parotid gland, which may overlap the values of pleomorphic adenoma.

14.1.4 Monitoring and Predicting Response to Treatment

In the era of personalized treatment, the imaging monitorization of treated head and neck cancer is critical. The early assessment of lack of response to chemoradiation will allow us to select candidates for salvage surgery before fibrous-inflammatory changes occur, limiting the chances of a successful outcome. Primary tumors with lower ADC values have been linked to complete response after chemoradiation (Fig. 14.8). Furthermore, significant increase in ADC values as early as 1 week after the beginning of therapy has been related to complete response. These high ADC values remain until the end of treatment. The relation between the observed ADC changes and the underlying pathophysiological processes is not clear. More cellular tumors, with lower ADC values, probably show a better response to radiation therapy due to less hypoxia, which is one of the major causes of radio-resistance (Fig. 14.8). Furthermore, tumors with higher pretreatment blood supplies will allow elevated oxygenation and accessibility to cytotoxic drugs, which allow increased necrosis and apoptosis to occur after treatment.

In a recent series by Vandecaveye et al., early ADC measurements performed 2 and 4 weeks after chemoradiation allowed a more accurate response prediction than volume calculation with anatomical MRI in patients with SCC followed up during 2 years. The increase in ADC values in tumors showing complete local response was significantly higher than in recurrences. In this series, the positive predictive value of the ADC increase of lymph nodes was lower for the measurements performed 2 weeks than the ones performed 4 weeks after the start of treatment. This was related to absorption of necrosis in a number of responding adenopathies, which caused an initial decrease in ADC, falsely suggesting a poor response. The authors stated that adenopathies may be preferably evaluated at a later time point during chemoradiation compared with primary tumors. Furthermore, the induction of extensive necrosis soon after chemoradiation on primary tumors was the cause of a false-positive result, falsely showing an increase of ADC value despite the presence of recurrent tumor in this series.

In all these series, mean ADC was the parametric used. As previously discussed in Chap. 3, lesional heterogeneity may not be correctly assessed with mean ADC. Probably more sophisticated means of mapping diffusivity changes, such as parametric ADC map or histogram analysis, will better reflect the different diffusion properties of a lesion, which are intimately ligated to their histological composition. Furthermore, these new approaches may better correlate with tumor response and patient survival, limiting the mentioned interpretation errors in the series by Vandecaveye et al.

14.1.5 Detection of Recurrence

Treatment of head and neck malignancies usually is multidisciplinary, including multi-fractioned radiotherapy, induction chemotherapy, chemoradiation, molecular targeted immunotherapy or even surgery. Follow-up imaging after treatment, especially after radiotherapy, of head and neck tumors is classically challenging due to loss of tissue planes, edema, and fibrous-inflammatory reaction with delayed scar formation (Fig. 14.8). The early depiction of recurrence, which usually occurs near the location of the primary tumor, is important to tailor the salvage treatment increasing the chances of a positive outcome (Fig. 14.5).

CT and MRI are limited in the distinction between irradiation effects and recurrent tumor. FDG PET-CT improves their results, mainly in the 4–6 months after radiation therapy, due to false-positive results related to inflammatory changes. In this scenario, DWI is a very useful and promising tool, as it has been able to make this distinction with a sensitivity, specificity, and accuracy of about 95% in several series. Furthermore, DWI can accurately detect early recurrence after radiation therapy due to its insensitivity to edema and fibrous-inflammatory reaction (Figs. 14.5 and 14.7). Besides, DWI has demonstrated less false positives than FDG PET-CT. Recurrent tumor or nodal disease show low ADC values compared to the high ones of posttherapeutic changes. DWI is reported to be especially useful in the differentiation between persistently enlarged inflammatory and tumoral lymph nodes with equivocal findings on CT, conventional MRI, or FDG-PET (Figs. 14.5 and 14.8).

14.2 Evaluation of Lymph Nodes With DWI

14.2.1 Evaluation of Cervical Lymph Nodes

Staging of head and neck malignancies is critical for therapeutic management. PET-CT is the gold standard in the characterization of cervical lymph nodes, although small lymph nodes may be lost with this technique which has limitations in the differentiation between inflammatory and metastatic lymphadenopathy. The ADC values of metastatic lymph nodes are significantly lower than benign ones (Fig. 14.9). In several series, DWI has been able to accurately distinguish between benign and malignant lymph nodes in the head and neck using ADC thresholds between 0.9 and 1.36×10^{-3} mm^2/s. In normal size lymph nodes, the lower the ADC value, the greater the chances to be metastatic in origin. This affirmation has demonstrated to be true even in lymph nodes between 4 and 9 mm. Only one series reported higher ADC in metastatic lymph nodes than in benign lymphadenopathy, probably due to the inclusion of necrotic regions in the ADC measurements. Besides, DWI increases the detection of small lymph nodes compared to morphological MRI sequences and other cross-sectional techniques, including PET-CT. The lymph node characterization is improved combining the ADC measurements with conventional MRI information, such as size, border irregularity, and degree of homogeneity for signal intensity on fat-suppressed T2-weighted images. Improvements in SNR, spatial resolution, and free artifact DWI acquisitions leave room for improvement in this task. To reduce partial volume effect and ADC reproducibility, some authors have proposed to use a high-resolution one-slice DWI acquisition in the area where the suspicious lymph nodes are located. In conclusion, DWI is probably the best imaging technique for nodal staging in the head and neck regions, and is able to accurately differentiate benign and malignant lymph nodes. Therefore, it enables a better therapeutic management of head and neck malignancies.

Potential pitfalls in the ADC measurements of lymph nodes are the presence of areas of necrosis or a fatty hilus. Although a fatty hilus is consider a criterion of benignity, as the fat shows very low ADC values, its inclusion in the ADC analysis may lower the mean ADC of a lymph node. In order to avoid this potential false-positive result, it is recommended to use DWI sequences with fat suppression. The presence of necrosis is very common in metastatic lymph nodes of SCC, and it may occur in lymphoma nodes in around a 25% of the cases. In lymphoma nodes, the nodal necrosis is secondary to apoptosis and not to death of tumor cells as in SCC metastatic nodes. As a general rule, it is recommended to exclude necrotic areas from ADC analysis to avoid a false increase in mean ADC (Fig. 14.5). Therefore, areas of high signal in ADC maps should be excluded of the ROI, which standard deviation should be reviewed in order to avoid ROIs with heterogeneous content, very probably due to necrosis. In the same way, a recent series has demonstrated that in nodes with necrosis, the well-known differences in ADC values between lymphoma and SCC were not achieved. Besides, the nodal necrosis in the lymphoma nodes showed significantly lower ADC values than SCC ones. The authors applied different ADC criteria for nodes with and without necrosis (threshold ADC values of 0.6×10^{-3} mm^2/s for entire nodes and 1.450×10^{-3} mm^2/s for focal defects), to significantly improve the diagnostic accuracy.

Inflammatory lymphadenopathy has demonstrated higher ADC values than malignant ones in several series, with mean ADC values around 1.7×10^{-3} mm^2/s. However, granulomatous disease such as sarcoidosis and Cat–scratch disease may show ADC values resembling malignancy. Nodal reactivity usually appears close to nodal metastases, which limits its clinical impact. Anyhow, caution is necessary as they may show ADC values similar to metastatic lymph nodes, due to their composition of a homogenous lymphoid infiltration, organized in a multitude of germinal centers, and the presence of fibrous stroma. The presence of a fatty hilus and other morphological signs of benignity may help in their distinction from nodal metastases.

Another lesion which usually shows low ADC values is parathyroid hyperplasia, due to its high proportion of glandular cells. Typical location enables its differentiation from lymph nodes.

14.2.2 DWI of Lymph Nodes in Chest, Abdomen, and Pelvis

As described above for head and neck neoplasm, the importance of nodal involvement in the diagnostic and evaluation of cancers of other body regions is well known because it is one of the most significant risk factors for local recurrence in the majority of tumors. Furthermore, characterization and differentiation between benign and malignant lymph nodes is critical for therapeutic management, mainly in candidates for chemoradiation. Posttreatment monitorization and prediction of response to treatment are the more challenging tasks for imaging in treated metastatic lymph nodes.

CT and MRI are usually the elective techniques in the nodal detection and characterization in the routine clinical practice. Both modalities are noninvasive, reproducible, and share the same morphological criteria in differentiating benign from malignant nodes, such as nodal size, shape, site, outline, density, or signal intensity. However, it is well documented that CT is more accurate in the detection of nodal calcifications, while MRI has the additional ability to assess nodal signal intensity, which in metastatic adenopathy commonly present similar features than those of the primary tumor. The addition of dynamic contrast-enhanced sequences has increased the sensibility and specificity in the characterization of malignant lymph nodes, although both of them remain low. Until the definitive approval for clinical use of the promising Ultrasmall Particles of Iron Oxide (USPIO), FDG PET-CT remains as the gold standard for pre- and post-treatment nodal assessment, although known limitations are a high false-positive rate due to concurrent lymphadenitis and problems to detect small metastatic lymph nodes.

In the last years, DWI has demonstrated its ability to detect even milimetric lymph nodes in all body regions (Fig. 14.10). Detection of small lymph nodes in the pelvis increases using fusion of DWI and T2-weighted sequence. The advantages of 3T for the detection of small lymph nodes have still to be fully explored. Furthermore, DWI has been tested in the differentiation between benign and malignant lymph nodes. Promising results using ADC measurements have been obtained for prostate, colorectal carcinoma and uterine cervical cancers (Figs. 8.6, 9.1 and 12.2). In all these series, metastatic lymph nodes demonstrated lower ADC values than benign ones, although with a great variability in the ADC values depending on the primary tumor and used DWI sequence. Anyhow, taking into consideration that the lymph nodes, benign and malignant, show bright signal with high *b* value, may present susceptibility artifacts or necrosis, or be very small or heterogeneous, their characterization based only on ADC measurements may be challenging. Some researchers have proposed to compare the ADC value and signal on DWI of the primary tumor and lymph nodes. Relative ADC values of metastatic lymph nodes compared to primary cervical and uterine tumors have been a useful tool for detection of nodal metastases.

In the upper abdomen, DWI also increases the detection of small lymph nodes, although there is scarce experience about characterization with ADC measurements. In this region, the respiratory motion, the peristalsis, and the presence of more artifacts and gastrointestinal tract are limiting factors, although in our experience, current

DWI-EPI sequences allow for accurate detection of lymph nodes (Figs. 11.2, 11.3 and 11.5).

Recent series have claimed a role for DWI in the characterization of mediastinal lymphadenopathy. Furthermore, Razek et al. propose a threshold ADC value of 1.85×10^{-3} mm^2/s for differentiating malignant nodes from benign ones. Pauls and colleagues compared DWI to PET-CT for N-staging of lung cancer. They found a moderately correlation between both techniques with a tendency for understaging with DWI.

With regard to lymphoma, WB-DWI has been compared to PET-CT for staging with excellent results. In a recent series, Kwee and colleagues demonstrated a significant difference in ADC values between lymphomatous lymph nodes and normal lymph with a sensitivity and specificity of 78.1% and 100%, respectively when using an optimal cutoff ADC value of 0.80. Besides, DWI also allows assessment of response to treatment in a similar manner to PET-CT, with increase of ADC values in responders (Fig. 16.8).

Case 14.1: Intraorbital Metastasis from Retroperitoneal Leiomyosarcoma

A 48-year-old female was submitted to surgery few years ago to remove a retroperitoneal leiomyosarcoma, which was in complete response. Now, she presented diplopia, vision loss, and suspected palsy of the left third cranial nerve. MRI was performed for further evaluation.

Comments

In the orbit, special difficulties to discriminate among different orbital masses are common in clinical and imaging diagnosis. There is typically clinical, radiological, and pathologic overlap among the most common lesions, such as lymphoma, inflammatory pseudotumor, atypical lymphocytic infiltrate, and metastases. Orbital metastases are uncommon, and when they are present, the patients often have a previous history of breast or lung primary tumors. In patients with sarcomas, metastases usually occurred to the skin and soft tissue and even in the lungs, but distant metastases are very rare, especially in the orbit. Therefore, as shown in this case, it is challenging to decide whether a little intraorbital mass is actually a metastasis.

MRI is clearly superior to CT for characterizing intraorbital metastases. CT can be better to evaluate bone or to detect calcifications. MRI is the elective technique for tumors without osseous invasion. It is preferred to CT for determining inflammation or compression of the optic nerve and extrinsic muscles or for evaluating eyeball structures.

There are limited reports of the DWI in the orbits, but several case series and case reports have shown feasibility and utility of DWI in evaluating orbital masses and optic nerve infarcts. The ADC values and DWI show a trend to higher accuracy than conventional MRI protocols alone for discriminating among benign and malignant orbital lesions. If the lesion is hypercellular, ADC is usually low, although some metastases may be relatively hypocellular and associated with significant surrounding edema.

By now, DWI and ADC measurements are challenging in the orbit, with clinical usefulness restricted to huge masses, as technical improvements are necessary for them to be applicable and reproducible techniques for the evaluation of small orbital lesions.

Imaging Findings

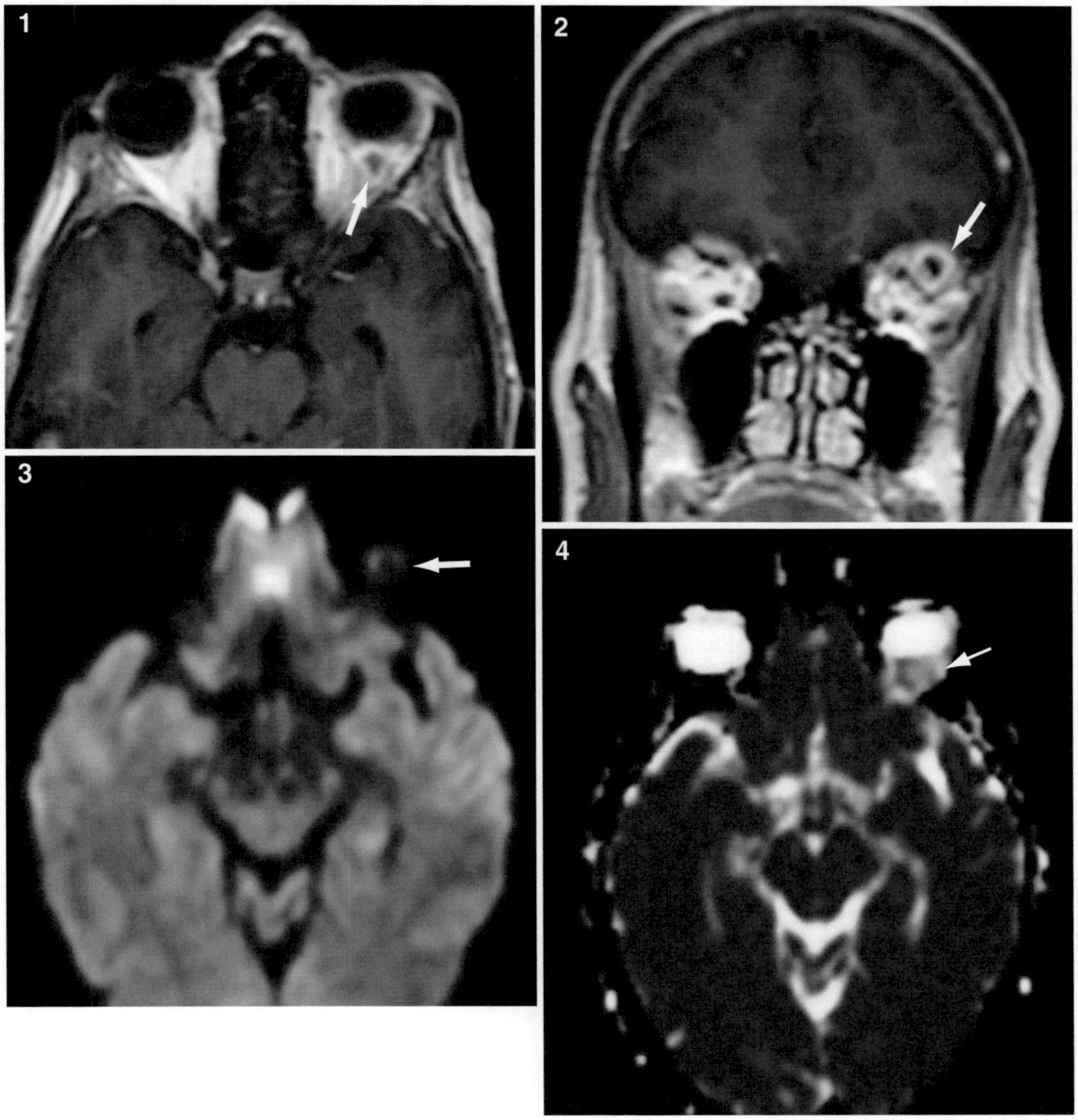

Fig. 14.1 **14.1.1**, **14.1.2** Transverse and coronal contrast-enhanced TSE T1-weighted images of the orbits show a left intraorbital nodule in the intraconal space. It shows posterior scleral invasion and it may not be adequately separated from the optic nerve and superior rectus muscle. The lesions shows a ring-like pattern of enhancement with central hypointensity (*arrows*). This appearance was not specific, as many masses in the orbit may have similar presentation, even an abscess. **14.1.3**, **14.1.4** DWI with a *b* value of 1,000 s/mm^2 and ADC map show a marked restriction of the lesion (*arrows*) that suggests hypercellularity and malignancy. Posterior surgical removal confirmed a metastasis from a retroperitoneal leiomyosarcoma

Case 14.2: Oropharynx Cancer with Nodal Metastases

A 68-year-old female with oropharyngeal dysphagia. She had difficulty swallowing and speaking and demonstrated swelling of left neck region. On laryngoscopy, a swollen area and partial obliteration of the left pyriform sinus was visualized. MRI was performed for further characterization. A posterior biopsy revealed a SCC.

Comments

Cancer of the oropharynx is expected to occur in approximately 4,000 persons per year in occidental countries. It is seen in men five to eight times more often than in women, with a peak incidence between sixth and eighth decades. Main risk factors include smoking and alcohol habits.

Base of the tongue tumors is less frequent than others and the most frequent histopathology is that of SCC. These cancers are the predominant primary extracranial head and neck malignancy in adults and have a high propensity to spread to adjacent lymph nodes, as shown in this case.

Tumors in the oral cavity and oropharynx differ in presentation and prognosis. The accurate definition of the local spread of tumor is crucial for the T-staging, as it defines the type of treatment. As the pattern of spread can be different, and for the necessity of correct N-staging before treatment planning, the imaging study is mandatory. MR and, to a lesser extent, CT and F-18 FDG PET-CT are the imaging modalities of choice for pretherapeutic workup of these lesions. Imaging protocols should be simple and reproducible, and should provide the key elements for treatment planning. Recently, DWI has incorporated oncological MRI protocols of head and neck regions. It allows an estimation of tissue cellularity and characterization of the origin of tumor according to ADC values. Bicompartmental analysis of DWI has been demonstrated to be feasible in brain, liver, pancreas, and muscle. Its performance in the head and neck region permits to estimate the tumoral perfusion without using contrast and a more realistic estimation of the tumoral diffusion, avoiding the perfusion effects.

Imaging Findings

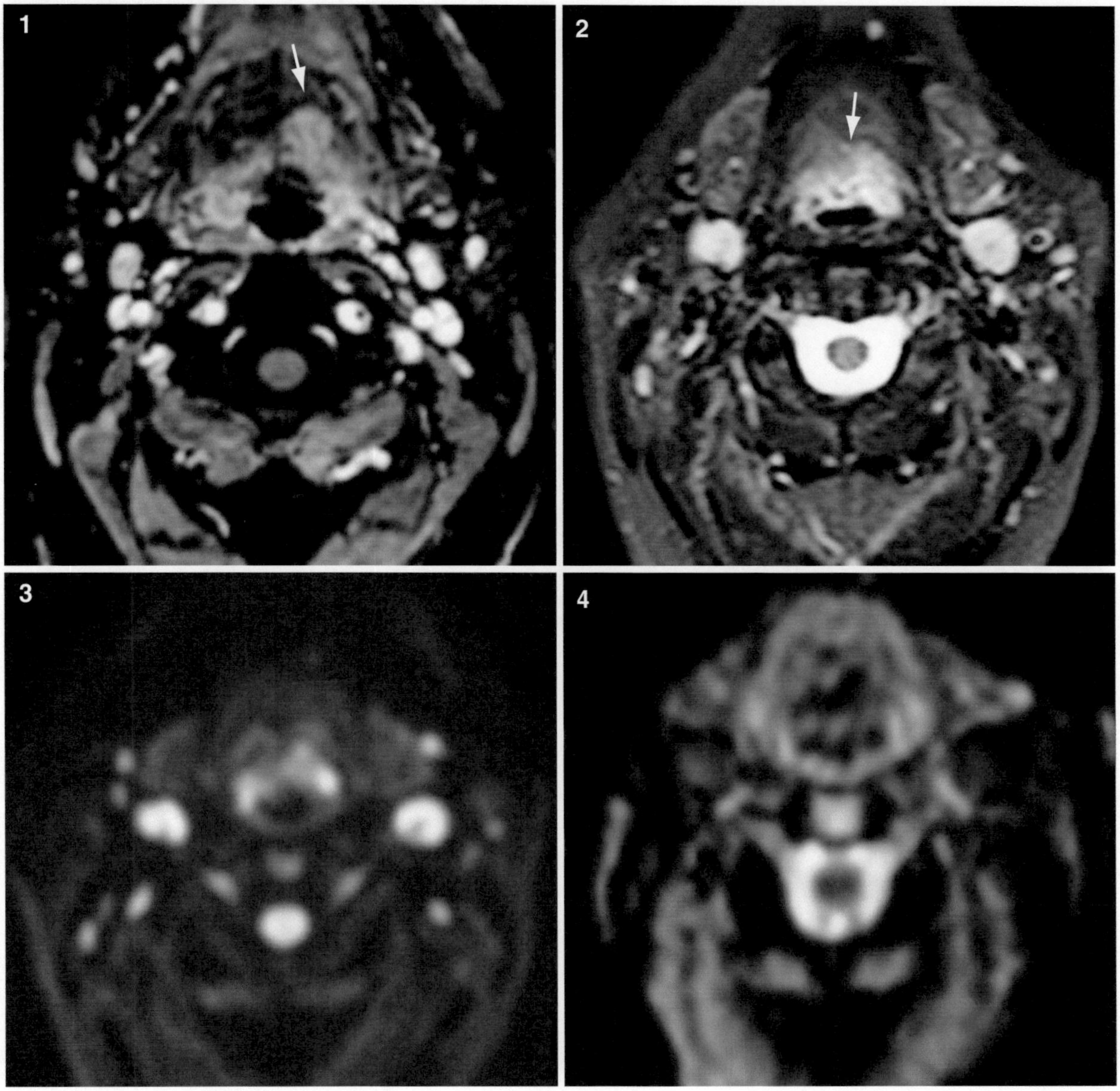

Fig. 14.2 **14.2.1, 14.2.2** Axial postcontrast THRIVE and STIR sequences confirmed an oropharynx mass (*vertical arrows*) that extended both to hypopharynx and left pyriform sinus. **14.2.3, 14.2.4** DWI with a *b* value of 1,000 s/mm^2 and ADC map in transverse plane show restriction of the mass consistent with malignancy. **14.2.5** Coronal MIP of DWI with a *b* value of 1,000 s/mm^2 with inverted gray scale enables the visualization of a left lymphadenopathy at II level, which also demonstrated restriction favoring a metastatic origin (*arrow*). **14.2.6, 14.2.7** A biexponential model of signal decay of the diffusion at a 3T magnet was used to obtain parametric maps of D (diffusion without perfusion, contamination) and perfusion fraction, respectively. **14.2.8** The signal decay of the diffusion of the mass is shown in the graph (x-axis represents the *b* values and y-axis the signal intensity). Notice the great difference between ADC (0.96×10^{-3} mm^2/s) and D (0.5×10^{-3} mm^2/s) values due to the effect of the mass perfusion. The perfusion fraction of the mass was high (35%), and it was estimated using only the signal decay of the diffusion for *b* values lower than 100 s/mm^2

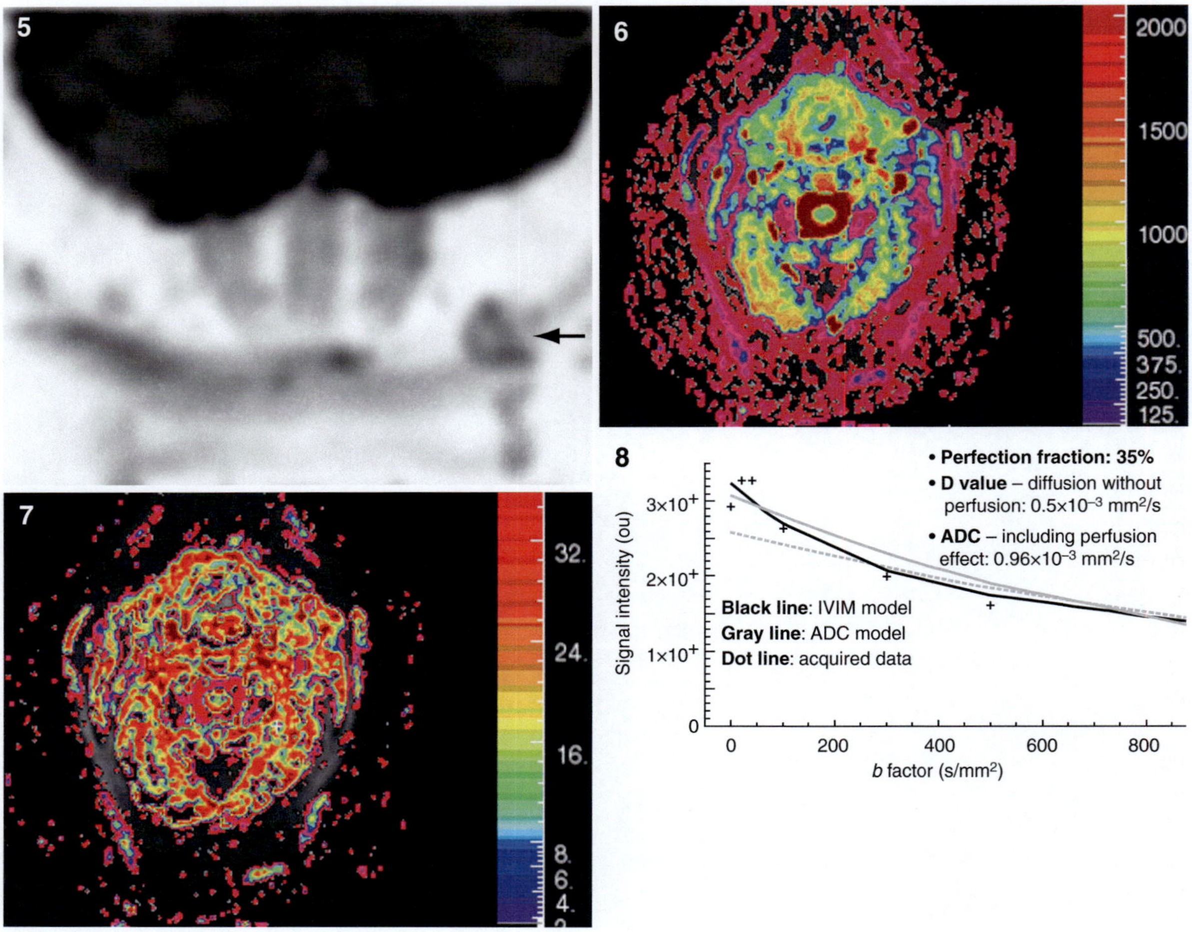

Fig. 14.2 (continued)

Case 14.3: Superficial Giant Neurofibroma

A 67-year-old female presented a huge palpable and asymmetric mass on the left side of the head and neck regions. A diagnosis of combined superficial and deep neurofibroma was established some years ago. She was submitted for a new MRI under the suspicion of lesional growth and malignant degeneration. MRI findings, posterior biopsy, and 2 year of imaging follow-up excluded a malignant nerve sheath tumor (MNST).

Comments

Neurofibromas are benign tumors that arise from connective tissue of nerve sheaths, especially the endoneurium. Plexiform types are composed of the same cell types as dermal ones, but have an expanded extracellular matrix. They may grow along the length of a nerve, involving multiple fascicles and branches, and extend into surrounding structures.

The highest incidence of neurofibromas occurs in patients with Neurofibromatosis type 1(NF-1). In this association, the neurofibromas are usually of the plexiform subtype, which often involve nerve plexi, thoracic nerve roots, and other structures deep in relation to the muscle fascia. They rarely have any evident superficial extension, as these lesions follow the course of major nerves. In occasions, neurofibromas occur superficially, in a cutaneous or subcutaneous location. In these cases, they can arise from peripheral nerves or to correspond to a superficial extension of a deeper plexiform neurofibroma.

Mautner VF et al. distinguish three growth patterns in these tumors: superficial, displacing, and invasive. The majority of invasive neurofibromas were found in the face and head and neck regions, causing functional deficits and disfigurement. The lifetime risk of developing malignant peripheral nerve sheath tumors from a benign plexiform neurofibromas is about 10%. Consecutive MRI studies are indicated, and even whole-body MRI has been proposed to monitor and calculate the total burden of neurofibromas in patients with NF1.

DWI and ADC values have demonstrated differences between benign and malignant lesion in the head and neck, with higher values of ADCs in benign lesion, although with some exceptions. Besides, morphological MRI is nonspecific in the differentiation between MNST and benign neurofibroma. Conversely, in a recent case report, DWI has proved to be able to differentiate between the malignant and benign regions of a retroperitoneal MNST. This suggests that the addition of DWI to routine MRI protocols may increase the accuracy in this distinction, although this must be confirmed in larger series.

Imaging Findings

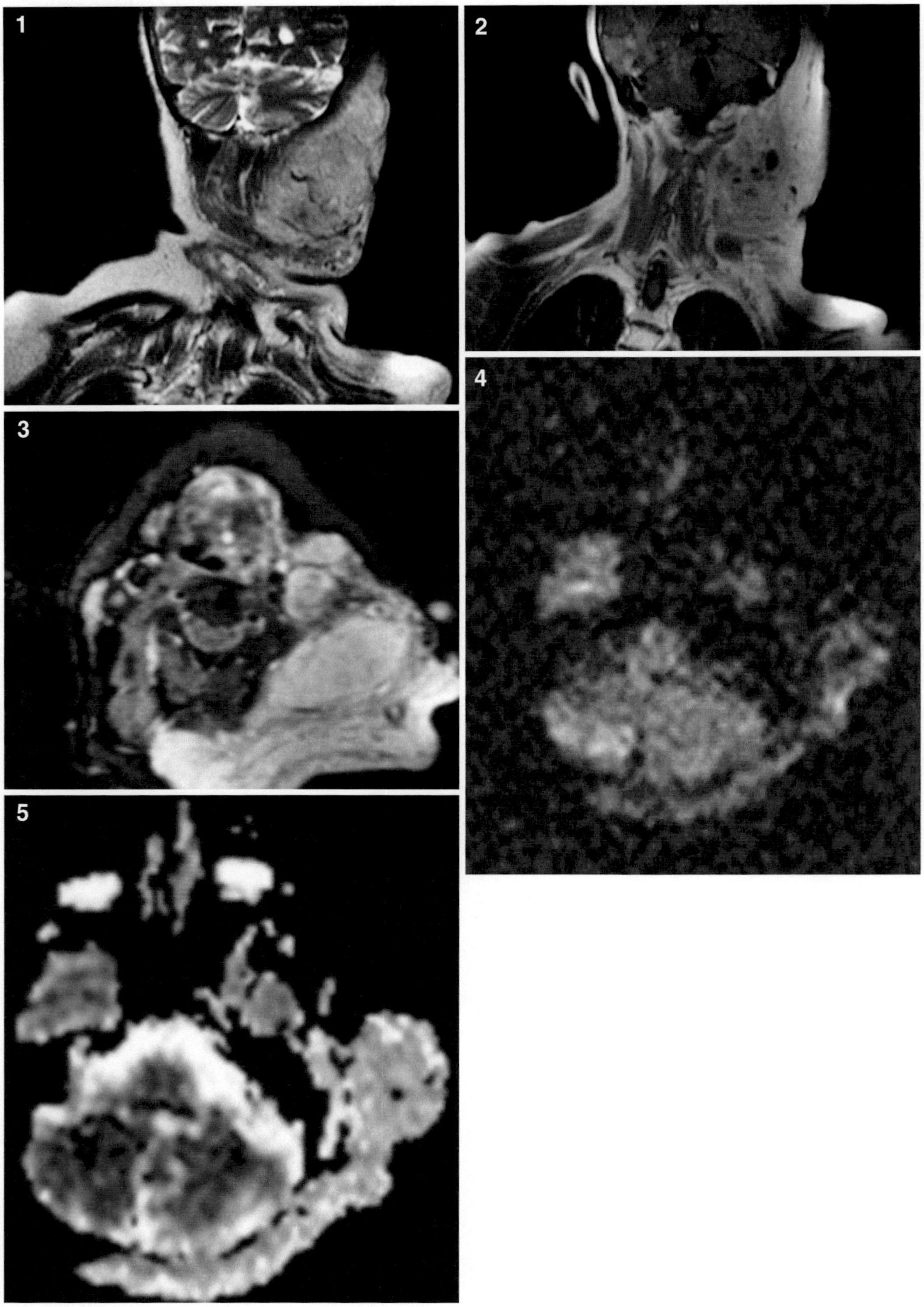

Fig. 14.3 **14.3.1–14.3.3** Coronal TSE T2-weighted, coronal post-contrast T1-weighted and transverse STIR images demonstrate a huge superficial and subcutaneous lesion, poorly delineated, with typical hyperintensity of neural tumors on T2-w and STIR sequences. The lesion shows a diffuse growing pattern on the left side of the head and neck regions with an intense and heterogeneous enhancement. It is not possible to definitively exclude malignancy. **14.3.4**, **14.3.5** DWI with a *b* value of 1,000 s/mm^2 and ADC map do not show intralesional restriction of the diffusion, excluding hypercellular areas. The mean ADC of the lesion was 1.9×10^{-3} mm^2/s

Case 14.4: Cervical Esophageal Cancer

A 71-year-old malnourished male with progressive dysphasia and normal laryngoscopy. A MRI was performed for further assessment and to rule out a mass.

Comments

The increase in incidence of esophageal cancer reflects a marked increase of adenocarcinoma. It is a leading cause of cancer mortality worldwide. Proximal esophageal cancer is usually diagnosed at an advanced stage, and the treatment is often limited to palliation. Surgery offers the best relief of dysphagia but it remains controversial, because a complete cure is unlikely even at the expense of laryngeal mutilation.

Classical techniques, like single or double contrast barium swallow, are still useful for identifying mucosal lesions, although they can provide little information about the depth of tumoral invasion in this area. Accurate preoperative staging and assessment of therapeutic response after neoadjuvant therapy are crucial. CT provides better delineation of tumor penetration through the esophageal wall and can identify invasion mainly into the tracheobronchial tree or aorta. However, CT is poor in predicting local invasion in malnourished or thin individuals, without fat planes. MRI is moderately useful in defining the extent of the primary tumor. The accurate definition of local peri-esophageal invasion is important for prognosis and therapeutic management. Tumors with evidence of aortic or tracheobronchial invasion on MRI or CT are considered to be unresectable. MRI benefits from a high sensitivity, although some false-positive findings have been described. There is scarce experience with DWI in esophageal cancer. The detection of the primary tumor, especially early tumors, is problematic. The rates of node metastasis were not optimal in a series by Sakurada and colleagues, with an average patient-based sensitivity and specificity of 77.8% and 55.6%, respectively.

The uses of neoadjuvant chemotherapy and radiation therapy are becoming widespread among patients with advanced stages. Response should be assessed as earlier as possible in the course of therapy. In this issue, MRI including DWI is finding an increasing role. Recently, DWIBS has shown similar potential than 18 F-FDG-PET for detecting postoperative recurrent squamous cell esophageal cancer and nodal metastases. Both recurrent tumors and nodal metastases showed low ADC values.

Imaging Findings

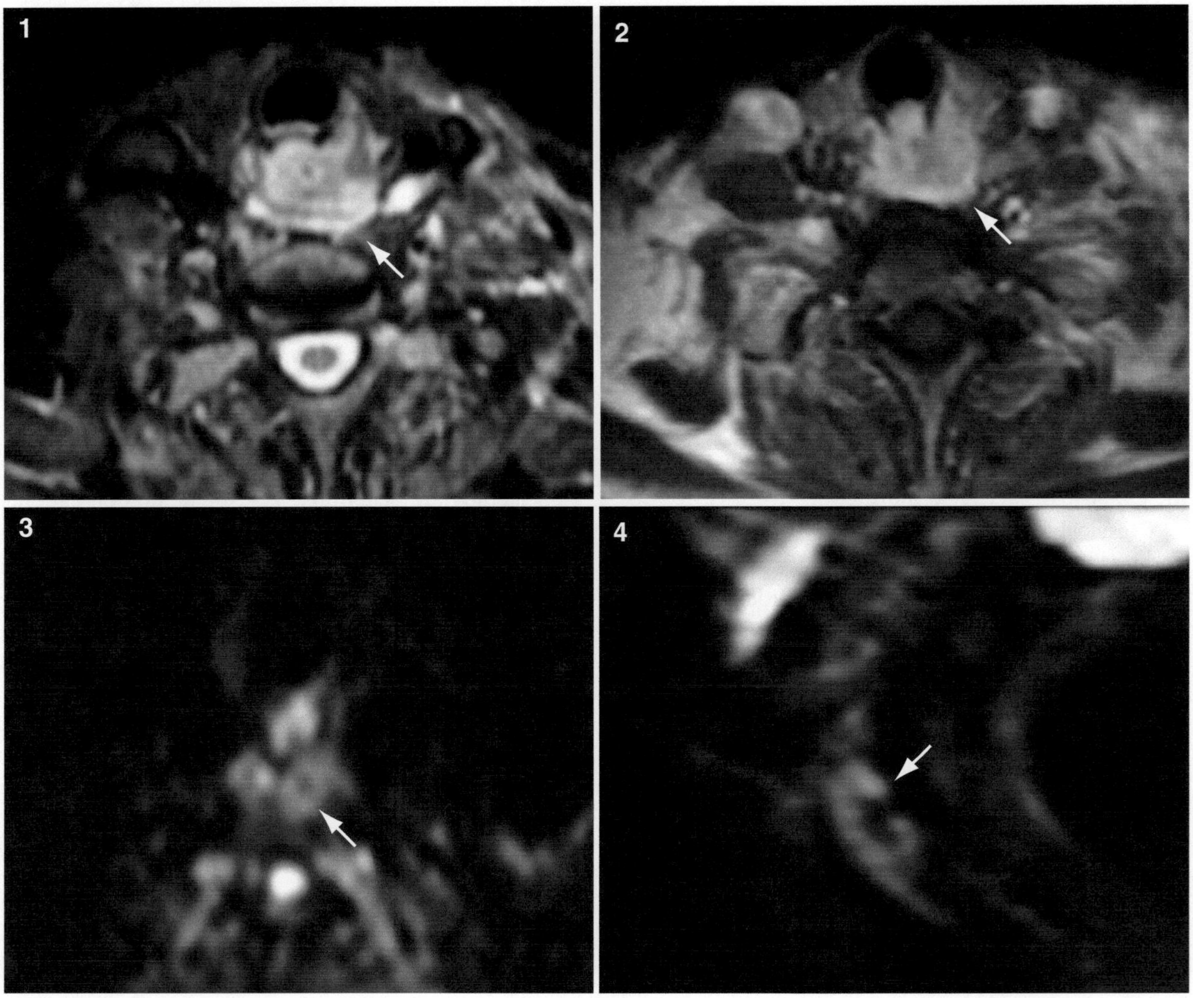

Fig. 14.4 **14.4.1** Transverse STIR image shows a poorly delineated esophageal lesion involving all mucosal layers. The lesion obliterates the lumen, infiltrates the prevertebral space (*arrows*), and invades the trachea. **14.4.2** Postcontrast axial fat-suppressed TSE T1-weighed sequence depicts invasion of posterior trachea, thyroid gland, left side mediastinum, and prevertebral space. There is doubtful involvement of the anterior aspect of cervical vertebrae. The carotid vessels are spared. **14.4.3** Transverse DWI with a *b* value of 1,000 s/mm^2 reveals a locally advanced tumor with tracheal and prevertebral space invasion (*arrow*). **14.4.4** Sagittal MPR of DWI confirms prevertebral invasion without osseous involvement (*arrow*)

Case 14.5: Recurrent Lingual Carcinoma

A 29-year-old female was submitted to our imaging center to perform a CT for follow-up of a previously resected and irradiated lingual carcinoma 2-years before. A biopsy of the enlarged soft tissue mass of left lingual region confirmed recurrence. MRI was performed to determine tumoral extension.

Comments

CT and MRI are nonspecific in the differentiation between recurrent tumor posttreatment changes in patients submitted to surgery, chemotherapy or mainly radiotherapy. Functional MRI techniques such as dynamic contrast MRI and DWI have shown to be useful in this task. DWI is able to detect recurrent tumor as areas of restricted diffusion and differentiate them form necrosis, apoptosis, or even edema. The depiction of recurrence of DWI is possible even in the acute posttherapeuthic setting, as it is not influenced by inflammatory changes or edema. This is a clear advantage over FDG PET, as inflammatory changes are a common cause of false-positive results.

ADC measurements allow quantification of the suspected areas of recurrence. As shown in this case, it is important avoid areas of necrosis or susceptibility artifact which may change the true ADC value of a lesion.

Imaging Findings

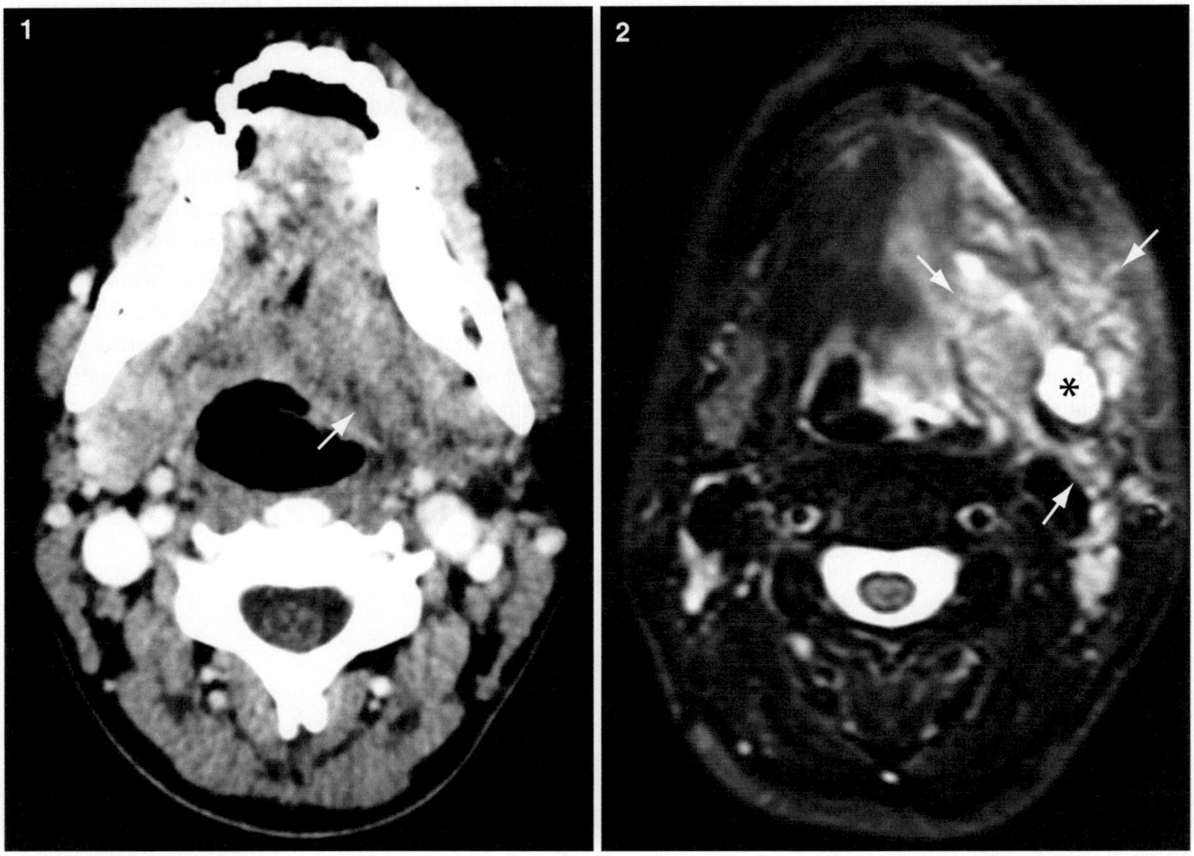

Fig. 14.5 **14.5.1** Enhanced CT shows enlargement and asymmetry of left lingual region (*arrow*). If these findings correspond either to recurrent tumor or posttreatment, changes cannot be defined. **14.5.2**, **14.5.3** Axial STIR and coronal TSE T2-weighted images show heterogeneous enlargement of the treated region (*arrows*) with diffuse edema and areas of necrosis (*asterisks*). **14.5.4**, **14.5.5** Axial dynamic postcontrast THRIVE at arterial and delayed phases show early central enhancement which become more diffuse on the delayed phase. The presence of early enhancement (*arrow*) favors recurrence. **14.5.6** ADC map demonstrates a central area of restricted diffusion with low signal corresponding to the area of recurrence (*asterisk*). On the left posterior aspect of the lesion, there is an area of high signal corresponding to necrosis, as previously confirmed in the dynamic series. **14.5.7–14.5.9** ROI positioning influence on ADC value. ADC value of the ROI including the whole lesion, as shown in Fig. **14.5.7**, was that of 1.7×10^{-3} mm^2/s. On Fig. **14.5.8**, the ROI was drawn, avoiding necrotic areas, including only the solid tumor recurrence with an ADC value of 1.3×10^{-3} mm^2/s. Finally, ADC value of necrosis was 2.6×10^{-3} mm^2/s as shown in Fig. **14.5.9**

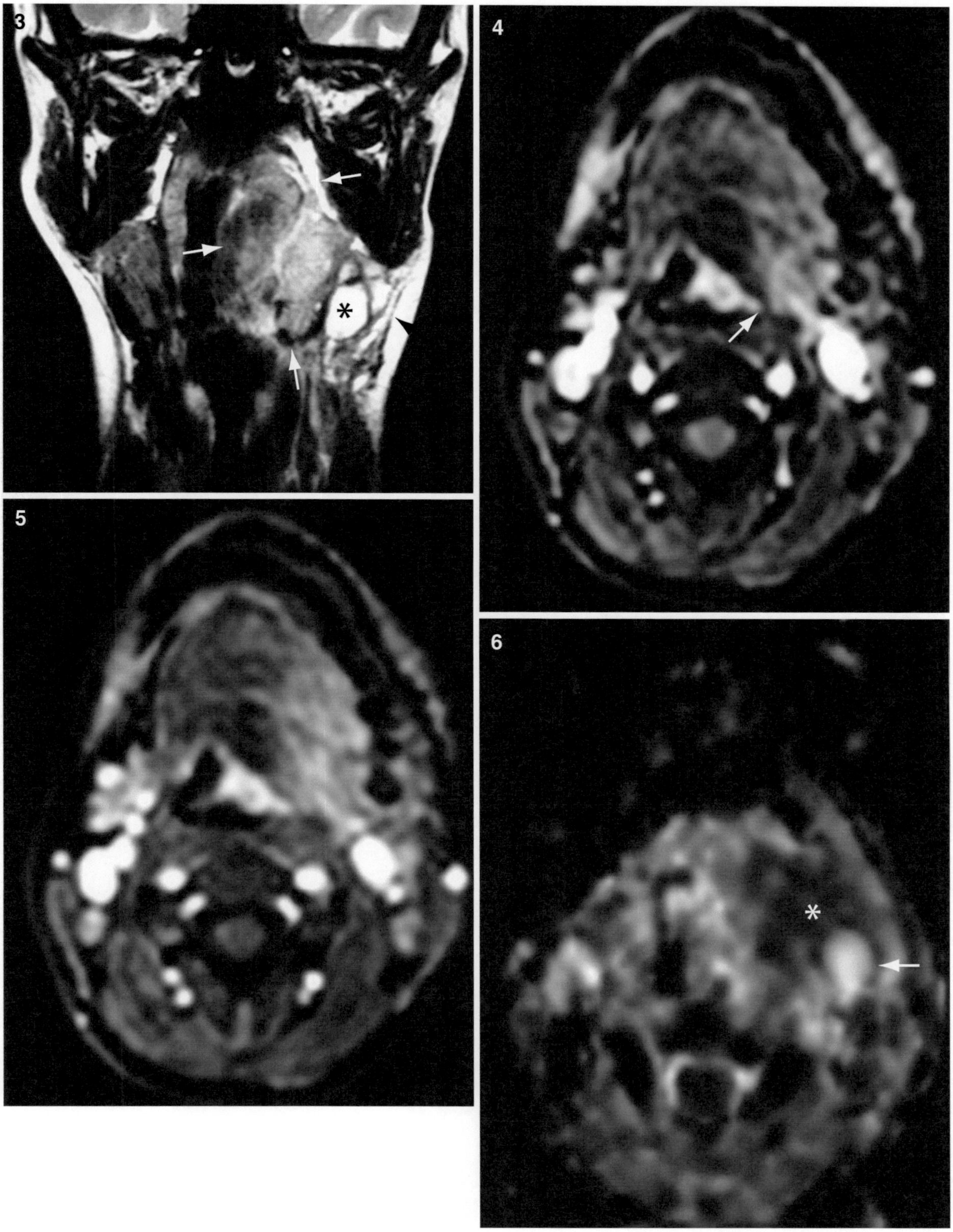

Fig. 14.5 (continued)

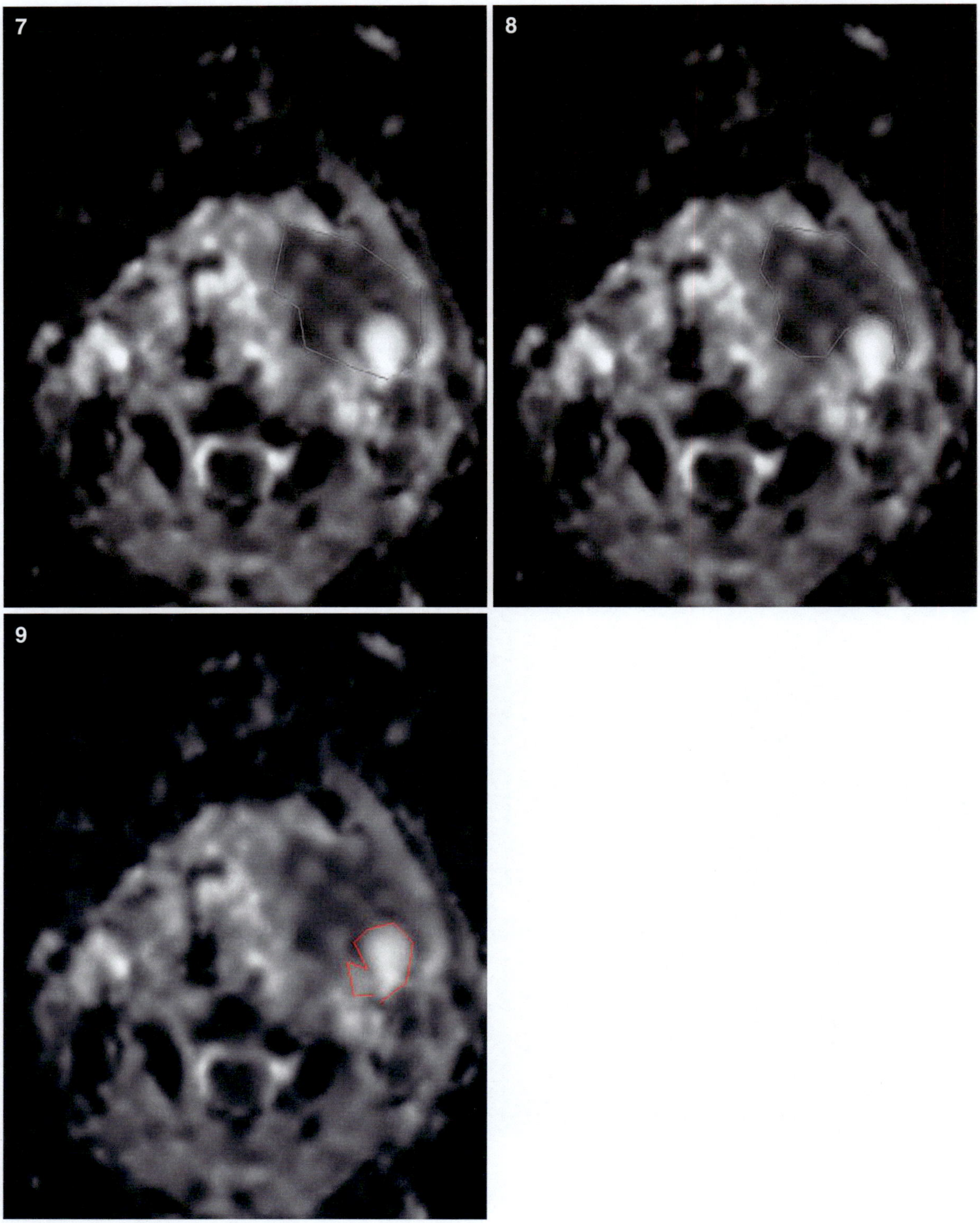

Fig. 14.5 (continued)

Case 14.6: Cellulitis and Sialadenitis of Parotid Gland with Abscess Formation

A 86-year-old female showed pain and left parotid enlargement for some weeks. She had facial erythema and parotid induration. The clinical diagnosis was uncertain. Therefore, MR examination was performed to exclude malignancy in a unilateral parotid process.

Comments

Infections caused for bacterial and viral agents are the most common processes of salivary abnormalities, and these are more frequent in the parotid gland than in the other salivary glands. The most common infecting agent is *Staphylococcus aureus*, but a great variety of microorganisms have been isolated in a parotid gland abscess.

Mainly in the brain, DWI is well accepted for diagnosing intracranial infectious diseases, in particular for brain abscess. Due to the high viscosity and cellularity of pus, there is restriction of water proton movement within the content of the abscess that causes areas of high signal on DWI and low signal on ADC maps. Because of this characteristic appearance, the utility of the DWI in this diagnosis is well recognized, and its use has spread to other localizations, as abscess in the head and neck regions.

On MRI, a parotid abscess usually presents as a glandular enlargement and diffuse hyperintensity with focal areas of higher signal intensity on T2-weighted images, representing edematous changes and fluid collections respectively. These fluid collections typically show ring enhancement on postcontrast T1-weighted sequences. Diffuse enlargement and edema sometimes may occur with focal lesion of different origin, and in those cases, DWI can be especially useful and valuable for making a diagnosis of parotid gland abscess.

Imaging Findings

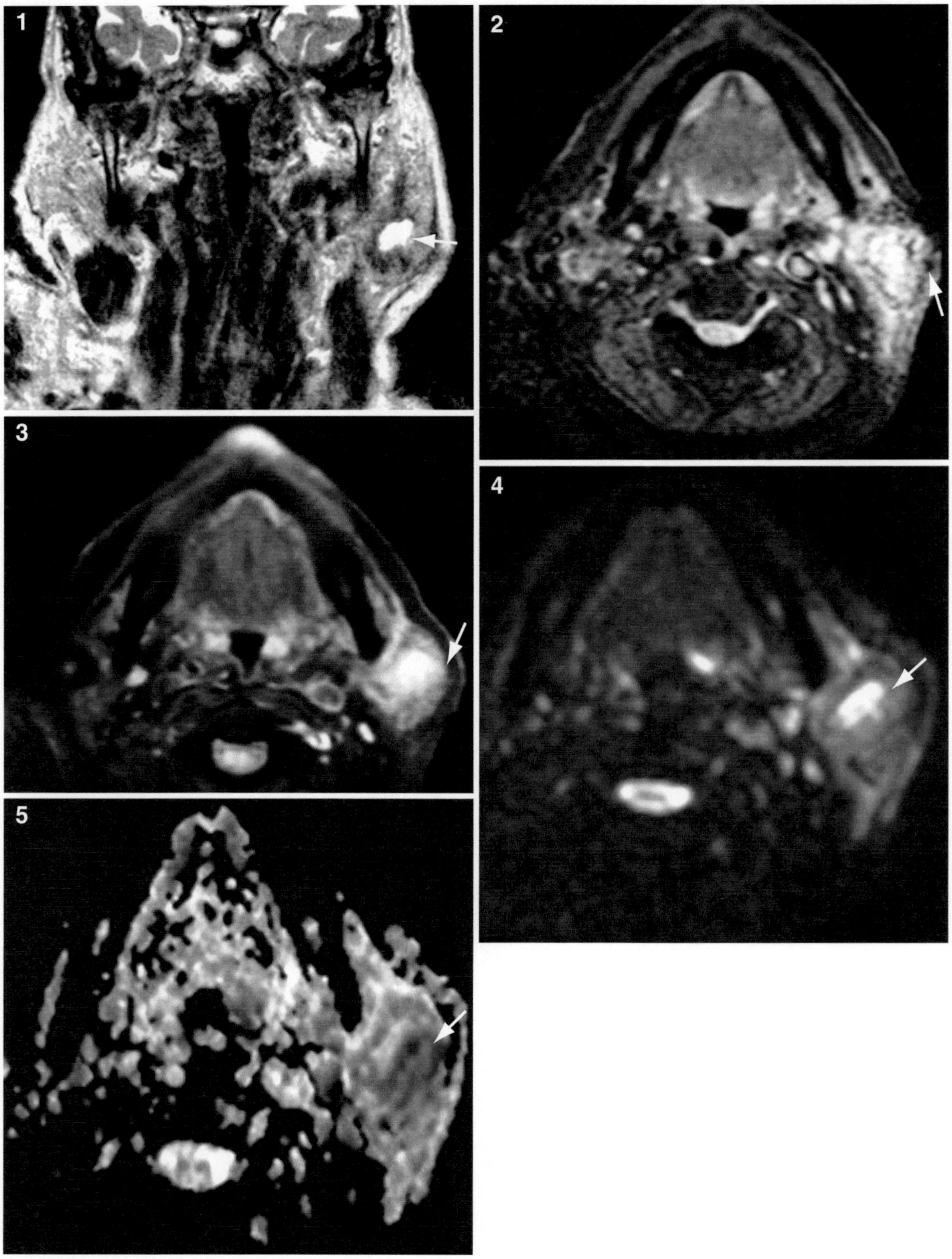

Fig. 14.6 **14.6.1** Coronal TSE T2-weighted image shows left parotid enlargement with diffuse hyperintensity and with an intraparotid area with higher hyperintensity favoring fluid content (*arrow*). **14.6.2** Transverse STIR confirms the diffuse hyperintensity of the left parotid gland, masseter muscle, and subcutaneous soft tissues in the preauricular region (*arrow*). **14.6.3** Axial postcontrast fat-suppressed TSE T1-weighted shows a diffuse and irregular enhancement of the left parotid gland and surrounding tissues with some areas without enhancement into the gland. **14.6.4**, **14.6.5** DWI with a *b* value of 1,000 s/mm^2 and ADC map in transverse plane demonstrate tiny central areas of restricted diffusion with decreased signal on ADC map into the left parotid gland (*arrows*) that support the diagnosis of an abscess. The surrounding tissues, which demonstrate diffuse swelling and edema on morphological sequences, do not show restriction of diffusion

Case 14.7: Nodal and Local Recurrence of Parotid Squamous Cell Carcinoma

A 74-year-old man with history of right parotid squamous cell carcinoma resected 5 years ago presented to our institution with several lymph nodes in both lateral neck regions. The patient was in study for lymphatic chronic leukemia (LLC) at that moment. A MRI was performed for characterization of these nodes and evaluation of extension in order to plan the therapeutic approach to follow.

Comments

In patients with cancer of head and neck regions, the detection of cervical nodes is crucial for an adequate treatment assessment. The patient's prognosis will also be determinated by the characterization of these nodes. The neck region is usually a crossroad for the lymphatic spread of many inflammatory and neoplasic processes, such as infection, granulomatous diseases, SCC, lymphoma, or malignancies of other origin. Classical morphological criteria on MRI sequences for characterization of lymph nodes included shape, size, extra capsular tumor spread, changes in signal intensity, or necrosis. The use of DWI sequences allows to determine the inner structure of these nodes by detecting alterations in water diffusion and microcirculation inside the node. Several studies had shown the utility of DWI in the head and neck areas to discriminate between benign and metastatic nodes, to detect micrometastases, or, even, to depict early apparent infiltration of normal nodes. According to several investigators, proposed cutoff ADC values to differentiate malignant from benign nodes range from 0.9×10^{-3} mm²/s to 1.3×10^{-3} mm²/s. ADC values range from 1×10^{-3} mm²/s to 1.4×10^{-3} mm²/s for reactive lymph nodes and 0.6×10^{-3} mm²/s to 0.9×10^{-3} mm²/s for metastatic ones from primary head and neck cancer or lymphoma.

Imaging Findings

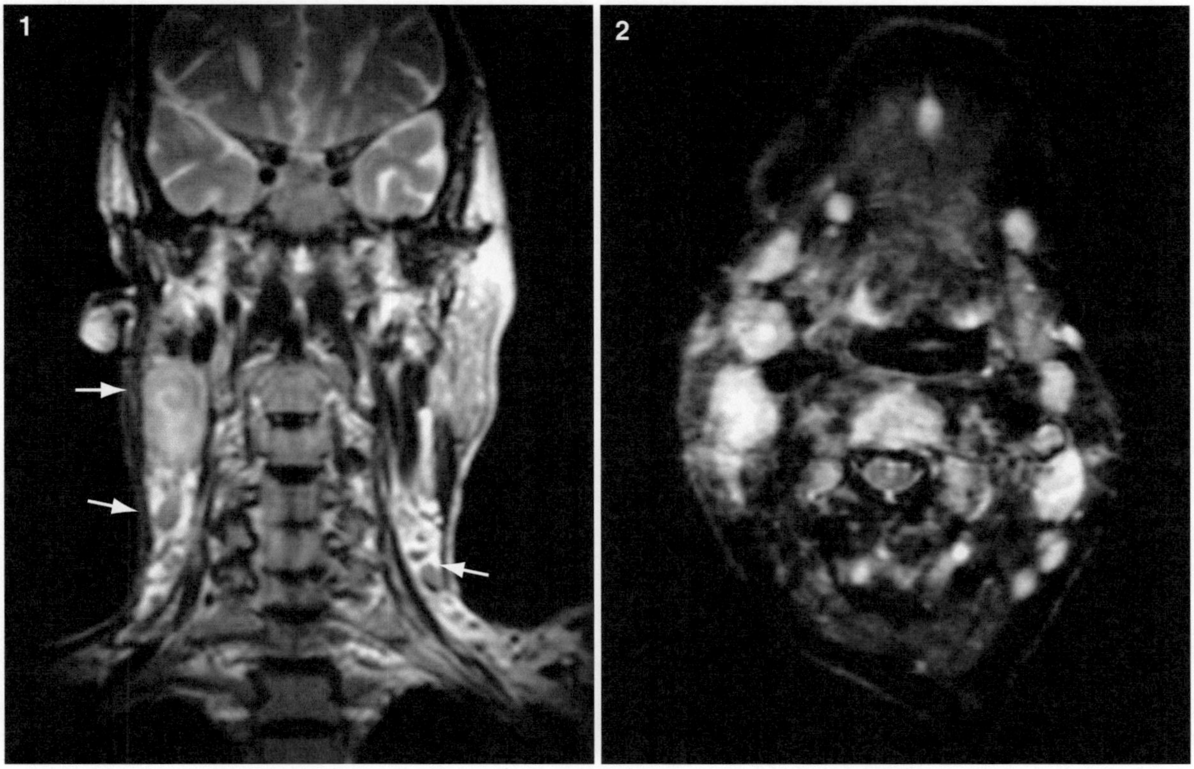

Fig. 14.7 **14.7.1**, **14.7.2** Coronal TSE T2-weighted and axial STIR images show a right large lymphoid mass at II-III neck levels and multiple bilateral small-sized nodes located in IA, IB and V levels (not shown). **14.7.3**, **14.7.4** These lymph nodes (*arrows*) showed restricted diffusion and low ADC values (*arrows*), between 0.6–0.8 × 10^{-3} mm²/s, favor a metastatic origin from a recurrent parotid carcinoma infiltration more than involvement by LLC, as surgically proved. **14.7.5–14.7.7** Axial STIR, DWI with a *b* value of 800 s/mm², and axial ADC map demonstrate heterogeneous appearance with areas of restricted diffusion of the right parotid cell (*arrows*) due to local recurrence

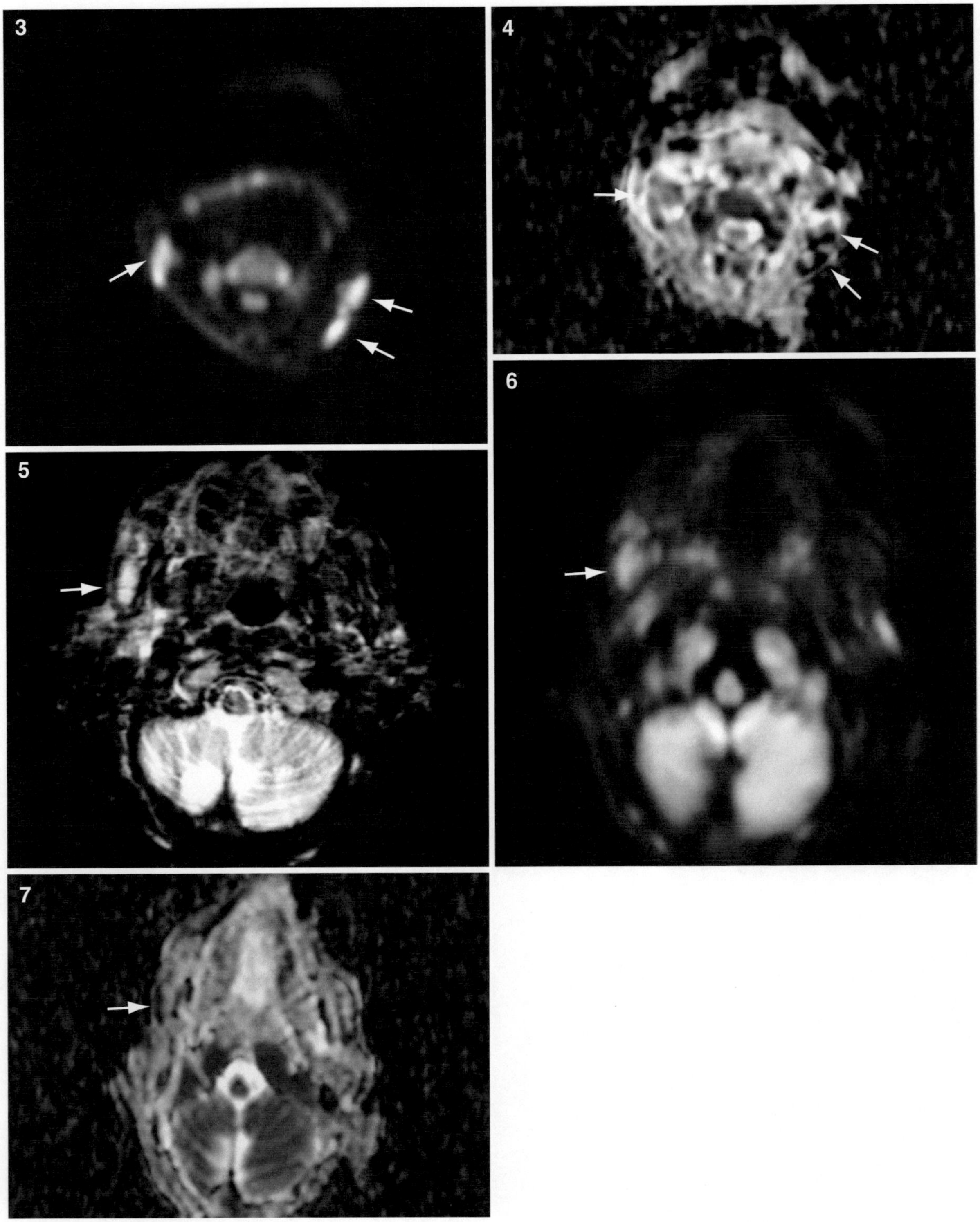

Fig. 14.7 (continued)

Case 14.8: Posttreatment Monitorization and Prediction of Response to Treatment of Occult Cavum Carcinoma with Metastatic Cervical Lymph Nodes

A 49-year year-old male showed a painful and growing deep right cervical mass during a month. Laryngoscopy was unremarkable. CT showed bilateral cervical lymph nodes with necrotic centers at levels IIb and III. MRI was performed for characterization and staging.

Comments

DWI is a powerful tool in the evaluation of head and neck malignancies. It allows for assessment of primary tumor and nodal staging in the same examination. As in this case, it is sometimes able to detect an occult primary neoplasm for other imaging techniques. Furthermore, DWI allows the accurate posttreatment monitorization of both primary tumor and nodal metastases. It has also been proposed for prediction of response to therapy. As in this case, primary tumors with low ADC values have more chances to completely respond to chemoradiation due to the absence of hypoxia, one of the main mechanisms of radio-resistance. In a similar manner, metastatic lymph nodes with low ADC values also generally show a better response to treatment.

Therefore, in this case, DWI allowed to find an occult primary tumor, to perform adequate nodal staging, predict response to treatment, and to assess the posttreatment response.

Imaging Findings

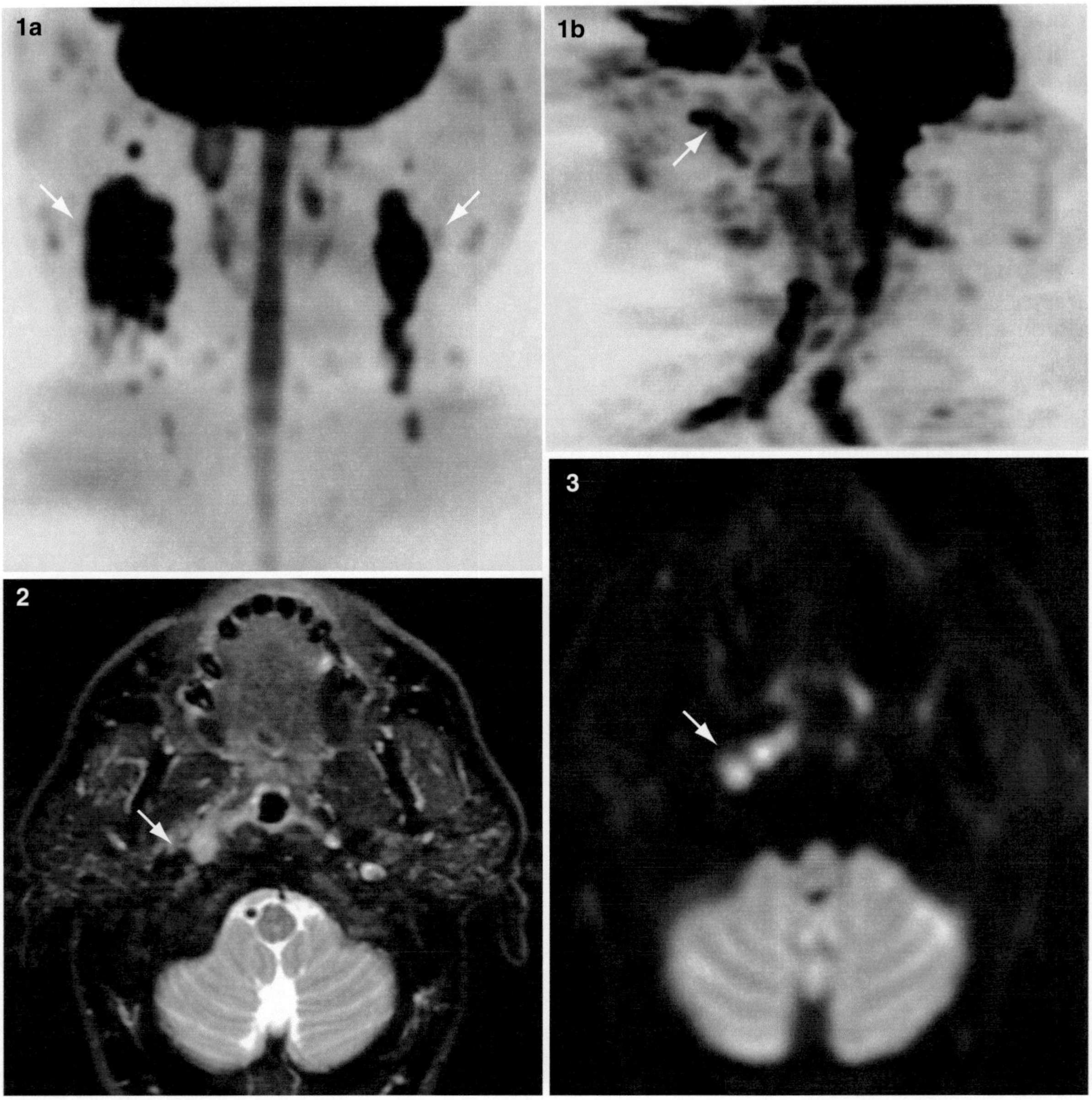

Fig. 14.8 **14.8.1a**, **14.8.1b** Coronal and sagittal MIP of a DWIBS sequence with *b* value of 1,000 s/mm^2 show bilateral enlarged lymph nodes (*arrows* on **14.8.1**) and a mass on the right lateral aspect of the cavum (*arrow* on **14.8.1b**) with restricted diffusion, favoring a primary neoplasm. **14.8.2–14.8.4** Axial STIR, SS EPI-DWI with a *b* value of 800 s/mm^2 and corresponding ADC map confirm the cavum neoplasm (*arrows*) with an ADC value of 0.6×10^{-3} mm^2/s, which was posteriorly confirmed as undifferentiated SCC. This low ADC value predicts favorable response to chemoradiation. **14.8.5**, **14.8.6** SS EPI-DWI with a *b* value of 800 s/mm^2 and corresponding ADC map demonstrate bilateral lymph nodes (*arrows*), some of them with central necrosis, showing predominantly restricted diffusion with ADC values of the solid component ranging between 0.6–0.8×10^{-3} mm^2/s. **14.8.7–14.8.10** Six months later, follow-up MRI after chemoradiation was performed. Axial SS EPI-DWI with a *b* value of 800 s/mm^2 and corresponding ADC map (**14.8.7**, **14.8.8**) demonstrate disappearance of the lymph nodes, except one right lymph node of 6 mm which was hyperintense on DWI (*arrow* on **14.8.7**), although in the ADC map revealed intermediate signal intensity (*arrow* on **14.8.8**) with an ADC value of 1.7 $\times 10^{-3}$ mm^2/s, favoring an inflammatory origin, as confirmed in posterior follow-up imaging. Superiorly, at the cavum level, STIR and DWI indicates complete response of the primary tumor, as there are neither residual masses nor areas of restricted diffusion (*arrows* on **14.8.9, 14.8.10**)

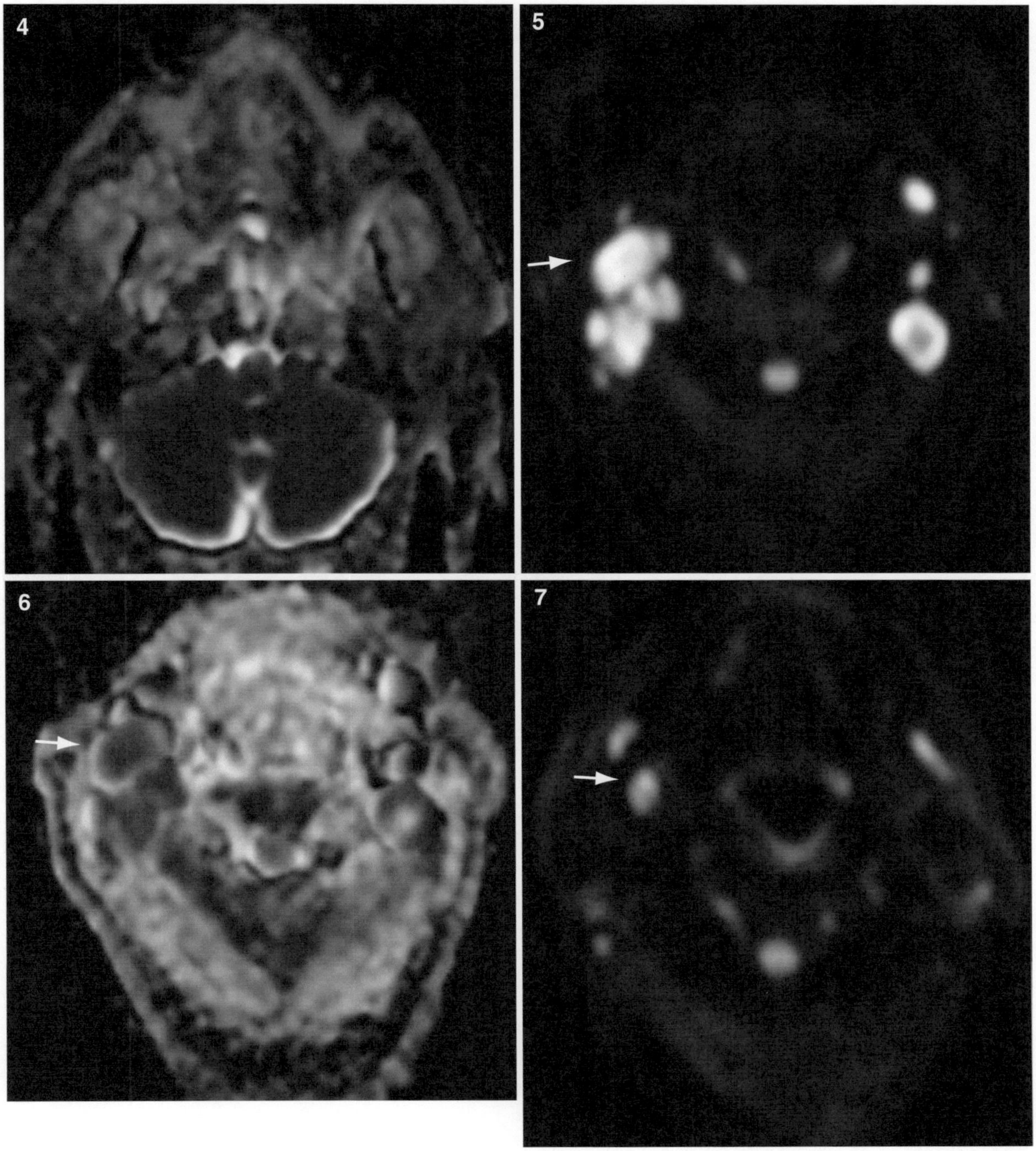

Fig. 14.8 (continued)

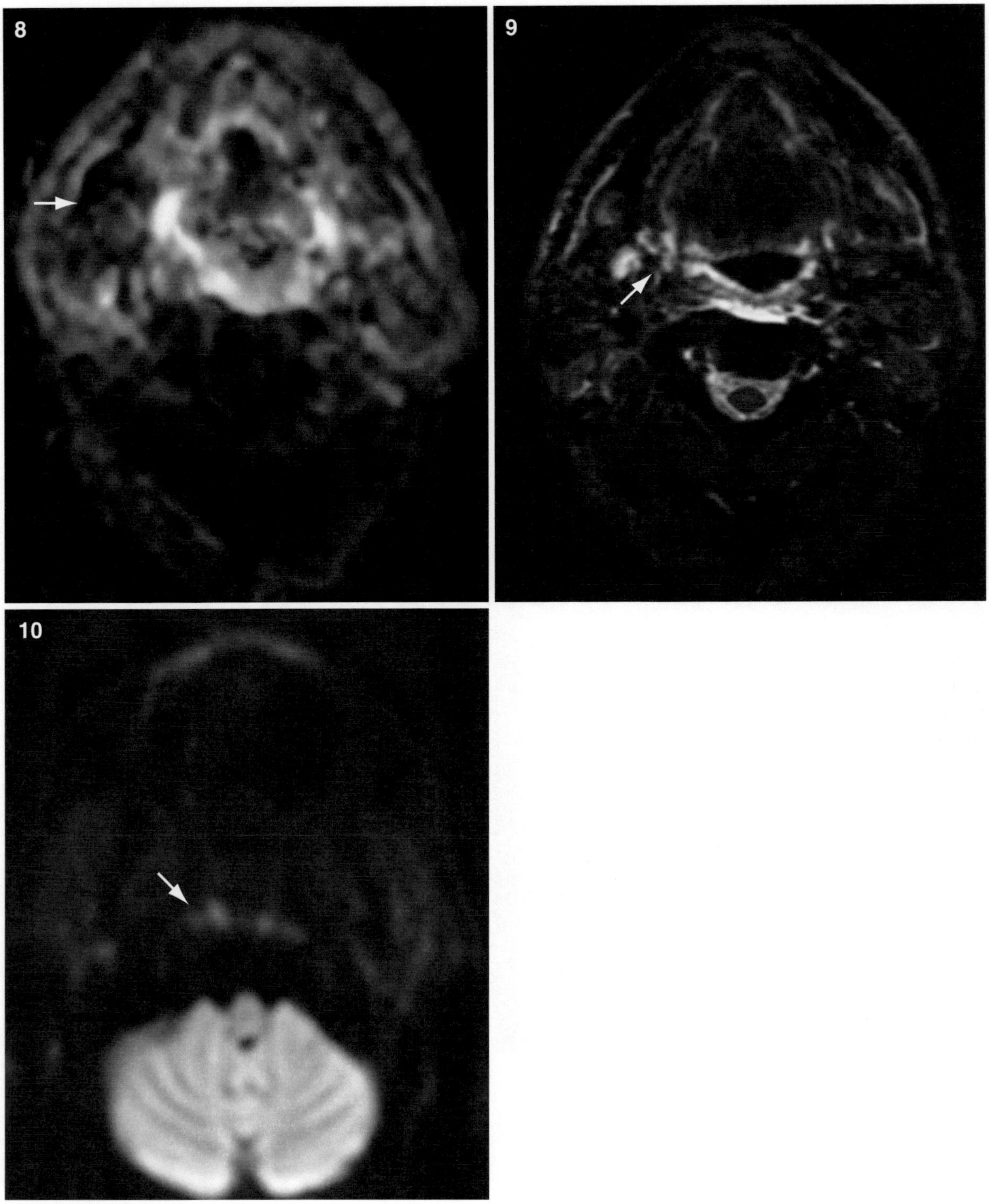

Fig. 14.8 (continued)

Case 14.9: Nodal Metastasis in the Neck from Squamous Cell Carcinoma

A 79-year-old smoker male was submitted for a neck MRI due to a right lateral mass in the neck. The mass was palpable and immobile. He did not have an undercurrent infection and he did suffer other important known disease. Whole-body CT was negative for a primary tumor. At last, histological examination of the major cervical lymph node was required to establish the diagnosis of poorly differentiated SCC.

Comments

The estimated number of European patients with newly diagnosed cancers of the oral cavity or pharynx is 9.8 per 100,000 inhabitants/year. SCC is the most common type of tumor among those in the oral cavity. They metastasize usually through the lymphatic system to cervical lymph nodes and some studies have revealed that the higher grading, the higher the risk of cervical metastasis. Metastasis of SCC to the neck with an occult primary is a recognized clinical and pathological entity. It is estimated that their incidence is an 81.1% of all the cases, although it is not the only tumoral type, because adenocarcinomas account for a 7.6% of the cases, the majority from tumors outside of the neck region. In these cases, the prognosis is poorer than for metastasis of unknown SCC. Most authors suggest an intensive treatment including radiotherapy and chemotherapy, and when it is possible salvage surgery.

The main differential diagnoses in these cases are lymphoma and inflammatory/infectious processes. When MR imaging is performed in a patient with lymphadenopathy due to suspected malignancy, the addition of a DWI technique can help to characterize the node. The differences in ADC values of head and neck lymph nodes have been well documented in the literature. ADC values are usually lower in nodal lymphomas than in metastatic lymph nodes from SCC, with a suggested cutoff point around 0.76×10^{-3} mm^2/s, according to several series. It should be taken into account that the ADC of highly or moderately differentiated cancers is greater than that of poorly differentiated ones, which may show overlap in their ADC values with lymphoma. ADC values of infectious processes are variable, but higher than in lymphoma. Most of infectious lymph nodes show ADC values greater than 1.7×10^{-3} mm^2/s. However, granulomatous disease such as sarcoidosis and Cat–scratch disease may show ADC values resembling malignancy.

Imaging Findings

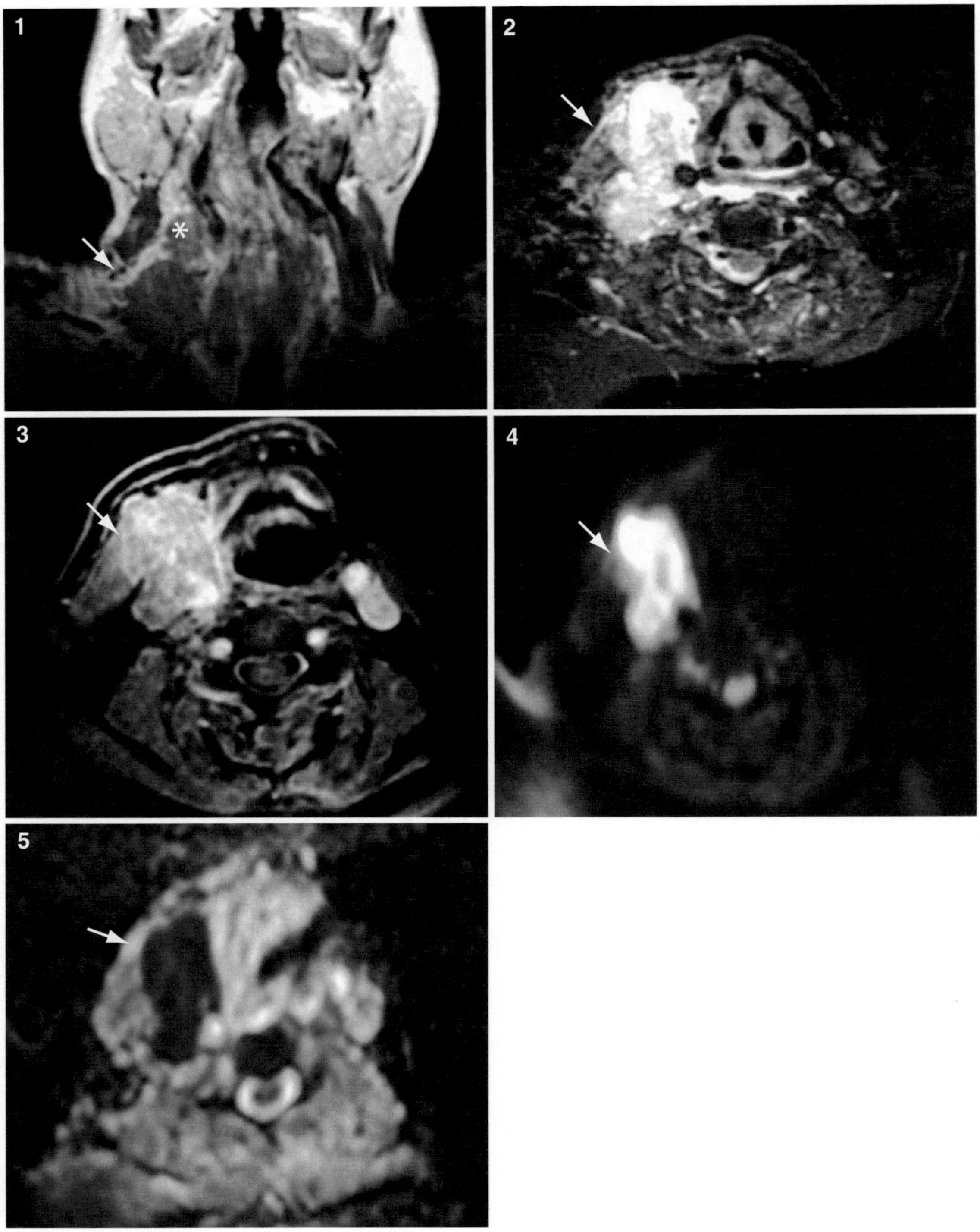

Fig. 14.9 **14.9.1** Coronal postcontrast T1-weighed image shows a large mass with heterogeneous enhancement and without necrosis, located in a lymphatic space on the right side of the neck (*arrow*). It is located in the II-III level. Another lymphadenopathy was present at the same ganglionar level on the same side (*asterisk*). **14.9.2, 14.9.3** Axial STIR and postcontrast fat-suppressed T1-weighted sequence confirm poor delimitation from adjacent structures and the extranodal spread of the lymphatic involvement (*arrows*). These findings and the size of the lymph nodes suggest malignancy. **14.9.4** Transverse DWI acquired using a *b* value of 800 s/mm^2 shows a markedly hyperintense lesion which is very hypointense on the corresponding ADC map. **14.9.5** The mean ADC value was 0.878× 10^{-3} mm^2/s. In this case, DWI favors SCC and the ADC value helped to distinguish it from lymphoma

Case 14.10: Vertebral, Nodal, and Peritoneal Metastases of Surgically Removed Endometrial Cancer

A 63-year-old female patient, who underwent surgery 6 years ago for endometrial cancer, was sent to our Department for pelvic MRI due to abdominal discomfort.

Comments

The use of DWI has become an important tool to assess the presence of node metastasis in female pelvic tumors. Ovarian and endometrial cancer also can spread into the peritoneum, which may easily be detected with DWI.

With morphological conventional MRI sequences, it is sometimes a challenge to determine if milimetric nodes, without malignancy size criteria (less than 6–8 mm), are infiltrated by packages of tumor cells. In these cases, DWI and ADC values can increase the capacity of detection and characterization, even more if fusion techniques are used.

ADC threshold values could be used to discriminate between hyperplasic and metastatic nodes, having these last ones mean ADC values usually lower than normal lymph nodes. However, further studies should be performed to establish adequate cutoff values.

Depiction and characterization of lymph nodes is crucial to discriminate between III b and III c stage, guiding the surgeons to selective node dissection and avoiding unnecessary extensive lymphadenectomy.

As in this case, fusion of DWI-T2 images can also help to correctly assess the presence of pelvic or peritoneal seeding and differentiate them, based on their localization or not from typical lymphatic chain territories.

Imaging Findings

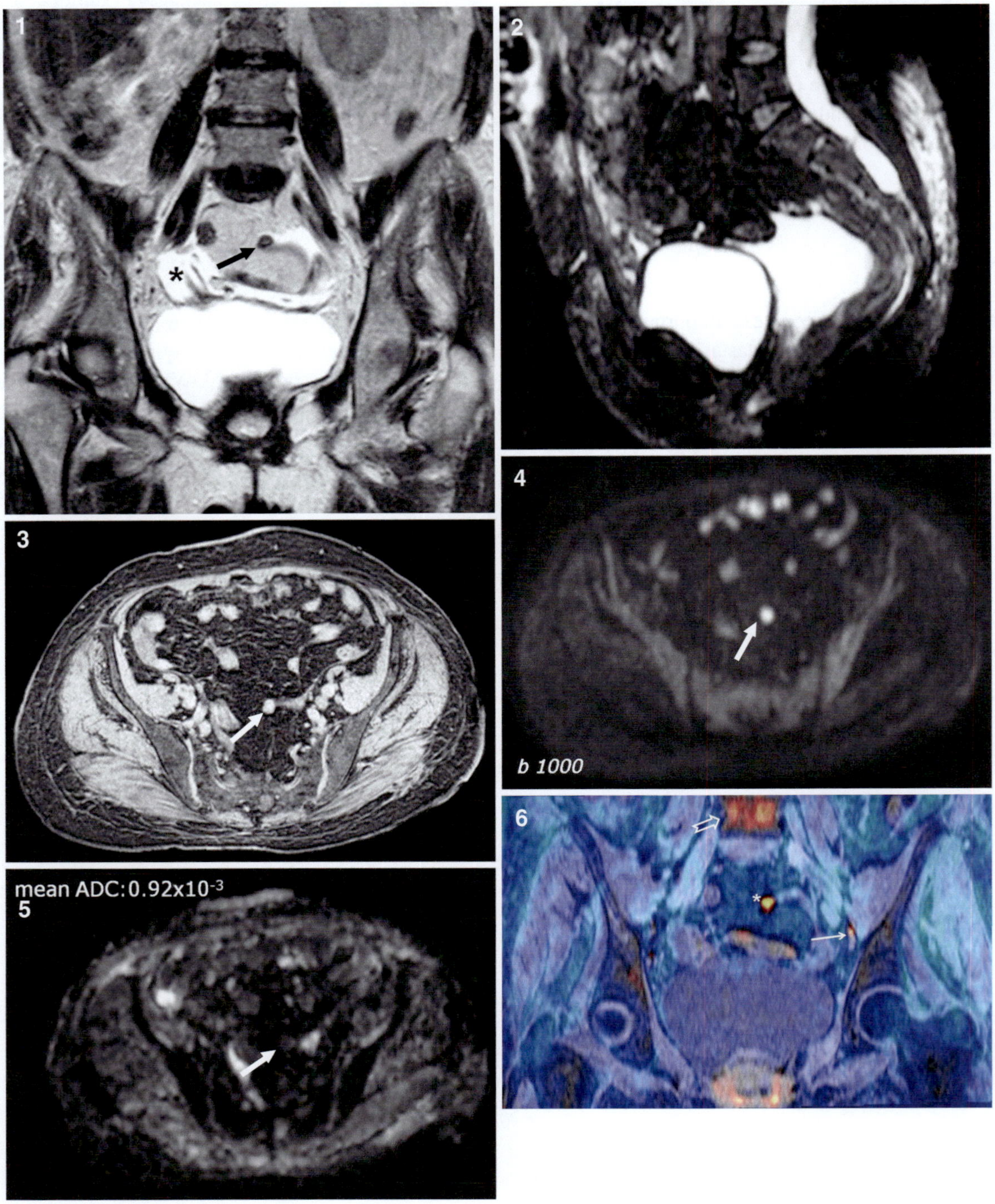

Fig. 14.10 Coronal TSE and sagittal fat-suppressed T2-weighted sequences (Figs. **14.10.1** and **14.10.2**, respectively) showed pelvic free fluid (*asterisk*) and a peritoneal nodule (*arrow*) consistent with peritoneal carcinomatosis, which is better depicted on axial postcontrast THRIVE as an enhancing lesion (*arrow*) Fig. **14.10.3**. This nodule shows restricted diffusion on DWI sequence with a *b* value of 1,000 mm²/s (Fig. **14.10.4**) and a mean ADC value of 0.92×10^{-3} mm²/s (Fig. **14.10.5**). Fig. **14.10.6** Coronal fusion image of DWI and T2-weighted sequences better depicts the peritoneal implant (*asterisk*), a tiny left iliac lymph node (*solid arrow*) and infiltration of L5 vertebral body (*empty arrow*). All of these lesions showed restricted diffusion and corresponded to metastases. Notice the absence of signal alteration of L5 in the sagittal SPIR TSE T2-weighted sequence (Fig. **14.10.2**)

Further Reading

Akduman EI, Momtahen AJ, Balci NC et al (2008) Comparison between malignant and benign abdominal lymph nodes on diffusion-weighted imaging. Acad Radiol 15:641–646

Aviv RI, Miszkiel K (2005) Orbital imaging: Part 2. Intraorbital pathology. Clin Radiol 60(3):288–307

Bindal R, Sawaya R, Leavens M et al (1994) Sarcoma metastatic to the brain: results of surgical treatment. Neurosurgery 35(2):185–191

Cai W, Kassarjian A, Bredella MA et al (2009) Tumor burden in patients with neurofibromatosis types 1 and 2 and schwannomatosis: determination on whole-body MR images. Radiology 250(3):665–673

Chawla S, Kim S, Wang S et al (2009) Diffusion-weighted imaging in head and neck cancers. Future Oncol 5(7):959–975

Chen YB, Liao J, Xie R et al (2011) Discrimination of metastatic from hyperplastic pelvic lymph nodes in patients with cervical cancer by diffusion-weighted magnetic resonance imaging. Abdom Imaging 36(1):102–109

Coutinho AC Jr, Krishnaraj A, Pires CE et al (2011) Pelvic applications of diffusion magnetic resonance images. Magn Reson Imaging Clin N Am 19(1):133–157

Eiber M, Beer AJ, Holzapfel K et al (2010) Preliminary results for characterization of pelvic lymph nodes in patients with prostate cancer by diffusion-weighted MR-imaging. Invest Radiol 45(1):15–23

Evans DG, Baser ME, McGaughran J, Sharif S, Howard E, Moran A (2002) Malignant peripheral nerve sheath tumours in neurofibromatosis 1. J Med Genet 39:311–314

Galban G, Mukherji S, Chenevert TL et al (2009) A feasibility study of parametric response map analysis of diffusion-weighted magnetic resonance imaging scans of head and neck cancer patients for providing early detection of therapeutic efficacy. Transl Oncol 2(3):184–190

Hamstra D, Lee K, Moffat A et al (2008) Diffusion magnetic resonance imaging: an imaging treatment response biomarker to chemoradiotherapy in a mouse model of squamous cell cancer of the head and neck. Transl Oncol 1(4):189–194

Harisinghani MG, Barentsz J, Hahn PF et al (2003) Noninvasive detection of clinically occult lymph node metastases in prostate cancer. N Engl J Med 19:2491–2499

Hermans R (2010) Diffusion-weighted MRI in head and neck cancer. Curr Opin Otoralyngol Head Neck Surg 18(2): 72–78

Herneth AM, Mayerhoefer M, Schernthaner R (2010) Diffusion weighted imaging: lymph nodes. Eur J Radiol 76(3): 398–406

Kakimoto N, Hiwatashi A, Larheim TA et al (2006) Diffusion-weighted imaging of an abscess in the parotid gland. Eur J Radiol Extra 60:11–14

Kapur R, Sepahdari AR, Mafee MF et al (2009) MR imaging of orbital inflammatory syndrome, orbital cellulitis and orbital lymphoid lesions: the role of diffusion-weighted imaging. Am J Neuroradiol 30:64–70

Kim JK, Kim KA, Park BW et al (2008) Feasibility of diffusion-weighted imaging in the differentiation of metastatic from nonmetastatic lymph nodes: early experience. J Magn Reson Imaging 28:714–719

Kim TJ, Kim HY, Lee KW et al (2009) Multimodality assessment of esophageal cancer: preoperative staging and monitoring of response to therapy. Radiographics 29:403–421

Kim S, Loevner L, Quon H et al (2009) Diffusion-weighted magnetic resonance imaging for predicting and detecting early response to chemoradiation Therapy of squamous cell carcinomas of the head and neck. Clin Cancer Re 15(3):986–994

King A, Ahuja A, Yeung D et al (2007) Malignant cervical lymphadenopathy: diagnostic accuracy of diffusion-weighted MR imaging. Radiology 245(3):807–813

Koc O, Paksoy Y, Erayman I et al (2007) Role of diffusion weighted MR in the discrimination diagnosis of the cystic and/or necrotic head and neck lesions. Eur J Radiol 62:205–213

Korf BR (1999) Plexiform neurofibromas. Am J Med Genet 89:31–37

Kowalski LP, Bagietto R, Lara JR et al (1999) Factors influencing contralateral lymph node metastasis from oral carcinoma. Head Neck 21(2):104–110

Kruse A, Grätz K (2009) Cervical metastases of squamous cell carcinoma of the maxilla: a retrospective study of 9 years. Head Neck Oncol 1:28

Kwee TC, Takahara T, Luijten PR, Nievelstein RA (2010) ADC measurements of lymph nodes: inter- and intra-observer reproducibility study and an overview of the literature. Eur J Radiol 75(2):215–220

Kwee TC, Ludwig I, Uiterwaal CS et al (2011) ADC measurements in the evaluation of lymph nodes in patients with non-Hodgkin lymphoma: feasibility study. Magma 24(1):1–8

LeBihan D, Breton E, Lallemand D et al (1988) Separation of diffusion and perfusion in intravoxel incoherent motion MR imaging. Radiology 168:497–505

Lim R, Jaramillo D, Young T, Chang Y et al (2005) Superficial Neurofibroma: a lesion with unique MRI characteristics in patients with neurofibromatosis Type 1. Am J Roentgenol 184:962–968

Lin G, Ho KC, Wang JJ et al (2008) Detection of lymph node metastasis in cervical and uterine cancers by diffusion-weighted magnetic resonance imaging at 3T. J Magn Reson Imaging 28(1):128–135

Lin C, Itti E, Luciani A et al (2010) Whole-body diffusion-weighted imaging in lymphoma. Cancer Imaging 10(Spec no A):S172–S178

Lowe LH, Stokes LS, Johnson JE et al (2001) Swelling at the angle of the mandible: imaging of the pediatric parotid gland and periparotid region. Radiographics 21(5):1211–1217

Maeda M, Maier S (2008) Usefulness of diffusion-weighted imaging and apparent diffusion coefficient in the assessment of head and neck tumors. J Neuroradiol 35(2):71–78

Maeda M, Kato H, Sakuma H et al (2005) Usefulness of apparent diffusion coefficient in line scan diffusion-weighted imaging for distinguishing between squamous cell carcinomas and malignant lymphomas of the head and neck. Am J Neuroradiol 26:1186–1192

Marx MV, Balfe DN (1987) Computed tomography of esophagus. Semin Ultrasound CT MR 8:316–348

Mautner VF, Hartmann M, Friedrich RE et al (2006) MRI growth patterns of plexiform neurofibromatosis type 1. Neuroradiology 48:160–165

Mautner VF, Asuagbor FA, Dombi E et al (2008) Assessment of benign tumor burden by whole-body MRI in patients with neurofibromatosis 1. Neuro Oncol 10(4):593–598

Mir N, Sohaib SA, Collins D et al (2010) Fusion of high b-value diffusion-weighted and T2-weighted MR images improves identification of lymph nodes in the pelvis. J Med Imaging Radiat Oncol 54(4):358–364

Montgamery RC, Ridge JA (1998) Radiologic staging of gastrointestinal cancer. Semin Surg Oncol 15:143–150

Moss AA, Schnyder P, Thoeni RF et al (1981) Esophageal carcinoma: pre-therapy staying by computed tomography. Am J Roentgenol 136:1051–1056

Niwa T, Aida N, Fujita K et al (2008) Diffusion-weighted imaging of retroperitoneal malignant peripheral nerve sheath tumor in a patient with neurofibromatosis type 1. Magn Reson Med Sci 7(1):49–53

Park SO, Kim JK, Kim KA et al (2009) Relative apparent diffusion coefficient: determination of reference site and validation of benefit for detecting metastatic lymph nodes in uterine cervical cancer. J Magn Reson Imaging 29:383–390

Razek AA, Megahed AS, Denewer A et al (2008) Role of diffusion-weighted magnetic resonance imaging in differentiation between the viable and necrotic parts of head and neck tumors. Acta Radiol 49:364–370

Roy C, Bierry G, Matau A et al (2010) Value of diffusion-weighted imaging to detect small malignant pelvic lymph nodes at 3T. Eur Radiol 20:1803–1811

Sakurada A, Takahaara T, Kwee TC et al (2009) Diagnostic performance of diffusion-weighted MRI in esophageal cancer. Eur Radiol 19:1461–1469

Schafer J, Srinivasan A, Mukherji S (2011) Diffusion magnetic resonance imaging in the head and neck. Magn Reson Imaging Clin N Am 19(1):55–67

Shen-Ping YU, Li H, Bo L et al (2010) Differential diagnosis of metastasis from non-metastatic lymph nodes in cervical cancers: pilot study of diffusion weighted imaging with background suppression at 3T magnetic resonance. Chin Med J 123(20):2820–2824

Smoker W, Gentry L, Yee N, Reede D, Nerad J (2008) Vascular lesions of the orbit: more than meets the eye. Radiographics 28:185–204

Srinivasan A, Dvorak R, Perni K et al (2008) Differentiation of benign and malignant pathology in the head and neck using 3T apparent diffusion coefficient values: early experience. Am J Neuroradiol 29:40–44

Sumi M, Nakamura T (2009) Diagnostic importance of focal defects in the apparent diffusion coefficient-based differentiation between lymphoma and squamous cell carcinoma nodes in the neck. Eur Radiol 19(4):975–981

Sumi M, Takagi Y, Uetani M et al (2002) Diffusion-weighted echoplanar MR imaging of the salivary glands. Am J Roentgenol 178(4):959–965

Sumi M, Sakihama N, Sumi T et al (2003) Discrimination of metastatic cervical Lymph Nodes with diffusion-weighted MR Imaging in patients with head and neck cancer. Am J Neuroradiol 24:1627–1634

Tshering Vogel DW, Zbaeren P et al (2010) Cancer of the oral cavity and oropharynx. Cancer Imaging 16(10):62–72

Tucker T, Friedman JM, Friedrich RE et al (2009) Longitudinal study of neurofibromatosis 1 associated plexiform neurofibromas. J Med Genet 46(2):81–85

Vandecaveye V, Dirix P, De Keyzer F et al (2010) Predictive value of diffusion-weighted magnetic resonance imaging during chemoradiotherapy for head and neck squamous cell carcinoma. Eur Radiol 20(7):1703–1714

Vandecaveye V, De Keyzer F, Hermans R (2008) Diffusion-weighted magnetic resonance imaging in neck lymph adenopathy. Cancer Imaging 8:173–180; 6(2): 81–85

Vandecaveye V, De Keyzer F, Nuyts S et al (2007) Detection of head and neck squamous cell carcinoma with diffusion weighted MRI after (chemo)radiotherapy: correlation between radiologic and histopathologic findings. Int J Radiat Oncol Biol Phys 67:960–971

Wang J, Takashima S, Takayama F et al (2001) Head and neck lesions: characterization with diffusion-weighted echoplanar MR imaging. Radiology 220:621–630

Yabuuchi H, Matsuo Y, Kamitani T et al (2008) Parotid gland tumors: can addition of diffusion-weighted MR imaging to dynamic contrast-enhanced MR imaging improve diagnostic accuracy in characterization? Radiology 249:909–916

Yasui O, Sato M, Kamada A (2009) Diffusion-weighted imaging in the detection of lymph node metastasis in colorectal cancer. Tohoku J Exp Med 218(3):177–183

Musculoskeletal Applications of DWI

15

Joan C. Vilanova, Sandra Baleato, and Elda Balliu

DWI provides complementary information to conventional morphological MRI sequences. DWI has found widespread use in neuroimaging, particularly in the diagnosis of acute brain ischemia. DWI of the musculoskeletal system shows different diffusion characteristics in normal tissues and musculoskeletal pathologies. The utility of DWI has been described for various musculoskeletal applications as bone marrow edema characterization (e.g., tumor metastasis, benign fracture, hematological diseases), bone and soft tissue tumors, infection, degenerative spondyloarthropathy, inflammatory arthropathy, and post-therapeutic monitorization. Besides, it may have a promising role in the evaluation of cartilage, intervertebral disk or bone necrosis, and musculoskeletal involvement of both oncological and non-oncological disease.

15.1 DWI Sequences

The most commonly used acquisition strategy for DWI is single-shot or multi-shot (segmented) EPI, because of its efficiency in terms of scan time. Its rapid acquisition makes this technique fast and less sensitive to patient motion, while large volume coverage is feasible. EPI usually achieves high signal-to-noise ratio (SNR) with low power deposition because several echoes are acquired after a single excitation pulse. In musculoskeletal applications, DWI-EPI sequences suffer less SNR gross geometrical distortions due to the long gradient-echo train and bone–soft tissue interfaces which are prone to susceptibility artifacts. It is necessary to use parallel imaging and the maximum gradient strength available in order to overcome these limitations. Multishot EPI allows us to reduce the susceptibility artifacts although it increases sensitivity to motion and scan time. Another approach is the use of single-shot fast-spin-echo (RARE or HASTE) sequences. These are also very fast sequences with less sensitivity to susceptibility artifacts. Their limitations are related to low SNR and blurring in phase-encoding direction. The application of PROPELLER or BLADE sequences to HASTE-DWI improves the robustness of the sequences. DWI based on SSFP sequences has also been used in the musculoskeletal system, mainly in the evaluation of the spine. This approach applies only a diffusion gradient in each TR (monopolar gradient) which leads to a diffusion weighting of consecutive echoes (spin echoes and stimulated echoes) under steady-state conditions. SSFP-DWI sequences are fast, insensitive to motion although ADC quantification is difficult. The most common one is called PSIF (reverse fast imaging with steady-state precession), which is a reversed FISP sequence. Even more, 3D DWI acquisitions have been designed for cartilage evaluation.

DWIBS technique, commonly used in whole-body diffusion approach, has shown an excellent sensitivity to detect metastases and other pathological bone marrow

J.C. Vilanova (✉)
Department of Radiology, Clínica Girona-Hospital Sta. Caterina, University of Girona, Girona, Spain
e-mail: kvilanova@comg.cat

S. Baleato
Department of Radiology, Complexo Hospitalario Universitario de Santiago, de Compostela, Spain
e-mail: baleatorum@hotmail.com

E. Balliu
Department of Radiology, Hospital Universitari Dr. J. Trueta, Girona, Spain
e-mail: eballiu@gmail.com

A. Luna et al., *Diffusion MRI Outside the Brain*,
DOI 10.1007/978-3-642-21052-5_15,

processes such as myeloma (Figs. 15.1, 16.1–16.6). This technique uses STIR to get an almost complete background suppression, although with limited SNR.

15.2 Clinical Applications

15.2.1 Bone Marrow Assessment

Bone marrow evaluation with DWI is feasible. Diffusion is greater in hematopoietic marrow than in fatty marrow and decreases in the skeleton with age. Fat content within the bone marrow increases with age and it is negatively correlated with ADC values, so fat marrow increases as ADC decreases. ADC values positively correlate with the cellularity of bone marrow, although unexpectedly, the ADC of fatty hypocellular marrow is lower than that of normal normocellular marrow of adults and hypercellular marrow of children. At a microscopic level, the large fatty cells constrain more the free diffusion of water than normal hematopoietic cells. Caution must be taken when using DWI to evaluate bone pathology in children, because areas of hypersignal are common in pelvic skeleton and lumbar spine. Increases of cells in a bone marrow without fat cells, due to bone marrow hyperplasia or tumoral infiltration, will parallely increase its signal intensity on DWI acquisitions with high *b* values and decrease its ADC values.

In spite of these complicated patterns of signal intensity variations that can be seen with different bone marrow stages, DWI has shown to be a very sensitive technique to detect bone marrow lesion, especially malignant ones, even before the morphological MRI sequences (Fig. 14.10). Even more, DWI was demonstrated to be superior to bone scintigraphy in bone metastases detection (Fig. 16.2). However, there are scarce reports of nonvertebral bone marrow to establish normal or pathological ADC values.

A potential clinical application for DWI is osteoporosis, as there is an increase in fatty marrow and a decrease in bone density and ADC values compared to normal marrow in osteoporotic patients. Although there are only a few reports in the literature and with some controversial results, DWI quantifications show the potential to help in the early identification of osteoporosis.

15.2.2 Evaluation of the Spine

The spine is a challenging anatomic region for DWI. Acquisition of robust DWI images with sufficient spatial resolution in a reasonable scan time is difficult. Artifacts can be induced by physiologic patient motion and pulsation of either the closely surrounding vasculature, or the cerebrospinal fluid. DWI EPI sequences suffer from gross geometrical distortions. Therefore, DWI SSTSE may be preferable in the spine due to better SNR and less image distortion at high *b* values.

Several reports have demonstrated that DWI provides excellent distinction between pathologic and benign vertebral fractures using a qualitative inspection (Fig. 15.2). On visual assessment, benign fractures are usually hypointense and malignant ones are hyperintense. In several series, this difference has been more obvious with the diffusion-weighted SSFP approach than with other pulse sequences. Bone metastases from prostate cancer normally present lower signal intensity than bone metastasis from other origin (Fig. 16.3). Osteosclerotic metastases also appear as hypointense areas on DWI due to their very low water content. Although ADC quantification may help in the differentiation of benign and malignant vertebral fractures, there is an overlap between the benign and malignant fractures values, which avoid the consideration of ADC values as a definitive tool in this differentiation. In a similar manner, treated bone metastases may appear low on DWI with high *b* values. The ADC values of normal vertebra range between 0.2 and 0.5×10^{-3} mm^2/s. This variation is due to different sequences and *b* values selected, and to the use, or not, of fat-saturation. Fat marrow shows a very low ADC, which decreases the ADC value of vertebrae if a fat-saturation pulse is not used. In vertebral fractures, the influence of fat decreases. Malignant fractures show lower ADC values (between 0.7 and 1×10^{-3} mm^2/s) than osteoporotic ones ($1\text{–}2 \times 10^{-3}$ mm^2/s). Inflammatory disease may show intermediate ADC values which make difficult its differentiation from other type of fracture on DWI (Fig. 15.3). Besides, there is overlap in ADC values between malignant involvement of bone marrow and tuberculosis spondylitis, as this one usually shows low ADC values (Fig. 16.1).

15.2.3 Soft-tissue Tumors

DWI may help in the differential diagnosis of soft tissue tumors as nonmyxoid malignant tumors show significantly lower ADC values than benign ones. In myxoid tumors, this differentiation is not achievable with DWI, probably due to the long T2 value of the myxoid extracellular matrix (Fig. 15.4). Even more,

DWI has demonstrated to be useful in the differentiation of chronic complicated hematomas from malignant soft tissue tumors (Fig. 15.5). In clinical practice, the differentiation of benign and malignant soft tissue tumors only based on ADC quantifications is not possible due to overlap in values between both groups, as not all malignant tumors are more cellular than benign ones and due to the influence of tumoral matrix. Besides, the use of the ADC without perfusion effect, avoiding b values under 100 mm^2/s, has been proposed in several series as a more reliable metric of diffusion than conventional ADC. This metric is called by some authors as perfusion-insensitive diffusion coefficient (PIDC). A most sophisticated approach, which has demonstrated to be feasible in the characterization of the anisotropy of the capillary network of muscle and in other organs such us liver and brain as well, would be to use the biexponential model of diffusion signal decay (IVIM approach).

In the recent and excellent review by Costa et al., a cutoff PIDC value of 1.1×10^{-3} mm^2/s was proposed to differentiate malignant from benign soft tissue tumors. Additional interesting observations in this review were: As it could be expected, small round blue cell tumors showed more restricted diffusion than the rest of malignant soft tissue tumors, specially lymphoma; abscesses and hematomas demonstrate more restricted diffusion in their central component than necrosis of malignant soft tissue tumors; both benign and malignant cartilaginous tumors show high ADC values, except mesenchymal chondrosarcoma; both subtypes of giant cell tumor, of the tendon sheath and diffuse-type, show restricted diffusion; benign and intermediate fibroblastic, myofibroblastic, and fibrohistiocytic soft tissue tumors show less restricted diffusion than malignant ones. All these data are concordant with previous literature, although due to scarce experience, they must be validated in larger series.

15.2.4 Postreatment Monitorization

DWI may become a noninvasive method for monitoring results of therapy. This diagnostic option is of great clinical interest, especially since preoperative neoadjuvant treatments, such as chemotherapy or hyperthermia, are becoming more widely applied in the musculoskeletal field. DWI may aid in therapy control, in the distinction between necrotic and viable tumor tissue and also in the differentiation between post-therapeutic soft tissue changes and tumor recurrence (Fig. 15.6). Both post-therapeutic soft tissue changes, such as hygromas and edematous or inflammatory changes after radiation therapy, and inflammatory changes, such as osteomyelitis, show a strong signal loss with increasing diffusion strength. The signal loss is significantly higher in post-therapeutic tissue changes than in viable tumor.

DWI has also been used to evaluate patients with osteosarcomas after chemotherapy, as the cellular necrosis induced by the treatment occurs before changes in volume and it is detectable with DWI. In a series by Oka and colleagues, ADC values of these tumors with less than 90% of necrosis after treatment (poor response group) demonstrated a mean increase of 25%, compared with the responding group (tumors with at least 90% necrosis after treatment) with a mean increase of ADC values of 95%. Minimal ADC values were significantly different between both groups, although this difference was not confirmed for mean ADC values. DWI has also allowed monitoring of anti-androgen therapy in bone metastases from prostate cancer. PSA level decrease corresponded well with an increase in mean ADC. Posttreatment monitorization of myeloma patients with bone involvement by means of DWI is probably feasible, as ADC values in patients with low M-component after successful therapy are significantly higher than in patients with high paraprotein levels, typically found in patients with acute recurrence. In treated myeloma and lymphoma, massive liquefactive necrosis in bone lesions may occur, increasing the signal intensity and ADC values of bone marrow, sometimes in a persistent manner, and others with a heterogeneous distribution, showing a predominantly high signal on ADC maps interspersed with areas of low ADC values. All these patterns suggest inactive disease. In a similar manner, DWI increases soon after chemotherapy in soft tissue sarcoma patients with successful response and decreased ADC correlates with lack of response and increase in tumor size. Posttreatment monitorization of inflammatory or degenerative diseases is also a potential benefit of DWI (Fig. 15.7).

The assessment of response to treatment may be performed using a qualitative or a quantitative approach. Visual assessment is easy to perform and works well for bone marrow in a majority of cases. This approach is the most commonly used in clinical practice for myeloma or bone metastasis patients evaluated with WB-DWI. Limitations of this approach are the presence of some potential pitfalls such as: the presence of edema after radiotherapy or surgery that can increase signal intensity of bone marrow on DWI or visualization of normal hypercellular structures. The use of ADC measurements and MRI morphological sequences can minimize these pitfalls. Another problematic scenario is the use of granulocyte-colony stimulating factor which is used along with chemotherapy to limit the appearance of neutropenia. This drug increases red bone marrow in the axial skeleton, which should not be interpreted as disease progression in oncological patients with bone lesions. Furthermore, the assessment of response to treatment in bone marrow with DWI is complex, as bone sclerosis and the increase of yellow marrow may occur at the same time, as recently pointed by Padhani and Koh. Both mechanisms, along with necrosis, apoptosis, and myelofibrosis, induce reductions of signal intensity on DWI and decrease of ADC value, which represent in fact a favorable response and not disease progression. This pattern is common in successfully treated breast and prostate carcinoma metastasis. These reductions in ADC value may also be detected in normal bone marrow due to the effect of cytotoxic drugs. Similarly, normal bone marrow also shows fatty atrophy secondarily to radiotherapy decreasing its signal on DWI with high *b* values.

15.2.5 Infection and Inflammation

Differentiating osteomyelitis from osseous tumors can be challenging, as osteomyelitis may display increased diffusion with low ADC values, mimicking malignancy (Figs. 15.8 and 15.9). The role of DWI in osteomyelitis is controversial, due to the overlap between ADC values of malignancy and infectious diseases.

DWI has been used for the detection of active inflammatory changes in the sacroiliac joints of patients with early axial spondyloarthritis; and also for early detection of rheumatoid arthritis (Fig. 15.10). In a report, ADC values in patients with sacroiliitis were significantly higher than those in patients with low back pain of mechanical origin. It was concluded that DWI may help to discern normal from involved subchondral bone. Other recently published reports have shown that DWI is an effective technique in quantifying changes in inflammation in skeletal lesions during the treatment of ankylosing spondylitis. The decrease in ADC values correlated with the effectiveness of treatment according to clinical and laboratory parameters, indicating the usefulness of DWI to assess treatment efficacy.

15.2.6 Bone Ischemia and Trauma

DWI also offers potential to assess the presence of avascular necrosis and posttraumatic bone bruise (Fig 13.8). While T2-weighted fat-suppressed images are commonly used to identify bone bruises, they may not be able to evaluate the severity of bone trauma. In fact, DWI can be used as a prognostic marker of skeletal ischemia before gross anatomic changes occur. It seems to be important to define the correct inclusion criteria for using DWI when trying to discern benign from malignant fractures. Acute fractures may be suitable for DWI before soft callus grows and diffusivity decreases. In cases of malignancy, therapy effects may lead to increased diffusivity. Therefore, DWI should be performed early in treatment, before therapy-related increase of diffusivity occurs and DWI results become false-negative.

15.2.7 Cartilage

A 3D-PSIR sequence has been used in the evaluation of cartilage, although it does not permit a quantitative measurement. In patients with matrix-associated autologous chondrocyte implantation, the diffusion was more restricted immediately after the surgery than in the late postoperative period. DWI may be included in multiparametric analysis of cartilage in the near future.

15.3 New Approaches to DWI of the Musculoskeletal System

Work remains to be done to test different types of optimized diffusion-weighted pulse sequences in musculoskeletal imaging. A new area of research is the application of the bicompartmental model of diffusion to the musculoskeletal system. This approach allows the separation of microcirculatory blood flow from molecular diffusion since both contribute to the random motion of water and the diffusion. For this purpose, different low *b* values should be applied in order to separate perfusion from diffusion and to overcome this effect. Multidirectional application of diffusion by means of diffusion tensor imaging (DTI) has shown to provide detailed information on muscle structural and functional changes (Fig. 4.6). DTI may have a role for visualizing muscle tears. Although, currently not universally applied, these applications of DWI offer great potential to enhance the diagnostic utility of MRI in musculoskeletal radiology.

Case 15.1: Bone Plasmacytoma

A 67-year-old male presented with right hip pain. MRI was indicated for further evaluation.

Comments

Plasmacytomas are malignant neoplasms characterized by the uncontrolled proliferation of cells of the immune system known as plasma cells. Solitary plasmacytoma (SP) represent only around 5% of plasma cell neoplasia. There are two main clinical presentations: solitary bone plasmacytoma (SBP) with a single bone lesion and solitary extramedullary plasmacytoma (SEP) with a soft tissue mass.

Clinical features of SBP are a median age of presentation of 55 years, that is, 7–10 years less than multiple myeloma (MM), a male to female ratio of 2:1, and a predominant axial skeleton involvement, especially of vertebrae. Plasmacytomas most commonly occur as an expansile lytic mass in the ribs, spine, pelvis, skull, and sacrum.

The relationship of SBP to multiple myeloma is controversial. Many authors believe that SBP is an early stage of a multiple myeloma, whereas others consider it as a distinct clinical entity. Recommendations on the diagnosis and management of SBP have been recently published by the Guidelines Working Group of the UK Myeloma Forum. Criteria for SBP are:

- Single area of bone destruction due to clonal plasma cells
- Normal marrow without clonal disease
- Normal results on a skeletal survey and MRI of the spine, pelvis, proximal femora, and humeri
- No anemia, hypercalcemia, or renal impairment attributable to myeloma
- Absent or low serum or urinary level of monoclonal protein and preserved levels of uninvolved immunoglobulins
- No additional lesions on MRI scan of the spine

Radiographic findings include a lytic, expansile osseous mass with possible soft tissue involvement. CT is the technique of choice to evaluate the extension of destruction of trabecular and cortical bone and to assess stability and fracture risk.

Bone scintigraphy, using 99m Tc-labeled bisphosphonates, is insensitive to diffuse or focal myeloma because there is no increased osteoblastic activity. 18-FDG-PET detects tumors according to their glucose demand. A recent study confirms that 18-FDG-PET can play a useful role in the evaluation of patients with solitary plasmacytoma who are candidates for definitive radiotherapy (RT) or who have been treated with RT.

MRI visualizes focal or diffuse myeloma infiltration of the marrow with high sensitivity and specificity. MRI might detect additional abnormalities and it has been reported that apparent SBP is considered as MM after a positive MRI scanning of the spine. Consequently, with present criteria of diagnosis including MRI scanning, the prognosis of SBP has improved in recent series. Differential diagnosis includes solitary metastasis and primary lymphoma of bone.

The role of DW-MRI for the assessment of disease in patients with myeloma has not been established; whole-body MRI provides a more detailed assessment of the pattern of bone marrow infiltration and strongly influences therapeutic strategies.

DCE–MRI in patients with bone marrow infiltration with myeloma has been used to detect and monitor changes in bone marrow microcirculation as a result of myeloma-induced angiogenesis and blood vessel permeability.

While the majority of patients with solitary plasmacytoma of bone develop myeloma after a median of 2–3 years, the overall median survival of 7–12 years is longer than that for patients diagnosed in the early phases of symptomatic myeloma.

Imaging Findings

Fig. 15.1 Frontal plain radiography of the pelvis (**15.1.1**) shows a lytic lesion in right iliac bone with cortical bone destruction. Anterior whole-body 99m with Technetium 99m images (**15.1.2**) reveals increased activity on both hip joints suggestive of inflammatory activity and a mild increased activity of the right iliac bone which is nonspecific. CT of the pelvis in soft tissue and bone windows, respectively, (**15.1.3**) confirms a rounded lytic lesion of the ilium with cortical disruption and soft tissue mass. Axial fat-suppressed FSE T2-weighted image (**15.1.4**) shows the infiltration of the soft tissue mass within the bone, and the presence of edema in the ilium. Coronal DWI of the pelvis (**15.1.5**) shows the high signal intensity of the tumor due to restricted diffusion

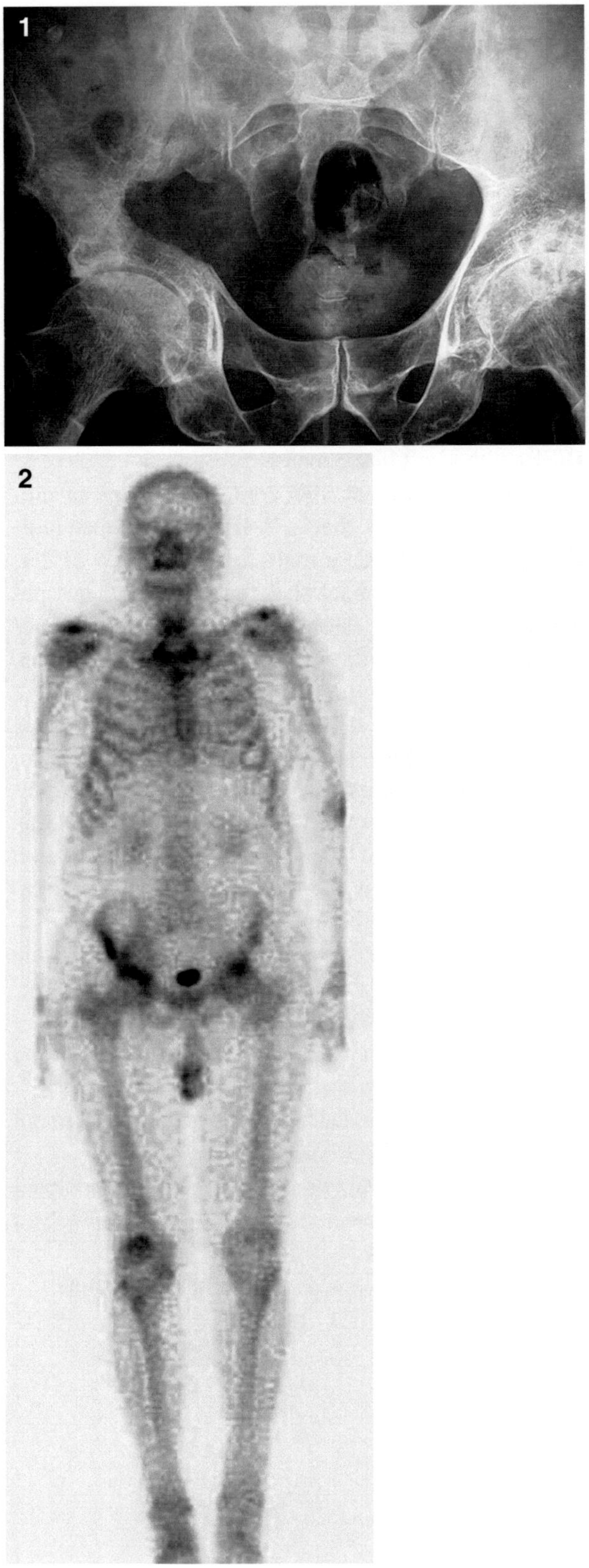

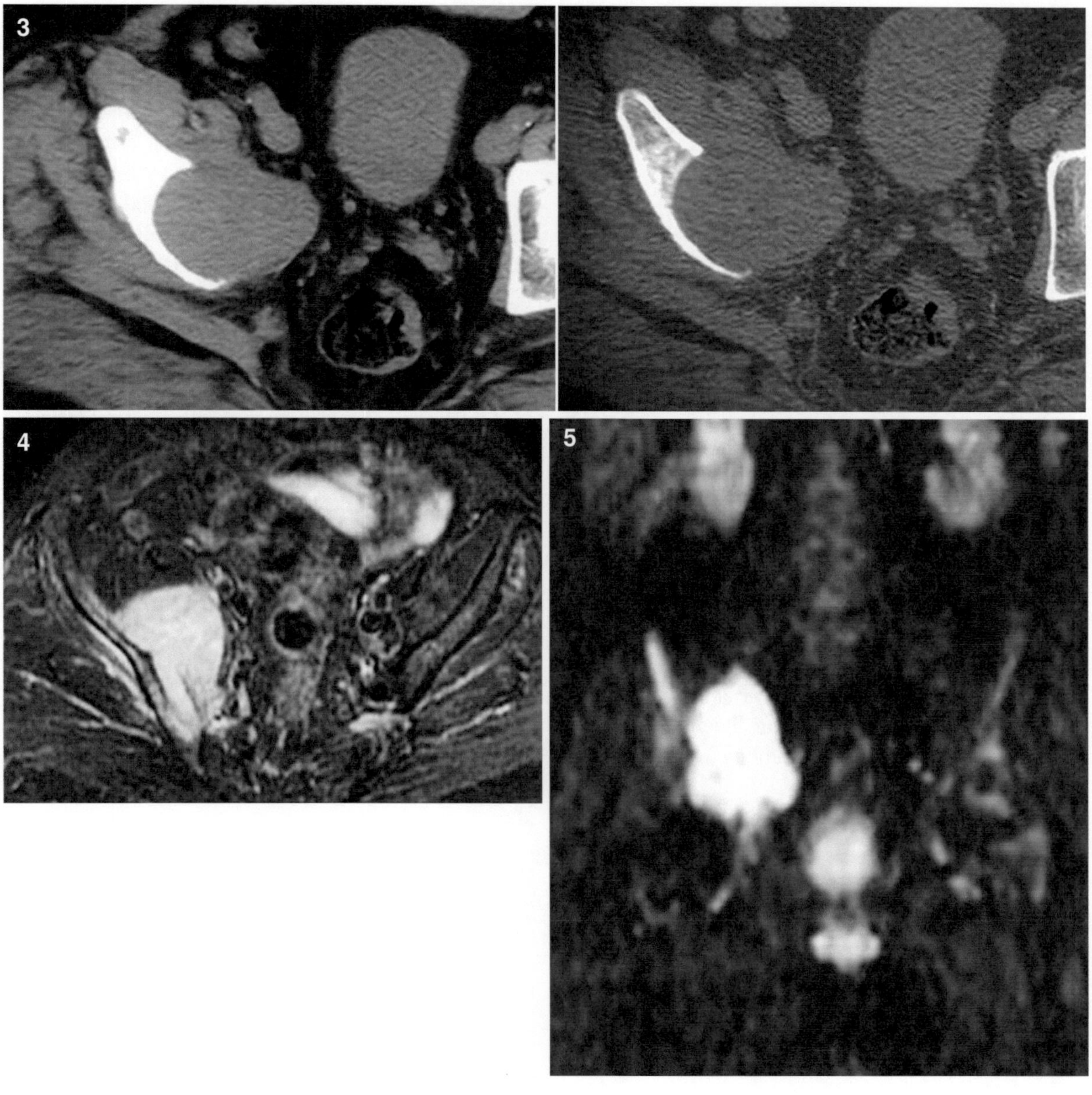

Fig. 15.1 (continued)

Case 15.2: Benign Vertebral Fracture

A 70-year-old male with a previous history of lung cancer. Bone scintigraphy revealed a doubtful metastasis at L1 level. MRI is requested to rule out metastases.

Comments

Skeletal metastases represent the most common malignant bone tumor. They occur mainly in adults and more frequently in the elderly. The most common metastases in men are those from prostate cancer (60%) and in women from breast cancer (70%). Clinical evaluation of patients with skeletal metastases needs of multimodal diagnostic imaging, by means of techniques capable to detect lesions, to assess their extension and localization, and eventually drive the biopsy (for histomorphological diagnosis).

Traditional imaging methods used in the detection and evaluation of metastatic bone disease lack either sensitivity (plain radiography) or specificity (bone scintigraphy). Currently, MRI has been shown to be the most sensitive imaging technique available for the detection of bone metastases.

Both osteoporotic and malignant vertebral collapses are frequent in elderly patients. In oncological patients, differentiation between acute benign and malignant vertebral fractures may sometimes be difficult, but it is important to distinguish it for different therapeutic managements.

On T1-weighted images, bone metastases tend to stand out as focal or diffuse hypointense lesions against a background of higher-signal-intensity bone marrow. Use of fat-suppressed FSE T2-weighted STIR techniques may further increase the conspicuity of metastatic lesions. Using conventional MRI (T1-weighted, T2-weighted and STIR sequences) and CT, it is frequently difficult to determine whether a collapsed vertebral body is the result of a metastatic or benign process.

Malignant solitary vertebral collapse tends to have an ill-defined margin, abnormal signal involvement of the pedicle, a marked and heterogeneous MRI enhancement pattern, and irregular nodular type paravertebral soft tissue lesions.

DWI has been shown to be useful to distinguish acute benign fractures from malignant or infectious bone lesions. Although ADC values of benign edema tend to be higher than those in malignant lesions, ADC values are not useful in order to differentiate malignancy from infection.

MRI is also useful to image the spine, vertebral bodies, paraspinal, and intraspinal soft tissues within the same examination, thus providing a noninvasive method to detect spinal cord compression.

Imaging Findings

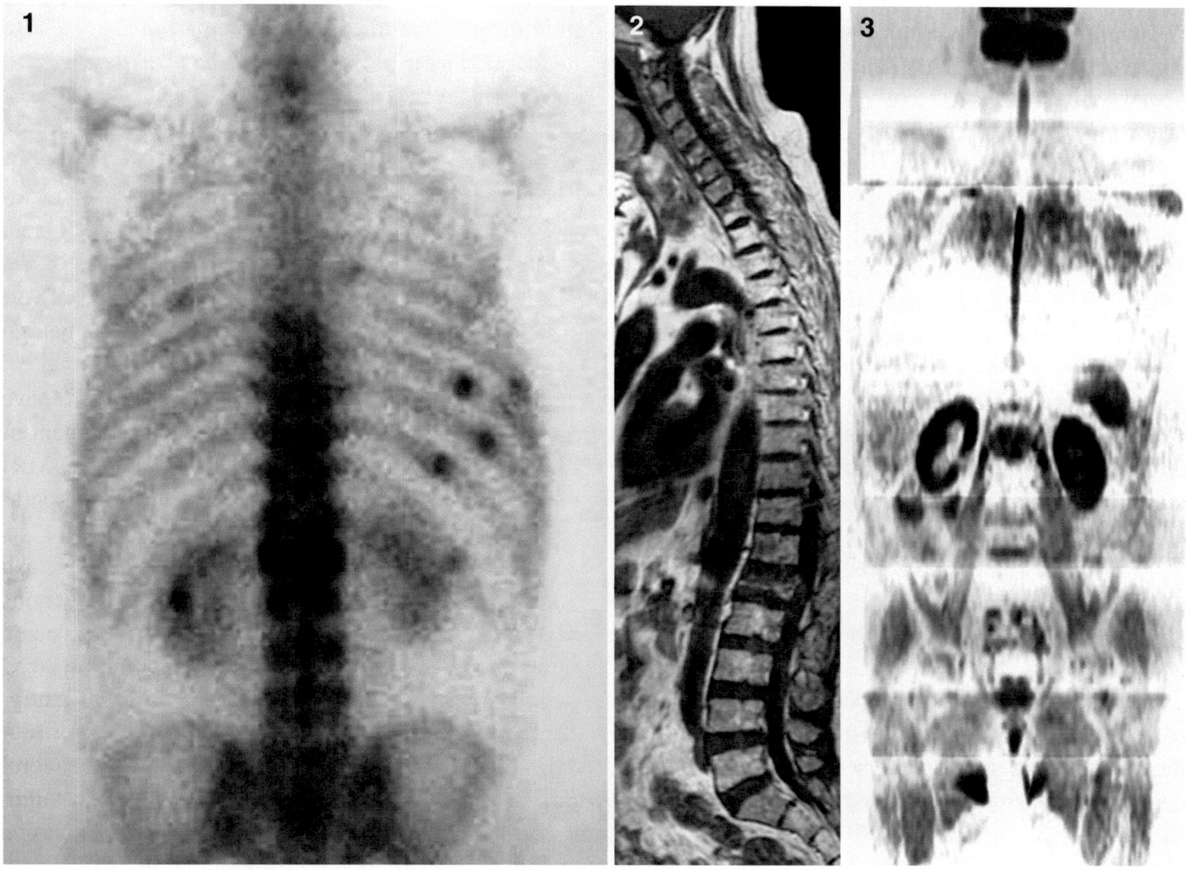

Fig. 15.2 Skeletal scintigram (**15.2.1**) shows increased tracer uptake within L1 vertebral body suggestive for metastasis (there is also uptake of several left ribs due to previous left rib fractures). Sagittal T1-weighted SE image (**15.2.2**) shows collapsed vertebral body with slight hypointense signal related to normal bone marrow at L1 level. Coronal MIP of the inverted gray scale DWI (**15.2.3**) shows low signal within L1 vertebral body. ADC value of the lesion was high (1.63×10^{-3} mm^2/s), consistent with a benign origin

Case 15.3: Spondylodiscitis

A 78-year-old-male presented with cervical pain and disturbances at swallowing. He had a previous history of larynx cancer.

Comments

The axial skeleton is frequently the site of septic osteomyelitis. However, other noninfectious conditions can simulate spinal infection. Infectious spondylodiscitis represents 4–7% of all cases of osteomyelitis. In the adult patient, the classic clinical features are back pain associated with fever, malaise, weight loss, and anorexia. Although neurologic deficits may occur later on in the disease process, they are not usually part of its early manifestation.

The lumbar spine is most frequently involved, (50% of cases) followed in frequency by the thoracic spine (35%). Cervical and sacral spine involvements are the least common ones.

A spinal infection may become established by hematogenous spread from distant septic foci, direct inoculation from spinal surgery or penetrating trauma, or direct extension from septic foci in adjacent soft tissues.

The most common infecting microorganism is *Staphylococcus aureus* (55–80% of cases). Granulomatous infections originated from *Mycobacterium tuberculosis*; brucellosis, fungi, and parasites are less common.

MRI is a powerful diagnostic tool that can be used to help evaluate spinal infection and distinguish between an infection and other clinical condition. MRI has a reported sensitivity of 96% and an accuracy of 94% in vertebral infections. Each part of the vertebra including the posterior elements, the disk, the epidural space, and the perivertebral soft tissues can be affected. Imaging findings associated with spinal infection include:

- Severe edema within the bone marrow of two vertebrae adjacent to the involved disk.
- Disk space narrowing. The signal intensity of the disk is reduced on T1-weighted images and is usually high on T2-weighted and STIR sequences. After contrast material administration, infected disks almost invariably enhance.
- Erosion or destruction of the vertebral endplates on T1-weighted images.
- Evidence of either paraspinal or epidural inflammatory tissue.

Sometimes when the manifestations of infection are atypical and the patient has a previous history of neoplasia, differentiation between metastasis and infection is not obvious. Infectious spondylitis and neoplastic disease can both cause alterations in the cortical or medullary bone and paravertebral soft tissues. DWI sequence is a new powerful tool for diagnosis of diseases which involve alterations in water mobility. In bone marrow, DWI has been proven to be a highly useful method for differentiating benign from malignant fractures. Unfortunately, several reports have demonstrated that DWI cannot distinguish between malignant and infectious processes as in both conditions, water diffusion is restricted and ADC values are low.

Imaging Findings

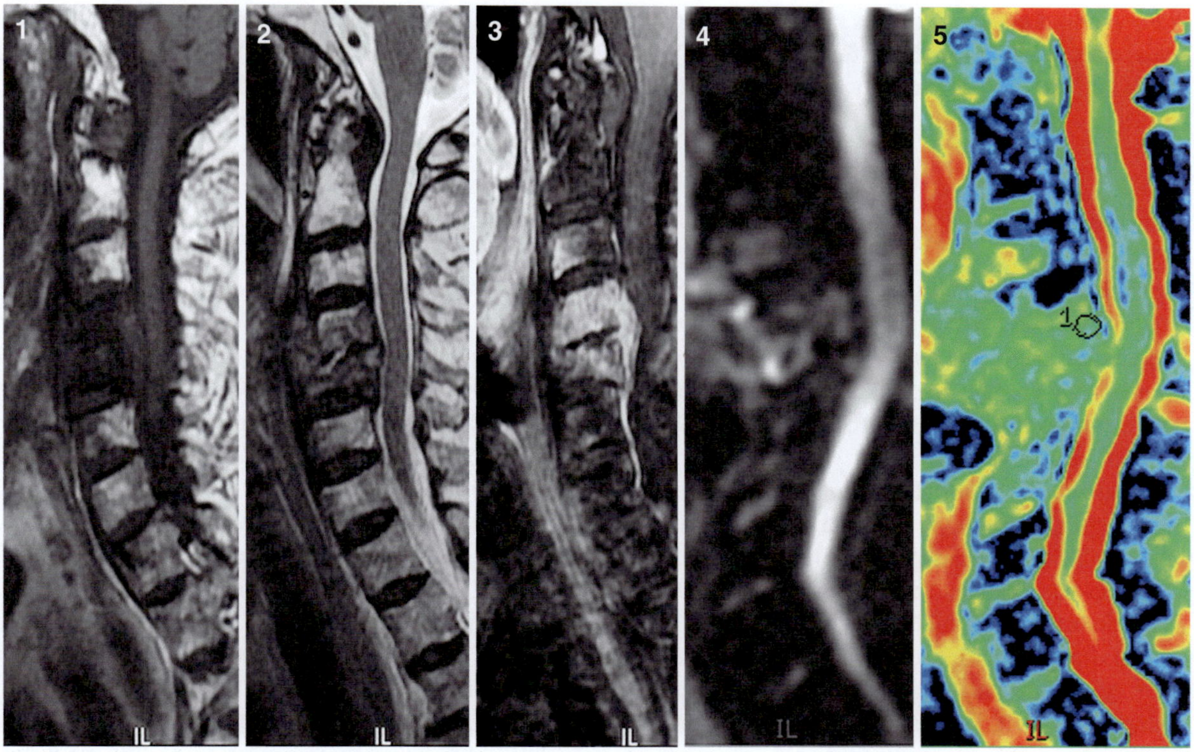

Fig. 15.3 Two contiguous vertebrae (C4 and C5) are involved showing low signal intensity on sagittal FSE T1-weighted images (**15.3.1**). The corresponding sagittal FSE T2-weighted images (**15.3.2**) show patchy hypointensity signal within C4 and C5 vertebrae bodies with anterior wedging of C5. The signal intensity of the disk is low in both sequences. Sagittal fat-suppressed FSE T1-weighted image after gadolinium injection (**15.3.3**) reveals marked enhancement within the vertebral bodies and a posterior soft tissue mass narrowing the spinal canal. Note that patients with spondylitis of cervical spine do have an increased risk for devastating complications including paraplegia or tetraplegia by the decreased ratio of the subarachnoid space to the volume of the spinal cord. Sagittal DWI (**15.3.4**) at a *b* value of 700 s/mm^2 shows high signal intensity representing restricted diffusion, which is confirmed with a low ADC value of 0.9×10^3 s/mm^2 (represented for *blue* and *green color* within the ROI) (**15.3.5**). Although, this low value can be also due to malignancy, in this case it represented infection

Case 15.4: Liposclerosing Myxofibrous Tumor

A 50-year-old male patient was diagnosed of a chondrosarcoma of the right distal femur. A PET-CT was requested for staging, which showed a suspected metastasis to the proximal left femur.

Comments

Liposclerosing myxofibrous tumor of bone (LSMFT) is a benign lesion with a complex histologic structure of uncertain origin and possibly related to intraosseous lipomas and fibrous dysplasia. Differential diagnosis between both entities based on pathological findings may not be possible.

Histologically LSMFT is characterized by a complex mixture of histologic elements, which may include lipoma, fibroxanthoma, myxoma, myxofibroma, fibrous dysplasia-like features, cyst formation, fat necrosis, ischemic ossification, and, rarely, cartilage.

The designation of "sclerosing" refers to the presence of intralesional bone formed or mineralized within altered fat. The term "myxofibrous" refers to the presence of fibrous or myxofibrous areas.

LSMFT has a relatively characteristic radiologic appearance and skeletal distribution. It is usually located in femur (85% of cases) with predilection for the intertrochanteric region. The age range is broad, usually adults. The tumors probably arise in childhood. Their appearance may evolve slowly over time. These lesions are usually incidental findings (40%) in asymptomatic patients. However, most patients present with pain (50%) and a lower percentage of patients present with pathologic fractures (10%).

Plain film shows a lytic, geographic, and well-defined lesion with a sclerotic margin. In some cases, mineralized matrix can be seen inside the lesion or a mild expansile remodeling. Both CT and MRI might not identify lipomatous tissue into the lesion, probably due to the small amount of fat and the abundance of myxofibrous tissue and fibro-osseous tissues.

On CT, areas of low attenuation values might be seen due to the presence of myxoid tissue, marginal sclerosis, and irregular globular mineralized matrix. On MRI, LSMFT is a well-defined lesion, hyperintense on T2-weighted sequences due to the myxoid content and it usually has a sclerotic rim.

The differential diagnosis of this lesion should include fibrous dysplasia and intraosseous lipoma. Usually CT and MRI can identify fat tissue within a lipoma. In some cases, the intraosseus lipoma may suffer involutional changes and the differential diagnosis on imaging is not possible. Fibrous dysplasia presents an intermediate or low signal on T2 MRI and minor sclerosis compared with LSMFT, but radiological distinction sometimes remains difficult.

Bone scintigrams usually reveal a mild or moderate tracer activity as occurs in patients with fibrous dysplasia. On PET imaging, benign bone lesions (i.e., fibrous dysplasia) typically do not show increased uptake of 18-FDG but in some cases, these lesions have an increased activity and may be confused with a malignant tumor or a metastasis.

DWI allows quantitative assessment of water diffusion in tissues. Malignant lesions show restricted diffusion due to higher cellularity and benign myxoid lesions show higher water diffusion. DWI with ADC map allows to differentiating metastases from benign myxoid tumors.

Asymptomatic patients may not need treatment. Treatment includes: curettage, bone grafting, or fixation. If pathological fractures occur, joint arthroplasty is required.

The image findings and the location of LSMFT are characteristic and almost allow a specific diagnosis by imaging, whereas on pathology or PET scans might mimic other lesions and even malignancy.

Imaging Findings

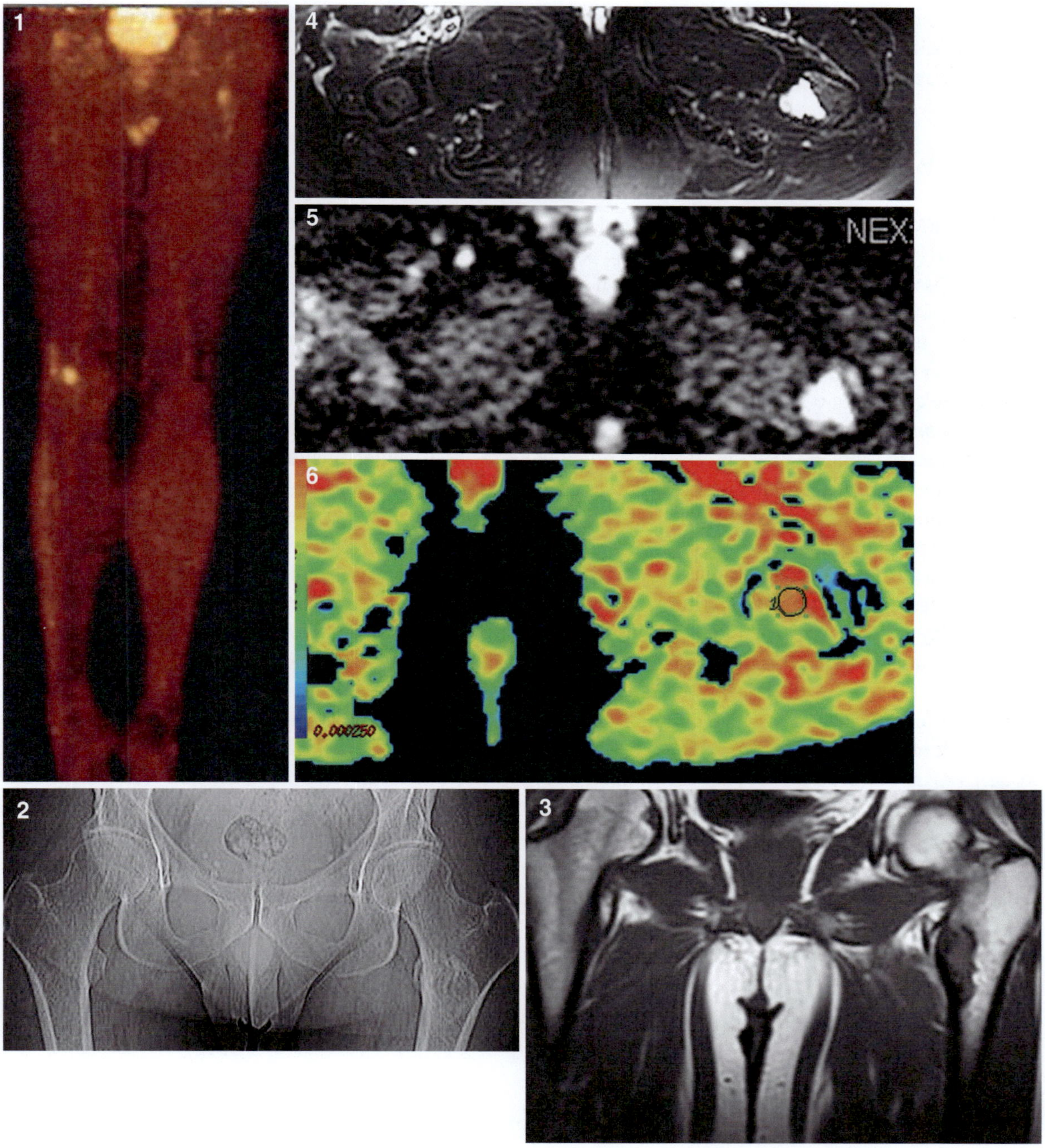

Fig. 15.4 PEC-CT (**15.4.1**) shows an increased activity in the distal metaphysis of right femur corresponding to the primary chondrosarcoma and a mild focal increased activity in the intertrochanteric region of left femur, suggestive of metastasis from primary chondrosarcoma. Plain film of the pelvis (**15.4.2**) shows a geographic lesion with well-defined sclerotic margin in the proximal left femur, centrally located in the intramedullary space, just above the lesser trochanter. The cortex appears intact without signs of cortical rupture. Coronal FSE T1-weighted image (**15.4.3**) shows intermediate signal intensity of the lesion. Axial fat-suppressed FSE T2-weighted image (**15.4.4**) reveals a high signal lesion with a well-defined margin, "the sclerotic rim," without internal fatty content. Axial DWI (**15.4.5**) demonstrates high signal intensity from the lesion within the left femur with high ADC value (2.14×10^{-3} mm^2/s) on the parametric map (**15.4.6**), represented with red color, and consistent with a benign tumor. High signal intensity on DWI with high *b* value, without low ADC value, was due to T2 shine-through effect

Case 15.5: Chronic Popliteal Cyst

A 71-year-old male referred pain on the popliteal fossa of the left knee. On inspection, there was a hard mass. No fever was referred.

Comments

A wide variety of masses may be visualized in the popliteal fossa of the knee. Differential diagnosis includes: lipoma, chronic hematoma, popliteal artery aneurysm, and other solid masses. Although, the most frequently encountered posterior knee mass is a popliteal cyst. This lesion most commonly goes through the capsule into the gastrocnemius-semimembranosus bursa, called Baker's cyst. It may extend in any direction, or rupture. Other cystic lesions might be found in other locations within the popliteal fossa.

Ultrasound is the imaging technique of choice to confirm the presence of a popliteal cyst and to allow to localizing and defining the extension of the cyst. While most popliteal cysts are small and asymptomatic, an expansile cyst may cause symptoms either by compression of adjacent structures or occasionally due to rupture or leakage. An enlarged cyst might extend in any direction. Popliteal cysts can rupture, allowing synovial fluid to dissect down the calf between the gastrocnemius and soleus, setting up an inflammatory process that can simulate deep venous thrombosis or even a neoplasm. It is important to early diagnose a ruptured Baker's cyst and to differentiate it from thrombophlebitis, a popliteal aneurysm, tumor, or muscle tear to determine the best treatment and avoid complications such as compartment syndrome.

MRI is the technique of choice to confirm the cystic nature of these lesions, to determine the correct etiology and diagnosis, to demonstrate associated internal derangement, and to identify the anatomical relationship to the joint and surrounding structures.

Popliteal cysts have a high water content and on MRI exhibit the typical signal features of fluid, hypointense on T1- weighted images, intermediate signal on proton density images, and hyperintense relative to the signal intensity of skeletal muscle on T2-weighted spin-echo, T2*-gradient-echo, and STIR images. Popliteal cysts may be septated and contain debris or loose bodies. Calcified loose bodies may arise in the knee joint due to trauma, an arthropathy, or synovial osteochondromatosis.

Popliteal cysts normally show peripheral wall enhancement as they are lined by synovium. If a central or irregular nodular gadolinium enhancement is present, it is necessary to exclude a synovial tumor.

DWI has been successful in the distinction of pus-like fluid collection from serous fluid in the brain, liver, and spine. DWI and ADC maps are robust MRI techniques that can be used for characterizing the water component and viscosity within the pathological tissue. Serous and pure water-like necrosis shows active water diffusion and a high ADC value. Conversely, purulent and pus-like fluid shows restricted water diffusion and a low ADC value due to the high viscosity and cellularity of the pus content. However, DWI should not be used as a stand-alone technique and should be combined with conventional and cross-sectional imaging techniques as an abscess may mimic a soft tissue tumor on DWI.

Imaging Findings

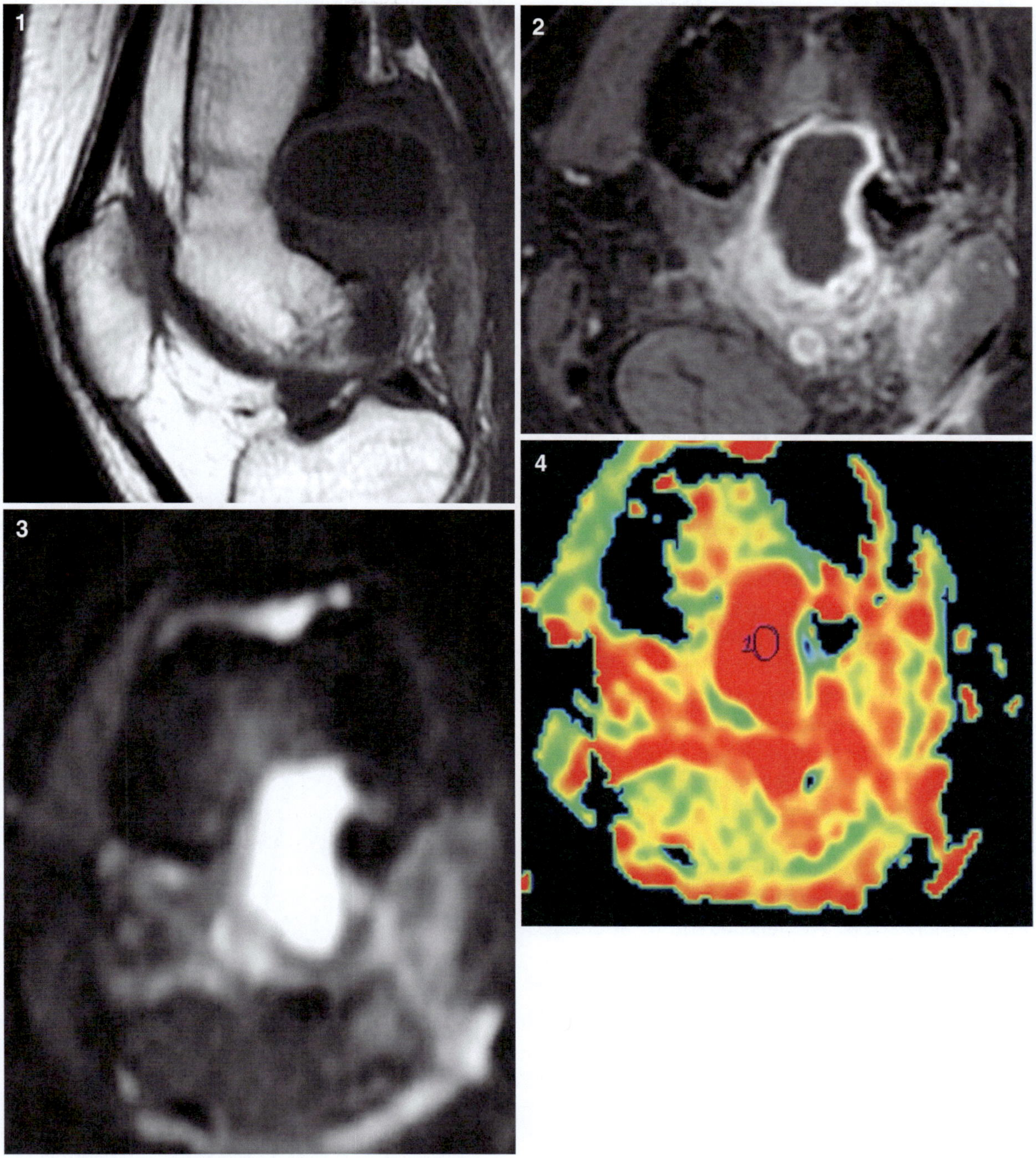

Fig. 15.5 Sagittal FSE T1-weighted image (**15.5.1**) demonstrates a hypointense lesion in the popliteal fossa with slight hyperintense margins. After gadolinium administration (**15.5.2**) peripheral enhancement is present on axial fat-suppressed FSE T1-weighted sequence. Axial DWI image (**15.5.3**) at a *b* value of 800 s/mm^2 shows a high signal intensity mass which could represent an abscess. However, the corresponding ADC map (**15.5.4**) reveals a high ADC value: 2.69×10^{-3} s/mm^2. Surgery demonstrated a noninfectious chronic fluid collection

Case 15.6: Recurrent Malignant Soft Tissue Tumor

A 76-year-old female presented with a soft tissue tumor in the Achilles tendon region. Past medical history was significant for a soft tissue low-grade leiomyosarcoma (T1, N0, M0) in the Achilles tendon region, diagnosed 5 years earlier, which was surgically treated with complete resection.

Comments

MRI is the method of choice in the diagnosis and follow-up of soft tissue tumors. The weakness of MRI is still its low specificity. After surgery or radiation of malignant soft tissue tumors, there is oftenly a marked change of signal in the adjacent normal tissue, due to edema or inflammation. With conventional MRI sequences, it can be difficult to distinguish tumor recurrences from post-therapeutic changes.

DWI sequence provides functional and microscopic information to supplement the static and macroscopic information provided by conventional sequences, because it reflects the random movement of water molecules. DWI may help in the differentiation between post-therapeutic soft tissue changes from viable tumor. It is due to the fact that tumors and post-therapeutic soft tissues changes have a different underlying tissue composition and water-proton distribution.

Up to now, only a few studies have evaluated the detection and differentiation of recurrence of solid soft tissue tumors and post-therapeutic soft tissue changes using DWI. The most common type of sequence employed has been a SSFP one, with very good image quality and short acquisition time, although they do not allow a quantitative evaluation.

Other types of DWI sequences allow the calculation of ADC, showing separation in values between recurrence and post-therapeutic soft tissue changes. Lesions with high cellularity, as recurrent tumors, present reduced diffusion of free water and therefore low ADC values. Conversely, lesions with low cellularity, as post-therapeutic soft tissue changes (inflammatory reactions after radiation therapy and hygromas) show higher values. Besides, preliminary data suggests that DWI may be useful to differentiate viable from necrotic tumors. Recently, some authors have investigated DWI as a tool to monitor response to therapy in patients with soft tissue tumors. Further studies with large series are necessary to confirm these affirmations.

Imaging Findings

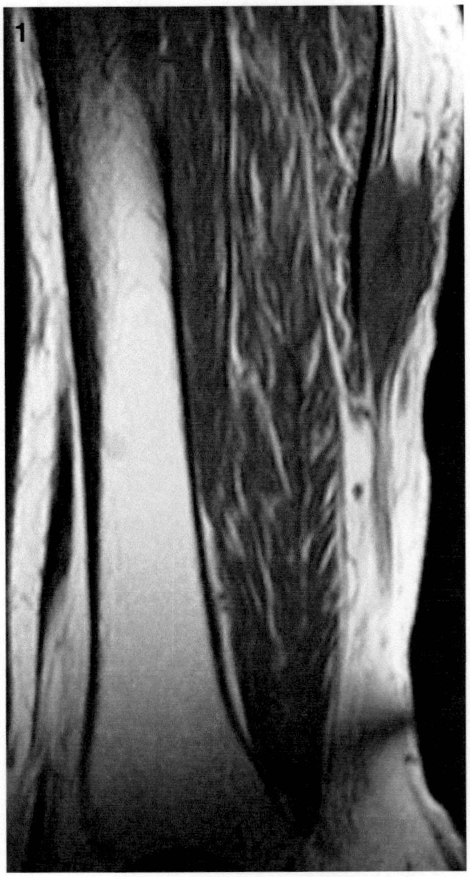

Fig. 15.6 Sagittal TSE T1-weighted (**15.6.1**), axial TSE T2-weighted (**15.6.2**), and axial postcontrast fat-suppressed TSE T1-weighted images (**15.6.3**) show a subcutaneous recurrent leiomyosarcoma. The gray scale ADC map on the sagittal plane (**15.6.4**) shows low signal of the lesion due to restricted diffusion (*arrow*). The ADC value was 0.9×10^{-3} mm²/s

Fig. 15.6 (continued)

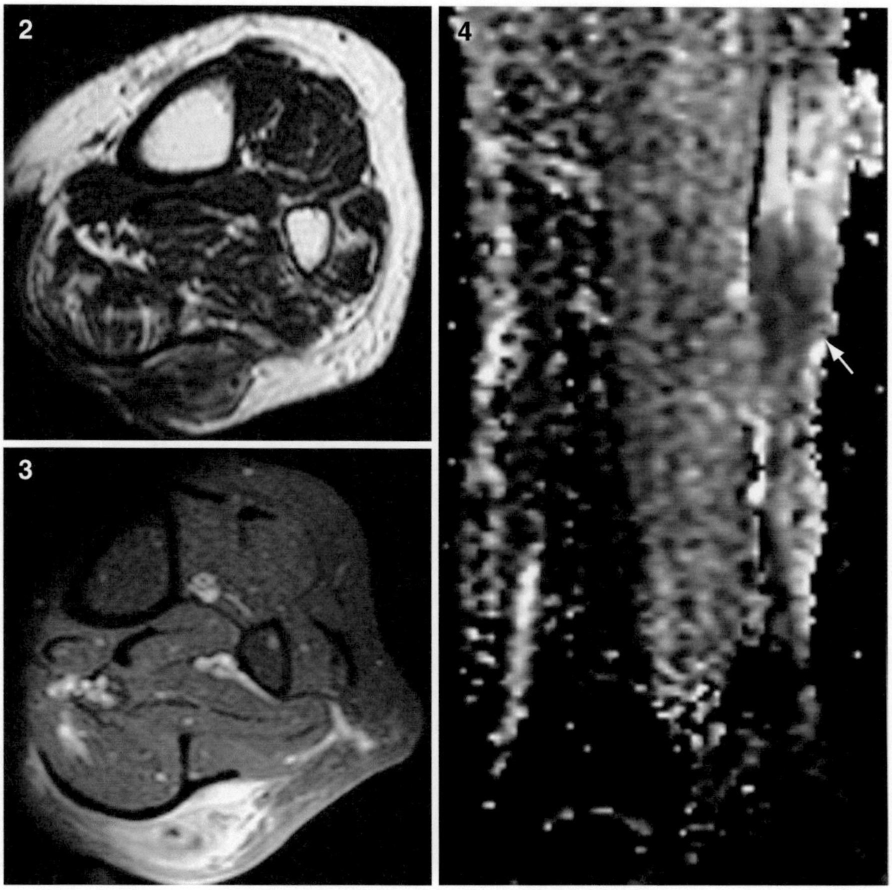

Case 15.7: Postsurgical Follow-up of Degenerative Disk Disease

A 37-year-old female presented with back pain for several years, which prevented her from normal life. Surgery was performed previously to solve instability from the lumbar spine. No symptoms were present immediately after surgery. Although 2 years after the procedure, the patient referred recurrent back pain.

Comments

Degenerative disease of the spine includes a wide spectrum of degenerative abnormalities. Degenerative changes of the spine may involve the disk space, the facet joints, or the supportive and surrounding soft tissues. Degenerative disk disease (DDD) is a chronic and multifactorial condition of the intervertebral disk that can manifest itself by axial pain, radiculopathy, myelopathy, and spinal stenosis. It constitutes an increasing cause of lumbar pain and morbidity in the industrialized world, with important socioeconomic implications.

The intervertebral disk (IVD) is a highly organized matrix laid down by relatively few cells in a specific manner. IVDs are composed of three distinct structural regions, the peripheral annulus fibrosus, which are abundant collagen fibers, the central nucleus pulposus rich in proteoglycan, and the cartilaginous endplates. The central gelatinous nucleus pulposus is contained laterally within the more collagenous annulus fibrosus and inferiorly and superiorly, by the cartilage endplates. The annulus consists of concentric rings or lamellae, with fibers in the outer lamellae continuing into the longitudinal ligaments and vertebral bodies. Both the annulus and the nucleus function in concert to provide the disk with mechanical stability. The composition and organization of the IVDs varies with age and location. The most dramatic changes in IVD with aging and degeneration are the loss of fluid pressurization and hydration, and the altered biochemical composition and matrix structure.

MRI provides excellent anatomic imaging of the spine and of a wide morphologic spectrum of disk abnormalities including: disk degeneration, disk bulging, disk protrusion, annular tears, vertebral degenerative bone marrow changes (Modic changes). However, the clinical significance of such abnormal findings is debatable, because in the majority of cases, the origin of the pain remains obscure.

Until today, the two major clinical procedures for treating disk degeneration are disk excision and spinal fusion. These treatment modalities have been disappointing because of altered spinal mechanics leading to subsequent degeneration at adjacent disk levels. Disk pathology treatment is shifting toward prevention and treatment of underlying etiologic processes at the level of the disk matrix composition and integrity.

In recent years, quantitative MRI techniques have been developed to noninvasively quantify the earliest degenerative changes that occur within the disk, such as DWI. Some reports have demonstrated a reduction of ADC values in the degenerated disk but also an overlap between ADC values of normal and degenerative disks. Larger studies should be performed to better understand the pathophysiology of disk degeneration in order to provide relevant information for a better outcome for the treatment of the degenerative discopathy.

Imaging Findings

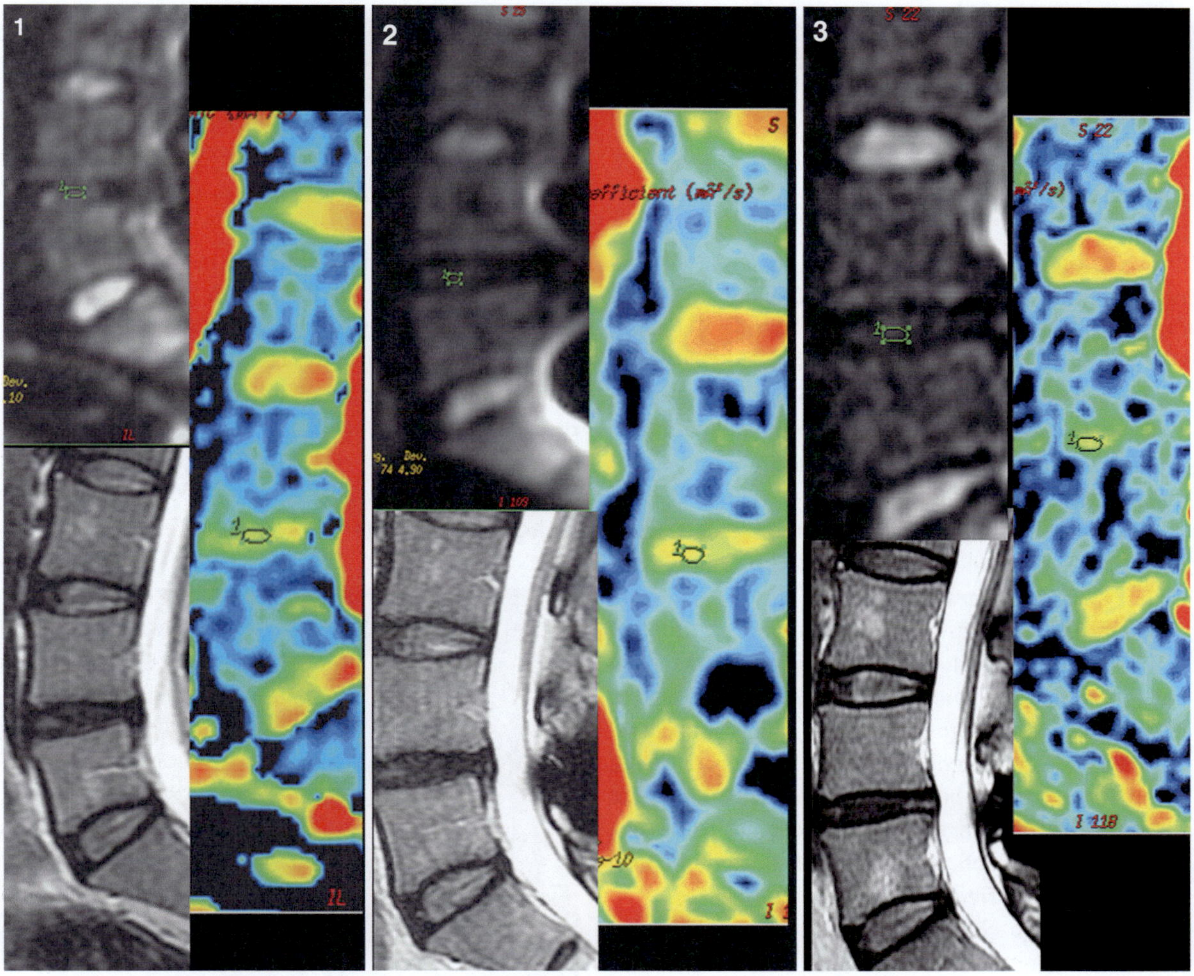

Fig. 15.7 Presurgical lumbar MRI (**15.7.1**) showed signs of degenerative disk disease in L4-L5 disk, consistent on low signal on sagittal FSE T2-weighted image (*bottom left image*) and on DWI (*upper left image*). On the parametric ADC map (*right image*), the ADC value was that of 1.4×10^{-3} mm²/s within the ROI placed at L4-L5 intervertebral disk. Three months after surgery the MRI (**15.7.2**) showed, on the same series of images as the previous one, an increase of the ADC up to 1.6×10^{-3} mm²/s, without morphological changes on T2-weighted image. One year later, the patient referred the same back pain, and the MRI (**15.7.3**) demonstrated a reduced ADC value of 1.4×10^{-3} mm²/s, consistent with treatment failure

Case 15.8: Diabetic Osteomyelitis and Neuropathic Foot

A 57-year-old male with diabetes and neuropathic arthropathy presented with clinical suspicion of infection.

Comments

Infectious complications of the foot are a major cause of morbidity and mortality in diabetic patients. Osteomyelitis of the foot is a challenging diagnosis and affects up to 15% of diabetic patients, often as the result of direct contamination from a soft tissue lesion. Early diagnosis of osteomyelitis in the diabetic foot is crucial because aggressive management, both medical and surgical, is required.

Diagnosis of osteomyelitis may be difficult because of the coexistence of chronic cellulitis, vascular insufficiency, and peripheral neuropathy.

Over 90% of cases of osteomyelitis of the foot of diabetic patient result from spread of infection from contiguous neurotrophic pedal ulcers. The ulcers tend to occur at sites of pressure over bony or joint prominences. In order of decreasing occurrence, the ulcers are found: below the metatarsal heads, at the tips of the toes, over deformed interphalangeal joints, under the calcaneus, and over the malleoli. These sites of ulceration correspond to the most frequent sites of osteomyelitis.

Radiographic changes are often not visible until 2–4 weeks after onset of infection, accounting in part for the low sensitivity of plain radiography. The specificity of plain radiography tends to be higher than its sensitivity but can be compromised by posttraumatic reactions, nonspecific periosteal reactions as seen in chronic venous stasis, and most commonly in Charcot's osteoarthropathy. CT is also used routinely although not considered accurate in this clinical setting. However, sequestra, cortical destruction, periosteal new bone, and intraosseous gas may be observed in CT images. Combined bone 99mTc-methylene diphosphonate and 111In-labeled white blood cell scintigraphy are highly sensitive procedures but may be hampered by coexisting pathologic processes such as neuroarthropathy, trauma, or cellulitis.

MRI is a powerful, noninvasive tool for determining the presence or absence of osteomyelitis in the diabetic patient with almost 100% sensitivity and specificity of 81%. The use of gadolinium improves delineation of soft tissue masses, but is not useful in distinguishing osteomyelitis from edema of acute neuropathic osteoarthropathy. The presence of an ulcer adjacent to the involved bone with cellulitis and a sinus tract, predominantly involving one bone, is one of the most specific sign for osteomyelitis. Besides, acute neuropathy usually affects multiple bones and joints at midfoot (metatarsophalangeal joints, Lisfranc's joint, and Chopart's joint) accompanied by usually intact skin and subcutaneous tissue.

DWI has been reported to be a useful tool in distinguishing reactive joint fluid from pyogenic abscess, and thus could be a powerful technique to differentiate between osteomyelitis and neuropathic osteoarthropathy whenever bone marrow edema and joint effusion is present.

Imaging Findings

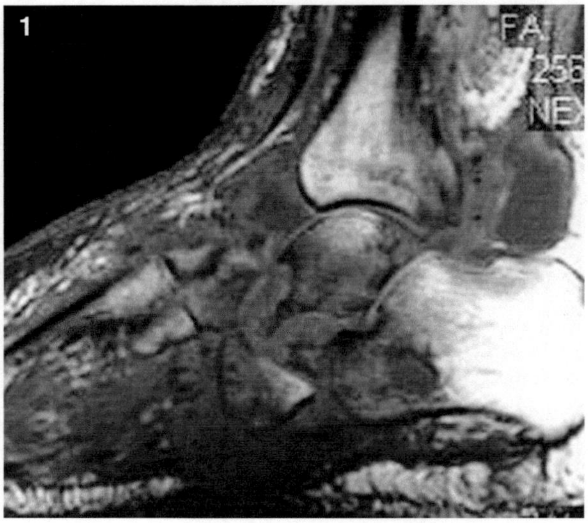

Fig. 15.8 Sagittal FSE T1-weighted (**15.8.1**) and corresponding STIR images (**15.8.2**) demonstrate a "Rocker-bottom" foot in a patient with diabetic neuroarthropathy. There is midfoot joint disruption and disorganization, bone marrow edema in the hindfoot with a central area of lower signal intensity on T1 weighted image, and fluid signal on STIR indicating an intraosseous abscess in the calcaneus. Joint effusion and a collection inside Kager's fat pad are present. Axial fat-saturated proton density image shows several soft tissue collections surrounding the ankle (**15.8.3**). Axial DWI (**15.8.4**) reveals a high signal intensity mass within the soft tissue adjacent to the tibial malleolus (*arrow*). ADC color map (**15.8.5**) shows blue color of the lesion (*arrow*) due to restricted diffusion related to an abscess. In opposition, the collection located in the Kager's fat pad with high signal on DWI but without restricted diffusion (no blue color) is related to a noninfectious fluid collection (*arrowheads*)

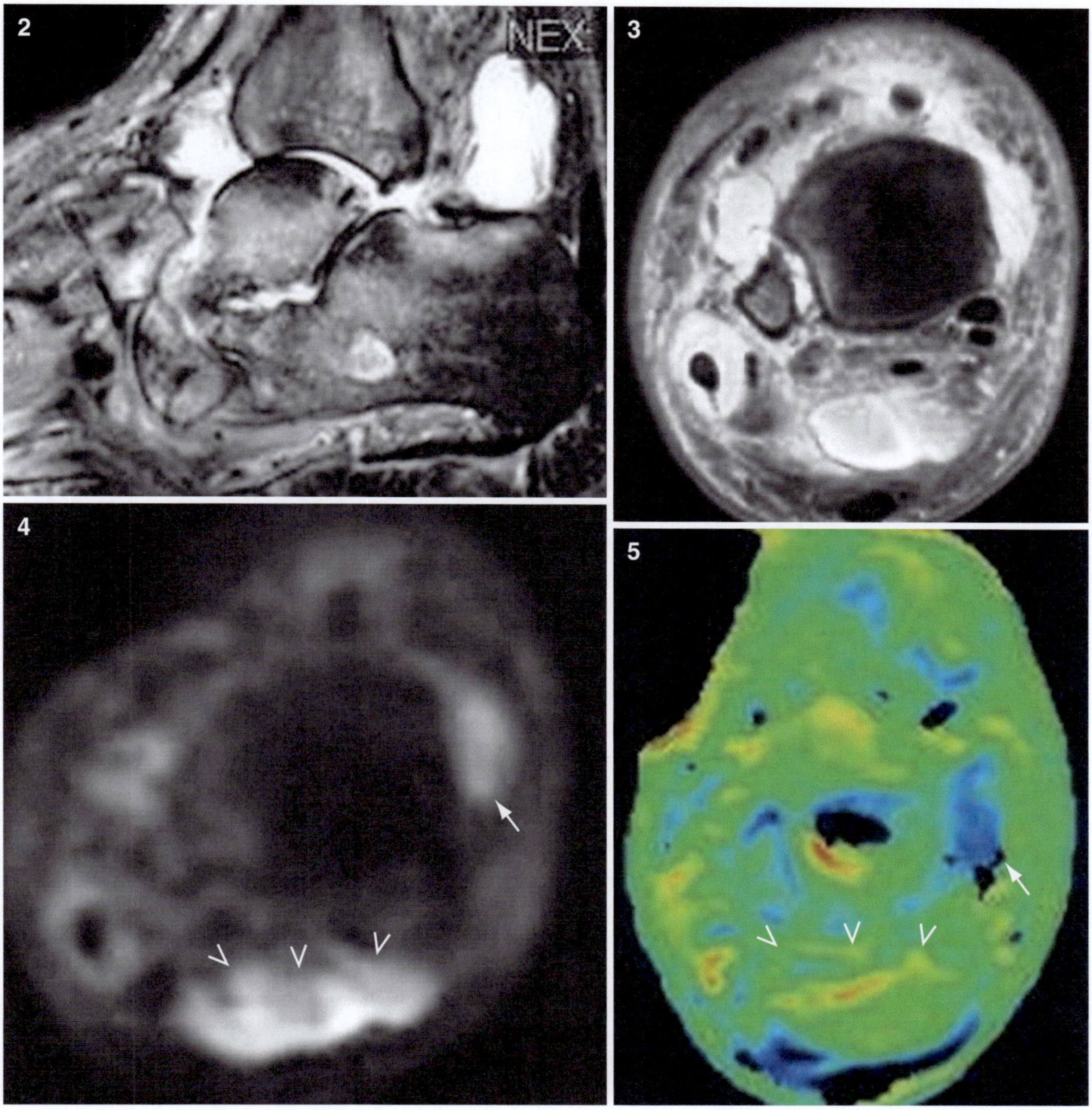

Fig. 15.8 (continued)

Case 15.9: Pelvic Abscesses Secondary to Symphysis Pubis Septic Arthritis and Osteomyelitis

A 67-year-old female patient complained of discomfort on her left pelvis. She referred mild fever on previous days. An ultrasound of the pelvis showed fluid collections nearby the urinary bladder, with suspicion of an ovarian origin. An MRI was requested for further assessment.

Comments

Bony infection or inflammation of the pubic area is rare. In the literature, these two conditions are commonly confused with each other. On the one hand, osteitis pubis is a noninfective inflammation of the symphysis pubis, without another distinct etiology. It has often been reported after urological or gynecological procedures, and it is also associated with trauma, rheumatic disorders, pregnancy, or overuse (usually in athletes). Symptoms mostly resolve spontaneously. On the other hand, osteomyelitis of the symphysis pubis has the same clinical signs, but it is infectious in nature. The differential diagnosis between both entities may be difficult.

Osteomyelitis of the symphysis pubis is relatively uncommon and represents less than 1% of all cases of hematogenous osteomyelitis.

The classic features are pain and tenderness over the pubis radiating into both groins, spasms of the adductor muscles and rectus abdominis, and a waddling gait. A number of predisposing risk factors have been identified. These include drug abusers, local trauma, pelvic surgery, childbirth, and abdominal pathology. Although the pathogenesis remains unclear, septic arthritis of the pubic symphysis is much more common in intravenous drug users, accounting for up to 9% of septic arthritis in this population. The joint involvement in parenteral drug abusers is unique, as they show a propensity for involvement of fibrocartilaginous rather than synovial joints.

Delay in diagnosis is common, primarily because of the uncommon site and rarity, and also because of the difficulty in making a differential diagnosis with urological, gynecological, and abdominal emergencies.

Radiological workup with plain X-rays, CT, MRI, and bone scan is helpful and may be diagnostic. Pelvic radiographs are relatively insensitive for the diagnosis of septic arthritis of the symphysis pubis, especially early in the course of disease. A three-phase technetium 99-methylene diphosphonate bone scan demonstrates increased activity on the affected areas in all phases.

MRI is extremely sensitive to detect septic arthritis and is more specific than conventional radiograph, CT, and bone scintigraphy. MRI is the technique of choice for evaluating the local extent of musculoskeletal infections.

On MRI, the involved joints reveal distension and high intensity signal on T2-weighted images of the joint capsule. The infectious process may extend into the adjacent bone causing osteomyelitis, which is typically identified on MRI as bone areas of low signal on T1-weighted images and hypersignal on T2-weighted images.

DWI is a new sequence in the diagnosis of abscesses in different sites of the body. An abscess is a localized collection of necrotic tissue, neutrophils, inflammatory cells, and bacteria caused by suppuration in a confined space that may become walled off by highly vascular connective tissue. On MRI, an abscess is usually a well-defined round containing fluid with low signal on T1-weighted images and high signal on T2-weighted sequences, and a surrounding rim that enhances following contrast administration. The abscess fluid does not enhance and the signal intensity of the fluid varies depending on the cellular and hemorrhagic components of the abscess.

On DWI, the abscesses are hyperintense and show low ADC values. The differential diagnosis of cystic lesions of the female pelvis includes endometriomas and hemorrhagic cysts. These hemorrhagic lesions may show "T2 blackout" effect which indicates hypointensity on DWI caused by hypointensity on T2-weighted images. T2 blackout is predominantly secondary to susceptibility effects.

Thus, whenever an infectious arthritis is suspected, DWI should be added to conventional MRI examination.

Imaging Findings

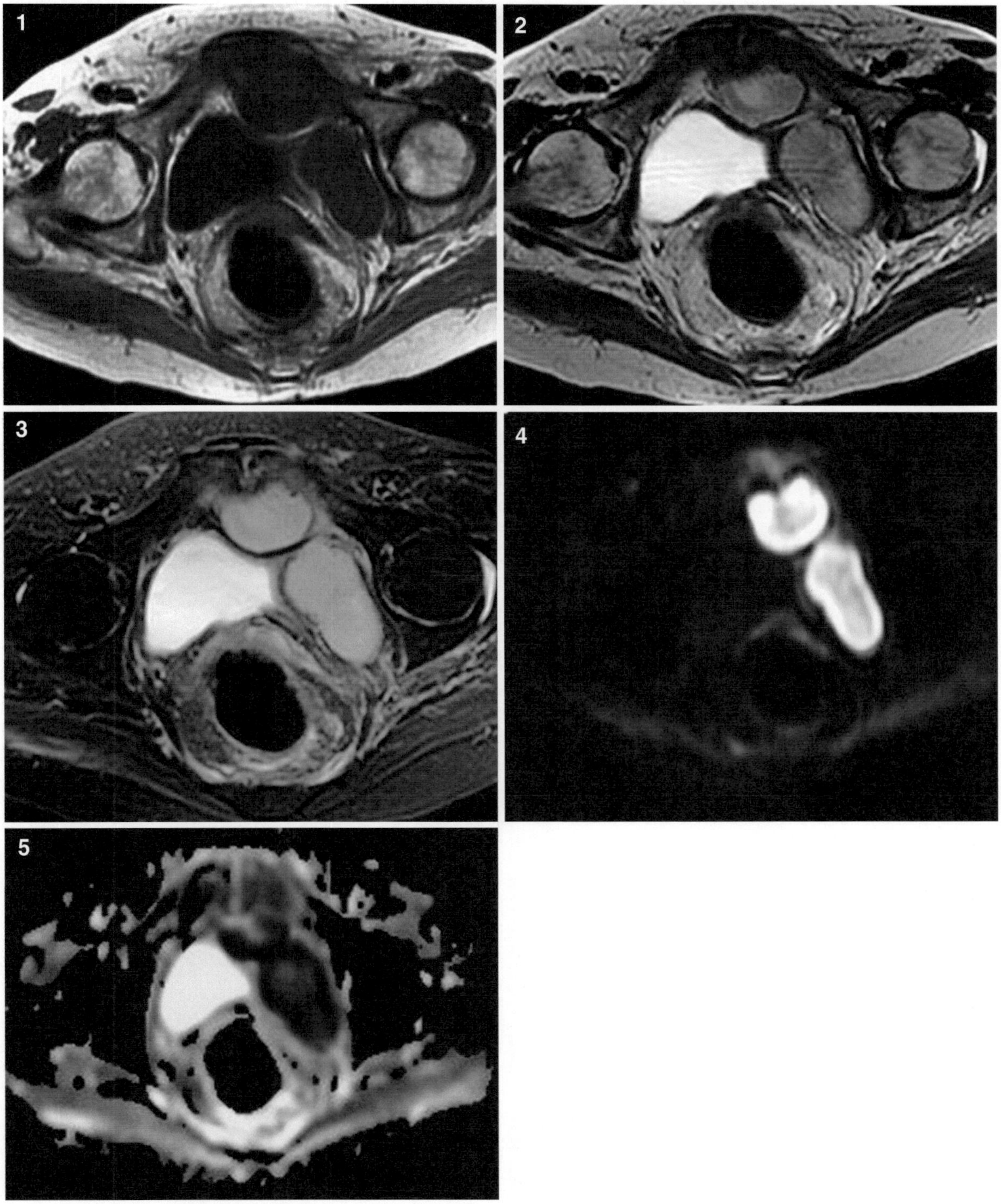

Fig. 15.9 Axial FSE T1-weighted image (**15.9.1**) shows two large pelvic fluid collections with higher signal intensity than the urinary bladder. The pubis symphysis presents hypointense signal compared with the normal bone marrow. Axial FSE T2-weighted images (**15.9.2**) shows the same lesions with less hyperintense signal than the urinary bladder. Corresponding axial fat-suppressed FSE T2-weighted image (**15.9.3**) reveals the same findings and mild bone edema in the pubic symphysis. Axial DWI (**15.9.4**) obtained with a *b* value of 1,000 s/mm^2 shows the high signal of the lesions due to restricted diffusion. Parametric ADC map in gray scale (**15.9.5**) confirms the restricted diffusion as low signal areas corresponding to abscesses

Case 15.10: Rheumatoid Arthritis

A 58-year-old female presents with stiffness and pain during movements of both wrists over several months. During the last weeks, bilateral swelling, especially on the left wrist, appeared.

Comments

Rheumatoid arthritis (RA) is an autoimmune disorder of unknown etiology characterized by symmetric, erosive synovitis, and sometimes multisystemic involvement. RA most commonly affects the small joints of the hands, wrists, knees, and feet. Swelling of the proximal interphalangeal (PIP) joints is one of the most common early signs of the disease. Bilateral and symmetrical swelling of the metacarpophalangeal (MCP) joints is also frequent. The distal interphalangeal (DIP) joints are usually not affected, which is a useful sign in discriminating RA from osteoarthritis or psoriatic arthritis.

Conventional radiography, the traditional gold standard for imaging in RA, is not able to detect early disease manifestations such as soft tissue changes and the earliest stages of bone erosion. Recent studies show that US is an excellent modality for depicting signs of soft tissue inflammation. It allows the detection of effusion, synovial proliferation, and tenosynovitis. However, MRI has been shown to be a highly sensitive technique for the detection of early inflammatory and destructive joint changes in RA and it is the only modality capable to detect bone marrow edema, which is a predictor of future bone erosions. Savnik et al. reported that erosions are visible on MRI in a median of 2 years before they are detectable on radiographs. The typical progression of RA that can be detected by MRI begins with synovitis, followed by bone marrow edema, and, finally, bony erosions.

Several authors have attempted to assess and quantify the disease manifestation in RA, i.e., the degree of synovial inflammation, bone marrow edema, erosions, and tenosynovitis.

Scoring systems and protocols, standardizing imaging of other joint regions, are still under development and will need to be tested in multicenter trials.

New technological advances such as the introduction of DWI, which depicts the motion of water molecules in biological tissue, are successfully applied in multiple pathologic conditions. A recently published article evaluates the role of DWI in the detection of early active sacroiliitis and showed that DWI sensitivity for detecting acute lesions in early sacroiliitis is similar to that of postcontrast T1-weighted images. Other reports have evaluated the effects of different therapies on enthesitis and osteitis, in active ankylosing spondylitis using DWI and DCE-MRI. They conclude that DWI has potential in the quantitative analysis of inflammatory skeletal lesions in patients with ankylosing spondylitis. Therefore, DWI is also useful for the assessment of treatment efficacy. Perhaps, DWI may be a useful tool in the early diagnosis and monitoring of the acute inflammatory lesions that occur in early RA, although this has still to be proven.

Fig. 15.10 Axial FSE T1-weighted with fat suppression and gadolinium injection (**15.10.1**) of the wrist demonstrates enhancement of the synovial membrane corresponding with synovitis and multiple carpal erosions. Note tenosynovitis of the flexor carpi radialis and the flexor pollicis longus. Coronal GE T2-weighted image (**15.10.2**) shows multiple erosions of the carpal bones, including scaphoid, lunate, capitate, and hamate. The membrane and synovial fluid appears hyperintense. Coronal STIR sequence (**15.10.3**) shows high signal due to bone marrow edema within the carpal bones. Axial DWI (**15.10.4**) reveals high signal and red color on corresponding ADC color map (**15.10.5**) within the peripheral synovium indicating inflammatory activity without true restricted diffusion. Therefore, high signal intensity on DWI is probably due to T2 shine-through effect

Imaging Findings

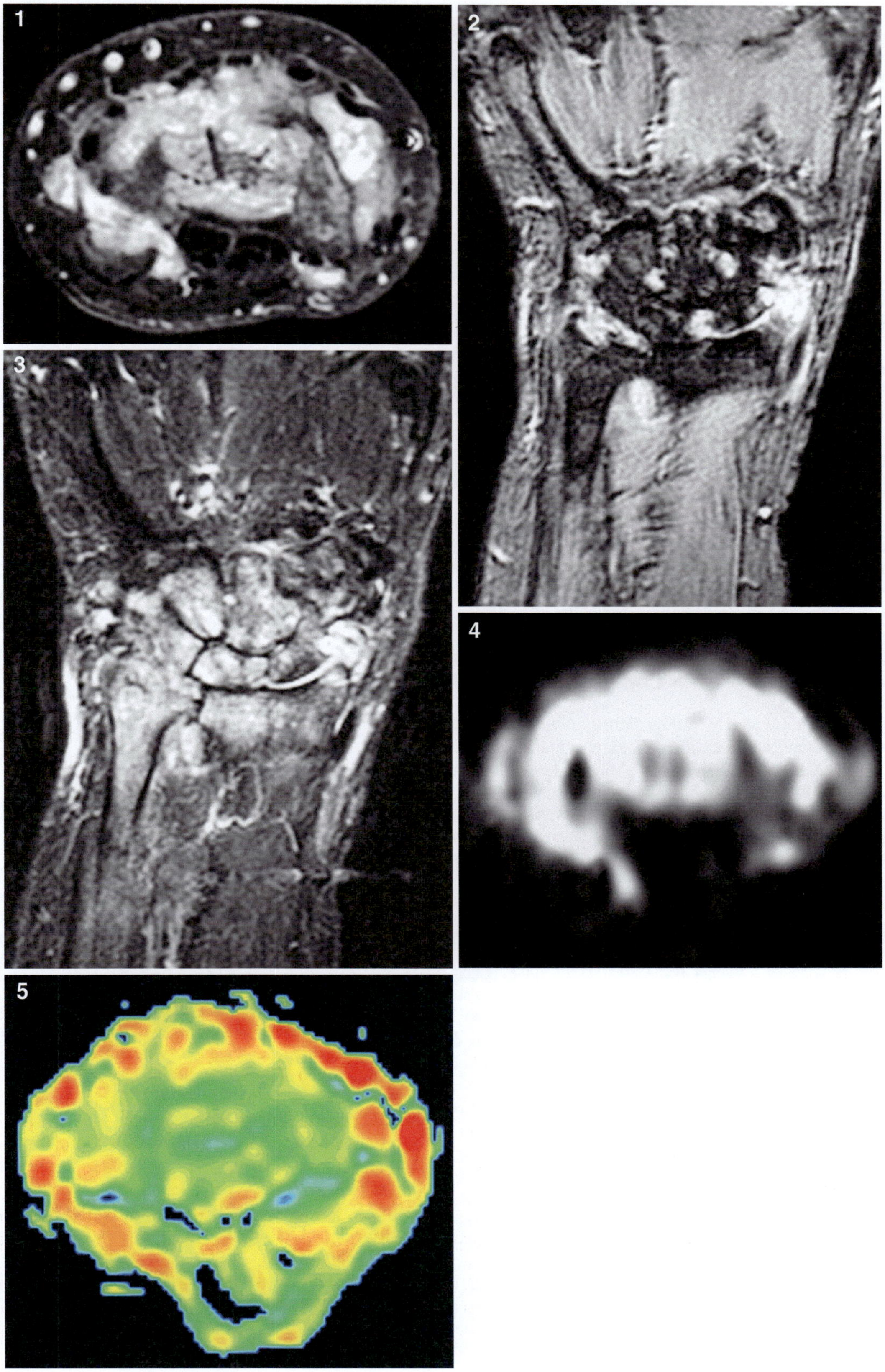

Further Reading

Alibek S, Cavallaro A, Aplas A et al (2009) Diffusion weighted imaging of pediatric and adolescent malignancies with regard to detection and delineation: initial experience. Acad Radiol 16:866–871

Andreisek G, White LM, Kassner A et al (2009) Diffusion tensor imaging and fiber tractography of the median nerve at 1.5T: optimization of b value. Skeletal Radiol 38:51–59

Andreisek G, White LM, Kassner A et al (2010) Evaluation of diffusion tensor imaging and fiber tractography of the median nerve: preliminary results on intrasubject variability and precision of measurements. Am J Roentgenol 194:W65–W72

Barcelo J, Vilanova JC, Riera E et al (2007) Diffusion-weighted whole-body MRI (virtual PET) in screening for osseous metastases. Radiología 49:407–415

Baur A, Reiser MF (2000) Diffusion-weighted imaging of the musculoskeletal system in humans. Skeletal Radiol 29:555–562

Baur A, Huber A, Arbogast S et al (2001) Diffusion-weighted imaging of tumor recurrencies and posttherapeutical soft-tissue changes in humans. Eur Radiol 11:828–833

Baur A, Dietrich O, Reiser M (2002) Diffusion-weighted imaging of the spinal column. Neuroimaging Clin N Am 12:147–160

Biffar A, Baur-Melnyk A, Schmidt GP et al (2010) Multiparameter MRI assessment of normal-appearing and diseased vertebral bone marrow. Eur Radiol 20(11):2679–2689

Bifar A, Dietrich O, Duerr HR et al (2010) Diffusion and perfusion imaging of bone marrow. Eur J Radiol 76:323–328

Biffar A, Soubron S, Dietrich O et al (2010) Combined diffusion-weighted and dynamic contrast-enhanced imaging of patients with acute osteoporotic vertebral fractures. Eur J Radiol 76:298–303

Bley TA, Wieben O, Uhl M (2009) Diffusion-weighted MR imaging in musculoskeletal radiology: applications in trauma, tumors, and inflammation. Magn Reson Imaging Clin N Am 17:263–275

Chan JH, Peh WC, Tsui EY et al (2002) Acute vertebral body compression fractures: discrimination between benign and malignant causes using apparent diffusion coefficients. Br J Radiol 75(891):207–214

Colagrande S, Carbone SF, Carusi LM et al (2006) Magnetic resonance diffusion-weighted imaging: extraneurological applications. Radiol Med 111:392–419

Costa FM, Ferreira EC, Vianna EM (2011) Diffusion-weighted magnetic resonance imaging for the evaluation of musculoskeletal tumors. Magn Reson Imaging Clin N Am 19(1):159–180

Dietrich O, Biffar A, Reiser MF et al (2009) Diffusion-weighted imaging of bone marrow. Semin Musculoskelet Radiol 13:134–144

Dudeck O, Zeile M, Pink D et al (2008) Diffusion-weighted magnetic resonance imaging allows monitoring of anticancer treatment effects in patients with soft-tissue sarcomas. J Magn Reson Imaging 27:1109–1113

Gaspersic N, Sersa I, Jevtic V et al (2008) Monitoring ankylosing spondylitis therapy by dynamic contrast-enhanced and diffusion-weighted magnetic resonance imaging. Skeletal Radiol 37:123–131

Glaser C (2005) New techniques for cartilage imaging: T2 relaxation time and diffusion-weighted MR imaging. Radiol Clin North Am 43:641–653, vii

Herneth AM, Ringl H, Memarsadeghi M et al (2007) Diffusion weighted imaging in osteoradiology. Top Magn Reson Imaging 18:203–212

Jaramillo D (2010) Whole-body MR imaging, bone diffusion imaging: how and why? Pediatr Radiol 40(6):978–984

Karampinos DC, King KF, Sutton BP et al (2010) Intravoxel partially coherent motion technique: characterization of the anisotropy of skeletal muscle microvasculature. J Magn Reson Imaging 31(4):942–953

Liu Y, Tang GY, Tang RB et al (2010) Assessment of bone marrow changes in postmenopausal women with varying bone densities: magnetic resonance spectroscopy and diffusion magnetic resonance imaging. Chin Med J (Engl) 123(12): 1524–1527

MacKenzie JD, Gonzalez L, Hernandez A et al (2007) Diffusion-weighted and diffusion tensor imaging for pediatric musculoskeletal disorders. Pediatr Radiol 37:781–788

Nagata S, Nishimura H, Uchida M et al (2008) Diffusion-weighted imaging of soft tissue tumors: usefulness of the apparent diffusion coefficient for differential diagnosis. Radiat Med 26(5):287–295

Nakanishi K, Kobayashi M, Nakaguchi K et al (2007) Whole-body MRI for detecting metastatic bone tumor: diagnostic value of diffusion-weighted images. Magn Reson Med Sci 6:147–155

Noseworthy MD, Davis AD, Elzibak AH (2010) Advanced MR imaging techniques for skeletal muscle evaluation. Semin Musculoskelet Radiol 14(2):257–268

Oka K, Yakushiji T, Sato H et al (2008) Ability of diffusion-weighted imaging for the differential diagnosis between chronic expanding hematomas and malignant soft tissue tumors. J Magn Reson Imaging 28:1195–1200

Oka K, Yakushiji T, Sato H et al (2010) The value of diffusion-weighted imaging for monitoring the chemotherapeutic response of osteosarcoma: a comparison between average apparent diffusion coefficient and minimum apparent diffusion coefficient. Skeletal Radiol 39:141–146

Padhani AR, Koh DM (2011) Diffusion MR imaging for monitoring of treatment response. Magn Reson Imaging Clin N Am 19(1):181–209

Pui MH, Mitha A, Rae WI et al (2005) Diffusion-weighted magnetic resonance imaging of spinal infection and malignancy. J Neuroimaging 15(2):164–170

Reeder SB, Mukherjee P (2009) Clinical applications of MR diffusion and perfusion imaging: preface. Magn Reson Imaging Clin N Am 17:xi–xii

Reischauer C, Froehlich JM, Koh DM et al (2010) Bone metastases from prostate cancer: assessing treatment response by using diffusion-weighted imaging and functional diffusion maps – initial observations. Radiology 257(2):523–531

Sommer G, Klarhöfer M, Lenz C et al (2011) Signal characteristics of focal bone marrow lesions in patients with multiple myeloma using whole body T1w-TSE, T2w-STIR and diffusion-weighted imaging with background suppression. Eur Radiol 21:857–862

Trattnig S, Domayer S, Welsch GW et al (2009) MR imaging of cartilage and its repair in the knee – a review. Eur Radiol 19(7):1582–1594

Vilanova JC, Barcelo J (2008) Diffusion-weighted whole-body MR screening. Eur J Radiol 67:440–447

16 Whole-Body Applications of DWI

Joan C. Vilanova, Sandra Baleato, Joaquim Barceló, and Antonio Luna

16.1 General and Technical Considerations

Whole-body MR imaging (WB-MRI) has been developed in recent years using different methods, either with a moving table platform in combination with the body-coil, or with a especially designed rolling table platform with multiple phase-array coils. Prior studies have shown the clinical impact of WB-MRI on bone marrow involvement, tumor staging, and screening. Furthermore, improvements in software and hardware allowed to evaluating the whole body on MRI in a short period of time. A WB-MRI protocol should include at least a T1-weighted sequence and a STIR one, which are highly efficient for the assessment of bone and soft tissues. Specific protocols of WB-MRI tailored to specific conditions and applications are necessary to fully explore the capabilities of this technique. For example, staging of colorectal carcinoma needs additional high resolution liver imaging to conventional WB-MRI sequences and a protocol for staging of prostate cancer should include extensive bone evaluation with sagittal and coronal T1-weighted and STIR sequences, including the whole spine and pelvis.

Besides, in the last decade, DWI has revealed a great potential for cancer and bone marrow imaging. Recent advances in MRI gradient technology allow the acquisition of DWI with a high *b*-factor, even in the body, thanks to the advent of fast imaging sequences like EPI, and parallel imaging techniques. Whole-body DWI (WB-DWI) is a recent application, which allows to perform multiple stations and a composite image of the entire body. In a short time, WB-DWI has shown a great potential and clinical value for both oncologic and nononcologic applications.

The examination protocol for WB-DWI relies on a STIR-EPI DWI sequence with or without parallel acquisition, most commonly known as Diffusion-weighted Whole-body Imaging with Background body Signal suppression (DWIBS). The design of this sequence was previously reviewed in Chap. 1 (Figs. 1.9 and 1.10). The patient is examined in the supine position and placed feet first into the bore of the magnet using either the body-coil or multiple phased-array coils with an automatic moving table.

A fast GE localizing pulse sequence is first performed in the coronal plane covering from the head to the calf in three anatomic regions. Our WB-DWI protocol includes a DWIBS acquisition in five-stations series (head and neck, thorax, abdomen, pelvis, and thighs) performed during free breathing. Diffusion gradients with two *b* values (0 and 500–1000 s/mm^2) are applied along the X, Y, and Z directions. The slice

J.C. Vilanova
Department of Radiology, Clínica Girona-Hospital Sta. Caterina, University of Girona, Girona, Spain
e-mail: kvilanova@comg.cat

S. Baleato
Department of Radiology, Complexo Hospitalario Universitario de Santiago, de Compostela, Spain
e-mail: baleatorum@hotmail.com

J. Barceló
Department of Radiology, Clínica Girona-Hospital Sta. Caterina, Girona, Spain
e-mail: jbarcelo@cetir.es

A. Luna
MRI section, Clínica Las Nieves, SERCOSA, Jaén, Spain
e-mail: aluna70@sercosa.com

A. Luna et al., *Diffusion MRI Outside the Brain*,
DOI 10.1007/978-3-642-21052-5_16, © Springer-Verlag Berlin Heidelberg 2012

thickness is between 4 and 6 mm with no gap and slices are acquired in an interleaved fashion. The acquisition is performed in the axial plane to minimize EPI distortion.

This sequence provides good background suppression, showing a high sensitivity to detect areas with restricted diffusion. It should be taking into account that normal hypercellular areas may show restricted diffusion, such us brain, spinal cord, peripheral nerves, salivary glands, gallbladder, small bowel and colorectal mucosa, lymphatic Waldeyer ring, spleen, lymph nodes, kidneys, adrenal glands, prostate, testes, penis, endometrium, ovaries, and bone marrow. A complete WB-MRI protocol with standard sequences, DWI, and dynamic 3D contrast-enhanced acquisition can be performed in less than 40 min.

The main limitations of DWIBS are the sensitivity to cardiac and respiratory motion and its reduced spatial resolution. Artifacts are induced by physiological patient motion and substantial magnetic susceptibility variations around the spine or thoraco-abdominal structures, due to the presence of bone, air, and vascular or cerebrospinal fluid pulsation. Breath-holding has not been employed in WB-DWI due to limitations in the slice thickness. The use of cardiac and respiratory triggering may help to reduce the motion related artifacts which are problematic for the evaluation of mediastinum and left hepatic lobe. The application of these motion control techniques is time consuming. Therefore, the use of free breathing is the most extended option for WB-DWI. In order to increase the SNR, multiple signal averaging is usually performed.

DWIBS is also feasible at 3T magnets, although the preliminary available data suggests larger susceptibility, distortion, and motion artifacts than those at 1.5T magnets. Advantages of increased SNR of DWIBS at 3T magnets should be further explored with the addition of advanced fat-suppression techniques as slice-selective gradient reversal and multi-source radiofrequency transmission technology.

The DWI data have to be processed on the workstation. The 3D data sets from the different axial series are combined, reformatted, and viewed along any axis as multiplanar reconstructions (MPR) or maximum intensity projections (MIP). The MPR images can be displayed as a whole-body image in the coronal plane. An inverse gray–white scale intensity scale is usually applied to the data sets for visual interpretation, which seems more familiar to clinicians, as they have some resemblance to the usual displays seen in scintigraphy or PET.

It is important to evaluate and try to combine the information from DWI with morphological series, as T1-weighted or STIR images, to accurately detect pathology or rule out artifacts from the DWI. This also helps to correctly locate the lesions with restricted diffusion, as DWIBS has an intrinsically low SNR. Furthermore, it is possible to perform fusion of WB-DWI and WB-MRI morphological series. The acquisition of low and high *b* values is time consuming but it allows us to calculate ADC maps, which are interesting for further characterization of lesions with restricted diffusion, as shown in the differentiation between acute benign fractures from malignant and infectious lesions (Fig. 16.1). Other authors prefer to perform DWIBS only with a high *b* value, which may be an interesting option in cases of screening for faster imaging.

16.2 Oncological Applications

WB-DWIBS has shown to increase the detection of malignant lesions and metastasis compared to morphological WB-MRI alone. DWI increases the detection of oncologic lesions in several organs and systems, with greater restriction of free water diffusion for the more aggressive ones. Areas of necrosis, cystic degeneration, and edema may reduce the tumoral restriction of diffusion. Initial studies describing WB-DWI have focused on the detection of osseous metastases in patients with primary malignancies that had the potential to metastasize to the skeletal system (Fig. 16.2). Several reports have demonstrated the value of adding DWI to WB-MRI protocols in the assessment of bone metastases. Furthermore, WB-MRI with DWIBS is superior to skeletal scintigraphy to detect bone metastases (Fig. 16.2). A series by Takenaka and colleagues concluded that WB-DWI was more specific than 18FDG PET-CT for bone metastases assessment in patients with non-small-cell lung cancer (NSCLC). WB-DWI has also shown to be as effective as 11C-choline PET-CT in the detection of bone metastases in prostate cancer patients. Entirely osteoblastic metastases are not adequately depicted on DWI (Fig. 16.3). Although this could represent a drawback for this whole-body technique, it has to be taken into account that an effective WB-MRI protocol should always include T1-weighted and STIR sequences, and osteoblastic lesions are well depicted on the T1-weighted images.

WB-DWI has also been described as a potential means to rapidly evaluate the therapeutic response in human bone marrow. A very recent report has demonstrated the potential of quantitative functional diffusion maps and ADC analysis for the assessment of tumor response of bone metastases to antiandrogen treatment in patients with advanced prostate cancer.

In a similar manner, the addition of DWIBS to whole-body staging protocols can improve the depiction of multiple myeloma lesions (Fig. 16.4). Furthermore, ADC values in patients with a low serum concentration of M-component (favoring inactive disease) are significantly higher than those in patients with a high M-component, which are present in patients with active multiple myeloma at initial diagnosis or acute recurrence.

One of the potentially powerful tools of WB-DWI is that it provides additional information of the extraskeletal areas. For this reason, the technique can be applied for extraskeletal tumor detection (Fig. 16.5), characterization, and staging (Fig. 16.6). DWIBS allows the detection of small metastatic foci in areas such as peritoneum or liver (Fig. 16.7). The detection of lymph nodes or pulmonary metastases is more challenging. Normal and pathological lymph nodes show restricted diffusion and are both highlighted on DWIBS. Although ADC measurements have recently shown promising results in the distinction of normal and metastatic lymph nodes of neck, pulmonary, and pelvic cancers, larger series are needed to validate these preliminary results. It is also helpful to take into account the predictable locations of normal lymph nodes in the different lymphatic chains. WB-DWI has shown excellent results in nodal and bone marrow staging of lymphoma and leukemia and it is a perfect tool for surveillance evaluation.

WB-DWI may also be used to locate unknown primary neoplasm (Fig. 16.7), in the assessment of response to treatment (Fig. 16.8), and in the evaluation of recurrent tumor (Fig. 16.9). WB-DWI is a fast manner to evaluate the response to treatment using a visual qualitative approach. As a general rule, areas with good response will show less signal on high *b* value images due to cell killing and areas of disease progression will demonstrate higher signal intensity and/or greater extent on high *b* value images. For better comparison between MIP or MPR reconstruction of two different WB-DWI studies, it is desirable to perform normalization of the source images of both studies and maintain similar window widths with respect to structures with unchanged diffusion properties. As the different patterns of response to therapy are complex physiological processes related to the type of drug, primary tumor, and patient, and there are several confounding factors for qualitative interpretation (e.g., T2 shine-through effect), it is preferable to always use ADC maps and morphologic information of WB-MRI to supplement the fast visual evaluation of DWI.

WB-MRI has also the potential to combine functional noninvasive techniques (diffusion, spectroscopy, and vascular imaging) to detect the response of tumors to antivascular therapies. Even more, DWI has been advocated in the prediction of response to treatment. All these applications are in a preliminary stage of clinical evaluation.

16.3 Comparison of WB-DWI to PET and PET-CT

Several series have compared the role of 18-FDG-PET or integrated PET-CT with WB-DWI in cancer imaging, although this comparison has been done in a limited number of patients or pathologies and with some important methodological shortcomings. As a general rule, PET-CT is superior for whole-body staging of different cancers when compared to either WB-MRI (without a DWI sequence) or WB-DWI alone, without using morphological sequences. As discussed above, protocols of WB-MRI must be adapted to extensively study the most common areas of metastases according to the dissemination pattern of the primary cancer studied and these protocols should always include both DWI and morphological sequences. WB-DWI does not use ionizing radiation and is faster than PET. Both techniques explore different properties of tumors, with a potential complementary role. WB-DWI shows higher spatial resolution than PET which may be of interest for detection of small lesions, such as tiny hepatic or peritoneal metastases. The evaluation of low-grade and well-differentiated tumors showing low 18F-FDG uptake may also benefit from the evaluation with WB-DWI. DWI has shown advantage over PET-CT in the evaluation of liver, peritoneum, bone marrow, and brain. In the evaluation of pulmonary metastases, the accuracy and sensitivity of both methods may be considered as similar, although small metastases may show low signal intensity on DWI. Furthermore, DWI yields less false-positive cases due to pulmonary inflammatory lesions than PET. The evaluation of nodal metastases is still challenging for both techniques. On the one hand, PET-CT cannot detect necrotic lymph nodes and submicroscopic metastases and it shows an important false-positive rate due to inflammatory lymphadenitis. On the other hand, the capabilities of DWI in the characterization of lymph nodes have still to be confirmed, although recent data opens a door to a clinical role in this task. Besides, free-breathing WB-DWI has shown limitations in the detection of mediastinal lymph nodes due to respiratory movement and cardiac pulsation related artifacts. Moreover, urothelial tumors may be obscured in PET studies due to the accumulation of 18F-FDG, which is not a limitation for WB-DWI. Evaluation of splenic or paracardiac lesions is better performed with PET than with WB-DWI (Fig. 16.9).

Recent data have shown a high grade of agreement for PET-CT and WB-DWI in the staging of diffuse large B-cell lymphoma, in the nodal staging of uterine cervical cancer, and in detection and nodal staging of colorectal carcinoma. In a recent series comparing WB-DWI and PET-CT in the staging of advanced malignant melanoma, WB-DWI showed a sensitivity and specificity of 82% and 97%, respectively, while PET-CT only achieved 72.8% and 92.7%, respectively. On the site-by-site analysis, WB-DWI was clearly superior in the evaluation of bone marrow, liver, subcutaneous, and intraperitoneal sites.

16.4 Non Oncological Applications

Clinical applications of WB-DWI are not limited to oncology (Fig. 16.10). Benign multifocal systemic conditions such as infectious and inflammatory diseases are a potential indication to perform it. In this sense, DWI, combined with dynamic contrast-enhanced MRI, has been proposed for the monitorization of ankylosing spondylitis therapy.

Case 16.1: Multifocal Bone Tuberculosis

A 22-year-old man presented with a right lobar pneumonia. A CT was performed demonstrating diffuse bone lesions in the thoracic spine. A WB-MRI was requested to rule out metastases or infectious process to the bone.

Comments

Tuberculosis (TB) remains a major cause of skeletal infection in many parts of the world. Skeletal involvement occurs in approximately 1–3% of patients with tuberculosis. Evidence of concurrent active intrathoracic tuberculosis is present in less than 50% of these patients. Osseous TB can be present with uni- or multifocal bony involvement. The spine is the most common site of osseous involvement by TB. However, multifocal involvement of the skeletal system in areas where TB is endemic is not a rare presentation, and its exact prevalence is still not well known. Multifocal skeletal TB is defined as osteoarticular lesions that occur simultaneously at two or more locations.

Diagnosis of extrapulmonary TB is often difficult. Although positive chest radiographic findings or a positive tuberculin skin test supports the diagnosis, negative results do not exclude extrapulmonary tuberculosis.

This condition may mimic malignant disease both clinically and radiographically and its differential diagnosis includes metastatic disease.

In the early phase of tuberculous osteomyelitis, plain films are frequently negative. Skeletal scintigraphy is usually more sensitive than radiological imaging and detects more asymptomatic lesions.

The sensitivity of 99Tcm skeletal scintigraphy for the detection of osteomyelitis, diskitis, and aseptic spine disease is high, but nonspecific. The combination of an agent for detecting inflammation (67 Ga citrate) and a metabolic agent (99m Tc-methylene diphosphonate) increases the diagnostic accuracy of scintigraphy. This method has shown a sensitivity of 90%, specificity of 78%, and an accuracy of 86% for vertebral osteomyelitis. However, it is unable to differentiate between tuberculous and pyogenic spondylitis.

With scintigraphic methods, precise assessment of the extent and localization of inflammatory spine processes is not possible and infection of bony elements and soft tissues cannot be differentiated. MRI is the modality of choice in the detection and staging of inflammatory disorders of spine. The multiplanar imaging capability of MRI greatly improves the detection of vertebral intraosseous abscesses, skip lesions, subligamentous spread of infection, and epidural extension commonly associated with tuberculous spondylitis.

WB-MRI using DWI sequences is a valuable tool for the diagnoses of diseases that involve alterations in water mobility. In the spine, DWI has proven to be a highly useful method for the differential diagnosis of benign and malignant compression fractures. However, several articles showed that ADC values may not be appropriate for differentiating between malignant and infective conditions. Infection usually shows restricted diffusion which is a potential source of error when evaluating oncological lesions.

Imaging Findings

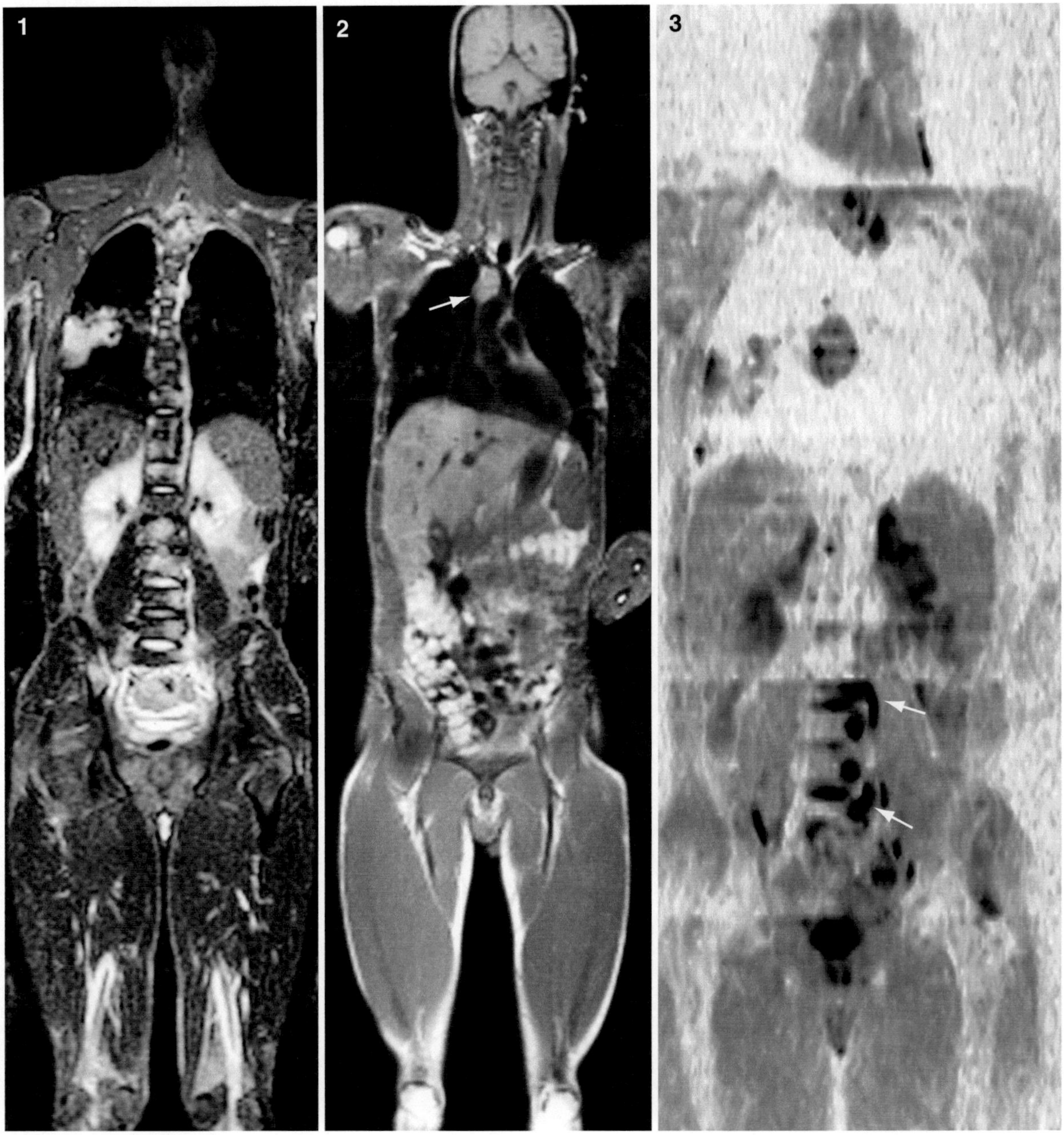

Fig. 16.1 Coronal STIR sequence (**16.1.1**) confirmed the infectious lesion of the right lung and the diffuse bone involvement of the spine. Coronal FSE T1-weighted image (**16.1.2**) showed the presence of mediastinal lymph nodes (*arrow*). WB-DWI with inverse gray-scale intensity (**16.1.3**) shows the right lobe lesion of the lung and the bone lesions in the lumbar spine, pelvis, and the paravertebral soft tissue involvement (*arrows*). Axial ADC color map at the level of T7 (**16.1.4**) shows the ROI within the vertebral body with a low ADC value (0.599×10^{-3} mm²/s) consistent with infectious process

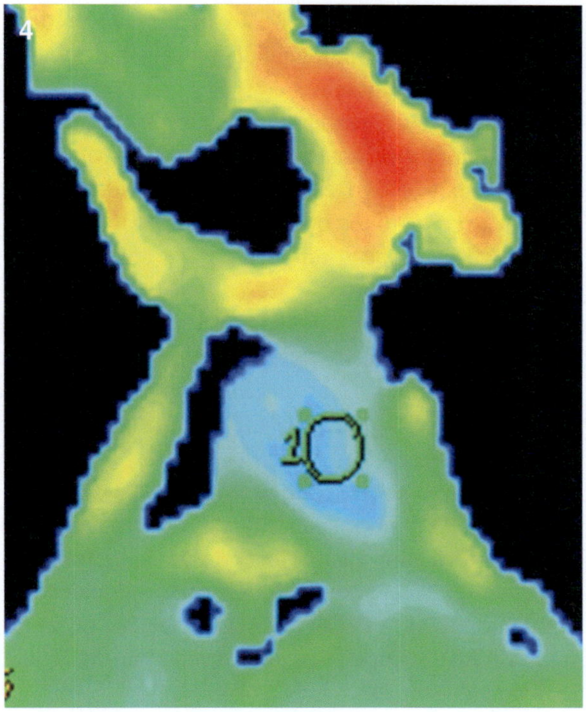

Fig. 16.1 (continued)

Case 16.2: Bone Metastases from Breast Cancer

A 67-year-old woman with a previous history of breast cancer 2 years ago presented with back pain within the lumbar spine. WB-DWI was performed for restaging.

Comments

Bone is the most common site of distant metastases from breast carcinoma. The presence of bone metastases affects patient's prognosis, quality of life, and the treatment planning. Between 30% and 85% of patients with metastatic breast cancer will develop bone metastases during the course of the disease. Bone also represents the first site of metastasis for 26–50% of patients with metastatic breast cancer. Breast cancer preferentially metastasizes to vertebrae and the pelvis, followed by ribs, skull, and femur, probably because the vertebrae are highly vascularized and contain 75% of the body's red marrow. Complications of bone metastasis include bone pain, pathologic fractures, hypercalcemia, and spinal cord compression.

The survival of patients with metastases is variable ranging from months to many years. It has previously been reported that 20% of patients with bone metastases survive more than 5 years, which emphasizes the wide variation in survival seen in this group of patients.

Imaging techniques, including skeletal scintigraphy, plain-film radiography, CT, MRI, PET, and single-photon-emission computed tomography (SPECT), are essential for the detection and management of bone metastases in breast cancer. However, no consensus has been reached about the optimal imaging modality for this purpose.

Skeletal scintigraphy (bone scan) is very sensitive in the detection of osseous metastases and is usually considered the first imaging study in asymptomatic patients. The sensitivity of radionuclide bone scintigraphy is dependent on the osteoblastic activity and up to half of all bone metastases from breast cancer tend to show osteolytic changes.

Radiographs are recommended for the assessment of abnormal radionuclide uptake or the risk of pathological fracture and as initial imaging studies in patients with bone pain. MRI or PET-CT can be considered for cases of abnormal radionuclide uptake that are not addressed by radiography.

However, new emergent imaging modalities such as WB-MRI might replace scintigraphy. WB-MRI uses fast pulse sequences over multiple anatomic stations to achieve a survey of the body from head to toe.

WB-MRI has been adopted for the evaluation of bone and bone marrow diseases and several studies have confirmed that the diagnostic accuracy using WB-MRI is higher than skeletal scintigraphy. Moreover, Schmidt et al. have shown that MRI has greater sensitivity than PET-CT for the detection of bone metastases.

DWI can be also used to detect metastatic disease. DWI and their corresponding ADC maps provide unique information that reflects tissue cellularity and organization. There are emerging studies demonstrating the value of WB-DWI for the detection of metastatic disease compared with conventional MRI and radionuclide studies.

The advantages of WB-DWI over skeletal scintigraphy include the fact that osteolytic bone lesions may not be tracer-avid and hence may be not visible on scintigraphy. Other advantages over skeletal scintigraphy and FDG-PET–CT are the WB-DWI capability of detection of small, subcentimetric lesions and its capability to provide additional information of extraskeletal involvement.

On DWI, all the lytic metastases show high signal intensity, with a higher ADC value than normal bone but lower than that of benign edema. However, WB-DWI must be performed along with conventional anatomical sequences because osteoblastic lesions may appear dark on high *b* value series, making their depiction difficult. Vilanova et al. proposed a new WB-MRI protocol with the addition of DWI sequences of the entire body to evaluate patients with suspected malignant or benign diffuse disease.

In conclusion, imaging plays an increasingly important role in the diagnosis as well as in the therapy and follow-up of breast cancer and metastatic disease. Whole-body MRI, including DWI sequences, can change patient management by detecting osseous and extraosseous metastases not seen on conventional imaging.

Imaging Findings

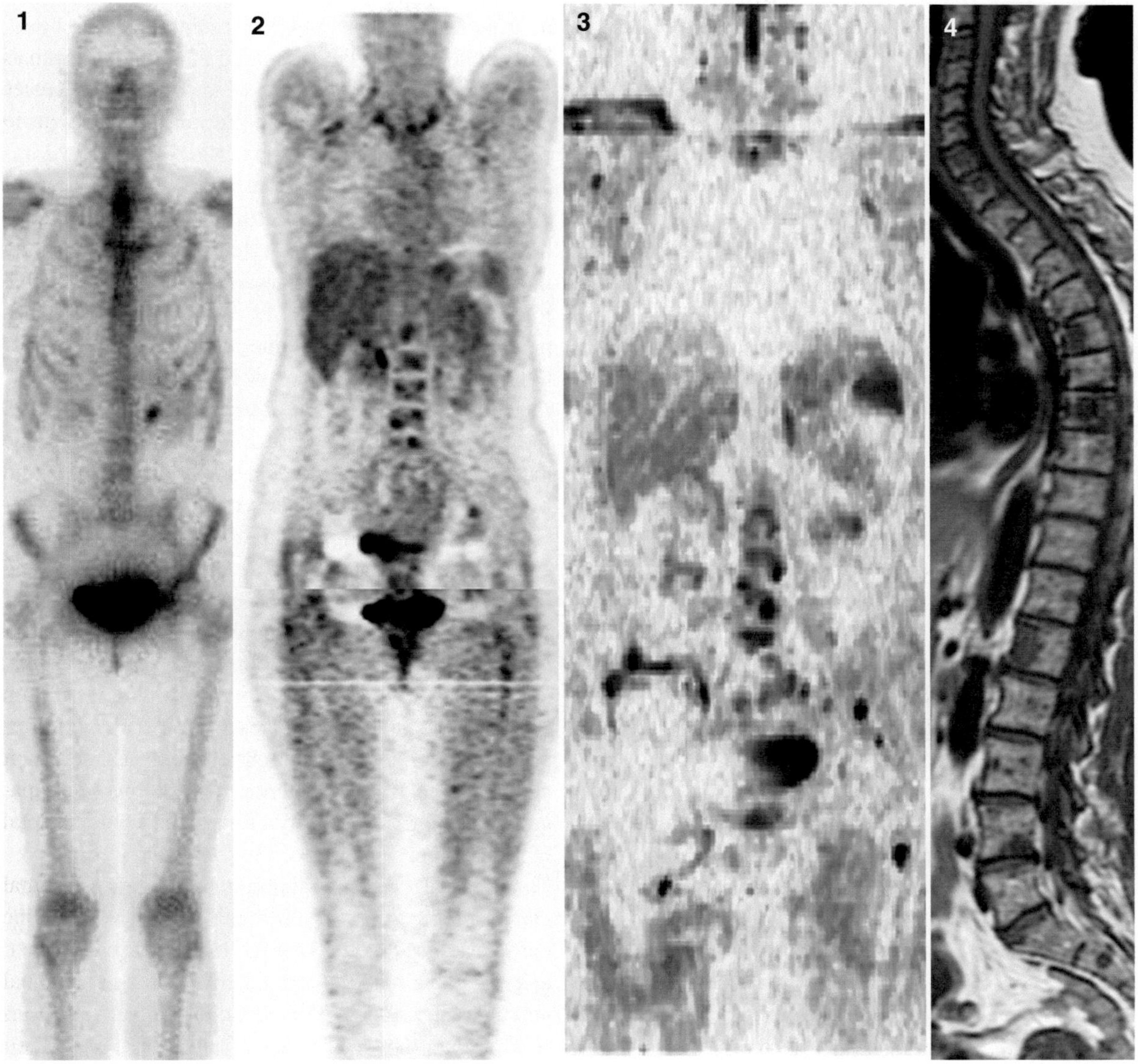

Fig. 16.2 Scintigraphy shows a unique metastasis at the second left rib (**16.2.1**). FDG-PET image (**16.2.2**) confirms the left rib metastasis and shows multiple bone metastases in the spine, pelvis, and left femur. Coronal WB-DWI with inverted gray scale (**16.2.3**) shows the same lesions as PET. Sagittal FSE T1-weighted of the whole spine (**16.2.4**) confirms the metastases of the vertebral bodies

Case 16.3: Bone and Lymph Node Metastases from Prostate Cancer

A 68-year-old-male with PSA of 21 ng/mL. WB-DWI was performed to rule out prostate cancer metastases.

Comments

Prostate adenocarcinoma (PCa) is the second most common cancer in men, accounting for one in nine of all new cancers. PCa is rarely diagnosed in men younger than 40 years, and it is uncommon in men younger than 50 years. Digital rectal examination and PSA evaluation are the two components necessary for a modern screening program. The upper limit of normal PSA is 4 ng/mL. When the PSA value is 21 ng/mL as in this case, metastatic disease must be excluded. PSA level is a strong indicator of stage and prognosis and is helpful in monitoring the response to therapy.

The mechanism for distant metastases in PCa is poorly understood. The cancer spreads to bone early, occasionally without significant lymphadenopathy. Metastatic clinical symptoms include weight loss and decrease of appetite, bone pain, with or without pathologic fracture, and lower extremity pain and edema due to obstruction of venous and lymphatic tributaries by nodal metastases. Uremic symptoms can occur from ureteral obstruction caused by local prostate growth or retroperitoneal adenopathy secondary to nodal metastases.

Skeletal metastases occur in approximately 90% of patients suffering from advanced prostate cancer, and the burden of bone disease directly correlates with survival. The detection of bone metastases indicates progression to lethal prostate carcinoma. The spread in bone also follows the distribution of adult red bone marrow – skull, thorax, pelvis, spine, proximal long bones – progressing to subsequently involve the adjacent cortical bone.

Imaging bone disease in prostate carcinoma frequently involves a cascade of studies that start with Tc99m methylene diphosphonate (Tc99mMDP) bone scintigraphy, backed up by plain film correlation and followed by MRI, CT, or even 18F-FDG or 11C-Choline PET/CT. Conventional planar bone scan has been extensively used in the detection of bone involvement because it offers the advantage of total body examination, low cost, and higher sensitivity for detection of bone metastases than plain-film radiography. However, MRI is potentially the technique of choice in evaluating prostate bone metastases as it is sensitive to early changes in bone marrow that precede the osteoblastic response in the bone matrix. Ketelsen et al. demonstrated that WB-MRI using native STIR and T1-weighted sequences was superior to bone scintigraphy for the detection of small bone metastases of prostate cancer. Lecouvet et al. revealed that MRI is capable to detect bone metastases in 37.5% of patients with negative or inconclusive bone scan and plain films.

Metastases to bone marrow lead to a lengthened T1 relaxation time and signal loss, which contrasts with the surrounding high signal of fatty marrow. The conspicuity of bone metastases can sometimes be increased by T2-weighted fat-suppressed sequences or STIR.

DWI starts playing an important role not only in the diagnosis of metastatic disease but also in the follow-up and monitoring of the response to treatment. DWI can identify differences in molecular water mobility in extracellular spaces, reflecting cellular organization and density, microstructure and microcirculation. Between the main challenges of DWI in oncologic patients are included: lymph nodal characterization and bone metastases detection. On the one hand, the generally higher cellularity of malignant lymph nodes facilitates their detection on high *b* value of diffusion. Thoeny et al. presented the first study on the value of DWI combined with ultrasmall superparamagnetic particles of iron oxide (USPIO) in patients with cancer of prostate or bladder with extension to normal-sized pelvic lymph nodes. They conclude that nodes with ADC values beyond 0.9×10^{-3} mm^2/s are malignant with a diagnostic accuracy of 79%. Nevertheless, future research should assess the validity of this technique.

On the other hand, several published studies have testified the potential of DWI in the detection of bone metastases. However, DWI should not be used in isolation but combined with conventional sequences, because osteoblastic metastases may be missed on DWI and are better visualized on T1-weighted imaging.

Imaging Findings

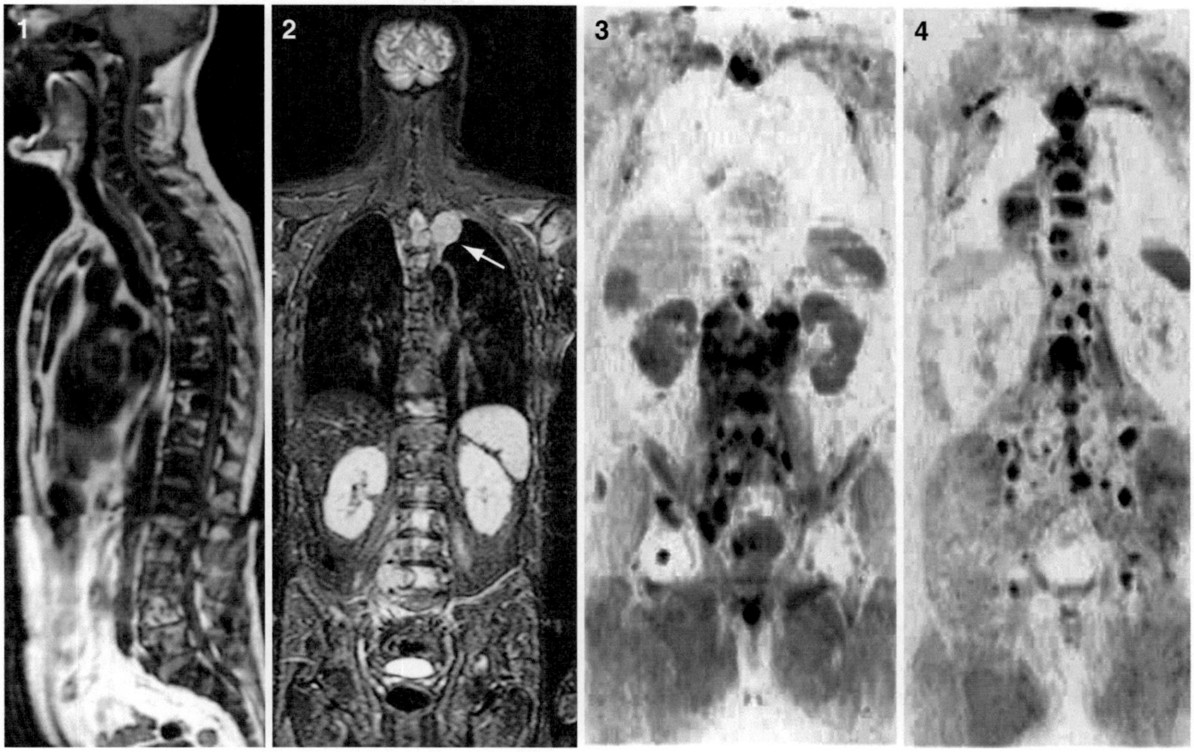

Fig. 16.3 Sagittal SE T1-weighted of the whole spine (**16.3.1**) shows low signal intensity foci along the spine, suggestive of osteoblastic metastases. Multiple areas of high signal intensity are shown in the spine on coronal STIR consistent with metastases, along with mediastinal nodal metastases (*arrow*) (**16.3.2**). Coronal MIP projections of a WB-DWI acquisition presented with inverted gray-scale (**16.3.3**, **16.3.4**) show multiples metastases in the bones depicted as low intensity lesions and extensive infradiaphragmatic lymph node involvement. Note that the normal bone marrow signal is suppressed

Case 16.4: Multiple Myeloma

A 51-year-old male complained of lumbar back pain. After a negative bone scan, a WB-MRI was performed.

Comments

Multiple myeloma is a generalized bone marrow disease caused by an infiltration of plasma cells. It is characterized by expansive growth of malignant plasma cell clones with consecutive destruction of the bony architecture. It accounts for 10–15% of all hematological malignancies and 1–2% of all cancers. The incidence of multiple myeloma varies by race and age. Clinically, approximately 10–40% of patients are asymptomatic at diagnosis, although bone pain is the most common symptom.

Predilection sites are not only the axial skeleton (spine and pelvis), but also the ribs, shoulder region, skull, and proximal femora. Therefore, whole-body imaging is needed to adequately assess the extent of disease.

In patients with myeloma, the basic diagnostic workup in many institutions includes radiographic examinations of the skull (two planes), the rib cage, the upper arms, the spine (two planes), the pelvis, and the upper legs. Typical radiographic findings include punched-out lytic lesions without any reactive sclerosis in the flat bones of the skull and pelvis. In the long bones, there is a range of appearances from endosteal scalloping and discrete small lytic lesions to larger destructive lesions. This diagnostic approach is still represented in the classic Salmon and Durie staging system of the disease, which assesses radiographic, immunohistochemical, and serological factors of the disease to determine the best therapy. Plain-film radiographs are routinely used for skeletal surveys; however, they are not sensitive enough to detect early osteolytic lesions. Newer imaging techniques like multislice CT, MRI, and whole-body PET offer improved diagnostic accuracy, enabling more precise staging and better management of this disease.

Modified diagnostic criteria published in 2006, the Durie-Salmon Plus Staging System, integrate WB-MRI, FDG-PET, and CT into routine staging. The role of imaging in the management of multiple myeloma is to assess the extent of intramedullary bone disease, to detect extramedullary foci, to evaluate the severity of disease at presentation, to identify and characterize complications, and to evaluate the response to treatment.

MRI has proven to be a valuable imaging tool for initial screening and follow-up in almost all types of multiple myeloma patients. MRI has the advantage of enabling bone marrow involvement to be evaluated and, therefore, it plays an important role in clinical decision making for patients with multiple myeloma.

WB-MRI has the potential to visualize the bone marrow directly and to determine abnormalities in bone marrow cell composition with high anatomic resolution. WB-MRI should be performed using sagittal SE T1-weighted sequences of the entire spine, coronal fat-suppressed T2-weighted or STIR sequences along with DWI of the head, thorax including the upper limbs, abdomen, pelvis, and thighs. Abnormalities in the bone marrow due to multiple myeloma typically show low signal intensity on T1-weighted sequences and high signal intensity on STIR or T2-weighted sequences. Diffuse involvement is best detected on unenhanced SE T1-weighted sequences, where it manifests as homogeneous signal reduction. Multiple myeloma lesions on DWI present restricted diffusion. ADC measurements have been correlated with serum markers of disease activity, with lower ADC values for active areas.

The differential diagnosis includes metastases, lymphomas, myeloproliferative diseases, or atypical hemangiomas. Treatment of multiple myeloma is complex and can include chemotherapy, radiation, and transplant. Areas with adequate response to therapy usually show increased T2 values.

Imaging Findings

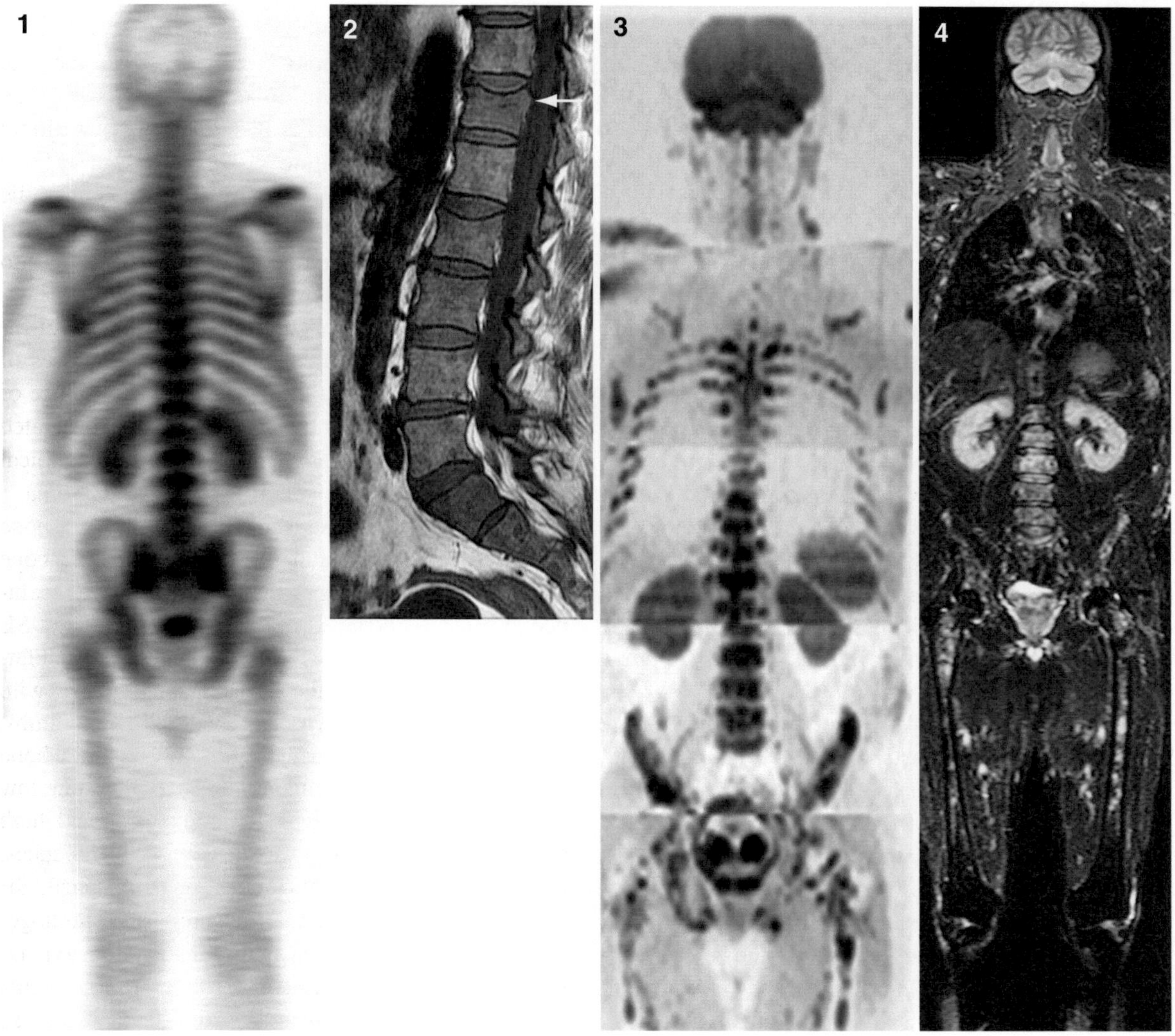

Fig. 16.4 Bone scintigraphy showed no abnormal uptake (**16.4.1**). Sagittal SE T1-weighted image showed diffuse and subtle low signal of all the vertebral bodies with some expansion at the posterior aspect of T12 level (*arrow*) (**16.4.2**). DWI-MRI (**16.4.3**) with inverted gray scale shows multiple lesions in the ribs, spine, pelvis, and femora (*arrows*). The corresponding STIR sequence from the whole-body MRI study (**16.4.4**) also demonstrates diffuse bone involvement in a similar manner

Case 16.5: Bone Metastases from Unknown Primary

A 31-year-old woman presented with left hip pain of one month's duration. A plain radiography and MRI were requested.

Comments

Bone is a common site of metastases for many primary malignant tumors; indeed, it is the third location after the liver and lungs. Metastases are the most frequent cause of bone tumors, accounting for 25% of cases. Furthermore, the spine represents the most frequent site of skeletal metastasis. Most metastatic lesions in the skeleton are encountered in middle-aged and elderly patients. Malignant cells can disseminate to the spine by various mechanisms: through the arterial system, through venous drainage, by cerebrospinal fluid, or by direct extension. Due to the rich blood supply of the vertebrae, the hematogenous route is the most common of these pathways.

Back pain is the most frequent initial complaint in patients with spinal metastatic disease. Pain, pathological fractures, and hypercalcemia are the major sources of morbidity of patients with bone metastases.

The diagnosis of bone metastases is crucial to determine the prognosis and to optimize therapy. Imaging of spinal metastatic disease may include radiography, myelography, bone scintigraphy, CT, and MRI. ^{99m}Tc-phosphonate-based skeletal scintigraphy is the standard method for the initial staging of bone tumors; its sensitivity ranges from 62% to 89%. MRI and PET can identify bone metastases. MRI is the only imaging technique that allows direct visualization of the bone marrow and its components.

Technical advances have enabled WB MRI examination using FSE T1-weighted, STIR, and DWI sequences in less than an hour.

Metastatic bone lesions can be described as osteolytic, osteoblastic, or mixed. On T1-weighted sequences, tumor spread is identified by replacement of normal marrow, resulting in an isointense or hypointense signal compared to muscle tissue. On STIR sequences, increased water content within tumor cells readily reveals bone tumors as lesions hyperintense to the surrounding normal marrow. In osteoblastic metastases, areas of low signal intensity on FSE T1-weighted images correspond to areas of low signal intensity on FSE T2-weighted images. On STIR, the appearance of osteoblastic metastases ranges from no signal in very dense sclerotic metastases to hyperintense signal in cases where more cellular components are present.

Unfortunately, T2-weighted and STIR sequences do not differentiate intracellular water signal intensity due to malignant disease from the interstitial water signal due to fracture edema. On DWI, these differences can be used to characterize tissue pathology. DWI highlights areas with restricted diffusion, such as it occurs in many malignant primary and metastatic tumors, and provides outstanding visualization of lymph nodes. DWI also provides functional information that can be used to detect and characterize bone metastases. DWI sequences typically demonstrate increased signal intensity in tumoral areas, edema, infections, highly cellular lymph nodes, as well as in lytic metastases. Moreover, differences in signal intensity on high *b* value acquisitions and ADC measurements have been proposed to differentiate bone metastases from benign edema. However, entirely osteoblastic metastases are not conspicuous on DWI.

Imaging Findings

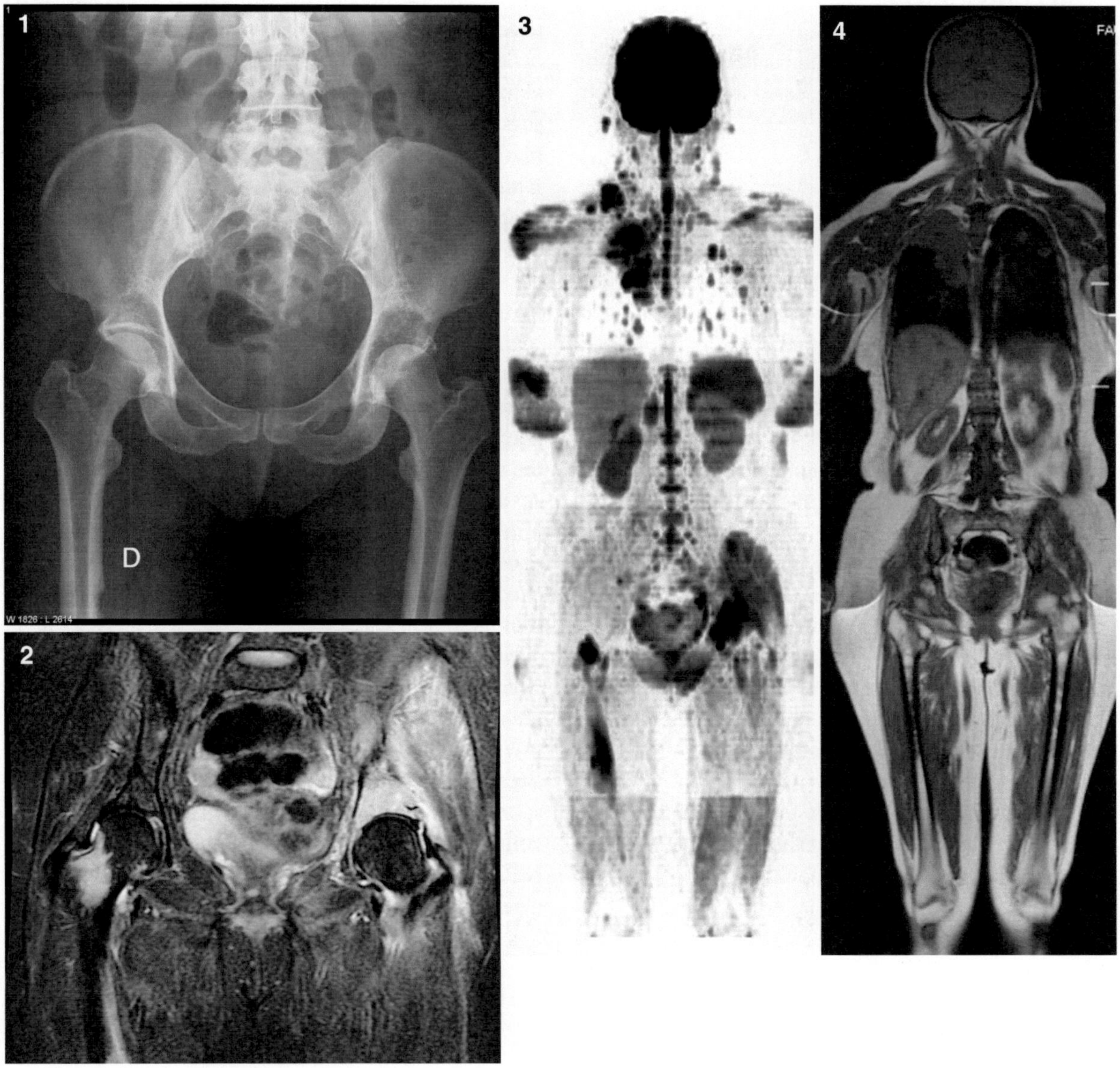

Fig. 16.5 Plain-film radiograph of the pelvis (**16.5.1**) shows a radiolucent lesion in the left acetabulum and another lytic bone lesion in the right femur. Both lesions are clearly depicted as areas of increased signal on coronal fat-suppressed T2-weighted MRI (**16.5.2**). Coronal MIP of DWIBS with inverted gray intensity scale (**16.5.3**) demonstrates a large apical right pulmonary mass as a low intensity area corresponding to a lung cancer. Notice also the presence of bilateral pulmonary, right adrenal gland, right supraclavicular lymph node, and bone pelvic and right femoral metastases. Corresponding coronal FSE T1-weighted image (**16.5.4**) also depicts the primary neoplasm in the right lung and the pulmonary and bone metastatic involvement

Case 16.6: Liver and Bone Metastases from Lung Cancer

A 67-year-old man with left lung cancer. Bone scintigraphy and WB-MRI were requested to rule out metastases and further staging.

Comments

Lung cancer is the leading cause of cancer deaths in the United States and worldwide. The two major forms of lung cancer are NSCLC (about 85% of all lung cancers) and small-cell lung cancer (about 15%). Accurate staging of lung cancer is requisite to choose the optimal therapeutic strategy and is very important for prognosis. Multimodality diagnostic imaging is currently used for detection, staging, and follow-up.

Most tumors are found on chest radiographs, although further evaluation with thoracic CT is performed to stage local disease. Chest CT scan defines the location, size, and anatomical characteristics of the tumor. Standard CT protocols, including the upper liver and adrenal glands, are also said to detect metastatic deposits in these organs in 3–10% of asymptomatic patients. Additional radiologic studies, including radionuclide bone scan, brain CT, or MRI, are typically used in selected patients to locate extrathoracic metastases. The most common sites of metastases from lung cancer are the brain, bone, liver, and adrenal glands.

Currently, whole-body 18-FDG-PET has become an extremely useful tool that combines high sensitivity and specificity for the detection of intrathoracic lymph node metastases or distant metastases and can help prevent unnecessary surgery. Lung cancer cells demonstrate increased cellular uptake of glucose and a higher rate of glycolysis when compared to normal cells. Besides, WB-MRI is widely used for diagnosis and characterization of diseases in all regions of the body and could be used as a tool in the staging of lung cancer. WB-MRI provides very exact morphological information, does not involve ionizing radiation, and allows scanning the whole body in a short acquisition time. Furthermore, several studies show that WB-DWI can be applied in the detection of small metastases in the body and bone. Recently, Nomori et al. have evaluated the accuracy of DWI in the detection of nodal metastases showing more accuracy than FDG-PET. DWI, combined with conventional sequences, is a new tool for the detection and evaluation of metastatic disease of lung cancer. Ohno and colleagues stated that WB-DWI with morphological whole-body sequences showed the same accuracy as PET-CT for M-staging of NSCLC. Conversely, WB-DWI alone was significantly worse than either morphological WB-MRI, with or without DWIBS sequence, or PET-CT. Most of the false-positives and false negatives with both techniques corresponded to brain and pulmonary lesions. Chen and colleagues found similar results in the M-staging of NSCLC for WB-DWI and PET-CT, although better detection rates were achieved with the last technique.

Imaging Findings

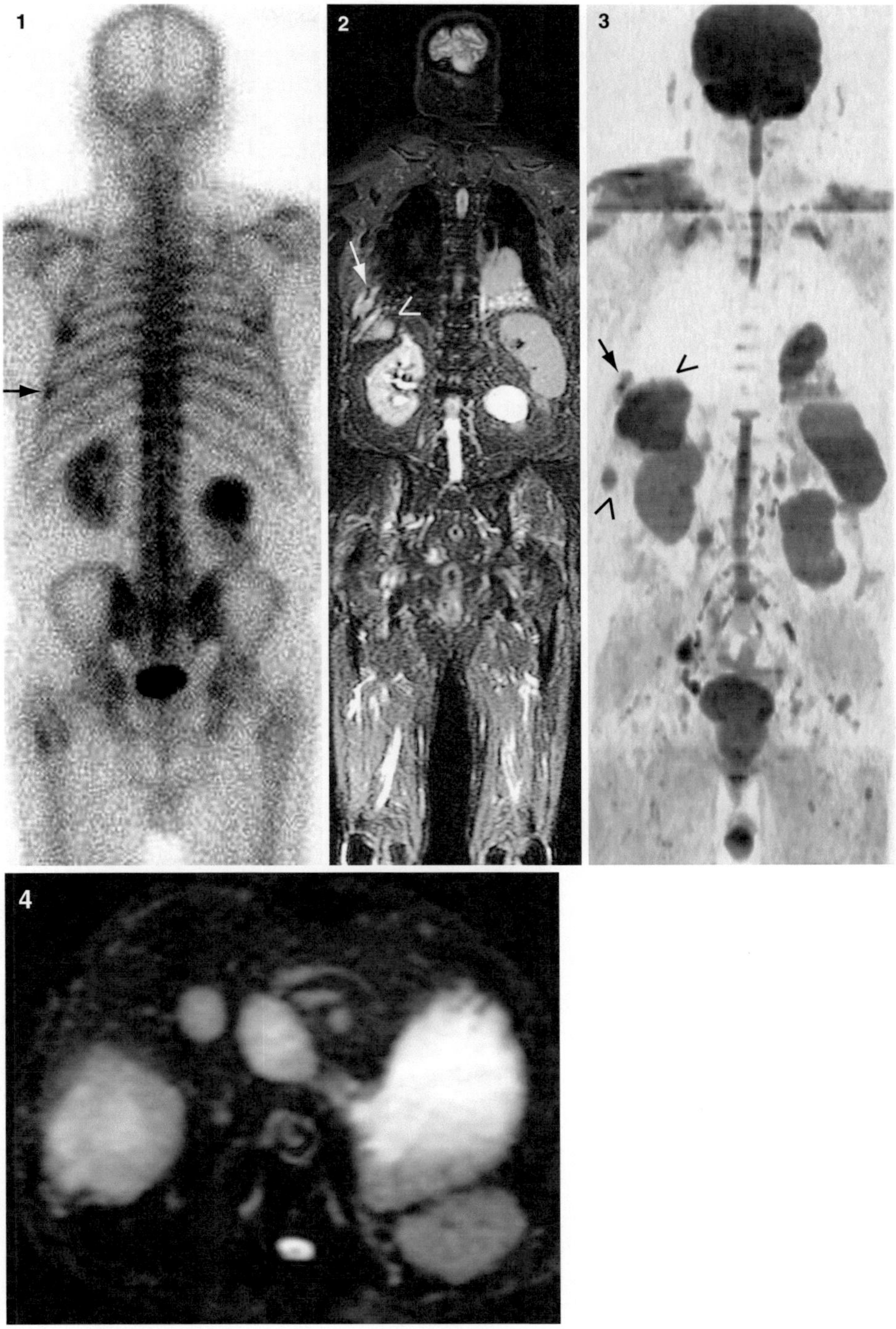

Fig. 16.6 Bone Scintigraphy (**16.6.1**) shows a possible posttraumatic lesion within the lateral aspect of the eighth right rib which was not consistent with metastasis (*arrow*). Coronal whole-body STIR (**16.6.2**) showed the primary left lung tumor with surrounding postobstructive pneumonitis and the previously mentioned lesion of the eighth right rib (*arrow*) consistent with a metastatic origin on MRI. Notice the presence of liver metastases as well (*arrowhead*). Coronal MIP of WB-DWI obtained with a *b* value of 600 s/mm^2 presented at inverted grayscale (**16.6.3**) confirms all the findings visualized on STIR. Axial DWI (**16.6.4**) at a *b* value of 0 s/mm^2 shows liver metastases in both hepatic lobes

Case 16.7: Search for the Primary Neoplasm in a Patient with Hepatic Metastases

A 67-year-old man with wasting syndrome. Ultrasound showed a cirrhotic liver with multiple focal liver lesions and portal thrombosis. A differential diagnosis between metastatic liver and diffuse hepatocarcinoma was proposed, favoring metastases. WB-DWI with dedicated liver sequences was performed for further characterization.

Comments

The feasibility and performance of WB-DWI for the detection of metastases and the staging of different types of tumor is well known, demonstrating a good correlation with PET-CT. Conversely, there is scarce experience in the capabilities of WB-DWI in the searching of primary tumors in patients with unknown primary. DWIBS should potentially be a powerful tool in this task due to its superb sensitivity in the detection of hypercellular lesions. Besides, tumor presenting with metastases are usually aggressive or undifferentiated ones, which also tend to show a greater degree of restricted diffusion, as it usually increases in a parallel manner to the grade of tumoral aggresiveness. In a series by Gu and colleagues, WB-DWI was able to detect the primary tumor in patients with metastases of unknown origin in 23 out of 24 patients. The other case corresponded to a benign tumor. Additionally, no definite primary lesion was found on WB-DWI in ten cases and only in one case, a primary tumor was found in the follow-up over half a year. Larger series are necessary to evaluate the role of DWIBS in the search of unknown primary tumors.

WB-DWI has shown advantage over PET-CT in the detection of small liver and peritoneal metastases. In the case presented, DWIBS allows us to accurately assess thoracic and abdominal metastases.

Imaging Findings

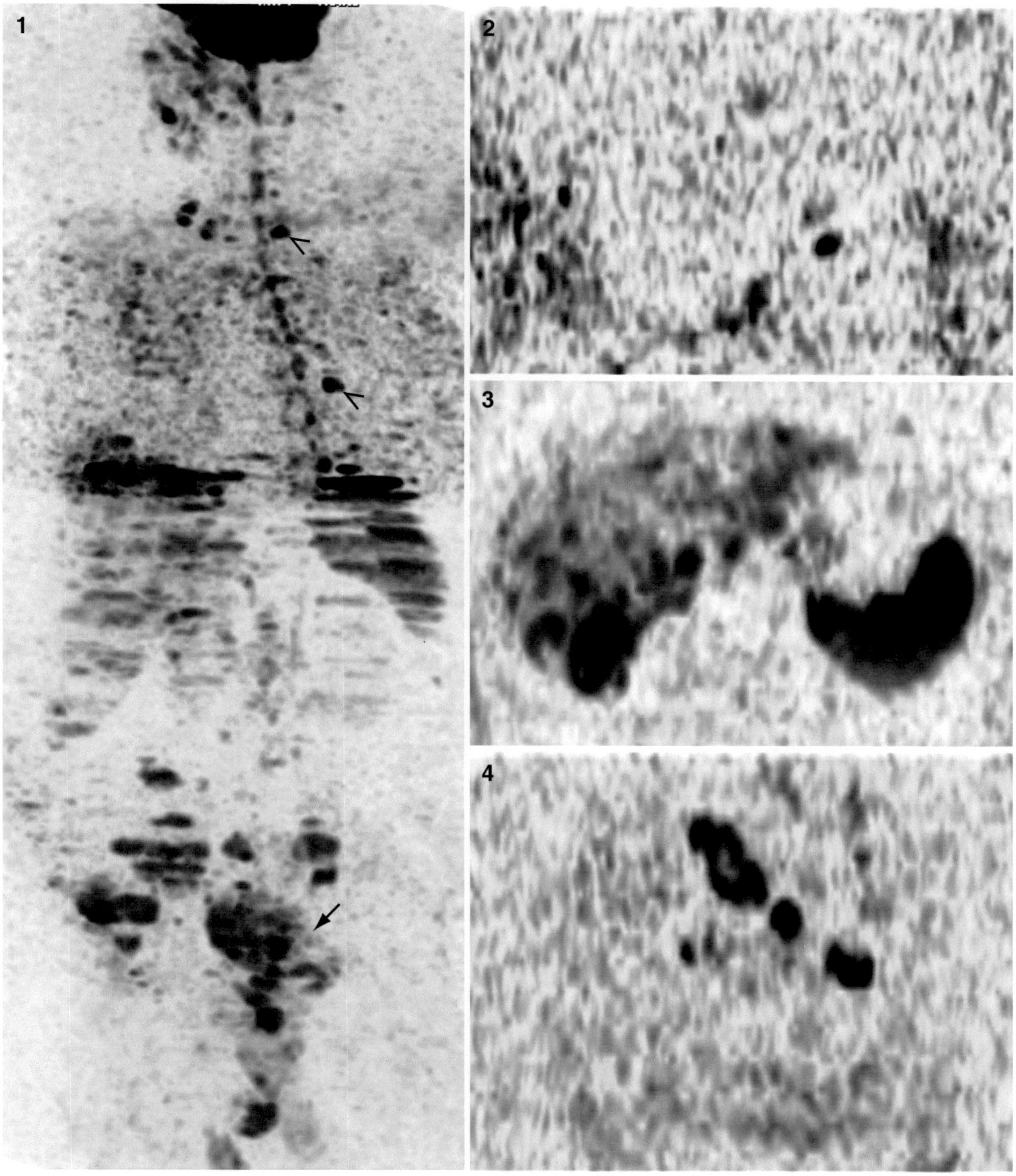

Fig. 16.7 Coronal MIP of a DWIBS sequence with *a b* value of 1000 mm^2/s shows multiple mediastinal lymph nodes (*arrowheads*), hepatic and peritoneal metastases, along with a mass with restricted diffusion within the pelvis corresponding to a primary sigmoid carcinoma (*arrow*) (**16.7.1**). Paired original DWIBS (**16.7.2–16.7.5**) and HASTE (**16.7.6–16.7.9**) images better demonstrate the presence of the primary tumor and mediastinal, hepatic, and peritoneal metastases. Notice the better depiction of the metastases on DWIBS compared with HASTE

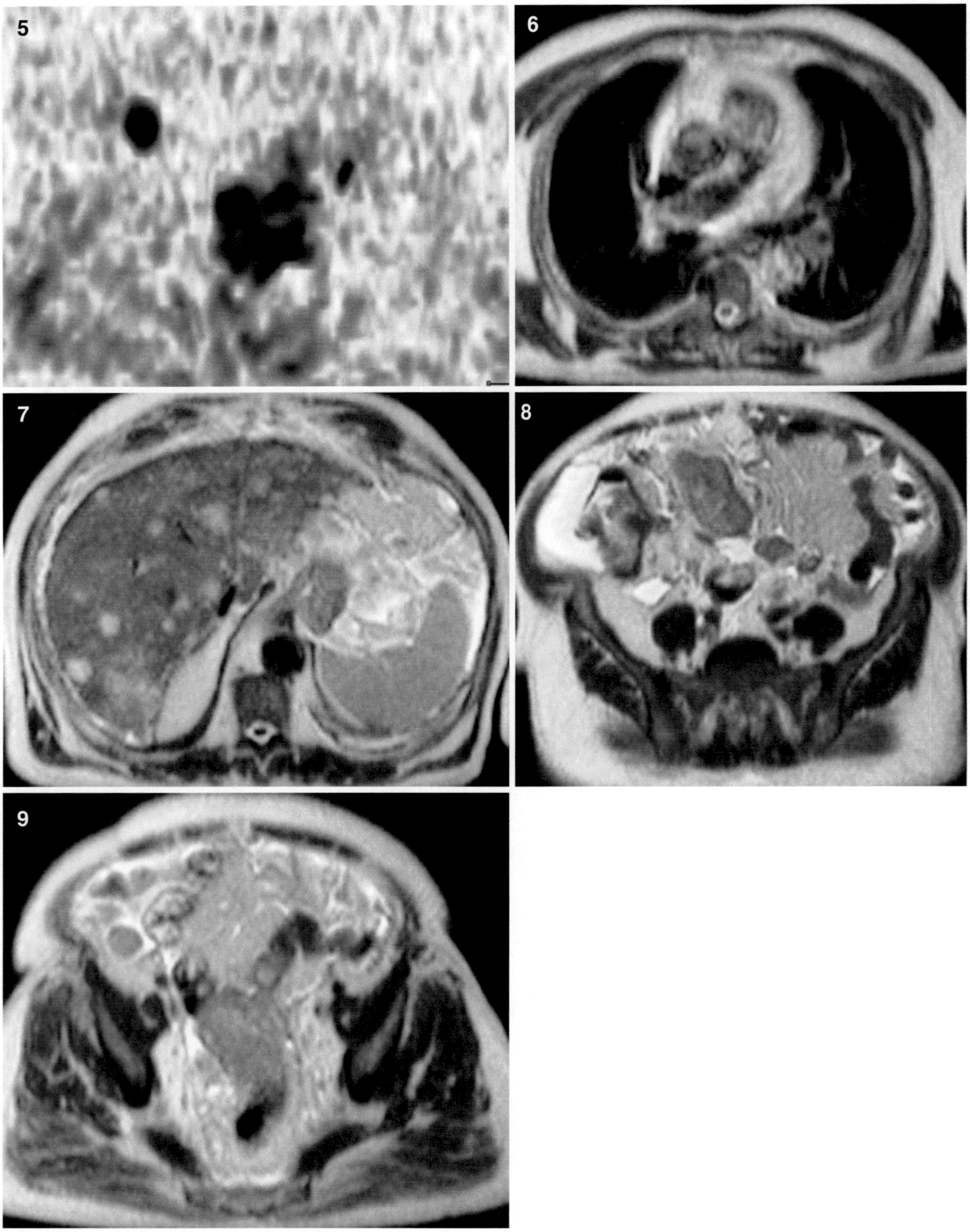

Fig. 16.7 (continued)

Case 16.8: Staging and Posttreatment Monitorization of Non-Hodgkin Lymphoma in a Pregnant Woman

A 27-year-old woman in the 16th week of pregnancy presented a fast growing mass in right supraclavicular space with positive biopsy for non-Hodgkin lymphoma. WB-DWI was performed for staging.

Comments

Malignant lymphomas are staged using the Ann Arbor staging system, except for childhood non-Hodgkin lymphomas that are staged using the Murphy staging system. Initial staging (at diagnosis) and restaging (after onset or completion of therapy or in cases of disease recurrence) is usually done by means of CT or combined 18-FDG-PET-CT.

Several reports have demonstrated the accuracy of WB-MRI and WB-DWI in the initial staging of both Hodgkin and non-Hodgkin lymphoma. Both techniques equal CT in the initial staging of lymphoma and correctly overstage relative to CT, with a possible advantage of using DWI, as it increases detection rates. DWIBS is able to highlight enlarged and normal-sized lymph nodes due to their hypercellularity against a suppressed background. This capability makes it a superb weapon for lymphoma detection and staging. Besides, ADC measurements have been demonstrated to accurately differentiate normal from lymphomatous enlarged lymph nodes. This difference has not been reported to our knowledge for normal-sized lymph nodes. Therefore, DWIBS is able to detect nodal involvement of lymphoma based in enlarged lymph nodes, which are better measured on anatomical sequences. WB-DWI has also been proposed for assessment of bone marrow involvement by lymphoma, although it should be performed along with T1-weighted and STIR sequences. Furthermore, a recent series showed excellent correlation in the staging of diffuse large B-cell lymphoma between WB-DWI and PET-CT, regarding both lymph node and organ involvement, using only a WB-DWI with spectral fat saturation and ADC measurements. Although PET-CT is the best imaging technique for the staging of lymphoma at this moment, WB-DWI should be considered a valid alternative, mainly in cases where the use of ionizing radiation must be managed with caution, such as in children or pregnant women.

PET-CT has also shown a role in the early and late therapy response assessment in lymphoma patients, due to the functional metabolic information PET provides. In a similar manner, DWI has shown its potential in the posttreatment monitorization of human non-Hodgkin lymphoma xenografts in mice, which has still to be confirmed in humans.

Imaging Findings

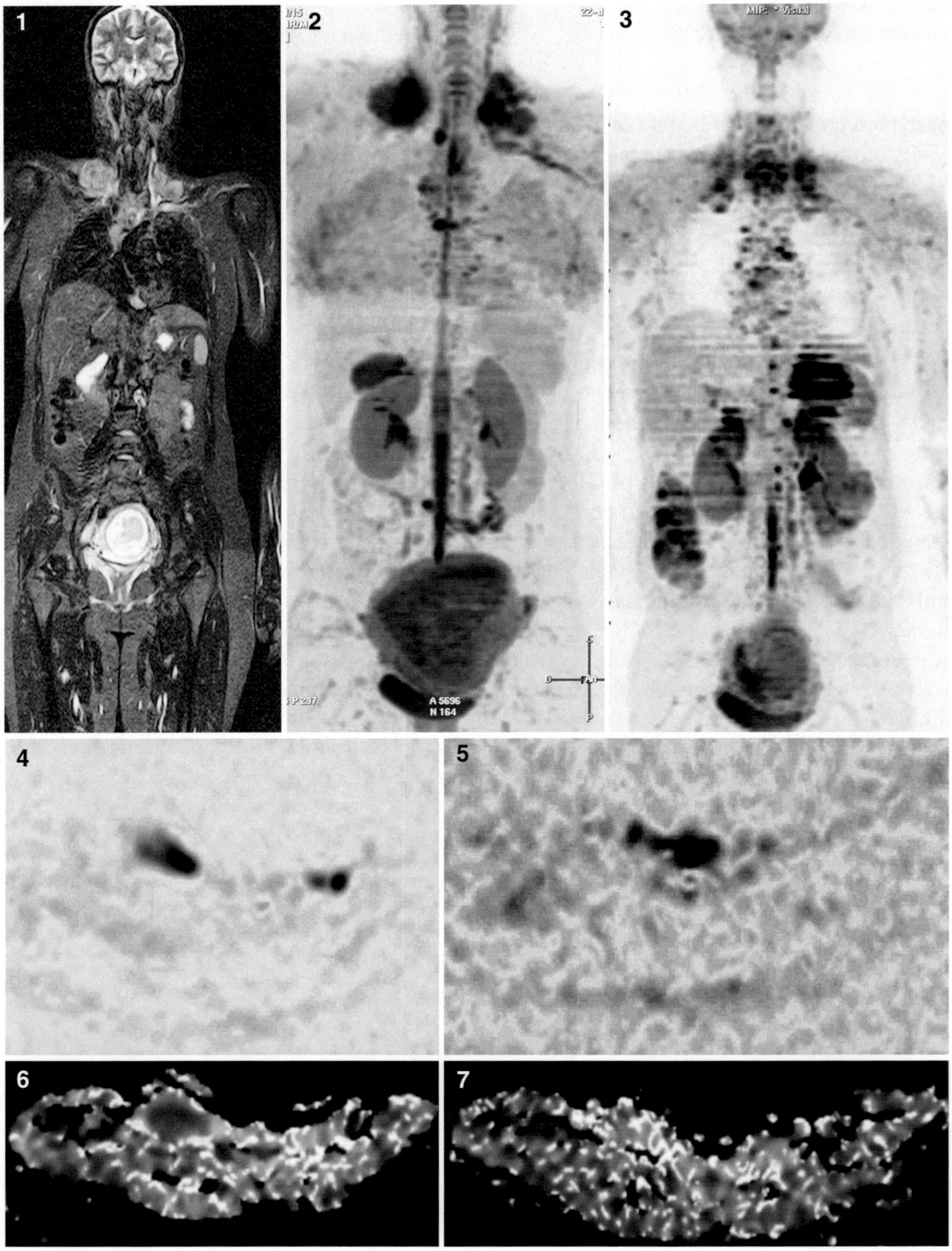

Fig. 16.8 Coronal WB-STIR shows bilateral supraclavicular nodal masses and mediastinal involvement (**16.8.1**). Coronal mini-MIP of a DWIBS with *a b* value of 400 mm²/s shows restricted diffusion of the masses of both supraclavicular spaces and mediastinum and additional involvement of left cervical and para-aortic lymph nodes (**16.8.2**). Posttreatment coronal mini-MIP of a DWIBS with *a b* value of 400 mm²/s allows accurate assessment of positive response to chemotherapy (**16.8.3**). The supraclavicular and mediastinal lymph nodes do not show restricted diffusion and have decreased in size. There is remnant left para-aortic lymph node active disease. Figures **16.8.4** and **16.8.5** show pretreatment and posttreatment DWIBS with *a b* value of 1000 mm²/s in the neck region confirming the absence of restriction of the supraclavicular masses after treatment. ADC measurements of the right supraclavicular mass increased from 1.1×10^{-3} mm²/s before treatment (**16.8.6**) to 3.71×10^{-3} mm²/s after chemotherapy (**16.8.7**)

Case 16.9: Unique Spleen Metastasis from Rectal Cancer

A 67-year-old female patient had previous surgery for rectal carcinoma (RC) stage T3N0M0. Three years after the intervention, the patient presented elevated levels of CarcinoEmbryonic Antigen (CEA). PET-CT and WB-DWI MRI were performed to exclude metastatic disease.

Comments

The presence of a hypermetabolic focus in the spleen in the PET-CT study in a patient with rectal cancer history raised the suspicion of metastasis, although the presence of a solitary splenic metastasis is unusual in patients with colorectal cancer (CRC). Finally, diagnosis after surgery and histological investigation confirmed the presence of a unique splenic metastasis.

Only 14 cases have been reported in the literature. Several hypotheses have attempted to explain the low incidence of splenic metastasis in patients with CRC. Both vascular and lymphatic routes have been proposed as the means of transmission. The exclusivity of this case is the small size of the lesion in contrast to the cases described in the literature. The treatment of choice is splenectomy.

On MRI, the presence of a hypointense focus on STIR in the spleen favors lymphoma or chronic infectious lesion, although metastases cannot be definitively excluded. Splenic metastases are better depicted on MRI by means of postcontrast dynamic series. Metastases are typically hypovascular on immediate postcontrast images, becoming isointense after the first postcontrast minute. In this case, the diagnostic clue was the increased metabolic uptake of the lesion in PET-CT, confirming that PET-CT is a useful technique for detecting splenic metastases, even small lesions, and performs better than other imaging techniques such as US, CT, and MRI. The differential diagnosis should consider the presence of an infectious focus due to the significant tracer uptake observed in PET-CT study, although in this case, there were not any clinical data suggesting infectious process.

DWI is not a valid technique to study the spleen, as it is hypercellular in normal conditions. Surprisingly, the lesion was hypointense against the high signal background of the hypercellular spleen on DWI because this splenic metastasis showed less cellularity than the normal spleen. In our experience, splenic metastasis may show more or less signal intensity than spleen on DWI with high *b* value. Moreover, there is lack of scientific series evaluating the role of DWI in splenic metastasis assessment.

The possibility of local recurrence at the suture line was considered based on CT findings, but the absence of tracer uptake on PET acquisition excluded this diagnosis. The DWI series also confirmed the absence of local recurrence.

Imaging Findings

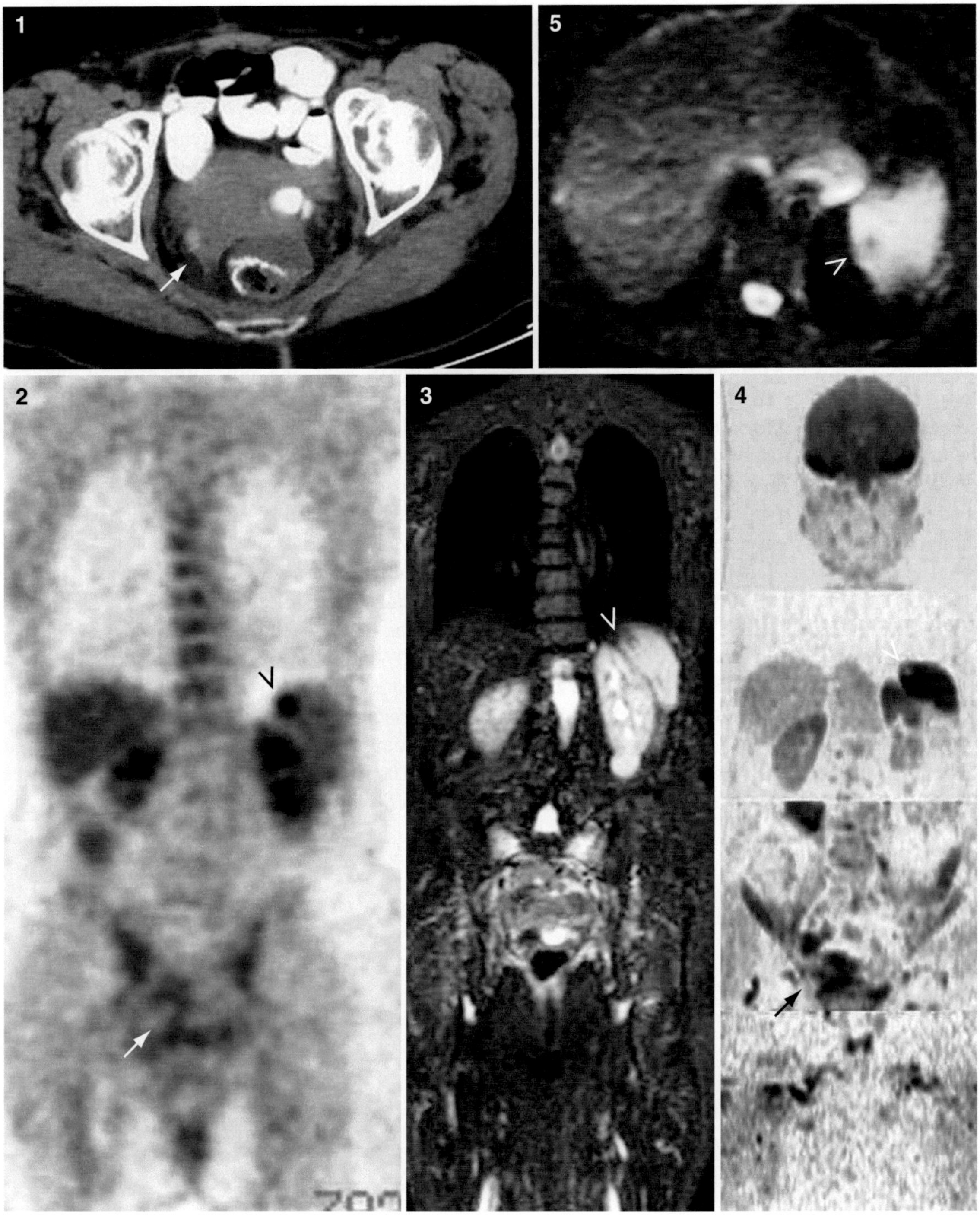

Fig. 16.9 Axial imaging on CT (**16.9.1**) shows postoperative pelvic changes after resection of rectal cancer (*arrow*). Coronal 18-FDG-PET (**16.9.2**) does not demonstrate signs of local tumor recurrence although a focal area of increased metabolic activity in the presacral region is visualized (*arrow*). Note the presence of a marked small hypermetabolic focus (SUVmax 7.6) in the medial border of the spleen (*arrowhead*). Coronal WB-MRI STIR sequence (**16.9.3**) reveals a nonspecific hypointense small lesion within the spleen consistent with metastasis (*arrowhead*). The corresponding coronal MPR of a WB-DWI with inverted contrast grayscale (**16.9.4**) demonstrates a small spleen lesion appearing as a white spot within the low signal spleen (*arrowhead*). Notice the absence of areas of restricted diffusion within the pelvis, excluding local recurrence (*arrow*). The native axial DWI-MR image (**16.9.5**) at a *b* value of 700 s/mm^2 through the upper abdomen confirms the low signal lesion at DWI (*arrowhead*)

Case 16.10: Neurofibromatosis Type 1

A 29-year-old male diagnosed of neurofibromatosis type 1 (NF-1). WB-DWI MRI was performed to assess the extension and number of peripheral plexiform neurofibromas and rule out malignant transformation.

Comments

NF-1 is a genetic disorder with an autosomal dominant transmission. Characteristic lesions of this syndrome are: cafe-au-lait spots, neurofibromas, Lisch nodules of the iris, and skinfold freckling. About 5% of patients with NF-1 develop malignant nerve sheath tumor (MNST), which arises from previous plexiform neurofibromas. Therefore, the active follow-up of NF-1 patients with peripheral plexiform neurofibromas is important. Neither CT nor MRI allow a correct differentiation of benign from MNST. On MRI, MNST usually has irregular margins, central necrosis, and shows incomplete fat-split sign. 18F-FDG PET has shown a higher uptake in MNST than in benign neurofibromas, permitting their distinction. Recently, DWI has been used in a case report for evaluation of a retroperitoneal MNST. DWI showed an interesting potential to distinguish the areas with malignant transformation from the benign areas of the tumor, as malignant areas showed significant lower ADC values. Besides, DWI has proven useful for the assessment of tumor cellularity in soft-tissue sarcomas, although there was only a tendency toward lower ADC in tumors with higher grading but no significant dependency.

WB-MRI has been recently proposed to determine tumor burden in patients with NF. As in the case shown, DWI is also useful for higher detection of plexiform neurofibromas compared to anatomical sequences (Figs. 16.10.1 and 16.10.2). The use of DWI with a low *b* value enhances the detection of neurofibromas, and only the ones with restricted diffusion on high *b* value acquisition should be considered as suspicious for malignant transformation (Fig. 16.10.3). In these suspicious lesions, ADC quantification enables further evaluation of cellularity. Only those lesions with low ADC should be considered for follow-up or biopsy, taking into account their appearance on the rest of sequences.

Imaging Findings

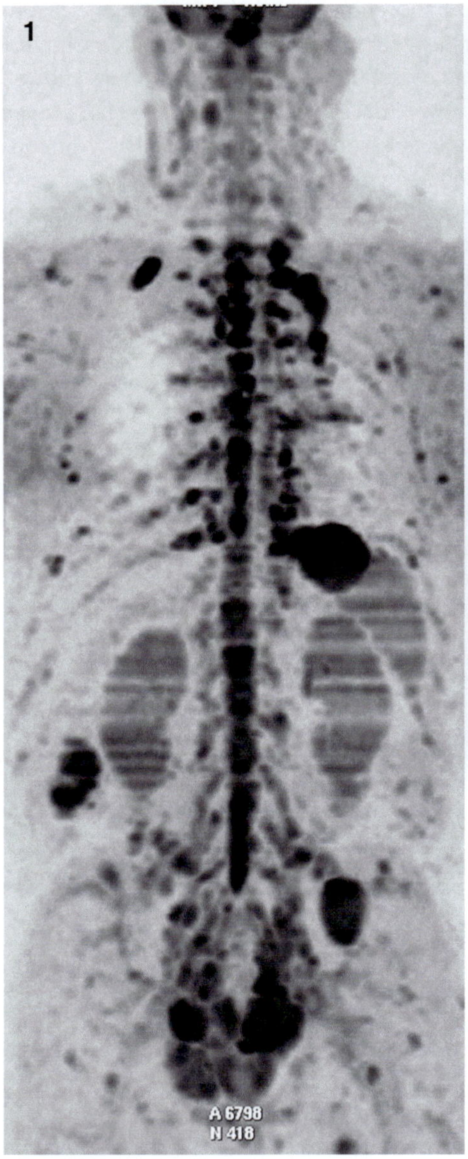

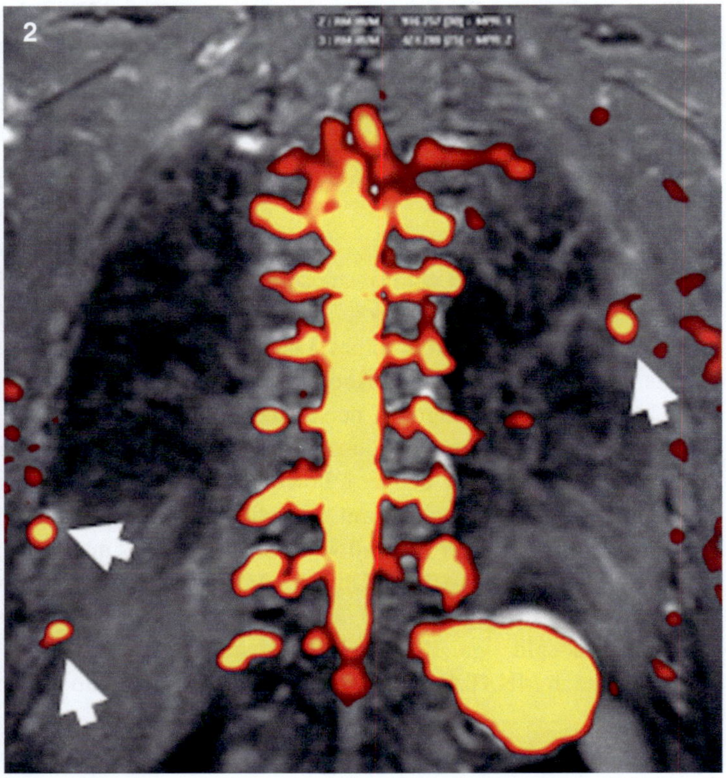

Fig. 16.10 WB-DWI with *a b* value of 0 s/mm^2 (**16.10.1**) shows multiple plexiform neurinomas in all body regions. The largest ones are located in: right parapharyngeal space, left upper mediastinum, left paravertebral thoracic region, immediately supradiaphragmatic on left hemithorax, between left psoas and iliacus muscles, and several confluent pelvic neurofibromas, the largest one within left abductor maximus. Fusion image of DWIBS with *b* 0 s/mm^2 and TSE T2-weighted sequence of the chest better depicts the plexiform neurofibromas involving thoracic nerve roots and intercostal nerves (*arrows*) (**16.10.2**). On DWIBS sequences with *a b* value of 1000 s/mm^2, only some of the pelvic and thoracic plexiform neurofibromas were visible (**16.10.3**). There were no signs of malignant degeneration in any of these lesions on either ADC quantification or morphological MRI sequences (not shown). ADC maps at the level of upper abdomen and pelvis (**16.10.4** and **16.10.5**, respectively) show several neurofibromas with ADC values between 1.7 and 2.3×10^{-3} mm^2/s

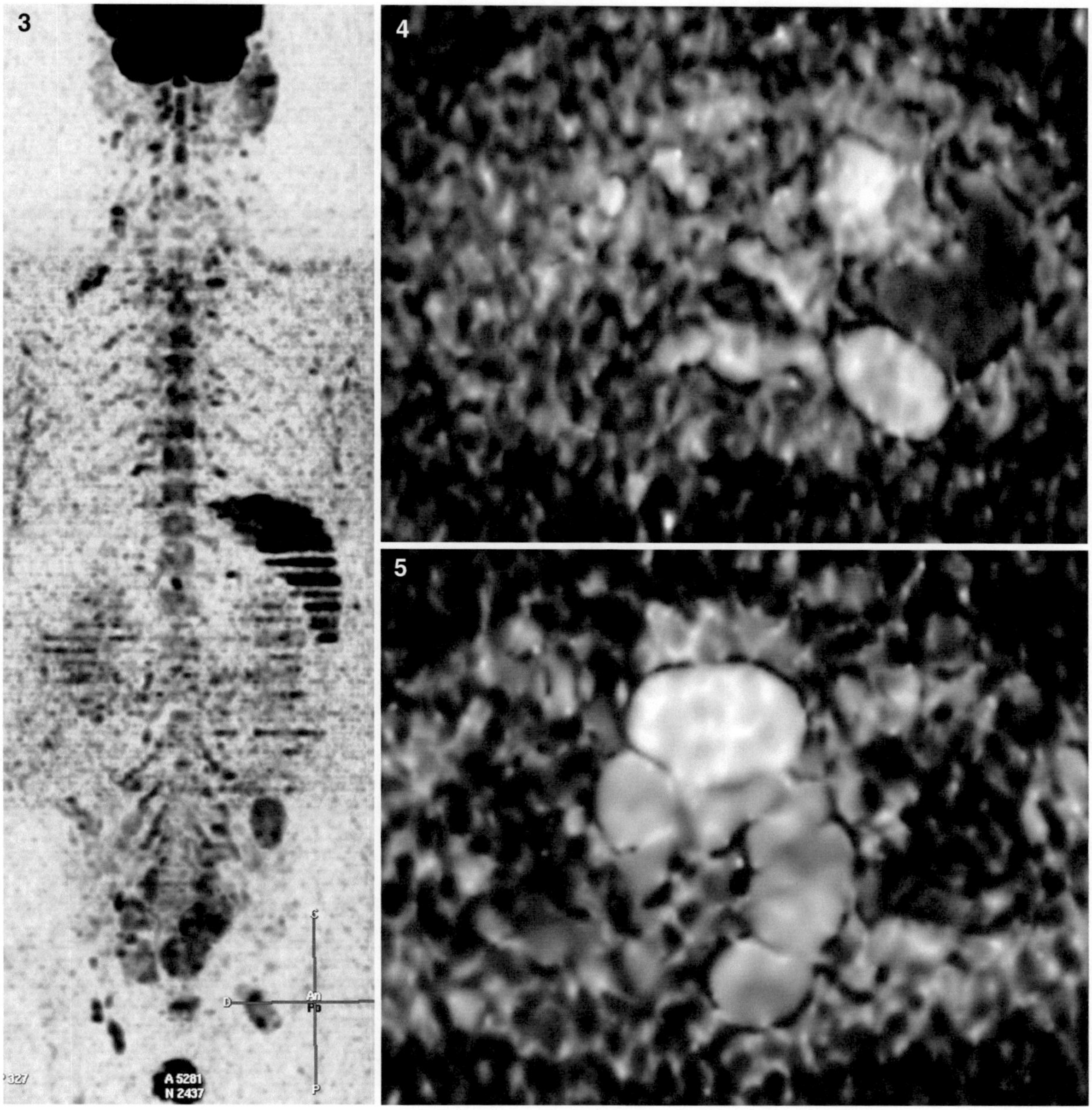

Fig. 16.10 (continued)

Further Reading

Balliu E, Vilanova JC, Peláez I et al (2009) Diagnostic value of apparent diffusion coefficients to differentiate benign from malignant vertebral bone marrow lesions. Eur J Radiol 69(3):560–566

Barcelo J, Vilanova JC, Riera E et al (2007) Diffusion-weighted whole-body MRI (virtual PET) in screening for osseous metastases. Radiología 49:407–415

Baur A, Reiser MF (2000) Diffusion-weighted imaging of the musculoskeletal system in humans. Skeletal Radiol 29:555–562

Bley TA, Wieben O, Uhl M (2009) Diffusion-weighted MR imaging in musculoskeletal radiology: applications in trauma, tumors, and inflammation. Magn Reson Imaging Clin N Am 17:263–275

Boussel L, Marchand B, Blineau N et al (2002) Imaging of osteoarticular tuberculosis. J Radiol 83(9 Pt 1):1025–1034

Cai W, Kassarjian A, Bredella MA et al (2009) Tumor burden in patients with neurofibromatosis types 1 and 2 and schwannomatosis: determination on whole-body MR images. Radiology 250(3):665–673

Chan JH, Peh WC, Tsui EY et al (2002) Acute vertebral body compression fractures: discrimination between benign and malignant causes using apparent diffusion coefficients. Br J Radiol 75(891):207–214

Chen W, Jian W, Li H et al (2010) Whole-body diffusion-weighted imaging vs. FDG-PET for the detection of non-small-cell lung cancer. How do they measure up? Magn Reson Imaging 28:613–620

Choi EK, Kim JK, Choi HJ et al (2009) Node-by-node correlation between MR and PET/CT in patients with uterine cervical cancer: diffusion-weighted imaging versus size-based criteria on T2WI. Eur Radiol 19:2024–2032

Dietrich O, Biffar A, Reiser MF et al (2009) Diffusion-weighted imaging of bone marrow. Semin Musculoskelet Radiol 13:134–144

Engin G, Acunaş B, Acunaş G et al (2000) Imaging of extrapulmonary tuberculosis. Radiographics 20(2):471–488

Gu TF, Xiao XL, Sun F et al (2008) Diagnostic value of whole body diffusion weighted imaging for screening primary tumors of patients with metastases. Chin Med Sci J 23(3):145–150

Herneth AM, Friedrich K, Weidekamm C et al (2005) Diffusion weighted imaging of bone marrow pathologies. Eur J Radiol 55(1):74–83

Heusner TA, Kuemmel S, Hamami ME et al (2010) Diagnostic value of DWI MRI compared to FDG PET/CT for whole body breast cancer staging. Eur J Nucl Med Mol Imaging 37(6):1077–1086

Huang MQ, Pickup S, Nelson DS et al (2008) Monitoring response to chemotherapy of non-Hodgkin's lymphoma xenografts by T(2)-weighted and diffusion-weighted MRI. NMR Biomed 21(10):1021–1029

Karchevsky M, Babb JS, Schweitzer ME (2008) Can diffusion-weighted imaging be used to differentiate benign from pathologic fractures? A meta-analysis. Skeletal Radiol 37(9):791–795

Ketelsen D, Röthke M, Aschoff P et al (2008) Detection of bone metastasis of prostate cancer –comparison of whole-body MRI and bone scintigraphy. Rofo 180(8):746–752

Kwee TC, Takahara T, Ochiai R et al (2009) Whole-body diffusion-weighted magnetic resonance imaging. Eur J Radiol 70(3):409–417

Kwee TC, Takahara T, Ochiai R et al (2010) Complementary roles of whole-body diffusion-weighted MRI and 18F-FDG PET: the state of the art and potential applications. J Nucl Med 51(10):1549–1558

Kwee TC, Takahara T, Vermoolen MA et al (2010) Whole-body diffusion-weighted imaging for staging malignant lymphoma in children. Pediatr Radiol 40(10):1592–1602

Kwee TC, van Ufford HM, Beek FJ et al (2009) Whole-body MRI, including diffusion-weighted imaging, for the initial staging of malignant lymphoma: comparison to computed tomography. Invest Radiol 44(10):683–690

Laurent V, Trausch G, Bruot O et al (2010) Comparative study of two whole-body imaging techniques in the case of melanoma metastases: advantages of multicontrast MRI examination including a diffusion-weighted sequence in comparison with PET-CT. Eur J Radiol 75(3):376–383

Lecouvet FE, Geukens D, Stainier A et al (2007) Magnetic resonance imaging of the axial skeleton for detecting bone metastases in patients with high-risk prostate cancer: diagnostic and cost-effectiveness and comparison with current detection strategies. J Clin Oncol 25(22):3281–3287

Lee KC, Bradley DA, Hussain M et al (2007) A feasibility study evaluating the functional diffusion map as a predictive imaging biomarker for detection of treatment response in a patient with metastatic prostate cancer to the bone. Neoplasia 9(12):1003–1011

Lin C, Luciani A, Itti E et al (2010) Whole-body diffusion-weighted magnetic resonance imaging with apparent diffusion coefficient mapping for staging patients with diffuse large B-cell lymphoma. Eur Radiol 20(8):2027–2038

Lisbona R, Derbekyan V, Novales-Díaz J, Veksler A (1993) Gallium-67 scintigraphy in tuberculous and nontuberculous infectious spondylitis. J Nucl Med 34(5):853–859

Low RN (2009) Diffusion-weighted MR imaging for whole body metastatic disease and lymphadenopathy. Magn Reson Imaging Clin N Am 17(2):245–261

Luboldt W, Küfer R, Blumstein N et al (2008) Prostate carcinoma: diffusion-weighted imaging as potential alternative to conventional MR and 11C-choline PET/CT for detection of bone metastases. Radiology 249(3):1017–1025

Luna A, Ribes R, Caro P et al (2006) MRI of focal splenic lesions without and with dynamic gadolinium enhancement. Am J Roentgenol 186(6):1533–1547

Luna A, Sanchez-Gonzalez J, Caro P (2011) DWI of the chest. Magn Reson Imaging Clin N Am 19:69–94

Mori T, Nomori H, Ikeda K et al (2008) Diffusion-weighted magnetic resonance imaging for diagnosing malignant pulmonary nodules/masses: comparison with positron emission tomography. J Thorac Oncol 3:358–364

Murtz P, Krautmacher C, Traber F, Gieseke J, Schild HH, Willinek WA (2007) Diffusion-weighted whole-body MR imaging with background body signal suppression: a feasibility study at 3.0 Tesla. Eur Radiol 17:3031–3037

Nakanishi K, Kobayashi M, Nakaguchi K et al (2007) Whole-body MRI for detecting metastatic bone tumor: diagnostic value of diffusion-weighted images. Magn Reson Med Sci 6:147–155

Niwa T, Aida N, Fujita K et al (2008) Diffusion-weighted imaging of retroperitoneal malignant peripheral nerve sheath tumor in a patient with neurofibromatosis type 1. Magn Reson Med Sci 7(1):49–53

Nomori H, Mori T, Ikeda K et al (2008) Diffusion-weighted magnetic resonance imaging can be used in place of positron emission tomography for N staging of non-small cell lung cancer with fewer false-positive results. J Thorac Cardiovasc Surg 135(4):816–822

Ohba Y, Nomori H, Mori T et al (2009) Is diffusion-weighted magnetic resonance imaging superior to positron emission tomography with fludeoxyglucose F 18 in imaging non-small cell lung cancer? J Thorac Cardiovasc Surg 138(2):439–445

Ohno Y, Koyama H, Onishi Y et al (2008) Non-small cell lung cancer: whole-body MR examination for M-stage assessment-utility for whole-body diffusion-weighted imaging compared with integrated FDG-PET/CT. Radiology 248(2):643–654

Ono K, Ochiai R, Yoshida T et al (2009) Comparison of diffusion-weighted MRI and 2-[fluorine-18]-fluoro-2-deoxy-D-glucose positron emission tomography (FDGPET) for detecting primary colorectal cancer and regional lymph node metastases. J Magn Reson Imaging 29:336–340

Oztekin O, Ozan E, Hilal Adibelli Z et al (2009) SSH-EPI diffusion-weighted MR imaging of the spine with low b values: is it useful in differentiating malignant metastatic tumor infiltration from benign fracture edema? Skeletal Radiol 38(7):651–658

Padhani AR, Koh DM (2011) Diffusion MR imaging for monitoring of treatment response. Magn Reson Imaging Clin N Am 19(1):181–209

Pui MH, Mitha A, Rae WI et al (2005) Diffusion-weighted magnetic resonance imaging of spinal infection and malignancy. J Neuroimaging 15(2):164–170

Reischauer C, Froehlich JM, Koh DM et al (2010) Bone metastases from prostate cancer: assessing treatment response by using diffusion-weighted imaging and functional diffusion maps – initial observations. Radiology 257(2):523–531

Schmidt GP, Reiser MF, Baur-Melnyk A (2009) Whole-body imaging of bone marrow. Semin Musculoskelet Radiol 13(2):120–133

Schnapauff D, Zeile M, Niederhagen MB et al (2009) Diffusion-weighted echo-planar magnetic resonance imaging for the assessment of tumor cellularity in patients with soft-tissue sarcomas. J Magn Reson Imaging 29(6):1355–1359

Sommer G, Klarhöfer M, Lenz C et al (2011) Signal characteristics of focal bone marrow lesions in patients with multiple myeloma using whole body T1w-TSE, T2w-STIR and diffusion-weighted imaging with background suppression. Eur Radiol 21(4):857–862

Stecco A, Romano G, Negru M et al (2009) Whole-body diffusion-weighted magnetic resonance imaging in the staging of oncological patients: comparison with positron emission tomography computed tomography (PET-CT) in a pilot study. Radiol Med (Torino) 114:11–17

Takenaka D, Ohno Y, Matsumoto K et al (2009) Detection of bone metastases in nonsmall cell lung cancer patients: comparison of whole-body diffusion-weighted imaging (DWI), whole-body MR imaging without and with DWI, whole-body FDG-PET/CT, and bone scintigraphy. J Magn Reson Imaging 30:298–308

Thoeny HC, Triantafyllou M, Birkhaeuser FD et al (2009) Combined ultrasmall superparamagnetic particles of iron oxide-enhanced and diffusion-weighted magnetic resonance imaging reliably detect pelvic lymph node metastases in normal-sized nodes of bladder and prostate cancer patients. Eur Urol 55(4):761–769

Vilanova JC, Barcelo J (2008) Diffusion-weighted whole-body MR screening. Eur J Radiol 67:440–447

Index

A. Luna et al., *Diffusion MRI Outside the Brain*,
DOI 10.1007/978-3-642-21052-5, © Springer-Verlag Berlin Heidelberg 2012